Liver Cell Carcinoma

FALK SYMPOSIUM 51

Liver Cell Carcinoma

EDITED BY

P. Bannasch
German Cancer Research Centre
Heidelberg
Federal Republic of Germany

D. Keppler
German Cancer Research Centre
Heidelberg
Federal Republic of Germany

G. Weber
Indiana University, School of Medicine
Indianapolis
USA

*Proceedings of the 51st Falk Symposium held at Freiburg im Breisgau,
Federal Republic of Germany, June 5–8, 1988*

KLUWER ACADEMIC PUBLISHERS
DORDRECHT / BOSTON / LONDON

Distributors

for the United States and Canada: Kluwer Academic Publishers, PO Box 358, Accord Station, Hingham, MA 02018-0358, USA
for all other countries: Kluwer Academic Publishers Group, Distribution Center, PO Box 322, 3300 AH Dordrecht, The Netherlands

British Library Cataloguing in Publication Data

Falk Symposium (51st, 1988) Frieburg im Breisgau,
   Germany
   Liver cell carcinoma.
   1. Man. Liver. Cancer
   I. Title II. Bannasch, P. (Peter) III. Keppler, D.
   (Dietrich) 1940– IV. Weber, G. (George)
   616.99'436

   ISBN 0-7462-0111-7

Copyright

Published in the United Kingdom by Kluwer Academic Publishers, PO Box 55, Lancaster, UK.

Kluwer Academic Publishers BV incorporates the publishing programmes of D. Reidel, Martinus Nijhoff, Dr W. Junk and MTP Press.

Typeset by Witwell Limited, Southport.

Printed in Great Britain by Butler and Tanner Ltd., Frome and London.

Contents

SECTION 2: HEPADNA VIRUSES AND HEPATOCARCINOGENESIS

SECTION 3: CHEMICALS AND HEPATOCARCINOGENESIS

CONTENTS

SECTION 4: BIOLOGY OF CHEMICAL HEPATOCARCINOGENESIS

SECTION 5: ALTERED GENE EXPRESSION IN LIVER CELL TUMOURS

SECTION 6: DIAGNOSIS AND THERAPY OF LIVER CELL CARCINOMA

Preface

These proceedings are based on the 51st Falk Symposium on 'Liver Cell Carcinoma', which was held in Freiburg from June 5–8, 1988. Ten years after the Falk Symposium No. 25 on 'Primary Liver Tumors' in Titisee, it appeared timely to meet again and discuss a decade's progress in basic and clinical research on liver cell carcinoma. The programme of the Symposium was comprehensive, leading from molecular biology of the hepatitis B virus and experimental and chemical hepatocarcinogenesis to epidemiology, morphology, biochemistry, early diagnosis, treatment, and possibilities of primary prevention of liver cell carcinoma. The participation of a large number of invited speakers covering these research areas was only made possible by the generous sponsorship of Dr Herbert Falk and the Falk Foundation to whom we are most grateful. The speakers' contributions provided an excellent basis for a critical discussion of new results in the context of well-founded knowledge and for building bridges between basic science and clinical research. The proceedings reflect their stimulating scientific input at the conference, and they represent an up-to-date-review on nearly all aspects of liver cell carcinoma. They deserve, and will hopefully find, many interested readers who may accept the challenge to study and combat this dreadful disease.

The Editors

List of Contributors

G. ACS
Department of Biochemistry
Mount Sinai School of Medicine
1 Gustave L. Levy Place
New York, NY. 10029
USA

G. N. ANDERSSON
Department of Pathology
Karolinska Institute
Huddinge Hospital, F-42
S-141 86 Huddinge
Sweden

S. O. ASBELL
Johns Hopkins Hospital
University of California, San Francisco
Albert Einstein Medical Center
Radiation Therapy Oncology Group
San Francisco
USA

R. BANERJEE
Department of Biochemistry
Mount Sinai School of Medicine
1 Gustave L. Levy Place
New York, NY. 10029
USA

P. BANNASCH
Institut für Experimentelle Pathologie
Deutsches Krebsforschungszentrum
Im Neuenheimer Feld 280
D-6900 Heidelberg
Federal Republic of Germany

S. BARDOCZ
Rowett Research Institute
Bucksburn
Aberdeen AB2 9SB
UK

R. BARTENSCHLAGER
Zentrum für Molekulare Biologie
Universität Heidelberg
Im Neuenheimer Feld 282
D-6900 Heidelberg 1
Federal Republic of Germany

G. BLAICH
Institute of Pharmacology and Toxicology
University of Würzburg
Versbacher Straße 9
D-8700 Würburg
Federal Republic of Germany

H. E. BLUM
Massachusetts General Hospital
Harvard Medical School
MGH Cancer Centre
Molecular Hepatology Laboratory
MGH East, 149 13th Street
Charlestown, MA 02129
USA

K. W. BOCK
Institute of Toxicology
University of Tübingen
Wilhelmstraße 56
D-7400 Tübingen
Federal Republic of Germany

F. X. BOSCH
Unit of Field and Intervention Studies
International Agency for Research on
    Cancer
150 Cours Albert Thomas
69372 Lyon Cédex 08
France

CH. BRECHOT
U 163, Institut Pasteur
28 rue du Dr Roux
75724 Paris Cédex 15
France

V. BRUSS
Department of Medical Microbiology
University of Göttingen
Kreuzbergring 57
D-3400 Göttingen
Federal Republic of Germany

W. BURSCH
Institut für Tumorbiologie-Krebsforschung
der Universität Wien
Borschkegasse 8a
A-1090 Wien
Austria

H. BUSCH
Department of Pharmacology
Baylor College of Medicine
One Baylor Plaza
Houston, Texas 77030
USA

R. K. BUSCH
Department of Pharmacology
Baylor College of Medicine
One Baylor Plaza
Houston, Texas 77030
USA

Z. -Y. CHEN
Department of Pathology
Medical Science Building
University of Toronto
Toronto, Ontario M5S 1A8
Canada

F. V. CHISARI
Department of Basic and Clinical
   Research
Research Institute of Scripps Clinic
10666 North Torrey Pines Road
La Jolla, CA 92037
USA

F. DEINHARDT
Max-von-Pettenkofer-Institut
Universität München
Pettenkoferstrasse 9a
D-8000 München 2
Federal Republic of Germany

V. J. DINDZANS
Medicine – Gastroenterology
University of Pittsburgh School of Medicine
1000 J Scaife
Pittsburgh, PA 15261

G. M. DUSHEIKO
Department of Medicine
Royal Free Hospital
Pond Street
London NW3 2QG
UK

H. ENZMANN
Institut für Experimentelle Pathologie
Deutsches Krebsforschungszentrum
Im Neuenheimer Feld 280
D-6900 Heidelberg
Federal Republic of Germany

L. C. ERIKSSON
Department of Pathology
Karolinska Institute
Huddinge Hospital, F-42
S-141 86 Huddinge
Sweden

E. FARBER
Department of Pathology
Medical Science Building
University of Toronto
Toronto, Ontario M5S 1A8
Canada

N. FAUSTO
Department of Pathology and Laboratory
   Medicine
Division of Biology and Medicine
Brown University Box G
Providence, RI 02912
USA

L. FESUS
Department of Biochemistry
University Medical School of Debrecen
H-40 12 Debrecen, PO Box 6
Hungary

LIST OF CONTRIBUTORS

A. FONAGY
Department of Pharmacology
Baylor College of Medicine
One Baylor Plaza
Houston, Texas 77030
USA

J. FREEMAN
Department of Pharmacology
Baylor College of Medicine
One Baylor Plaza
Houston, Texas 77030
USA

P. GALLE
Zentrum für Molekulare Biologie
Universität Heidelberg
Im Neuenheimer Feld 282
D-6900 Heidelberg 1
Federal Republic of Germany

J. S. GAVALER
Medicine – Gastroenterology
University of Pittsburgh
School of Medicine
1000 J Scaife Hall
Pittsburgh, PA 15261
USA

M. A. GERBER
Department of Pathology
Tulane University School of Medicine
1430 Tulane Avenue
New Orleans, Louisiana 70112
USA

W. H. GERLICH
Department of Medical Microbiology
University of Göttingen
Kreuzbergring 57
D-3400 Göttingen
Federal Republic of Germany

W. GEROK
Universitäts-Klinikum
Medizinische Klinik
Hugstetter Straße 55
D-7800 Freiburg/Br.
Federal Republic of Germany

H. R. GLATT
Institute of Toxicology
University of Mainz
Obere Zahlbacher Straße 67
D-6500 Mainz
Federal Republic of Germany

H. GRUNICKE
Institut für Medizinische Chemie und
  Biochemie
Universität Innsbruck
Fritz-Pregl-Straße 3
A-6060 Innsbruck
Austria

W. GUNTER
Institut für Medizinische Chemie und
  Biochemie
Universitat Innsbruck
Fritz-Pregl-Straße 3
A-6020 Innsbruck
Austria

H. J. HACKER
Institut für Experimentelle Pathologie
Deutsches Krebsforschungszentrum
Im Neuenheimer Feld 280
D-6900 Heidelberg
Federal Republic of Germany

L. HARRIS
Department of Pathology
Medical Science Building
University of Toronto
Toronto, Ontario M5S 1A8
Canada

J. HAZELWOOD
Department of Pharmacology
Baylor College of Medicine
One Baylor Plaza
Houston, Texas 77030
USA

K. -H. HEERMANN
Department of Medical Microbiology
University of Göttingen
Kreuzbergring 57
D-3400 Göttingen
Federal Republic of Germany

W. HELLIGER
Institut für Medizinische Chemie und
  Biochemie
Universität Innsbruck
Fritz-Pregl-Straße 3
A-6020 Innsbruck
Austria

D. HENNING
Department of Pharmacology
Baylor College of Medicine
One Baylor Plaza
Houston, Texas 77030
USA

O. HINO
Department of Pathology
Cancer Institute
Kami-Ikebukuro
Toshima-ku
Tokyo 170
Japan

M. HOERNER
Department of Medicine
University of Heidelberg
Bergheimerstr. 58
D-6900 Heidelberg
Federal Republic of Germany

P. H. HOFSCHNEIDER
Virusforschung
Max-Planck Institut für Biochemie
D-8033 Martinsried bei München
Federal Republic of Germany

M. HÖHNE
Department of Pathology and Toxicology
University of Göttingen
Robert-Koch-Str. 40
D-3400 Göttingen
Federal Republic of Germany

W. JILG
Max-von-Pettenkofer-Institut
Universität München
Pettenkoferstrasse 9a
D-8000 München 2
Federal Republic of Germany

S. KARPEN
Department of Biochemistry
Mount Sinai School of Medicine
1 Gustave L. Levy Place
New York, NY 10029
USA

H. KAUFMAN
Nuclear Medicine Service/115
VA Medical Center
1st Avenue at East 24th Street
New York, NY 10010
USA

D. KEPPLER
Deutsches Krebsforschungszentrum
Im Neuenheimer Feld 280
D-6900 Heidelberg
Federal Republic of Germany

M. C. KEW
Department of Medicine
Witwatersrand University Medical School
York Road
Parktown 2193
Johannesburg
South Africa

J. L. KLEIN
Johns Hopkins Hospital
University of California, San Francisco
Albert Einstein Medical Center
Radiation Therapy Oncology Group
San Francisco
USA

F. KLIMEK
Institut für Experimentelle Pathologie
Deutsches Krebsforschungszentrum
Im Neuenheimer Feld 280
D-6900 Heidelberg
Federal Republic of Germany

B. KOMMERELL
Department of Medicine
University of Heidelberg
Bergheimerstr. 58
D-6900 Heidelberg
Federal Republic of Germany

LIST OF CONTRIBUTORS

R. KOSHY
Virusforschung
Max-Planck Institut für Biochemie
D-8033 Martinsried bei München
Federal Republic of Germany

B. KRAUPP
Institut für Tumorbiologie-Krebsforschung
der Universität Wien
Borschkegasse 8a
A-1090 Wien
Austria

B. KRONE
Department of Medical Microbiology
University of Göttingen
Kreuzbergring 57
D-3400 Göttingen
Federal Republic of Germany

CH. KUHN
Zentrum für Molekulare Biologie
Universität Heidelberg
Im Neuenheimer Feld 282
D-6900 Heidelberg 1
Federal Republic of Germany

K. LAPIS
Ist. Institute of Pathology and
   Experimental Cancer Research
Semmelweis Medical University
Üllöi ut 26
Budapest
1085 — Hungary

D. LARZUL
U 163, Institut Pasteur
28 rue du Dr Roux
75724 Paris Cédex 15
France

G. LEE
Department of Pathology
Medical Science Building
University of Toronto
Toronto, Ontario M5S 1A8
Canada

ST. A. LEIBEL
Memorial Sloan-Kettering Cancer Center
1275 York Avenue
New York, NY 10021
USA

P. L. LEICHNER
Johns Hopkins Hospital
University of California, San Francisco
Albert Einstein Medical Center
Radiation Therapy Oncology Group
San Francisco
USA

G. LENGYEL
Department of Biochemistry
Mount Sinai School of Medicine
1 Gustave L. Levy Place
New York, NY 10029

J. LIEHR
Department of Pharmacology and
   Toxicology
The University of Texas Medical Branch
Market and 11th Street
Galveston, TX 77550
USA

W. L. LIN
Department of Pharmacology
Baylor College of Medicine
One Baylor Plaza
Houston, Texas 77030
USA

L. MAKOWKA
Surgery – Transplantation
Cedars Sinai Hospital
8700 Beverly Boulevard
Room 8215
Los Angeles, CA 90048
USA

R. A. MALT
Surgical Services Department
Massachusetts General Hospital
3 Acorn Street
Harvard Medical School
Boston, Massachusetts 02114
USA

D. MAYER
Institut für Experimentelle Pathologie
Deutsches Krebsforschungszentrum
Im Neuenheimer Feld 280
D-6900 Heidelberg
Federal Republic of Germany

J. E. MEAD
Department of Pathology and Laboratory
  Medicine
Division of Biology and Medicine
Brown University Box G
Providence, RI 02912
USA

M. METZLER
Institute of Pharmacology and Toxicology
University of Würzburg
Versbacher Straße 9
D-8700 Würzburg
Federal Republic of Germany

N. MUÑOZ
Unit of Field and Intervention Studies
International Agency for Research on
  Cancer
150 Cours Albert Thomas
69372 Lyon Cédex 08
France

E. NAKAJIMA
U 163, Institut Pasteur
28 rue du Dr Roux
75724 Paris Cédex 15
France

M. NASSAL
Zentrum für Molekulare Biologie
Universität Heidelberg
Im Neuenheimer Feld 282
D-6900 Heidelberg 1
Federal Republic of Germany

Y. NATSUMEDA
Laboratory for Experimental Oncology
Indiana University School of Medicine
702 Barnhill Drive
Indianapolis, Indiana 46223
USA

M. NIEPMANN
Zentrum für Molekulare Biologie
Universität Heidelberg
Im Neuenheimer Feld 282
D-6900 Heidelberg 1
Federal Republic of Germany

F. OESCH
Institute of Toxicology
University of Mainz
Obere Zahlbacher Straße 67
D-6500 Mainz
Federal Republic of Germany

S. OFFENSPERGER
Universitäts-Klinikum
Medizinische Klinik
Hugstetter Straße 55
D-7800 Freiburg/Br.
Federal Republic of Germany

W. B. OFFENSPERGER
Universitäts-Klinikum
Medizinische Klinik
Hugstetter Straße 55
D-7800 Freiburg/Br.
Federal Republic of Germany

K. OKUDA
1st Department of Internal Medicine
Chiba-University
School of Medicine
1-8-1, Inohana
Chiba City 280
Japan

E. OLÁH
Department of Molecular Biology
National Oncological Institute
Ráth György Str. 7–9
H-1525 Budapest
Hungary pf. 21

M. ORATZ
Nuclear Medicine Service/115
VA Medical Center
1st Avenue at East 24th Street
New York, NY 10010
USA

LIST OF CONTRIBUTORS

ST. E. ORDER
Johns Hopkins Hospital
University of California, San Francisco
Albert Einstein Medical Center
Radiation Therapy Oncology Group
San Francisco
USA

R. PICHLMAYR
Klinik für Abdominal- und
 Transplantationschirurgie
Medizinishce Hochschule Hannover
Konstanty-Gutschow-Strasse 8
D-3000 Hannover 61
Federal Republic of Germany

P. PRICE
Department of Biochemistry
Mount Sinai School of Medicine
1 Gustave L. Levy Place
New York, NY 10029
USA

B. PUSCHENDORF
Institut für Medizinische Chemie und
 Biochemie
Universität Innsbruck
Fritz-Pregl-Straße 3
A-6020 Innsbruck
Austria

H. M. RABES
Institute of Pathology
University of Munich
Thalkirchner Straße 36
D-8000 München 2
Federal Republic of Germany

G. RADZIWILL
Zentrum für Molekulare Biologie
Universität Heidelberg
Im Neuenheimer Feld 282
D-6900 Heidelberg 1
Federal Republic of Germany

B. A. REDDY
Department of Pharmacology
Baylor College of Medicine
One Baylor Plaza
Houston, Texas 77030
USA

J. S. RINAUDO
Department of Pathology
Medical Science Building
University of Toronto
Toronto, Ontario M5S 1A8
Canada

Ch. E. ROGLER
Department of Medicine
Marion Bessin Liver Research Center
Albert Einstein College of Medicine
1300 Morris Park Avenue
New York 10461
USA

W. M. ROOMI
Department of Pathology
Medical Science Building
University of Toronto
Toronto, Ontario M5S 1A8
Canada

M. A. ROTHSCHILD
Nuclear Medicine Service/115
VA Medical Center
1st Avenue at East 24th Street
New York, NY 10010
USA

J. ROTSTEIN
College of Medicine
University of Illinois
Chicago, Illinois
USA

ST. SCHAEFER
Department of Medical Microbiology
University of Göttingen
Kreuzbergring 57
D-3400 Göttingen
Federal Republic of Germany

Z. SCHAFF
Ist. Institute of Pathology and Experimental
 Cancer Research
Semmelweis Medical University
Üllöi ut 26
Budapest
1085 — Hungary

H. SCHALLER
Zentrum für Molekulare Biologie
Universität Heidelberg
Im Neuenheimer Feld 282
D-6900 Heidelberg 1
Federal Republic of Germany

P. J. SCHEUER
Department of Histopathology
Royal Free Hospital
Pond Street, Hampstead
GB-London NW3 2QG
UK

L. SCHLADT
Institute of Toxicology
University of Mainz
Obere Zahlbacher Straße 67
D-6500 Mainz
Federal Republic of Germany

C. SCHLETTERER
Institut für Medizinische Chemie und
   Biochemie
Universität Innsbruck
Fritz-Pregl-Straße 3
A-6020 Innsbruck
Austria

H. -J. SCHLICHT
Zentrum für Molekulare Biologie
Universität Heidelberg
Im Neuenheimer Feld 282
D-6900 Heidelberg 1
Federal Republic of Germany

S. S. SCHREIBER
Nuclear Medicine Service/115
VA Medical Center
1st Avenue at East 24th Street
New York, NY 10010
USA

R. SCHULTE-HERMANN
Institut für Tumorbiologie-Krebsforschung
der Universität Wien
Borschkegasse 8a
A-1090 Wien
Austria

G. SEELMANN-EGGEBERT
Institut Für Experimentelle Pathologie
Deutsches Krebsforschungszentrum
Im Nevenheimer Feld
D-6900 Heidelberg
Federal Republic of Germany

M. SEIFER
Department of Medical Microbiology
University of Göttingen
Kreuzbergring 57
D-3400 Göttingen
Federal Republic of Germany

H. K. SEITZ
Department of Medicine
University of Heidelberg
Bergheimerstr. 58
D-6900 Heidelberg
Federal Republic of Germany

M. A. SELLS
Department of Biochemistry
Mount Sinai School of Medicine
1 Gustave L. Levy Place
New York, NY 10029
USA

E. SEMPLE
Department of Pathology
Medical Science Building
University of Toronto
Toronto, Ontario M5S 1A8
Canada

D. A. SHAFRITZ
Department of Medical and Cell Biology
Marion Bessin Liver Research Center
Departments of Medicine and Cell Biology
Albert Einstein College of Medicine
Bronx, New York 10461
USA

M. SHVARTSMAN
Department of Biochemistry
Mount Sinai School of Medicine
1 Gustave L. Levy Place
New York, NY. 10029
USA

U. A. SIMANOWSKI
Department of Medicine
University of Heidelberg
Bergheimerstr. 58
D-6900 Heidelberg
Federal Republic of Germany

K. SNELL
Department of Biochemistry
University of Surrey
Guildford Surrey, GU2 5XH
UK

Th. E. STARZL
Surgery – Transplantation
University of Pittsburgh School of Medicine
3601 Fifth Ave, 5W Falk Clinic
Pittsburgh, PA 15213
USA

G. B. STILLWAGON
Johns Hopkins Hospital
University of California, San Francisco
Albert Einstein Medical Center
Radiation Therapy Oncology Group
San Francisco
USA

M. SUNG
Department of Biochemistry
Mount Sinai School of Medicine
1 Gustave L. Levy Place
New York, NY 10029
USA

J. A. SWENBERG
Department of Biochemical Toxicology
  and Pathology
Chemical Industry Institute of Toxicology
P. O. Box 12 137
Research Triangle Park, NC 27709
USA

H. TALASZ
Institut für Medizinische Chemie und
  Biochemie
Universität Innsbruck
Fritz-Pregl-Straße 3
A-6060 Innsbruck
Austria

K. TEUBNER
Universitäts-Klinikum
Medizinische Klinik
Hugstetter Straße 55
D-7800 Freiburg/Br.
Federal Republic of Germany

V. THIERS
U 163, Institut Pasteur
28 rue du Dr Roux
75724 Paris Cédex 15
France

H. THOMAS
Institute of Toxicology
University of Mainz
Obere Zahlbacher Straße 67
D-6500 Mainz
Federal Republic of Germany

S. N. THUNG
Department of Pathology
Tulane University School of Medicine
1430 Tulane Avenue
New Orleans, Louisiana 70112
USA

I. TIMMERMANN-TROSIENER
Institut für Tumorbiologie-Krebsforschung
der Universität Wien
Borschkegasse 8a
A-1090 Wien
Austria

P. TIOLLAIS
U 163, Institut Pasteur
28 rue du Dr Roux
75724 Paris Cédex 15
France

U. -B. TORNDAL
Department of Pathology
Karolinska Istitute
Huddinge Hospital, F-42
S-141 86 Huddinge
Sweden

A. M. TRITSCHER
Institut of Pharmacology and Toxicology
University of Würzburg
Versbacher Straße 9
D-8700 Würzburg
Federal Republic of Germany

D. H. VAN THIEL
Department of Medicine – Gastroenterology
University of Pittsburgh School of Medicine
1000 J Scaife,
Pittsburgh PA 15261
USA

G. VATJA
Department of Biochemistry
Mount Sinai School of Medicine
1 Gustave L. Levy Place
New York, NY 10029
USA

E. WALTER
Universitäts-Klinikum
Medizinische Klinik
Hugstetter Straße 55
D-7800 Freiburg/Br.
Federal Republic of Germany

E. WEBER
Institut für Experimentelle Pathologie
Deutsches Krebsforschungszentrum
Im Neuenheimer Feld 280
D-6900 Heidelberg
Federal Republic of Germany

G. WEBER
Laboratory for Experimental Oncology
Indiana University School of Medicine
702 Barnhill Drive
Indianapolis, Indiana 46223
USA

G. WEISS
Institut für Medizinische Chemie und
 Biochemie
Universität Innsbruck
Fritz-Pregl-Straße 3
A-6060 Innsbruck
Austria

G. M. WILLIAMS
Department of Medical Sciences
Naylor Dana Institute for Disease and
 Prevention
American Health Foundation
1 Dana Road
Valhalla, NY 10595
USA

H. G. WILLIAMS-ASHMAN
Ben May Institute
University of Chicago
5841 S. Maryland Avenue
Chicago, IL 60637
USA

M. WOLLERSHEIM
Virusforschung
Max-Planck Institut für Biochemie
D-8033 Martinsried bei München
Federal Republic of Germany

Y. YAMADA
Laboratory for Experimental Oncology
Indiana University School of Medicine
702 Barnhill Drive
Indianapolis, Indiana 46223
USA

D. YOUNG
Department of Medicine
Marion Bessin Liver Research Center
Albert Einstein College of Medicine
1300 Morris Park Avenue
New York 10461
USA

P. ZAHM
Virusforschung
Max-Planck Institut für Biochemie
D-8033 Martinsried
Federal Republic of Germany

H. ZERBAN
Institut für Experimentelle Pathologie
Deutsches Krebsforschungszentrum
Im Neuenheimer Feld 280
D-6900 Heidelberg
Federal Republic of Germany

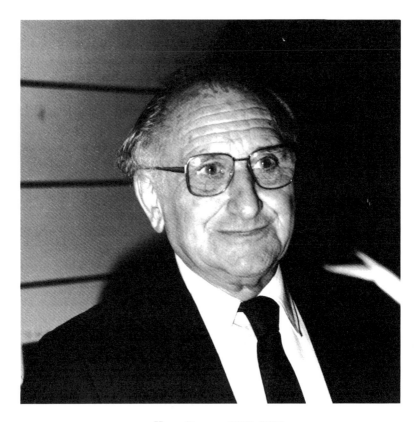

Hans Popper 1903–1988

In Memoriam Hans Popper, MD (Vienna) PhD (Illinois)

Dr Hans Popper died in New York City on May 6, 1988, one month before the Symposium on Liver Cell Carcinoma was held in Freiburg. The symposium and these proceedings were dedicated to his memory. Hans Popper had a decisive influence on the planning of this meeting which dealt with a topic that was in the focus of his interests during the last years of his life. He and the editors of this volume gathered in June of 1987 in Titisee to finalize the programme in a vivid discussion. Hans Popper, then at the age of 83, was the one among us who argued for *more* molecular biology in this symposium, as one key to modern hepatology.

International hepatology lost its dominating personality. The Falk Foundation and scientific organizers of Falk Symposia lost Hans Popper's advice and his exciting ideas based on enormous knowledge and on his awareness of good research going on in laboratories around the world. His passing is an irreplaceable loss to his colleagues and friends, to his family, as well as these symposia.

Hans Popper was born into one of Vienna's privileged Jewish families on November 24, 1903, the only son of a physician. He was a medical student not only in Vienna but also at the Sorbonne in Paris and in Oxford. He was trained in biochemistry with Van Fuerth, in pathology with Maresch, and in internal medicine with Eppinger. In 1925, as a student in Vienna, he published his first paper on the action of adrenaline on glycogenolysis in yeast, showing for the first time hormonal action in a microorganism. Later in Vienna he developed and described the measurement of the creatinine clearance.

The productive and happy period in Vienna was terminated in 1938 when the Third Reich forced him to depart quickly to the United States of America. He started a new career from the beginning in Chicago, working at the Graduate School of the Cook Country Hospital. Within a few short years he assembled a hepatology research group and became Scientific Director of the Hektoen Institute for Medical Research from 1943 to 1957. In 1957 he moved to the Mount Sinai Hospital in New York City to succeed Paul Klemperer as Director of the Department of Pathology. Hans Popper played a key role in the foundation of Mount Sinai Medical School where he was Dean and President. Despite the load of administrative work he continued as the hospital's pathologist and as a leading experimental hepatologist. He coined the term *cholestasis* and proposed mechanisms uniting biochemical and pathological concepts. Since his 'retirement' in 1973, Hans Popper was the Gustave L. Levy Distinguished Service Professor, and he was working in his office until February of 1988 — unless he was lecturing in Europe, China, South America, or elsewhere.

Among his 15 honorary doctorates from universities around the world, there is one from Vienna given in 1965 and one from the University of Freiburg in 1984. Hans Popper was a member of the National Academy of Sciences of the USA since 1976 and in the same year he became an elected member of the Deutsche Akademie der Naturforscher Leopoldina zu Halle.

Hans Popper accomplished so much because of enormous energy, highly efficient use of his time, and a total period of time devoted to creative research in hepatology of about 63 years. His memory was outstanding up to the age of 84 — at least as far as science and his friends were concerned. He remained curious and was always ready to learn about new developments in science and exciting new ideas. Last but not least, he shared his knowledge and his ideas with his colleagues.

The Symposium on Liver Cell Carcinoma reminded us on many occasions of Hans Popper's ideas and influence, as well as of his absence.

Dietrich Keppler

Introduction: a decade's progress in basic and clinical research on liver cell carcinoma

P. BANNASCH

A decade ago, in his presidential introduction to the Falk Symposium No. 25 on Primary Liver Tumours in Titisee, the late Hans Popper stressed the increasing importance of liver tumours[1]. There appeared to be some need in 1977 to justify that a whole symposium was dedicated to a disease which was relatively rare in the Western world, and for which neither effective therapy nor promising preventive measures were available. Since then the vision of Hans Popper on the increasing importance of primary liver tumours in both biomedical research and practical medicine has so much become reality that we are not asked for further vindication of a symposium with this topic. Actually, our knowledge on the aetiology, pathogenesis, early diagnosis, therapy and possibilities of primary prevention of liver tumours has so rapidly expanded during the past two decades[2] that we will not be able to deal with all types of primary liver tumours at this symposium. The Scientific Organizing Committee felt that we should rather concentrate on liver cell carcinoma which is by far the most prevalent type of primary liver tumour in man.

As to the aetiology of the hepatocellular carcinoma which is on a worldwide basis one of the most frequent malignant neoplasms, three main risk factors are presently discussed, namely the hepatitis B virus (HBV), the aflatoxins, and alcohol abuse. There is indeed strong epidemiological evidence, which will be presented in detail in the first Session of this Symposium, for an important role of HBV in the pathogenesis of human liver cancer[3]. However, the precise mechanism by which HBV infection might lead to neoplastic transformation of hepatocytes is still far from clear[4]. It has been estimated that the lag period between HBV infection and the appearance of hepatocellular carcinoma takes 30–50 years[5], and that only 1 out of 200 infected newborns develops the disease. An interaction of HBV infection with chemical cofactors, particularly the aflatoxins, has been postulated by several authors. In a recent multivariate epidemiological analysis involving 10 smaller subregions of Swaziland, aflatoxin exposure emerged as a more potent determinant of the variation in liver cancer incidence than the prevalence of HBV infection[6]. This and other studies published in the last few years prompted the International Agency for Research on Cancer in Lyon only recently to list the aflatoxins, the strong carcinogenic potential of which had been known from animal experiments for a long time, as human carcinogens[7].

A big step forward in the further elucidation of the role of viruses and their possible interaction with chemical carcinogens in hepatocarcinogenesis was achieved when animal models of hepadna-virus-induced liver cancer were established in the past decade. Since the discovery of Summers and his co-workers in 1978[8] of a virus similar to human HBV associated with hepatitis and hepatoma in the woodchuck, comparable viruses were found in other species, such as ground squirrels and ducks, and grouped together with human HBV as hepadna-viruses[2]. The molecular biology of these viruses will be discussed in considerable detail.

It is an explicit goal of this Symposium to bring together the different views on viral and chemical hepatocarcinogenesis which evolved during the past decade due to the different methodological approaches used and the different groups of scientists involved in these research areas. Thus, chemical carcinogenesis will be the next main topic of this meeting. In view of the very long and ever increasing list of chemicals which have been shown to produce liver cancer in experimental animals, especially in rodents, we will focus our discussion on some important points. Predominantly those chemical risk factors will be considered which are likely to have relevance for human liver cancer, such as aflatoxins or steroids (including the combined oral contraceptives). The importance of the nitrosamines as possible risk factors for liver cancer in man was emphasized at the Titisee meeting 10 years ago[1]. Another group of chemicals attracted considerable attention in the discussion on hepatocarcinogenesis in recent years: these compounds which are very variable from a structural point of view modulate tumour development and may either inhibit or enhance this process without showing interactions with DNA which are considered to be decisive for initiation of chemical carcinogenesis[9]. In the concept of an interaction between viral and chemical factors in hepatocarcinogenesis the enhancing effect of such compounds, some of which are widely distributed in our environment, should not be neglected. We have also included a contribution on the possible role of alcohol in the aetiology of liver cancer, although we realize that the risk from alcohol is difficult to assess since alcoholic beverages contain a variety of ingredients the majority of which are either unknown or have not properly been evaluated as to their carcinogenicity.

Metabolic activation of chemical carcinogens and the interaction of their reactive metabolites with cellular macromolecules was treated in considerable detail at the Titisee Conference in 1977[1] the spiritus rector of which was Herbert Remmer, one of the pioneers in the field. In the forthcoming meeting the principles of these mechanisms and the progress made since then will be discussed.

As to the pathobiology of hepatocarcinogenesis the bulk of information still comes from studies in rodents treated with various chemical carcinogens[9-12]. There has been a remarkable improvement of the level of information in the past two decades. From the histological level research moved to the cellular and molecular level when modern cytomorphological, cytochemical, cytogenetic, molecular genetic and microbiochemical methods became available. In addition to cellular proliferation, a large number of phenotypic cellular changes were identified in prestages of hepatocellular tumours, and hepatic preneoplasia was more precisely defined. Changes in drug or carbohydrate metabolism and alterations in cell surface receptors will be presented in some detail. The same holds true for the attractive concept that apoptosis as a genetically controlled cell death might play an important role. Alterations in the expression of oncogenes were detected during chemically induced hepatocarcinogenesis, but it remains to be clarified whether they are related to neoplastic transformation or cell proliferation in general.

A whole session of the Symposium is devoted to altered gene expression in liver cell tumours as inferred from a large body of information collected over the years in detailed studies on metabolic changes in transplantable hepatomas. The understanding of the numerous metabolic changes which looked puzzling at first glance has been forwarded by the molecular correlation concept proposed by George Weber years ago[13]. It is of particular interest that many findings in transplantable hepatomas appear in a new light since similar metabolic aberrations were found in pre-neoplastic liver lesions[10]. Another important aspect of this research area is the knowledge provided for an enzyme-targeted chemotherapy of cancer.

Finally, diagnosis, therapy, and possibilities of primary prevention of liver cell cancer in man will be discussed. Remarkable progress has been made in recent years in diagnostic imaging techniques, such as angiography, computed tomography, and ultrasonography[2]. In combination with more conventional diagnostic approaches, such as histological evaluation of fine needle biopsies, detection of serum α-fetoprotein and immunohistochemical procedures, these methods considerably improved early diagnosis of liver cancer and stimulated a new interest in the pathology of early cancer or cancer pre-stages. In the treatment of liver cancer the situation is much less hopeless than a decade ago due to new procedures in surgery, liver grafting and percutaneous intratumoral injection of absolute alcohol as proposed by Okuda and his colleagues in Japan[2]. However, the overall result of the treatment of liver cancer is still disappointing. Therefore, primary prevention appears to be the most important aim of our research if we are to win the fight against hepatocellular carcinoma[14]. The last contribution of our conference will, hopefully, give an optimistic outlook on the possibilities of primary prevention of liver cancer by vaccination against the hepatitis B virus.

References

1. Remmer, H., Bolt, H., Bannasch, P. and Popper, H. (eds.) (1978). *Primary Liver Tumors* (Lancaster: MTP Press)
2. Okuda, K. and Ishak, K. G. (eds.) (1987). *Neoplasms of the Liver* (Tokyo, Berlin, Heidelberg, New York, London, Paris: Springer-Verlag)

3. Beasley, R. P., Hwang, L. -Y., Lin, C. -C. and Chien, C. S. (1981). Hepatocellular carcinoma and hepatitis B virus. A prospective study of 22,707 men in Taiwan. *Lancet, 2*, 1129–33

4. Tiollais, P., Pourcel, C. and Dejean, A. (1985). The hepatitis B virus. *Nature, 317*, 489–95

5. Zur Hausen, H. (1986). Intracellular surveillance of persisting viral infections. *Lancet, 2*, 489–91

6. Peers, F., Bosch, X., Kaldor, J., Linsell, A. and Pluijomen, M. (1987). Aflatoxin exposure, hepatitis B virus infection and liver cancer in Swaziland. *Int. J. Cancer, 39*, 545–53

7. IARC (1987). Monographs on the Evaluation of the Carcinogenic Risk of Chemicals to Humans, Suppl. 7, Chemicals, Occupational Exposures and Cultural Habits Associated with Cancer in Humans, Vols. 1–42 (Lyon: International Agency for Research on Cancer)

8. Summers, J., Smolec, J and Snyder, R. L. (1978) A virus similar to human hepatitis B virus associated with hepatitis and hepatoma in woodchuck. *Proc. Natl. Acad. Sci USA. 75*, 4533–7

9. Pitot, H. C. (1988). Hepatic neoplasia: chemical inducation. In Arias, J. M., Jakoby, W. B., Popper, H. Schachter, D. and Shafritz, D. A. (eds.) The Liver, *Biology and Pathobiology*, pp. 1125–46 (New York: Raven Press)

10. Bannasch, P. (1988). Phenotypic cellular changes as indicators of stages during neoplastic development. In Inversen, O. H. (ed.) *Theories of Carcinogenesis*, pp. 231–49 (Washington: Hemisphere Publishing Corporation)

11 Farber, E. and Sarma, D. S. R. (1987). Hepatocarcinogenesis: A dynamic cellular perspective. *Lab. Invest. 56*, 4–22

12. Roberfroid, M. B. and Préat, V. (eds.) (1988) *Experimental Hepatocarcinogenesis.* (New York, London: Plenum Press)

13. Weber, G. (1977). Enzymology of cancer cells. Parts 1 and 2. *N. Engl. J. Med.*, 296, 486–93, 541–51

14. Bannasch, P. (ed.)(1987). *Cancer Risks: Strategies for Elimination* (Berlin, Heidelberg, New York, London, Paris, Tokyo, Springer-Verlag)

Section 1:
Epidemology and
Morphology

1
Epidemiology of hepatocellular carcinoma

F. X. BOSCH and N. MUÑOZ

INTRODUCTION

The estimates of the fraction of hepatocellular carcinoma (HCC) which is due to hepatitis B virus (HBV) infection vary between 60 and 90% in high-risk countries and 1–50% in low- to intermediate-risk countries. The development of more sensitive assays to determine the presence of HBV markers might change these proportions in the future; the evidence to date, however, has consistently documented that a substantial proportion of HCC cases in low-risk countries occurs in individuals without any serological HBV markers and, further, that only a fraction of persistent HBV carriers eventually develop HCC. The occurrence of HBV-negative HCC cases, as well as the progression from chronic HBV infection to HCC, has to be explained by other factors.

In most studies, the magnitude of the relative risk (RR) among hepatitis B surface antigen (HBsAg) carriers is between 10 and 20, indicating that the association is indeed one of the strongest ever demonstrated, and that the role of other risk factors has therefore to be assessed after adjusting for the effects of the HBV. In addition to HBV, aflatoxin, alcohol consumption, tobacco smoking and long-term use of oral contraceptives have been identified as risk factors for HCC. One of the major difficulties in quantifying the contribution of aflatoxins (AF) to the causation of HCC has been the lack of appropriate markers of exposure at the individual level. Alcohol consumption plays a major role in low-risk countries, and long-term users of oral contraceptives seem to be at increased risk of HCC. Steroid hormones might be involved in the causation of HCC and perhaps explain the male predominance in the HBsAg carrier rate and in the incidence of HCC. Some studies have found an association between cigarette smoking and HCC, but the effect was only clearly demonstrated among HCC cases negative for HBsAg. Other industrial chemicals have also been reported in association with HCC, but their contribution is difficult to estimate due to the rarity of the exposure, which is largely restricted to occupationally exposed groups in developed countries at low risk for HCC.

HEPATOCELLULAR CARCINOMA AND RISK FACTORS

Hepatitis B virus (HBV)

The association between HCC and HBV has been extensively reviewed[1-6]. At the international level there is a strong positive correlation between the incidence of, or mortality from, HCC and the prevalence of HBsAg carriers[1]. However, this study, like other correlation studies, is based on routinely collected data at the level of the general population, and one should expect a large variation in the level of misclassification in HCC reporting. More important, correlation studies cannot properly adjust for other variables that might be associated with HCC (usually only one is considered), and no temporal relationship can be established between exposure and disease when both factors are assessed cross-sectionally.

Case-control studies in high- and low-risk populations have shown that the RR associated with the presence of HBsAg in the sera ranges from 10 to infinity, with most studies ranging from 10 to 20[7-14]. Table 1 summarizes the results of some of these studies in terms of the relative risk (RR) and its 95% confidence intervals (95% CI) and the corresponding estimates of the attributable risk (AR).

The consistency of the findings and the size of the RR strongly indicate that the association is causal. However, because case-control studies are also cross-sectional surveys on HBV markers in a set of cases and controls, they

Table 1 Case-control studies on HBsAg and HCC

Study population	Relative risk (95% CI)		Attributable[a] risk (%)	Reference No.
High-risk areas				
Senegal	12.4	(7.7–19.3)	56.3	7
South Africa	12.6	(7.7–20.1)	56.7	8
Hong Kong	21.3	(10.1–45.9)	78.5	9
People's Republic of China	17.0	(4.3–99.4)	77.9	10
Philippines	10.8	(5.3–20.9)	63.9	11
Intermediate-risk area				
Greece	13.7[b]	(8.0–23.5)	38.8[c]	12
Low-risk area				
USA[d]	48.4	(1.5–∞)	4.5	13
USA[d]	28.6	(3.8–∞)	2.7	14

[a]Unless specified, the prevalence of HBsAg in the general population is that reported among the control group
[b]Weighted for the presence of cirrhosis
[c]Estimated prevalence rate of HBsAg in the general population of 5%
[d]Relative risk and attributable risk estimated for this review from the original data using a correction for continuity. Estimated prevalence rate of HBsAg in the general population of 0.1%

cannot provide evidence on the temporal relationship between exposure and disease (e.g. if HBV markers were more readily detected in HCC cases or if HBV infection were to develop more readily in HCC cases than in controls).

Cohort studies have compared the occurrence of HCC among HBsAg carriers with that of a non-carrier control population or with HCC rates in the general population[2, 7, 15-17]. Some of these are summarized in Table 2. The estimates of the RR vary from 7 to over 100, with the 95% CI ranging from 2 to 212. These prospective cohort studies provide unequivocal proof that the HBV infection precedes the development of HCC.

Table 2 Cohort studies on HBsAg carriers

Study population	RR or SMR[a] (95% CI)	Attributable risk	Reference No.
Taiwan	104.0 (51.0–212.0)	93.9	2
Japan	10.4 (5.0–19.1)	12.7	15
Japan, Osaka	6.6 (4.0–10.2)	10.1[b]	16
USA, New York	9.7 (2.0–28.3)	1.0[c]	7
England and Wales	42.0 (14.0–100.0)	4.0[c]	17

[a]RR: relative risk; SMR: standardized mortality ratio
[b]Estimated prevalence rate of HBsAg in the general population of 1.0%
[c]Estimated prevalence rate of HBsAg in the general population of 0.1%.

That this association is specific as well as strong is suggested by the lack of association of HBV with other cancers[7] and with metastatic liver cancer[18].

The epidemiological evidence for HBV in HCC is strong, consistent and has been demonstrated using various study designs. Causality is now widely accepted[19], and several intervention studies and public health programmes aimed at preventing HBV infection by means of vaccination have been activated. Intervention trials will try to demonstrate that HBV vaccination of newborns in high-risk countries could prevent the occurrence of HCC later in life. In Africa, the Gambia Hepatitis Intervention Study (GHIS) is gradually introducing HBV vaccine into the Expanded Programme of Immunization (EPI) to achieve complete coverage of the country in a four-year period. During the period in which the vaccine is being introduced, all newborns are carefully registered. By the end of the fourth year, a cohort of about 120000 newborns will have been identified. About half of the cohort will have received the standard EPI vaccines and the other half will have received these plus the HBV vaccine. Long-term follow-up of this cohort will be achieved through a national cancer registry, and the incidence of HCC will be compared between the children vaccinated against HBV and those not so protected[20]. In China a large trial in the Quidong region is introducing HBV vaccine into the vaccination programme of a group of randomly-selected communes, while some other communes remain as controls. Long-term follow-up will assess the impact of HBV vaccination on the incidence and mortality from HCC (Sun Tsung-Tang, personal communication, 1987). It is expected that these projects will provide the final proof of causality.

Several other countries at high risk for HBV infection have already adopted public health policies of HBV vaccination of all newborns[21]. The impact of such policies on HCC will have to be evaluated in a less accurate way, namely by monitoring time trends of HCC incidence or mortality rates against the trend in HBV vaccine coverage rates.

Aflatoxin (AF)

Aflatoxins are mycotoxins elaborated by *Aspergillus flavus* and *Aspergillus parasiticus* fungi. Human exposure can occur following ingestion of contaminated food or by consumption of products derived from animals that have consumed AF-contaminated feeds. The main sources of AF in most countries are peanuts, peanut derivatives and corn although, under appropriate conditions, any foodstuff could host the growth of the mould and the production of toxins. There is strong evidence that AF has a carcinogenic effect in many animal species, including primates. AFB_1 is the most potent of the four major types[22].

The evidence for humans is less strong because of the crudeness of the methods used for assessing exposure at the individual level. The epidemiological evidence available is limited to several population correlation studies[23-27] and two case-control studies[9,28]. More accurate follow-up projects are now being conducted[29].

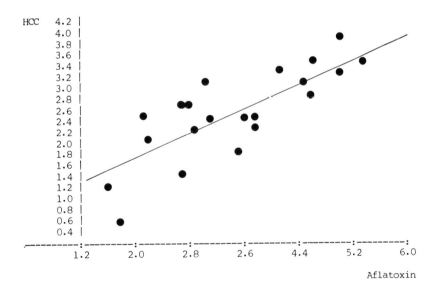

Figure 1 Correlation (correlation coefficient, $r = 0.79$) between incidence of HCC in males over 15 years of age (log incidence/100000/year) and estimates of aflatoxin B_1 exposure (Log ng/kg body weight/day). Data are for: Thailand (1972)[23]; Kenya (1973)[24]; Swaziland (1976, 1987)[25,26]; Mozambique and Transkei (1985)[27]

Figure 1 summarizes the findings of the five most comparable correlation studies. Although the techniques used to estimate AF exposure and to determine or to estimate HCC incidence rates vary from study to study, the overall correlation in these countries is highly significant.

It should be noted that these studies were all conducted in high-risk countries for HCC and that information on exposure to AF is scarce for extensive areas of the world, particularly for the past 10 to 20 years. These include areas in Latin America where some differences in HCC incidence rates are observed[30] and extensive areas in Africa and Asia. Data from Europe and North America indicate that, at least in recent years, AF exposure is rare and of low intensity[31].

The same methodological caveats that were discussed concerning the correlation studies between HBV and HCC apply to these studies, particularly the inability to adjust fully for HBV status. However, since random misclassification of exposure tends to reduce the level of association (e.g. the size of the RR or the correlation coefficients), the evidence reported by these studies is indeed compatible with a strong association.

Only two case-control studies have been reported in which AF exposure has been estimated for HCC patients and controls. In these, the methods used to assess AF exposure were dietary questionnaires, food tables, and some measurements on the AF contents of common foodstuffs in the local markets. These methods are clearly very crude in the sense that, (i) since only a fraction of a given foodstuff is contaminated, consumption of the food item does not accurately reflect exposure to AF, and (ii) questionnaires tend to reflect 'recent' diets, which are likely to be influenced by disease status and underlying time trends in AF contamination.

In the Philippines, RRs of 17.0 and 13.9 were reported for individuals classified as receiving 'very heavy' or 'moderately heavy' overall mean loads of AF, as compared to those receiving a light mean load ($p < 0.05$). The effect of AF was higher among heavy alcohol consumers, RR = 35.5, and a dose–response was demonstrated[28]. This study provided suggestive evidence for the association between AF and HCC and for the interaction between alcohol and AF. Unfortunately, no adjustment was made for HBV status.

A study in Hong Kong[9] did not show an effect of AF as measured by the frequency of consumption of corn and beans, the two major sources of AF in foodstuffs in Hong Kong[23].

Joint effects of aflatoxin and hepatitis B virus in hepatocellular carcinoma: The Swaziland studies

In Swaziland, two studies have been conducted on the risk factors for HCC. In 1976 a correlation was found between HCC incidence rates in males and dietary exposure to AF in the four main geographical regions of the country[25]. In 1987 a second study was conducted to assess specifically the relationship between AF exposure, HBV infection and the incidence of HCC[26]. The methods used in 1987 to sample diets throughout the country were fairly similar to those used in 1976. AF intake was measured in about

3000 dietary samples from a representative cross-section of households across the country. The prevalence of hepatitis B markers was determined in a group of about 3000 consecutive blood donors, and HCC incidence was recorded through a national system of hospital-based cancer registration. Across the four broad geographic regions, there was a more than five-fold variation in the estimated daily intake of AF, ranging from 3.1 to 17.5 μg. The proportion of HBV-exposed individuals was very high (86% in men), but varied relatively little by geographic region; the prevalence of HBsAg carriers was 23% in men, and varied from 21% to 28%. HCC incidence varied over a five-fold range and was strongly associated with estimated levels of AF in the diet. In an analysis involving ten smaller sub-regions, AF exposure emerged as a more important determinant of the variation in HCC incidence than the prevalence of HBsAg. In other words, in a model in which the incidence rates of HCC among males are described by the level of exposure to AF and the prevalence of HBsAg in the population, once the level of AF in diet was taken into account, the addition of the prevalence rate for HBsAg was no longer significant at the 5% level. However, in this study, the estimates of AF exposure were made at the population level and did not take into account individual variation. Moreover, for some food items (e.g. groundnuts eaten outside the main meal), the quantities consumed were not directly weighed. Thus, variations in AF exposure between the geographical areas should be viewed as crude approximations. In addition, it is important to note that these results were based on 52 cases only. However, the likely under-reporting of HCC to the registry did not seem to account for differences observed by geographic region, since no such variations were observed for cancers of other sites or for all cancers, and the medical facilities are evenly distributed in Swaziland.

The association found between AF and HCC in this study does not contradict a strong effect of the HBsAg carrier status on HCC; indeed, within the study period, a case-control study was also conducted and an RR of 19.0 (95% CI = 2.5–149.3) was found for HBsAg carriers. The corresponding AR was 80.5%. Although virtually all of the HCC cases had been exposed to HBV, only half were positive for HBsAg, as determined using the standard serological assays. That suggests that a proportion of the HCC cases, ranging from 20% to perhaps 50%, would not be explained by HBV, and AF could be acting as an independent risk factor for HCC, rather than simply as a co-factor to HBV.

In Swaziland there was an opportunity to evaluate the impact of a Rural Development Area (RDA) programme in reducing human exposure to AF. The RDA programme was introduced gradually in the country as from 1973. By 1983 the different areas of the country could be mapped with regard to the impact of the RDA into four categories, corresponding to 'no input', 'minimal input', 'maximal input for about four years' and 'maximal input for about ten years'. The programme was a complex investment scheme aimed at increasing the standard income of rural families. The means used under the RDA included, among other things, the improvement of farming and storing practices. All samples from both 1972–73 and 1982–83 surveys were then recoded as to their source into one of the four RDA groups. Table 3 shows the

Table 3 Effects of the establishment of the Rural Development Areas (RDA) Programme on the proportion of human diets contaminated with aflatoxin (AF) in Swaziland. Surveys conducted in 1972 and 1982. Number of samples analyzed and proportion of AF-positive samples are shown

| Food type | Input of the RDA Programme | | | | | | | |
| | None | | Moderate | | High | | Very high | |
	1972	1982	1972	1982	1972	1982	1972	1982
Diet[a]	288	360	288	560	384	559	96	287
	(4.2%)	(1.7%)	(5.9%)	(4.6%)	(8.9%)	(3.9%)	(8.3%)	(2.5%)
Other[b]	123	170	119	263	170	263	43	130
	(4.1%)	(7.1%)	(5.0%)	(9.5%)	(8.2%)	(6.1%)	(7.0%)	(4.6%)
Total	411	530	407	823	554	822	139	408
	(4.1%)	(4.1%)	(5.7%)	(6.2%)	(8.7%)	(4.6%)[c]	(7.9%)	(3.2%)[d]

[a]Maize meal and vegetable sauce
[b]Includes samples of maize gruel (166), peanuts (165), fermented milk (150), sour porridge (176), and beer (169)
[c]$p < 0.01$
[d]$p < 0.05$

crude comparison between the proportion of AF-contaminated samples by RDA. The table suggests that some improvement occurred in the ten-year period in the regions where the development programme concentrated its efforts. Unfortunately, it was not possible to attempt other evaluations on the impact of this reduction in AF contamination on the occurrence of HCC.

Other studies carried out in Mozambique[27] and in some regions in China[32-34] have also suggested that variations in HCC incidence may be better explained by differences in exposure to AF rather than by differences in the prevalence of HBV markers. Although these studies are highly suggestive, they share the major limitations of correlation studies. More accurate markers of exposure to AF at the individual level should therefore be used to assess fully the contribution of AF to the development of HCC. As a general rule, if only markers of recent exposure are available, the most appropriate study design would be a prospective follow-up including repeated sampling from every subject. This is the case for the urine assays available and also for the recently developed assays measuring AF–albumin adducts in sera.

Tobacco and alcohol in the presence of hepatitis B virus

A moderate excess of HCC has been observed in the data from some of the major cohort studies on smoking and cancer[16,35,36] and, in one of these[36], there was an indication of a possible interaction between cigarette smoking and alcohol consumption in the causation of HCC; the data were not, however, adjusted for HBV status. The association of HCC with cigarette smoking has been strongly suggested in a case-control study conducted in Greece, but the

9

effect could only be observed among HBsAg negative HCC cases[12]. In this study, a dose–response relationship was also found. The possible association between HCC and cigarette smoking is likely to be of low strength, as indicated by the fact that in countries heavily exposed to cigarette smoking the secular trend of HCC has not paralleled the trends of smoking prevalence or the trends in occurrence of lung cancer, the human cancer which shows the strongest association with cigarette smoking. In addition, due to the strength of the association of HCC with HBV, large-scale studies will be needed to quantify the contribution of smoking and its possible interaction with the virus.

At least thirteen cohort studies have been reported on the association between alcohol consumption and HCC. Some of them are cohorts of individuals identified because of known high exposure to alcoholic beverages. A recent IARC monograph has reviewed the topic and concluded that there is evidence that the risk for HCC is significantly increased by alcohol consumption and that a dose–response relationship could be established[37].

These results should be interpreted taking into consideration the fact that most of them have assessed the occurrence of HCC on the basis of death certificates, which are known to be unreliable as diagnostic sources of HCC. In addition, cohort studies that are not specifically designed to evaluate risk factors for HCC cannot adjust for the relevant potential confounders, particularly HBV infection.

Table 4 summarizes the findings of five case-control studies in which cigarette smoking, alcohol consumption and HBV status were assessed.

Table 4 Effects of cigarette smoking and alcohol drinking on HCC in the presence of HBV markers: case-control studies

| Study population | Relative risk for[a] | | HBV status | Reference No. |
	tobacco	alcohol		
Greece	2.4[b]	Not significant	Effect found only in HBsAg-negative HCC cases	12
USA	Not significant	3.3	Effect found for all HCC irrespective of HBV status	14
Japan	6.3	8.0[b]	All subjects were HBsAg carriers	16
USA	2.6	4.2	HBV exposure sought in the medical record only	38
Hong Kong	3.3[c]	Not significant	Effect found only in HBsAg-negative HCC cases	9

[a]Figures are relative risk for tobacco or alcohol, significant at the 0.05 level after adjustment for the remaining two factors
[b]Dose–response was also significant
[c]The relative risk for heavy smokers was 8.1 (95% CI = 1.5–91.9) for individuals aged ≥50 years

The interpretation of these results has been discussed[39], taking into consideration the size of the study, particularly the number of HCC cases who were negative for HBsAg and the relative prevalences of the three factors in the study population. In summary, alcohol consumption confers an increased risk and, in some developed countries, it is likely to be the major cause of HCC. Cigarette smoking might be associated with HCC, but the association is difficult to demonstrate. Any of these factors might be of increasing public health concern if they are introduced on a large scale to countries which already have high rates of HBV exposure and HCC incidence.

Oral contraceptives

The occurrence of benign liver adenomas among oral contraceptive (OC) users has been reported repeatedly in case reports, and an increased risk among users has been found in two case-control studies. Case reports of HCC among OC users have also been published[40]. More recently, three case-control studies of HCC have been reported. A study in the USA based on a group of 11 cases and 22 controls reported a significant difference in their average duration of OC use[41]. Two other case-control studies in the UK, one based on 26 cases the other on 19 cases, have found that the risk for HCC among women who had used OCs for eight years or more was significantly increased, and there was an indication of a dose–response relationship with duration of exposure[42,43]. In one of these studies[42], the increased risk was also present among the 22 HCC cases who were negative for HBV markers.

These data should be interpreted with caution in view of the rather small size of the studies involved and, therefore, the impossibility of controlling for possible confounders. An analysis of the time trends in mortality from HCC in England and Wales showed a small but consistent increase in young women starting to occur in the last decade. However, the trend was not found for other countries with similar patterns of OC use[44].

The overall evidence so far available appears to indicate an association between OCs and HCC. Further studies on this hypothesis should be envisaged, bearing in mind that:

(i)   In only a few countries have large numbers of women been exposed to OCs for long periods of time (i.e. longer than eight years), starting 20 to 30 years ago when OCs first became available in the 60s. These cohorts of women might just be attaining the necessary latency period, and will be the first to show an increase in the incidence of HCC, if the association with OCs is in fact true.

(ii) Since the formulation of OCs and their patterns of use have changed several times, the results from one country might not be applicable to others.

(iii) As basic information on the epidemiology of the possible association between OCs and HCC is lacking, new studies should be powerful enough to be able to address issues such as age at first OC exposure and reproductive and menstrual life.

CONCLUSION

Chronic HBV infection is responsible for a very large fraction of HCC cases in the world, and intervention studies/public health programmes using the HBV vaccine have been fully endorsed by WHO since 1983. AFs play a role in the Third World, but it is not yet possible to quantify the risk. In developed countries the relevance of AF is likely to be marginal; alcohol consumption is probably the main risk factor, and cigarette smoking may make some contribution to the risk. Long-term use of OCs is likely to confer an increased risk. If the latency period is just now beginning to elapse for large numbers of women, the surveillance of OC users in the years to come might become a public health issue.

References

1. Szmuness, W. (1978). Hepatocellular carcinoma and the hepatitis B virus: evidence for a causal association. *Prog. Med. Virol.*, **24**, 40–69
2. Beasley, R. P. (1982). Hepatitis B virus as the etiologic agent in hepatocellular carcinoma – epidemiologic considerations. *Hepatology*, **2**, 21S–26S
3. Trichopoulos, D., Kremastinou, J. and Tzonou, A. (1982). Does hepatitis B virus cause hepatocellular carcinoma? In Bartsch, H. and Armstrong, B. (eds), *Host Factors in Human Carcinogenesis*, IARC Sci. Publ. No. 39, pp. 317–32. (Lyon: International Agency for Research on Cancer)
4. Blumberg, B. S. and London, W. T. (1985). Hepatitis B virus and prevention of primary cancer of the liver. *J. Natl. Cancer Inst.*, **74**, 267–73
5. Nishioka, K. (1985). Hepatitis B virus and hepatocellular carcinoma: postulates for an etiological relationship. *Adv. Viral Oncol.*, **5**, 173–99
6. Muñoz, N. and Bosch, F. X. (1987). Epidemiology of hepatocellular carcinoma. In Okuda, K. and Ishak, K. G. (eds), *Neoplasms of the Liver*, pp. 3–19. (Tokyo: Springer)
7. Prince, A. M., Szmuness, W., Michon, J., Desmaille, J., Diebolt, G., Linhard, J., Quenum, C. and Sankale, M. (1975). A case-control study of the association between primary liver cancer and hepatitis B infection in Senegal. *Int. J. Cancer*, **16**, 376–83
8. Kew, M. C., Desmyter, J., Bradburne, A. F. and Macnab, G. M. (1979). Hepatitis B virus infection in southern African blacks with hepatocellular cancer. *J. Natl. Cancer Inst.*, **62**, 517–20
9. Lam, K. C., Yu, M. C., Leung, J. W. C. and Henderson, B. E. (1982). Hepatitis B virus and cigarette smoking: risk factors for hepatocellular carcinoma in Hong Kong. *Cancer Res.*, **42**, 5246–8
10. Yeh, F. S., Mo, C. C., Luo, S., Henderson, B. E., Tong, M. J. and Yu, M. C. (1985). A serological case-control study of primary hepatocellular carcinoma in Guangxi, China. *Cancer Res.*, **45**, 872–3
11. Lingao, A. L., Domingo, E. O. and Nishioka, K. (1981). Hepatitis B virus profile of hepatocellular carcinoma in the Philippines. *Cancer*, **48**, 1590–5
12. Trichopoulos, D., Day, N. E., Kaklamani, E., Tzonou, A., Muñoz, N., Zavitsanos, X., Koumantaki, Y. and Trichopoulou, A. (1987). Hepatitis B virus, tobacco smoking and ethanol consumption in the etiology of hepatocellular carcinoma. *Int. J. Cancer*, **39**, 45–9
13. Yarrish, R. L., Werner, B. G. and Blumberg, B. S. (1980). Association of hepatitis B virus infection with hepatocellular carcinoma in American patients. *Int. J. Cancer*, **26**, 711–15
14. Austin, H., Delzell, E., Grufferman, S., Levine, R., Morrison, A. S., Stolley, P. D. and Cole, P. (1986). A case-control study of hepatocellular carcinoma and the hepatitis B virus, cigarette smoking, and alcohol consumption. *Cancer Res.*, **46**, 962–6
15. Iijima, T., Saitoh, N., Nobutomo, K., Nambu, M. and Sakuma, K. (1984). A prospective cohort study of hepatitis B surface antigen carriers in a working population. *Gann*, **75**, 571–3
16. Oshima, A., Tsukuma, H., Hiyama, T., Fujimoto, I., Yamano, H. and Tanaka, M. (1984).

Follow-up study of HBsAg positive blood donors with special reference to effect of drinking and smoking on development of liver cancer. *Int. J. Cancer,* **34**, 775–9

17. Hall, A. J., Winter, P. D. and Wright, R. (1985). Mortality of hepatitis B positive blood donors in England and Wales. *Lancet,* **1**, 91–3

18. Trichopoulos, D., Tabor, E., Gerety, R. J., Xirouchaki, E., Sparros, L., Muñoz, N. and Linsell, A. (1978). Hepatitis B and primary hepatocellular carcinoma in a European population. *Lancet,* **2**, 1217–19

19. WHO (1983). *Prevention of Liver Cancer,* Technical Report Series, Vol. 691. (Geneva: World Health Organization)

20. The Gambia Hepatitis Study Group (1987). The Gambia Hepatitis Intervention Study. *Cancer Res.,* **47**, 5782–7

21. Chen, D. S., Hsu, N. H. M., Sung, J. L., Hsu, T. C., Hsu, S. T., Kuo, Y. T., Lo, K. J. and Shih, Y. T. (1987). A mass vaccination program in Taiwan against hepatitis B virus infection in infants of hepatitis B surface antigen-carrier mothers. *J. Am. Med. Assoc.,* **257**, 2597–603

22. Busby, W. F. and Wogan, G. N. (1984). *Aflatoxins.* In Searle, C. E. (ed.), *Aflatoxins in Chemical Carcinogens,* 2nd edn, pp. 945–1136 (Washington D.C.: American Chemical Society)

23. Shank, R. C., Gordon, J. E., Wogan, G. N., Nondasuta, A. and Subhamani, B. (1972). Dietary aflatoxins and human liver cancer: III. Field survey of rural Thai families for ingested aflatoxins. *Fd. Cosmet. Toxicol.,* **10**, 71–84

24. Peers, F. G. and Linsell, C. A. (1973). Dietary aflatoxins and liver cancer. A population based study in Kenya. *Br. J. Cancer,* **27**, 473–84

25. Peers, F. G., Gilman, G. A. and Linsell, C. A. (1976). Dietary aflatoxins and human liver cancer. A study in Swaziland. *Int. J. Cancer,* **17**, 167–76

26. Peers, F., Bosch, X., Kaldor, J., Linsell, A. and Pluijmen, M. (1987). Aflatoxin exposure, hepatitis B virus infection and liver cancer in Swaziland. *Int. J. Cancer,* **39**, 545–53

27. Van Rensburg, S. J., Cook-Mozafarri, P., van Schalkwyk, D. J., van der Watt, J. J., Vincent, T. J. and Purchase, I. F. (1985). Hepatocellular carcinoma and dietary aflatoxin in Mozambique and Transkei. *Br. J. Cancer,* **51**, 713–26

28. Bulatao-Jayme, J., Almero, E. M., Castro, C. A., Jardeleza, T. R. and Salamat, L. A. (1982). A case-control dietary study of primary liver cancer risk from aflatoxin exposure. *Int. J. Epidemiol.,* **11**, 112–19

29. IARC (1987). *Biennial Report, 1986–87,* pp. 46–7. (Lyon: International Agency for Research on Cancer)

30. Parkin, M. (1986) *Cancer Occurrence in Developing Countries,* IARC Sci. Publ. No. 75, pp. 133–89. (Lyon: International Agency for Research on Cancer)

31. FAO/WHO/UNEP (1988). *Report on Second International Conference on Mycotoxins, Bangkok, 28 Sept.–2 Oct. 1987.* (Rome: Food and Agriculture Organization)

32. Sun, T. T. and Chu, Y. Y. (1984). Carcinogenesis and prevention strategy of liver cancer in areas of prevalence. *J. Cell. Physiol. (Suppl.),* **3**, 39–44

33. Sun, T. T., Chu, Y. R., Hsia, C. C., Wei, Y. P. and Wu, S. M. (1986). Strategies and current trends of etiologic prevention of liver cancer. *Biochem. Molec. Epidemiol. Cancer,* 283–92

34. Yeh, F. S., Mo, C. C. and Yen, R. C. (1985). Risk factors for hepatocellular carcinoma in Guangxi, People's Republic of China. *Natl. Cancer Inst. Monogr.,* **69**, 47–8

35. Garfinkel, L. (1980). Cancer mortality in non-smokers. Prospective study by the American Cancer Society. *J. Natl. Cancer Inst.,* **65**, 1169–73

36. Hirayama, T. (1981). A large-scale cohort study on the relationship between diet and selected cancers of digestive organs. In Bruce, W. R., Correa, P., Lipkin, M., Tanenbaum, S. and Wilkins, T. (eds), *Gastrointestinal Cancer: Endogenous Factors,* Banbury Report 7, pp. 409–26. (Cold Spring Harbor: CSH Press)

37. IARC (1988) *Alcohol and Alcoholic Beverages.* IARC Monographs on the Evaluation of the Carcinogenic Risk of Chemicals to Humans, Vol. **44** (Lyon: International Agency for Research on Cancer), in press

38. Yu, M. C., Mack, T., Hanisch, R., Peters, R. L., Henderson, B. E. and Pike, M. C. (1983). Hepatitis, alcohol consumption, cigarette smoking and hepatocellular carcinoma in Los Angeles. *Cancer Res.,* **43**, 6077–9

39. Bosch, F. X. and Muñoz, N. (1988). Prospects for epidemiological studies on hepatocellular cancer as a model to assess viral and chemical interactions. In Bartsch, H., Hemminki, K. and O'Neill, I. K. (eds), *Methods for Detecting DNA Damaging Agents in Humans:*

Applications in Cancer Epidemiology and Prevention, IARC Sci. Publ. No. 89. (Lyon: International Agency for Research on Cancer), pp. 427–39

40. IARC (1987). *Sex Hormones (II)*, IARC Monographs on the Evaluation of the Carcinogenic Risk of Chemicals to Humans, Vol. **21**, pp. 114–15. (Lyon: International Agency for Research on Cancer)
41. Henderson, B. E., Preston-Martin, S., Edmondson, H. A., Peters, R. L. and Pike, M. C. (1983). Hepatocellular carcinoma and oral contraceptives. *Br. J. Cancer,* **48**, 437–40
42. Neuberger, J., Forman, D., Doll, R. and Williams, R. (1986). Oral contraceptives and hepatocellular carcinoma. *Br. Med. J.,* **292**, 1355–7
43. Forman, D., Doll, R. and Peto, R. (1983). Trends in mortality from carcinoma of the liver and the use of oral contraceptives. *Br. J. Cancer,* **48**, 349–54
44. Forman, D., Vincent, T. J. and Doll, R. (1986). Cancer of the liver and the use of oral contraceptives. *Br. Med. J.,* **292**, 1357–61

2
Pathologic types of hepatic tumours

P. J. SCHEUER

INTRODUCTION

In this chapter the pathological features of major types of liver neoplasms and nodules will be briefly reviewed. Lesions have been included either because they are common, or because their diagnosis and differentiation from other lesions presents particular problems (Table 1). Much of the review is concerned with hepatocellular neoplasms, because these form the subject of many of the chapters which follow.

FOCAL NODULAR HYPERPLASIA

This is a localized nodule, the nature of which has long been debated. It is not considered to be a true neoplasm. Regarded by many as a hamartoma, it has recently been suggested that it may also represent a hyperplastic response to a locally abnormal blood supply[1]. It is found at all ages and in both sexes, and is commonest in adult women. A relationship to oral contraceptives has been postulated but is unlikely; however, these drugs may be responsible for increased size and vascularity[2]. Most examples are found incidentally.

Macroscopically, focal nodular hyperplasia forms a rounded, solitary, well-

Table 1 Major liver tumours

Benign	Malignant
Focal nodular hyperplasia[a]	Hepatoblastoma
Liver-cell adenoma	Hepatocellular carcinoma
Bile-duct adenoma	Bile-duct carcinoma
Haemangioma	Angiosarcoma
	Epithelioid haemangioendothelioma

[a]Not considered to be a neoplasm.

15

circumscribed mass several centimetres in diameter. A central scar may be seen, from which fibrous septa radiate to dissect the parenchymal component, which is composed of relatively normal liver tissue. However, portal tracts are lacking. There are no well-formed bile ducts, but groups of proliferated duct-like structures are common[3]. Cholestasis is often seen in the form of canalicular bile thrombi, liver-cell rosettes and accumulation of copper and copper-associated protein. An important diagnostic feature, distinguishing focal nodular hyperplasia from the histologically very similar lesion of cirrhosis, is the presence of disproportionately large, thick-walled and structurally abnormal arteries (Figure 1).

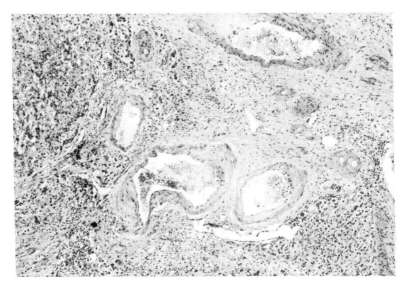

Figure 1 *Focal nodular hyperplasia.* Part of a central scar containing thickened blood vessels. Nodular parenchyma is also seen. Haematoxylin and eosin (H & E), × 56

Focal nodular hyperplasia must be distinguished from the very different condition of *nodular regenerative hyperplasia*, in which hyperplastic parenchymal nodules are found throughout the liver, often in association with portal hypertension and with a variety of systemic diseases[4].

LIVER-CELL ADENOMA

A causal relationship with contraceptive steroids is well established for this benign neoplasm[5]. Liver-cell adenomas may present with abdominal pain resulting from haemorrhage with or without rupture. Haemoperitoneum is a serious complication.

Liver-cell adenomas are solitary or occasionally multiple nodules, lying within more or less normal liver tissue. They may be incompletely encapsulated, or separated from adjacent liver only by their growth pattern. Histologically they are composed of normal-looking liver cells arranged in a trabecular pattern. Fatty change may be seen. There are prominent blood vessels but no portal tracts (Figure 2), an important distinguishing feature from normal liver. The nuclei of the liver cells in an adenoma usually show little variation in size or staining. When nuclei are pleomorphic and hyperchromatic, or when large nucleoli are present, an alternative diagnosis of well-differentiated hepatocellular carcinoma should be considered. Malignant change in liver-cell adenoma has been reported, but histological appearances are sometimes deceptive in so far as clinical behaviour is often benign[6].

Areas of vascular dilatation, haemorrhage and necrosis are commonly found in liver-cell adenomas. In contrast to focal nodular hyperplasia there is no central scar, but fibrosis may result from previous haemorrhage or necrosis.

A few examples of liver-cell adenomas are seen in men, or in children of either sex. In the rare adenomatosis, there are multiple nodules in the liver[7,8].

HEPATOCELLULAR CARCINOMA

Epidemiological, clinical, therapeutic and biological aspects of this important tumour are extensively discussed elsewhere in this volume. Most examples of hepatocellular carcinoma arise in cirrhotic liver but some, such as the fibrolamellar variant described below, are usually found in the absence of cirrhosis. For full discussion of aetiological factors and macroscopic features the reader is referred to larger texts[5,9,10].

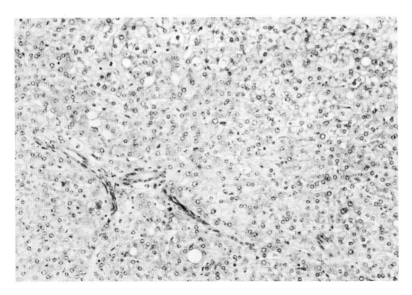

Figure 2 *Liver-cell adenoma.* The parenchyma appears near-normal except for the absence of portal tracts. H & E, × 140

Table 2 Classification of hepatocellular carcinoma.
(Modified from Anthony, 1987[5])

Structure	Cells	Special forms
Trabecular	Liver cell-like	Fibrolamellar
Pseudoglandular	Clear cell	Sclerosing
Compact	Pleomorphic	Minute, encapsulated
		Pedunculated

Different tissue patterns and cellular appearances are found in hepatocellular carcinomas, as well as separate variants with particular clinical and histological characteristics (Table 2).

Tissue patterns

The most common and characteristic form is the *trabecular* pattern (Figure 3). Tumour cells are arranged in anastomosing plates separated by a sinusoidal network. The structure thus resembles that of normal liver, but the trabeculae are usually wider and less regular. An abnormal reticulin pattern, almost always with marked reduction in the amount of reticulin, helps to distinguish well-differentiated trabecular carcinoma from non-neoplastic liver tissue. Bile secretion is found in a minority of tumours.

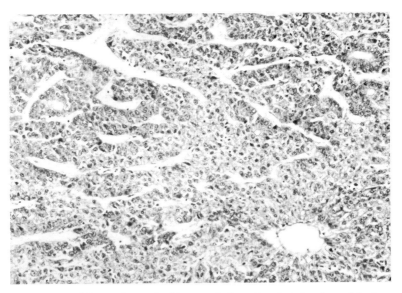

Figure 3 *Hepatocellular carcinoma.* In this example the pattern is trabecular and the tumour cells resemble hepatocytes. H & E, × 140

In the *pseudoglandular* or *adenoid* pattern, the tumour cells form gland-like structures around lumens which may contain bile and are analogous to bile canaliculi. A trabecular and sinusoidal pattern can usually be found in parts of the tumour, confirming the diagnosis and distinguishing it clearly from bile-duct cancer (cholangiocarcinoma). It should be noted that the characteristic secretory product of the latter is mucin rather than bile.

Compact or *solid* carcinomas are occasionally seen, having neither trabecular nor pseudoglandular form.

Cellular characteristics

In most hepatocellular carcinomas the tumour cells resemble non-neoplastic hepatocytes in having a cuboidal or polygonal shape, abundant cytoplasm and centrally placed nuclei. Clear-cell areas may be found (Figure 4), or whole tumours composed of such cells. The appearance is attributed to a high content of glycogen, dissolved out during processing. Some carcinomas are pleomorphic, with bizarre giant nuclei and multinucleated tumour cells.

Many different inclusions may be found within the cells of a hepatocellular carcinoma. These include globular hyaline bodies, fat and typical Mallory bodies[11]. Alpha-1-antitrypsin bodies are sometimes seen in tumour cells, not denoting alpha-1-antitrypsin deficiency.

In difficult cases, immunocytochemical investigation may help to establish the diagnosis of hepatocellular carcinoma. Antigens demonstrable in a proportion of cases include alpha-fetoprotein, alpha-1-antitrypsin and alpha-

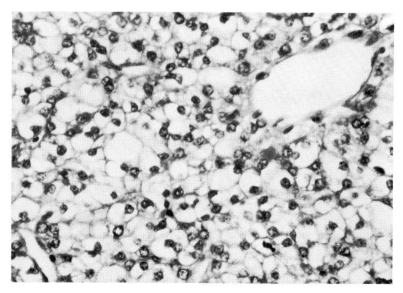

Figure 4 *Hepatocellular carcinoma.* Clear cell type, with large tumour cells having pale-staining cytoplasm. H & E, × 350

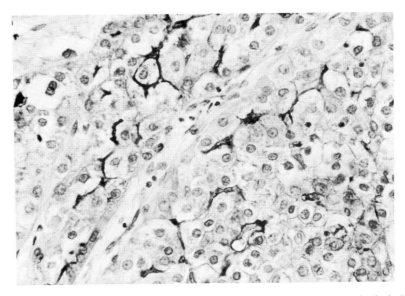

Figure 5 *Hepatocellular carcinoma.* Structures analogous to normal bile canaliculi display carcinoembryonic antigen (CEA). Specific immunoperoxidase, × 350

1-antichymotrypsin among others[12,13]. Carcinoembryonic antigen is found in bile canalicular structures (Figure 5), which also bind several lectins[14].

Fibrolamellar carcinoma

This variant of hepatocellular carcinoma has highly characteristic histological features[15,16]. It is usually not associated with cirrhosis, and is found most often in adolescents and young adults. Groups of large eosinophilic tumour cells rich in mitochondria are separated by septa of fibrous tissue (Figure 6). The cells often contain pale-staining inclusions, and may contain copper and copper-associated protein[17,18]. Bile secretion is sometimes seen, as in hepatocellular carcinoma in general.

Other forms of hepatocellular carcinoma

A fibrous stroma is found in tumours associated with hypercalcaemia, the so-called *sclerosing hepatic carcinoma*[19]. Some of these may be of bile-duct rather than hepatocellular origin. Their relationship to fibrolamellar carcinoma is not yet clear. *Minute* or *encapsulated hepatocellular carcinomas*[20] are found in Japan and other parts of the Far East. *Pedunculated hepatocellular carcinoma* has been described mainly in older patients[5]. In children, hepatocellular carcinoma has to be distinguished from *hepatoblastoma*. This tumour may be entirely epithelial, or contain a variety of

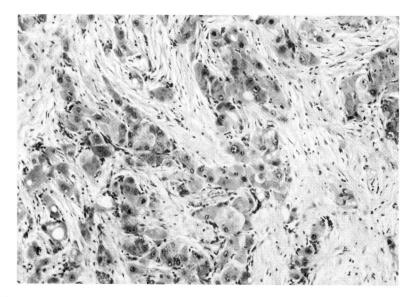

Figure 6 *Hepatocellular carcinoma, fibrolamellar type.* Groups of large, deeply-stained tumour cells resembling hepatocytes are separated by abundant fibrous stroma. Many of the cells contain pale inclusions. H & E, × 140

mesenchymal elements[21]. The pathological features of hepatoblastoma will not be further discussed here.

TUMOURS OF BILE-DUCT ORIGIN

Bile-duct adenomas are small subcapsular nodules composed of ducts set in a fibrous stroma. *Carcinoma of bile-ducts,* or cholangiocarcinoma, is an adeno-carcinoma with variable mucin secretion, arising anywhere in the extra- or intra-hepatic biliary tree. These tumours are not further dealt with in the present review. Carcinoma may also arise in cysts and other congenital biliary abnormalities.

TUMOURS OF VASCULAR ORIGIN

Simple *haemangiomas* are a common incidental finding. They rarely cause symptoms. *Angiosarcoma* is a rare, highly malignant tumour, notable for its association with several carcinogenic agents including arsenic, Thorotrast and vinyl chloride[22]. Histologically, the tumour is composed of elongated cells with a characteristic growth pattern of sinusoidal infiltration (Figure 7). Surviving liver-cell trabeculae may give a false impression that the tumour is of hepatocellular origin. Occasionally, angiosarcoma and hepatocellular car-cinoma co-exist.

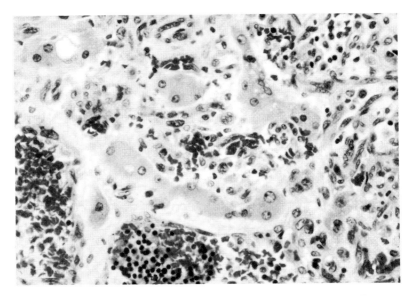

Figure 7 *Angiosarcoma.* Elongated, deeply-stained tumour cells are seen growing between non-neoplastic liver-cell trabeculae. H & E, × 350

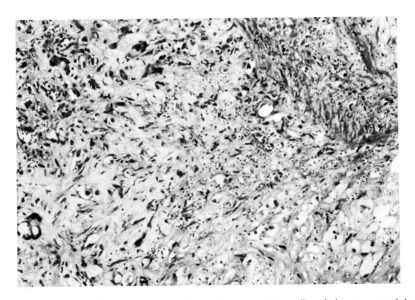

Figure 8 *Epithelioid haemangioendothelioma.* An area of dense fibrosis is seen, containing irregular groups of deeply-stained tumour cells. A vein (top right) has been invaded by tumour. H & E, × 140

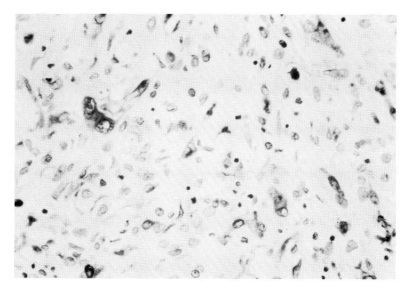

Figure 9 *Epithelioid haemangioendothelioma.* The section has been stained with antibody to Factor VIII-related antigen. Some tumour cells are positive. Specific immunoperoxidase, × 350

Epithelioid haemangioendothelioma[23] is also included in this survey because it may, as its name implies, be mistaken for an epithelial neoplasm. It has a very variable, sometimes good prognosis. Multiple areas of tumour infiltration in the liver often have a regular lobular or acinar distribution. There is an abundant fibrous stroma in which groups of tumour cells are embedded, some of them with lumens and thus reminiscent of bile-duct carcinoma (Figure 8). However, in many instances staining for the vascular marker Factor VIII-related antigen demonstrates the endothelial nature of the tumour (Figure 9). Vascular invasion is a prominent feature, leading to possible confusion with veno-occlusive disease.

Acknowledgements

I am grateful to Mr Francis Moll for help with the illustrations and to Mrs Nell Lam for preparing the manuscript.

References

1. Wanless, I. R., Mawdsley, C. and Adams, R. (1985). On the pathogenesis of focal nodular hyperplasia of the liver. *Hepatology,* **5**, 1194–1200
2. Nime, F., Pickren, J. W., Vana, J., Aronoff, B. L., Baker, H. W. and Murphy, G. P. (1979). The histology of liver tumors in oral contraceptive users observed during a national survey by the American College of Surgeons' Commission on Cancer. *Cancer,* **44**, 1481–9

3. Butron Vila, M. M., Haot, J. and Desmet, V. J. (1984). Cholestatic features in focal nodular hyperplasia. *Liver,* **4**, 387–95
4. Stromeyer, F. W. and Ishak, K. G. (1981). Nodular transformation (nodular 'regenerative' hyperplasia) of the liver. A clinicopathologic study of 30 cases. *Hum. Pathol.,* **12**, 60–71
5. Anthony, P. P. (1987). Tumours and tumour-like lesions of the liver and biliary tract. In MacSween, R. N. M., Anthony, P. P. and Scheuer, P. J. (eds), *Pathology of the Liver,* 2nd edn, pp. 574–645. (Edinburgh: Churchill-Livingstone).
6. Anthony, P. P. (1975). Hepatoma associated with androgenic steroids. *Lancet,* **1**, 685–6
7. Lui, A. F. K., Hiratzka, L. F. and Hirose, F. M. (1980). Multiple adenomas of the liver. *Cancer,* **45**, 1001–4
8. Flejou, J-F., Barge, J., Menu, Y., Degott, C., Bismuth, H., Potet, F. and Benhamou, J-P. (1985). Liver adenomatosis. An entity distinct from liver adenoma? *Gastroenterology,* **89**, 1132–8
9. Nakashima, T. and Kojiro, M. (1987). *Hepatocellular Carcinoma.* (Tokyo: Springer-Verlag)
10. Okuda, K. and Ishak, K. G. (eds) (1987). *Neoplasms of the Liver.* (Berlin: Springer-Verlag)
11. Nakanuma, Y. and Ohta, G. (1986). Expression of Mallory bodies in hepatocellular carcinoma in man and its significance. *Cancer,* **57**, 81–6
12. Thung, S. N., Gerber, M. A., Sarno, E. and Popper, H. (1979). Distribution of five antigens in hepatocellular carcinoma. *Lab. Invest.,* **41**, 101–5
13. Ordonez, N. G. and Manning, J. T. (1984). Comparison of α-1-antitrypsin and α-1-antichymotrypsin in hepatocellular carcinoma: an immunoperoxidase study. *Am. J. Gastroenterol.,* **79**, 959–63
14. Machinami, R. and Oono, Y. (1987). Carcinoembryonic antigen and lectin binding in the bile canalicular structures of hepatocellular carcinoma. *Virchows Arch. [A],* **412**, 111–18
15. Berman, M. M., Libbey, P. and Foster, J. H. (1980). Hepatocellular carcinoma. Polygonal cell type with fibrous stroma – an atypical variant with a favorable prognosis. *Cancer,* **46**, 1448–55
16. Craig, J. R., Peters, R. L., Edmondson, H. A. and Omata, M. (1980). Fibrolamellar carcinoma of the liver: a tumor of adolescents and young adults with distinctive clinicopathologic features. *Cancer,* **46**, 372–9
17. Lefkowitch, J. H., Muschel, R., Price, J. B., Marboe, C. and Braunhut, S. (1983). Copper and copper-binding protein in fibrolamellar liver cell carcinoma. *Cancer,* **51**, 97–100
18. Vecchio, F. M., Federico, F. and Dina, M. A. (1986). Copper and hepatocellular carcinoma. *Digestion,* **35**, 109–14
19. Omata, M., Peters, R. L. and Tatter, D. (1981). Sclerosing hepatic carcinoma: relationship to hypercalcemia. *Liver,* **1**, 33–49
20. Okuda, K., Musha, H., Nakajima, Y., Kubo, Y., Shimokawa, Y., Nagasaki, Y., Sawa, Y., Jinnouchi, S., Kaneko, I., Obata, H., Hisamitsu, T., Motoike, Y., Okazaki, N., Kojiro, M., Sakamoto, K. and Nakashima, T. (1977). Clinicopathologic features of encapsulated hepatocellular carcinoma. A study of 26 cases. *Cancer,* **40**, 1240–5
21. Lack, E. E., Neave, C. and Vawter, G. F. (1982). Hepatoblastoma. A clinical and pathologic study of 54 cases. *Am. J. Surg. Pathol.,* **6**, 693–705
22. Thomas, L. B., Popper, H., Berk, P. D., Selikoff, I. and Falk, H. (1975). Vinyl-chloride-induced liver disease. From idiopathic portal hypertension (Banti's syndrome) to angiosarcomas. *N. Engl. J. Med.* **292**, 17–22
23. Ishak, K. G., Sesterhenn, I. A., Goodman, Z. D., Rabin, L. and Stromeyer, F. W. (1984). Epithelioid hemangioendothelioma of the liver: a clinicopathologic and follow-up study of 32 cases. *Hum. Pathol.,* **15**, 839–52.

3
Immunohistochemistry in the diagnosis of hepatocellular carcinoma

S. N. THUNG AND M. A. GERBER

INTRODUCTION

Immunohistochemical studies of tumour cell markers are useful in the diagnosis and classification of tumours, in predicting prognosis and tumour response to therapy, and in detecting pre-neoplastic conditions and early cases. Refinement of the techniques, particularly the introduction of the peroxidase-antiperoxidase (PAP)[1] and the avidin-biotin complex (ABC) methods[2], allows the demonstration of antigens in formalin-fixed, paraffin-embedded material. Hepatocellular carcinoma (HCC) synthesizes a variety of normal, abnormal, aberrant and ectopic proteins which can be considered as tumour markers. Most of these antigens are preserved during routine processing and may be helpful in differentiating hepatocellular carcinoma from other primary tumours of the liver or from metastatic neoplasms to the liver.

TUMOUR MARKERS

Alpha-fetoprotein

The usefulness and limitation of serological tests for alpha-fetoprotein (AFP) in the diagnosis and follow-up of HCC have been well documented[3,4]. Recent studies suggest that AFP derived from HCC may be differentiated from AFP from non-tumorous liver based on differences in glycosylation as determined by lectin binding[5,6] or on unique epitopes which may be detected with monoclonal antibodies[7]. AFP has been demonstrated in the cytoplasm of HCC cells[8-10]. The presence of AFP in the cytoplasm of tumour cells of the liver indicates their hepatocellular origin, if metastatic germ-cell tumour, which may produce AFP, is excluded.

The question of AFP expression in pre-neoplastic hepatocytes has received

25

much less attention. AFP has been detected in morphologically normal hepatocytes and also in some dysplastic cells in the non-tumorous portion of cirrhotic liver of patients with HCC[11,12]. It is of great interest that elevation of serum AFP is found in patients with hepatic regeneration following acute or chronic hepatitis, but not after partial hepatectomy, which suggests that expression of AFP reflects altered regeneration[13,14]. Clearly, studies with monoclonal antibodies to different species of AFP are needed to determine the relation of AFP expression in hepatocytes to malignant transformation.

Other export proteins

Hepatocellular carcinoma cells often retain the function of their normal counterpart and synthesize a large number of plasma proteins. These proteins have been demonstrated in HCC by immunohistochemical methods. Albumin, alpha-1-antitrypsin, alpha-1-antichymotrypsin and carcinoembryonic antigen (CEA) are found in the majority of HCC[8,15,16]. Alpha-1-antitrypsin and CEA are present also in cholangiocarcinomas and metastatic adenocarcinomas and therefore are less specific markers for HCC. Ferritin is observed both in neoplastic and non-neoplastic liver tissue[17,18]. Tumour-specific isoferritin[19,20] has been defined and may have diagnostic importance. HCC may also produce fibronectin[21], fibrinogen[22], abnormal prothrombin[23], vitamin A binding proteins[24], as well as copper metallothionein associated with copper accumulation in the tumour cells[25,26].

Hepatitis B virus antigens

There is a strong association between hepatitis B virus infection and the development of HCC[27,28]. The expression of hepatitis B surface antigen (IIBsAg) and hepatitis B core antigen (HBcAg) has been studied extensively by histochemical (Shikata's orcein, Victoria blue or aldehyde fuchsin stains) and immunohistochemical methods[29]. HBsAg is demonstrable in the cytoplasm of a few scattered tumour cells in a small percentage (usually <20%) of HBV-associated HCC. HBsAg and, less commonly, HBcAg are detected more readily in the surrounding liver, both in the immediate vicinity of and at a distance from the tumour[8,29].

Tumour-specific antigens

Progress has been made recently in the production of monoclonal antibodies to cell-surface antigens of human HCC cell lines. the monoclonal antibodies react to cell-surface proteins of HCC with molecular weights of 50000 and 70000 daltons[30,31]. These reagents may be useful for the serological diagnosis, histological identification, imaging and immunotherapy of HCC.

Blood-group antigens

Blood-group ABH and Lewis determinants are expressed not only in blood cells but also in a variety of epithelial cells[32]. Aberrant expression of blood-group antigens has been previously observed in human cancers[33-35]. These changes, studied immunohistochemically[35,36], include: the deletion of A, B and Lewis[a, b] antigens; the accumulation of precursor determinants such as H and I substances; the abnormal distribution and co-expression of Lewis antigens; and the neosynthesis of incompatible blood-group antigens, i.e. A antigen in patients with blood type O or B. In the liver, blood-group antigens are detectable in biliary epithelium, but not on hepatocytes. HCC cells, however, in some cases, expressed H and Lewis antigens[37]. Recently Jovanovic *et al.* studied the expression of Lewis[X] and Lewis[Y] in cholangiocarcinomas and hepatocellular carcinomas and found preferential expression of these two blood-group antigens in cholangiocarcinomas[38].

Cytoskeletal proteins

Intermediate filament typing yields information on the histogenetic origin of neoplasms because tumours continue to express the major intermediate

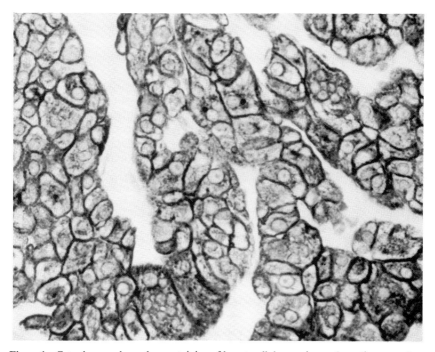

Figure 1 Cytoplasm and membrane staining of hepatocellular carcinoma by antiserum to low-molecular-weight cytokeratin polypeptides. (Immunoperoxidase, counterstained with haematoxylin, × 100)

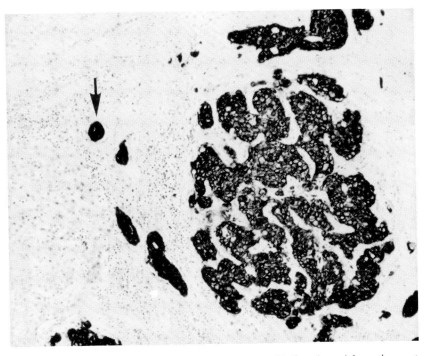

Figure 2 Staining of cholangiocarcinoma and bile-duct epithelium (arrow) by antiserum to high-molecular-weight cytokeratin polypeptides. Hepatocytes and inflammatory cells are unstained. (Immunoperoxidase, counterstained with haematoxylin, × 40)

filament-type characteristic of the cell of origin. Cytokeratins are intermediate filament proteins that form part of the cytoskeleton of epithelial cells[39]. They belong to a family of at least 19 distinct polypeptides with molecular weights ranging from 40000 to 70000 daltons. Antibodies directed against these dissimilar polypeptides react differently with hepatocytes and bile-duct epithelium. Antibodies directed against low-molecular-weight cytokeratin polypeptides react with normal hepatocytes and bile-duct epithelium, while antibodies to higher-molecular-weight polypeptides stain only bile-duct epithelium. Consequently, antibodies to these distinct cytokeratin polypeptides are useful in differentiating hepatocellular from cholangiolar carcinomas[40–42] (Figures 1 and 2).

Acknowledgements

We are grateful to Norman Katz for photographic assistance and to John Morgan for keyboarding this manuscript.

References

1. Sternberger, L. A. (1979). In *Immunocytochemistry*, 2nd edn. New York: (John Wiley & Sons).
2. Hsu, S. N., Raine, L. and Fanger, H. (1981). Use of avidin–biotin–peroxidase complex (ABC) in immunoperoxidase technique. A comparison between ABC and unlabeled antibody (PAP) procedures. *J. Histochem. Cytochem.*, **29**, 577–80
3. Wespic, H. T. and Kirkpatrick, A. (1979). Alpha-fetoprotein and its relevance to human disease. *Gastroenterology*, **77**, 787–96
4. Chen, D.-S., Sung, J.-L., Sheu, J.-C., Lai, M.-Y., How, S.-W., Hsu, H.-C., Lee, C.-S. and Wei, T.-C (1984). Serum alpha-fetoprotein in the early stage of human hepatocellular carcinoma. *Gastroenterology*, **86**, 1404–9
5. Fujise, K., Nagamori, S., Hasumura, S., Homma, S., Sujino, H. and Kameda, H. (1983). Heterogeneity of alpha-fetoprotein with concanavalin A-binding properties in serum and ascites from patients of liver cancer and liver cirrhosis. *Jpn. J. Gastroenterol.*, **80**, 2362–6
6. Aoyagi, Y., Suzuki, Y., Isemura, M., Soga, K., Ozaki, T., Ichida, T., Inoue, K., Sasaki, H. and Ichida, F. (1984). Differential reactivity of alpha-fetoprotein with lectins and evaluation of its usefulness in the diagnosis of hepatocellular carcinoma. *Jpn. J. Cancer Res.* (Gann), **75**, 809–15
7. Bellet, D. H., Wands, J. R., Isselbacher, K. J. and Bohuon, C. (1984). Serum alpha-fetoprotein levels in human disease: perspectives from a highly specific monoclonal radio-immunoassay. *Proc. Natl. Acad. Sci. USA*, **81**, 3869–73
8. Thung, S. N., Gerber, M. A., Sarno, E. and Popper, H. (1979). Distribution of five antigens in hepatocellular carcinoma. *Lab. Invest.*, **41**, 101–5
9. Goodman, Z., Ishak, K., Langloss, J. M., Sesterhenn, I. A. and Rabin, L. (1985). Combined hepatocellular–cholangiocarcinoma. A histological and immunohistochemical study. *Cancer*, **55**, 124–35
10. Imoto, M., Nishimura, D., Fukuda, Y., Sugiyama, K., Kumada, T. and Nakano, S. (1985). Immunohistochemical detection of alpha-fetoprotein, carcinoembryonic antigen and ferritin in formalin–paraffin sections from hepatocellular carcinoma. *Am. J. Gastroenterol.*, **80**, 902–6
11. Gerber, M. A., Thung, S. N. and Popper, H. (1980). Localization of fetal antigens in relation to HBsAg in hepatocytes. In Bianchi, L., Gerok, W., Sickinger, K. and Stalder, G. A. (eds), *Virus and the Liver*, pp. 205–8. (Lancaster: MTP Press)
12. Roncalli, M., Borzio, M., Debiagi, G., Servida, E., Cantaboni, A., Seroni, M. and Taccagmi, G. L. (1985). Liver cell dysplasia and hepatocellular carcinoma: a histological and immunohistochemical study. *Histopathology*, **9**, 209–21
13. Alpert, E. and Feller, E. R. (1978). Alpha-fetoprotein (AFP) in benign liver disease: evidence that normal liver regeneration does not induce AFP synthesis. *Gastroenterology*, **74**, 856–8
14. Watanabe, A., Shiota, T., Hayashi, S. and Nagashima, H. (1984). Serum alpha-fetoprotein in fulminant hepatitis and hepatic regeneration following partial hepatectomy. *Biochem. Med.*, **32**, 132–7
15. Kojiro, M., Parada, L. F. and Weinberg, R. A. (1983). Tumorigenic conversion of primary embryofibroblasts requires at least two cooperating oncogenes. *Nature*, **304**, 576–7
16. Ordonez, N. G. and Manning, J. T. (1984). Comparison of alpha-1-antitrypsin and alpha-1-antichymotrypsin in hepatocellular carcinoma: an immuno-peroxidase study. *Am. J. Gastroenterol.*, **79**, 959–63
17. Cohen, C., Berson, S. D., Shulman, G. and Budgeon, L. R. (1984). Immunohistochemical ferritin in hepatocellular carcinoma. *Cancer*, **53**, 1931–5
18. Imoto, M., Nishimura, D., Fukuda, Y., Sugiyama, K., Kumada, T. and Nakano, S. (1985). Immunohistochemical detection of alpha-fetoprotein, carcinoembryonic antigen and ferritin in formalin–paraffin sections from hepatocellular carcinoma. *Am. J. Gastroenterol.*, **80**, 902–6
19. Alpert, E. and Coston, R. L. (1973). Carcinofoetal human liver ferritins. *Nature*, **242**, 194–5
20. Asakawa, H. and Mori, W. (1985). Isoferritins from tumorous and non-tumorous human liver. *Jpn. J. Cancer Res.* (Gann), **76**, 95–8
21. Jagirdar, J., Ishak, K. G., Colombo, M., Brambilla, C. and Paronetto, F. (1985). Fibronectin patterns in hepatocellular carcinoma and its clinical significance. *Cancer*, **56**, 1643–8

22. Stromeyer, F. W., Ishak, K. G., Gerber, M. A. and Mathew, T. (1980). Ground glass cells in hepatocellular carcinoma. *Am. J. Clin. Pathol.,* **74**, 254–8

23. Liebman, H. A., Furie, B. C., Tong, M. J., Blanchard, R. A., Lo, K.-J., Lee, S.-D., Coleman, M. S. and Furie, G. (1984). Decarboxy (abnormal) prothrombin as a serum marker of primary hepatocellular carcinoma. *N. Engl. J. Med.,* **310**, 1427–31

24. Ikezaki, K., Ueda, H., Koyanogi, T., Kuwano, M., Ando, K., Sato, S., Takenaka, K. and Inokuchi, K. (1985). Cellular vitamin A-binding proteins in liver tumors and adjacent tissues. *Cancer,* **55**, 2405–10

25. Lefkowitch, J. H., Muschel, R., Price, J. B., Marboe, E. and Braunhut, S. (1983). Copper and copper-binding proteins in fibrolamellar liver cell carcinoma. *Cancer,* **51**, 97–100

26. Haratake, J., Horie, A., Nakashima, A., Takeda, S. and Mori, A. (1986). Minute hepatoma with excessive copper accumulation. *Arch. Pathol. Lab. Med.,* **110**, 192–4

27. Beasley, R. P. (1982). Hepatitis B virus as the etiologic agent in hepatocellular carcinoma— epidemiologic considerations. *Hepatology,* **2**, 21S–26S

28. Gerber, M. A. and Thung, S. N. (1985). Molecular and cellular pathology of hepatitis B. *Lab. Invest.,* **52**, 572–90

29. Gerber, M. A., Thung, S. N. and Popper, H. (1983). Viral hepatitis and hepatocellular carcinoma. In Deinhardt, F. and Deinhardt, J. (eds), *Viral Hepatitis: Laboratory and Clinical Science,* pp. 317–31. (New York: Marcel Dekker)

30. Carlson, R. I., Ben-Porath, E., Shouval, D., Strauss, W., Isselbacher, K. J. and Wands, J. R. (1985). Antigenic characterization of human hepatocellular carcinoma. *Gastroenterology,* **86**, 1404–7

31. Shouval, D., Eilat, D., Carlson, R. I., Adler, R., Livini, N. and Wands, J. R. (1985). Human hepatoma-associated cell surface antigen: identification and characterization by means of monoclonal antibodies. *Hepatology,* **5**, 347–56

32. Szulman, A. E. (1960). The histological distribution of blood group substances A and B in man. *J. Exp. Med.,* **111**, 785–800

33. Hakomori, S. (1985). Aberrant glycosylation in cancer cell membranes as focused on glycolipids: Overview and perspectives. *Cancer Res.,* **45**, 2405–14

34. Finan, P. J. Wright, D. G., Lennox, E. S., Sacks, S. H. and Bleehen, N. M. (1983). Human blood group isoantigen expression on normal and malignant-gastric epithelium studied with anti-A and anti-B monoclonal antibodies. *J. Natl. Cancer Inst.,* **70**, 679–85

35. Ernst, C., Atkinson, B., Wysocka, M., Blazczyk, M., Herlyn, M., Sears, H., Steplewski, A. and Koprowski, H. (1984). Monoclonal antibody localization of Lewis antigen in fixed tissue. *Lab. Invest.,* **50**, 394–400

36. Hirohashi, S., Ito, Y., Kodama, T. and Shimosato, Y. (1984). Distribution of blood group antigen A, B, H, and I (Ma) in mucous-producing adenocarcinoma of human lung. *J. Natl. Cancer Inst.,* **72**, 1299–1305

37. Okada, Y., Arima, T., Togawa, K., Nagashima, H., Jinno, K., Moriwaki, S., Kunitomo, T., Thurin, J. and Koprowski, H. (1987). Neoexpression of ABH Lewis blood group antigens in human hepatocellular carcinomas. *J. Natl. Cancer Inst.,* **78**, 19–28

38. Jovanovic, R., Jagirdar, J., Thung, S. N. and Paronetto, F. Blood group-related antigens Lewis[x] and Lewis[y] in the differential diagnosis of cholangiocarcinoma and hepatocellular carcinoma. *Arch. Pathol. Lab. Med.,* in press

39. Sun, T. T. and Green, H. (1978). Keratin filaments of cultured human epidermal cells: formation of intermolecular disulphide bonds during terminal differentiation. *J. Biol. Chem.,* **235**, 2053–60

40. Fischer, H., Altmannsberger, M., Weber, K. and Osborn, M. (1987). Keratin polypeptides in malignant epithelial liver tumors. Differential diagnostic and histogenetic aspects. *Am. J. Pathol.,* **127**, 530–7

41. Pastolero, G., Wakabayashi, T., Oka, T. and Mori, S. (1987). Tissue polypeptide antigens— a marker antigen differentiating cholangiolar tumor from other hepatic tumors. *Am. J. Clin. Pathol.,* **87**, 168–73

42. Lai, Y. S., Thung, S. N., Gerber, M. A., Chen, M. L. and Schaffner, F. Expression of cytokeratins in normal and diseased livers and in primary liver carcinomas. *Arch. Pathol. Lab. Med.,* in press

4
Morphology of hepadna virus-induced hepatocellular carcinoma in animals

M. A. GERBER, S. N. THUNG AND H. POPPER

INTRODUCTION

In contrast to chemical hepatocarcinogenesis[1], only few experimental models of viral hepatocarcinogenesis have been available for study in the past[2]. Recently however, hepatocellular carcinoma (HCC) has been observed in several mammalian and avian species associated with chronic infection by hepadna viruses[3,4]. These viruses belong to a family of closely-related DNA viruses which besides hepatitis B virus (HBV) of man include woodchuck hepatitis virus (WHV) of *Marmota monax*[5], ground squirrel hepatitis virus (GSHV) of *Spermophilus beecheyi*[6], duck hepatitis B virus (DHBV) of *Anas domesticus*[7] and other ducks, heron hepatitis B virus in gray herons (H. Will, personal communication), tree squirrel hepatitis B virus[8], and probably others. Preliminary observations in several other species including snakes suggest that hepadna viruses may be widely distributed in the animal kingdom[4]. These viruses share close genomic, structural, antigenic and biological similarities such as a narrow host range, a significant tropism for hepatocytes, and frequent development of chronic infections associated with development of chronic hepatitis and HCC. In fact, the mechanisms of genome replication and DNA sequence homology indicate that hepadna viruses are phylogenetically related to retroviruses[4]. Development of HCC has been observed in woodchucks, ground squirrels, and ducks after infection in the wild or in the laboratory with the respective viruses. These models of viral hepatocarcinogenesis will permit the type of investigations so effectively carried out on animal models of chemical carcinogenesis. The shorter life span of animals susceptible to hepadna virus infections and of their hepatocytes in comparison to humans reduces the time of evolution of chronic hepatitis and HCC and facilitates prospective and follow-up studies of diseases which last decades in man. In this report, we will describe the morphologic features during the development of HCC in hepadna virus-infected animals with particular reference to the histogenesis and pathogenesis of the disease.

HCC IN VARIOUS SPECIES

HCC in woodchucks

Among the currently available animal models of hepadna virus-induced hepatocarcinogenesis, the development of HCC in woodchucks has been studied most extensively[9-11]. After infection of newborn woodchucks by WHV in the laboratory, all animals which became carriers of surface antigen developed HCC within 17–36 months[11]. Liver biopsy specimens obtained at 12 months revealed mild infiltration of portal tracts by scattered lymphocytes, slight focal increase of sinusoidal cells, and scattered hepatocytes with ground glass cytoplasm which stained with Victoria blue. These histologic features were similar to those seen in healthy asymptomatic human carriers of HBsAg. However, in contrast to human carriers, the woodchuck livers also contained nodules up to 0.2 mm in diameter composed of larger hepatocytes with basophilic or vacuolated cytoplasm. Liver specimens obtained at 18 months or later, revealed distinct hepatocytic nodules measuring up to 0.2 cm in diameter and consisting of basophilic hepatocytes in plates more than one cell thick. The surrounding parenchyma was compressed and infiltrated by inflammatory cells. Gradual transition from these neoplastic nodules to frank HCC was observed. The carcinomas were trabecular in type and contained hematopoietic cells which often were atypical. The degree of anaplasia of HCC varied throughout, but was more conspicuous in the central portions.

In contrast to newborn woodchucks, adult woodchucks developed features of acute viral hepatitis within 5–12 weeks of laboratory infection[9]. Most of the animals (19 of 21) seroconverted to anti-WHs and did not develop evidence of HCC. Two woodchucks became chronic carriers and subsequent biopsy specimens revealed chronic persistent hepatitis, hepatocytic nodules, scattered dysplastic hepatocytes and HCC with features similar to those described above. In all woodchuck carriers, the inflammatory reaction increased conspicuously at the time when HCC was recognized and resembled chronic active hepatitis, accompanied by atypical hematopoietic cells, mainly megakaryocytes. The necro-inflammatory reaction appeared to be more severe in the vicinity of the tumour. Similar observations have been made in woodchucks which were infected in the wild. The following features distinguish the woodchuck lesions from chronic HBV infection with HCC in man: (a) association of carcinoma with active hepatic necroinflammation (including conspicuous plasma cell reaction), but not with cirrhosis; (b) conspicuous neoplastic nodules and transition to carcinoma; (c) hematopoietic cells, often atypical, in the tumour and in the surrounding liver; (d) presence of serologic markers of active viral replication[9].

Based on these findings, the following points are emphasized:

(1) The development of HCC in all woodchucks which became chronic carriers after closely monitored laboratory infection indicates that WHV is directly carcinogenic in the absence of exogenous carcinogens such as aflatoxin[11]. In contrast, HCC was not observed in adult or newborn laboratory-infected woodchucks which developed anti-WHs or in non-infected animals. Thus, permanent carriage of WHV or WHsAg appears to

be a significant risk factor for the development of HCC. These observations support the large body of evidence that HBV is oncogenic in man[12,13].

(2) Histologic studies of the chronically infected woodchucks revealed an apparent continuum from normal liver to hyperplastic and dysplastic hepatocytes over well-differentiated neoplastic nodules to frank hepatocellular carcinomas.

(3) Before or at the time of discovery of the carcinoma, a necro-inflammatory reaction developed in the surrounding liver often accompanied by atypical hematopoietic cells. It is not clear whether the inflammation is a promoting factor effecting proliferation of hepatocytes or a secondary response to tissue injury by the expanding tumour. We have made similar observations in Yupik Eskimos with chronic HBV infection in southwestern Alaska, where as a result of a screening program HCC is frequently detected in early stages in the absence of cirrhosis[14]. The peri-carcinomatous liver also showed a necro-inflammatory reaction and continuous transition from hyperplasia and dysplasia to increasing anaplasia in the centre of the tumours (Fig. 1).

HCC in ground squirrels

In Beechey ground squirrels infected with GSHV, acute hepatitis and carrier stage sometimes associated with Victoria blue positive hepatocytes, has been seen[15,16]. HCC has developed in over four years old animals with chronic GSHV infection (Fig. 2). The livers exhibited hyperplastic nodules with gradual transition to carcinoma, necro-inflammation around the tumours, and sometimes hematopoietic cells as observed in woodchuck livers.

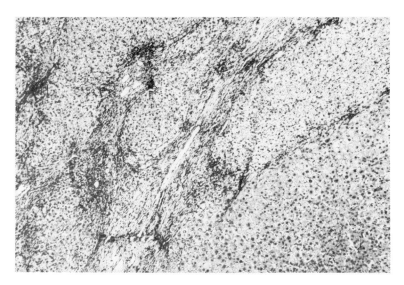

Figure 1 Hepatocellular carcinoma (lower right) in Alaskan Eskimo. The tumour is surrounded by fibrosis and an intense necro-inflammatory reaction (hematoxylin and eosin, × 80).

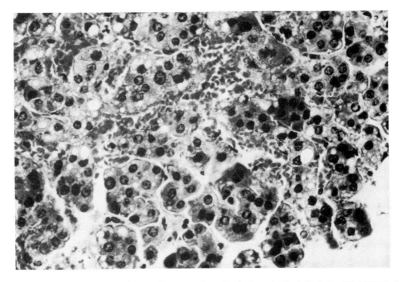

Figure 2 Hepatocellular carcinoma in ground squirrel chronically infected with GSHV. The trabecular carcinoma is identical to that seen in man and woodchucks (hematoxylin and eosin, × 320)

HCC in Chinese ducks

A variety of liver diseases including HCC has been observed in Chinese ducks, but the relation to chronic infection by DHBV has not been established[17-19]. One duck with HCC with integrated DHBV DNA and chronic active hepatitis in the surrounding liver has been described[16]. The investigations of chronically-infected ground squirrels and Chinese ducks are still at an early stage.

FUTURE DIRECTIONS

Woodchucks with chronic hepadna virus infection represent the first readily reproducible model of viral hepatocarcinogenesis. This and additional models in ground squirrels and ducks will allow a large variety of investigations so far not possible and will supplement our knowledge in an area which until now was derived primarily from experiments in chemical carcinogenesis. Many unsolved questions can be addressed such as the evolution of chronic viral hepatitis and hepatocellular carcinoma, their molecular basis, the histo- and pathogenesis, and possible therapeutic interventions. Similarities and dissimilarities to human disease can be analyzed such as the precursor lesions[20] and the continuum in hepatocarcinogenesis, and the possible role of necro-inflammation and hematopoietic cells in promoting the development of HCC. Finally, we can analyze the growth pattern of HCC which appears to be bi-directional with gradual centripetal transition from precursor lesions to HCC and its subsequent centrifugal expansion, possibly related to growth factors. Conclusions from these new animal models of hepatocarcinogenesis may apply to cancer in other organs.

References

1. Farber, E. and Sarma, D. S. R. (1987). Hepatocarcinogenesis: a dynamic cellular perspective. *Lab. Invest., 56*, 4–22
2. Lapis, K. (1977). Histologic and ultrastructural aspects of virus-induced primary hepatocellular carcinoma and transplantable hepatomas of viral origin in chickens. *J. Tox. Environ. Health,* 5, 469–501
3. Summers, J. (1981). Three recently described animal virus models for human hepatitis B virus. *Hepatology,* 1, 179–83
4. Robinson, W. S. and Marion, P. L. (1988). Biological features of hepadna viruses. In Zuckerman, A. J. (ed.), *Viral Hepatitis and Liver Disease.* pp. 449–58. (New York: Alan R. Liss, Inc.)
5. Summers, J., Smolec, J. M. and Snyder, R. (1978). A virus similar to human hepatitis B virus associated with hepatitis and hepatoma in woodchucks. *Proc. Natl. Acad. Sci, USA,* 75, 4533–7
6. Marion, P. L., Oshiro, L., Regnery, D. C., Scullard, G. H. and Robinson, W. S. (1980). A virus in Beechey ground squirrels that is related to hepatitis B virus of man. *Proc. Natl. Acad. Sci. USA,* 77, 2941–5
7. Mason, W. S., Seal, G. and Summers, J. (1980). Virus of Pekin ducks with structural and biological relatedness to human hepatitis B virus. *J. Virol.,* 36, 829–36
8. Feitelson, M. A., Millman, I. and Blumberg, B. S. (1986). Tree squirrel hepatitis B virus: antigenic and structural characterization. *Proc. Natl. Acad. Sci. USA,* 83, 2994–7
9. Popper, H., Shih, J. W. -K., Gerin, J. L., Wong, D. C., Hoyer, B. H., London, W. T., Sly, D. L. and Purcell, R. H. (1981). Woodchuck hepatitis and hepatocellular carcinoma: correlation of histologic with virologic observations. *Hepatology,* 1, 91–8
10. Snyder, R. L., Tyler, G. and Summers, J. (1982). Chronic hepatitis and hepatocellular carcinoma associated with woodchuck hepatitis virus. *Am. J. Pathol.,* 107, 422–5
11. Popper, H., Roth, L., Purcell, R. H., Tennant, B. C. and Gerin, J. L. (1987). Hepatocarcinogenicity of the woodchuck hepatitis virus. *Proc. Natl. Acad. Sci. USA,* 84, 866–70
12. Popper, H., Shafritz, D. A. and Hoofnagle, J. H. (1987). Relation of the hepatitis B virus carrier state to hepatocellular carcinoma. *Hepatology,* 7, 764–72
13. Gerber, M. A., Thung, S. N. and Popper, H. (1983). Viral hepatitis and hepatocellular carcinoma. In Deinhardt, F. and Deinhardt, J. (eds), *Viral Hepatitis.* pp. 327–41. (New York: Marcel Dekker, Inc.)
14. Popper, H., Thung, S. N., McMahon, B. J., Lanier, A. P., Hawkins, I. and Alberts, S. R. (1987). Evolution of hepatocellular carcinoma associated with chronic hepatitis B virus infection in Alaskan Eskimos. *Arch. Pathol. Lab. Med.,* 112, 498–504
15. Marion, P. L., Knight, S. S., Salazar, F. H., Popper, H. and Robinson, W. S. (1983). Ground squirrel hepatitis virus infection. *Hepatology,* 3, 519–27
16. Marion, P. L., van Davelaar, M. J., Knight S. S., Salazar, F. H., Garcia, G., Popper, H. and Robinson, W. S. (1986). Hepatocellular carcinoma in ground squirrels persistently infected with ground squirrel hepatitis virus. *Proc. Natl. Acad. Sci. USA,* 83, 4543–6
17. Omata, M., Yokosuka, O., Imazeki, F., Matsuyama, Y., Uchiumi, K., Ito, Y., Mori, J. and Okuda, K. (1984). Transmission of duck hepatitis B virus from Chinese carrier ducks to Japanese ducklings: a study of viral DNA in serum and tissue. *Hepatology,* 4, 603–7
18. Yokosuka, O., Omata, M., Zhou Y.-Z., Imazeki, F. and Okuda, F. (1986). Duck hepatitis B virus DNA in liver and serum of Chinese ducks: integration of viral DNA in a hepatocellular carcinoma. *Proc. Natl. Acad. Sci. USA,* 82, 5180–4
19. Omata, M., Hirota, K., Takano S., Yokosuka, O. and Okuda, K. (1987). Hepatocarcinogenesis in the duck. *J. Cell. Biochem. (Suppl.),* 11D, 13–17

20. Gerber, M. A. (1986). Recent studies on the developing human hepatocellular carcinoma. *Cancer Surveys,* **5,** 741–63

5
Role of cirrhosis in hepatocarcinogenesis

M. C. KEW

INTRODUCTION

Substantial progress has been made during recent years in elucidating the aetiology and pathogenesis of human hepatocellular carcinoma (HCC). Three major and several minor causal associations of the tumour have been identified. Of the former, persistent hepatitis-B virus (HBV) infection, which may be implicated as an initiator of as much as 80% of HCC world-wide[1], and cirrhosis, which co-exists with HCC in 56–90% of patients in both high- and low-incidence regions of the tumour[2], can most convincingly be incriminated. Although there is both epidemiological and experimental evidence linking the mycotoxin, aflatoxin, to HCC, the extent and importance of this association remain to be determined[3].

Although cirrhosis and HCC frequently co-exist, they do not have parallel geographical distributions. In most parts of the world HCC is rare or uncommon, and cirrhosis is far more prevalent. However, throughout Africa south of the Sahara and in many parts of the Far East HCC occurs commonly and may exceed cirrhosis in incidence. Despite being present in a similar proportion of HCC patients in different geographical regions, there is mounting evidence that the relation between cirrhosis and the tumour differs between high- and low-risk regions of the tumour[2]. This evidence will be presented before discussing the varying roles of cirrhosis in hepatocarcinogenesis in the different regions.

DIFFERENCES BETWEEN HIGH- AND LOW-INCIDENCE REGIONS OF HEPATOCELLULAR CARCINOMA

Presentation and prognosis

In regions with a low incidence of HCC, patients who develop the tumour frequently do so against a background of long-standing symptomatic cirrhosis[4–6]. This sequence of events is rare in patients in high-incidence regions, in almost all of whom the co-existing cirrhosis is asymptomatic (or if symptoms are present they are overshadowed by those of the tumour) and is discovered coincidentally either during investigation of the symptoms and signs attributable to the tumour or at necropsy[7–10]. Indirect support for this important difference in presentation is provided by the observations that in low-incidence regions, patients with co-existing HCC and cirrhosis are on average 8–10 years older than those with HCC in a non-cirrhotic liver and those with cirrhosis alone[5,11–15]. By contrast, African and Chinese patients with co-existing HCC and cirrhosis are the same age as those with HCC without cirrhosis and those with cirrhosis alone[16–17].

Further evidence for the advanced stage of the associated cirrhosis in low-risk populations is provided by the finding that HCC patients with cirrhosis are more likely than those with HCC alone to be jaundiced, to have ascites, and to bleed from oesophageal varices[11]. These clinical features of hepatic dysfunction and prolonged portal hypertension are no more common in African and Chinese patients with both HCC and cirrhosis than in those with HCC alone (Kew, unpublished data). The deleterious effect that the advanced cirrhosis in low incidence populations has on hepatic function is confirmed by the biochemical findings in these patients. Melia and his colleagues reported from Britain that HCC patients with cirrhosis were far more likely than those without cirrhosis to have a prolonged prothrombin time, a low serum albumin concentration, and raised serum bilirubin and serum aspartate aminotransferase levels[11]. By contrast, southern African Blacks with HCC with and without cirrhosis have similar hepatic function, with the exception of a slightly lower serum albumin concentration in patients with cirrhosis (29.0 ± 5.5g% versus 30.7 ± 5.9g%) (Kew, unpublished data).

HCC in the presence of cirrhosis is far more common (5–11:1) in men than women in both high- and low-incidence regions of the tumour[5,11,15,16,18]. In high-risk regions, male predominance is also present but is less striking (4:1) when HCC occurs in a non-cirrhotic liver[15,16], but in low-risk regions, the sex ratio in HCC patients without cirrhosis is almost parity[5,11,18].

In regions with a low incidence of HCC, patients with co-existing HCC and cirrhosis have a poorer prognosis and they survive for an appreciably shorter period than do those with the tumour alone[11]. In high-risk regions, the prognosis is equally poor whether or not cirrhosis co-exists with HCC, and the survival of these patients is so short that the difference (4 weeks versus 6 weeks) is not biologically significant (although it is statistically significant) (Kew, unpublished data).

The presence or absence of associated cirrhosis has a striking effect on the size of the tumour in populations at low risk of HCC. Thus, in an analysis of North American patients, the mean weight of the tumorous liver was 2530 g in the presence of cirrhosis and 3810 g when the tumour arose in a non-cirrhotic liver[19]. In high-incidence regions, HCCs are generally much larger than those occurring in low-incidence regions. However, the presence or absence of co-existing cirrhosis has a less obvious influence on tumour size. For example, in southern African Blacks with HCC and cirrhosis, the mean weight of the tumour is 3692 g, while in those without cirrhosis it is 4195 g (Kew, unpublished data).

Serum alpha-fetoprotein levels

In regions with a low incidence of HCC, serum alpha-fetoprotein concentrations are more likely to be raised to a diagnostic level in patients with co-existing cirrhosis and HCC than in those with the tumour alone, e.g. 71% compared with 36% ($P < 0.001$) in a British study[11]. This difference does not occur in African patients, as shown by the figures of 68.5% and 68.0% for HCC patients with and without cirrhosis, respectively, in southern Africa (Kew, unpublished data).

Type and aetiology of co-existing cirrhosis

In Africans and Chinese with HCC the co-existing cirrhosis is almost invariably of the macronodular variety[16,17,19–21]. These patients often show serological markers of current or past HBV infection and HBsAg and HBcAg can frequently be detected in the cirrhotic liver. A history of alcohol abuse is uncommon and features of alcoholic liver disease are rarely seen. Other causes of cirrhosis, such as hereditary haemochromatosis, Wilson's disease, primary biliary cirrhosis and α_1-antitrypsin deficiency are almost never encountered in Black and Chinese patients with HCC. The histological features of centrolobular fibrosis and chronic venous congestion resulting from long-standing membranous obstruction of the inferior vena cava are found in a small proportion of African (and Japanese) patients with HCC[22].

The picture is very different in regions with a low risk of HCC where the associated cirrhosis may be either micronodular or macronodular[12,13,23,24]. Whether micronodular or macronodular, histological features of alcoholic liver disease are often evident. Chronic alcohol abuse is unquestionably the most important cause of the associated cirrhosis in these regions. In some patients in these regions no obvious cause for the cirrhosis is apparent, and in others tissue and serological evidence of HBV infection is present. Hereditary haemochromatosis is another important cause of cirrhosis in low incidence regions, although the frequency with which it is reported to occur is influenced by patient selection[25]. Primary biliary cirrhosis, Wilson's disease and α_1-antitrypsin deficiency are occasionally found.

The young age of African patients with HCC, whether or not cirrhosis is present, and with cirrhosis alone suggests that the causative agent or agents of both diseases are operative at an early age. By contrast, the advanced age of the corresponding patients in regions with a low risk of HCC favours exposure to the relevant aetiological factors during adult life. In alcoholic cirrhosis the time elapsing between diagnosis of cirrhosis and recognition of HCC is longer than it is for other forms of cirrhosis[14]. Given that Oriental patients become infected with the virus at the same age as Africans[1], the reason for the very prolonged induction period of the tumour in these patients has not been explained.

It has long been known that a proportion of cirrhotic patients will either develop a clinically-recognized HCC or will exhibit at necropsy a tumour not detected during life. The frequency with which this occurs also varies between high and low risk regions of the tumour, although the main determinants appear to be the type and aetiology of the cirrhosis rather than the geographical location *per se*[2]. The risk is greatest with macronodular cirrhosis, irrespective of its aetiology. In Africans and Chinese the prevalence of tumour formation in a macronodular cirrhotic liver (which is thought almost always to be of viral origin) is of the order of 44–55%[19,26,27]. In low-incidence regions, macronodular cirrhosis, whatever the cause (including alcohol abuse, which is an important cause of this type of cirrhosis in first-world countries), the risk of HCC supervention may be high as 33%[28]. Micronodular cirrhosis carries a lower risk of subsequent tumour formation, figures of 3–10% being usual[9,23,24]. The risk of HCC formation in patients with hereditary haemochromatosis is intermediate between that of macronodular and micronodular cirrhosis, incidences of between 17 and 25% being usually quoted[25].

Hepatitis-B virus status

In Africans and Chinese there is a very close association between HCC and chronic HBV infection, 70–90% of patients showing markers of current infection and most of the remainder markers of past infection[1]. In Africans, there is no difference in the prevalence of any HBV markers between HCC patients with and without cirrhosis[20,29,30]. For example, in a series of southern African Blacks with this tumour, HBsAg was present in the serum of 60.5% of those with cirrhosis but also in 52.8% of those without cirrhosis ($P > 0.05$)[30]. Anti-HBc alone was present in a further 16.8%, anti-HBs in 11.6%, HBeAg in 17.0% of the HBsAg-positive patients and anti-HBe in 48.3% of the HBsAg-positive patients with HCC and cirrhosis; the corresponding figures in those without cirrhosis were 15.6%, 7.7%, 10.8% and 63.9%, with none of the differences being statistically significant[30]. The picture is somewhat different in Chinese patients in whom HBsAg is found in fewer HCC patients with a non-cirrhotic liver (38%) than with a cirrhotic liver (88%) ($P < 0.001$)[16]. However, the former figure indicates that a substantial proportion of patients with HCC alone may have HBV-related HCC.

In populations with a low incidence of HCC chronic HBV infection is rare. Analyses of HCC patients in these regions have consistently shown that those without co-existing cirrhosis have a prevalence of HBs antigenaemia which is much lower than that of patients with cirrhosis, e.g. in 14 and 37%, respectively ($P < 0.01$), of British patients[11], and in 9.2 and 19%, respectively ($P < 0.01$), of Austrian patients[14], or of active HBV infection — 26 and 67%, respectively ($P < 0.001$) — in Greek patients[31]. Nevertheless, as with Chinese patients, the lower prevalence of current HBV infection is still appreciably higher than that found in the general population in these countries.

In populations at high risk of HCC development, HBV infection is more common in patients with both the tumour and cirrhosis than in those with cirrhosis alone, e.g. 83 and 62%, respectively, in Chinese patients in Hong Kong[16]. In low-risk populations, the incidence of HBV infection is found to be the same in patients with cirrhosis alone and those with cirrhosis and HCC[14]. In Hong Kong Chinese the relative risk of a male carrier of HBV developing cirrhosis has been estimated to be 16:1 and of developing HCC combined with cirrhosis 50:1[16].

The extact nature of the relation between cirrhosis and HCC is uncertain and an aetiological role for cirrhosis has not been proven. However, from a consideration of the many differences between high- and low-risk populations of HCC with respect to the association between the tumour and cirrhosis, it is apparent that the relation between the two pathological conditions is not unitary but rather takes one of two possible forms.

RELATION BETWEEN HEPATOCELLULAR CARCINOMA AND CIRRHOSIS IN HIGH-INCIDENCE REGIONS OF THE TUMOUR

Any explanation for the role played by cirrhosis in hepatocarcinogenesis in populations with a high risk of HCC must account for the observations that the vast majority of these patients show markers of current or past HBV infection and that between 60 and 85% have co-existing macronodular cirrhosis which is usually HBV-related[2], as well as explaining the features already outlined. The likely explanation for the link between HCC and cirrhosis in these populations is that one (or possibly more than one) agent is the cause of both pathological conditions, and HBV is unquestionably the main suspect[2]. There is now compelling epidemiological and molecular biological evidence linking persistent infection with this virus to HCC[1]. Persistent HBV infection is also known to be an important, although variable, cause of cirrhosis throughout the world. If HCC and macronodular cirrhosis are both caused by chronic HBV infection, one would expect the geographical distribution of the two conditions to run parallel, and there is ample epidemiological evidence for this[19,26]. HBV may be both the initiator of malignant transformation and the cause of the associated necro-inflammatory hepatic disease, in the form of chronic active hepatitis, chronic lobular hepatitis, or cirrhosis. The necro-inflammatory disease may act as a promoter to HBV-initiated hepatocarcinogenesis by increasing the hepatocyte turnover rate. Cells in mitosis are more susceptible to integration of viral DNA because the human DNA is temporally single-stranded. After a variable but usually prolonged period, HCC will develop. At about the same rate but independently and without producing obvious symptoms, the necro-inflammatory hepatic disease progresses to cirrhosis or resolves with residual fibrosis. Occasionally chronic active hepatitis is still present at this time or it may have regressed to a chronic persistent hepatitis. The resulting cirrhosis is almost always asymptomatic at the time the tumour becomes symptomatic and is diagnosed. Why HBV causes cirrhosis in some patients, HCC in others, and both diseases in yet others is not known. It is conceivable that a proportion of the patients who have necro-inflammatory disease early on could resolve completely, accounting for some of the patients with HBV-related HCC in whom the non-neoplastic hepatic tissue is normal.

Other patients with persistent HBV infection proceed to HCC formation without cirrhosis developing. Hepadna viruses (of which HBV is one) have been shown to be oncogenic in their own right[32], and this may be relevant in these particular patients. More likely, however, other promoters, such as aflatoxin, play a role in these patients. Finally, to explain the occurrence of HCC that is not HBV-related (whether or not cirrhosis co-exists) other carcinogens need to be considered. Non-A, non-B hepatitis viruses may be important in this respect, as may aflatoxin or other naturally-occurring chemical carcinogens. Because aflatoxin exposure does not cause cirrhosis in humans, it is unlikely that this agent acting alone plays a major role in human hepatocarcinogenesis.

RELATION BETWEEN HEPATOCELLULAR CARCINOMA AND CIRRHOSIS IN LOW-INCIDENCE REGIONS OF THE TUMOUR

The explanation for the role played by cirrhosis in hepatocarcinogenesis in low-incidence regions of HCC must take into account the evidence that the cirrhosis precedes the onset of the tumour by several to many years. From a consideration of the interrelation between cirrhosis and HCC in these populations it becomes apparent that cirrhosis *per se* is the major aetiological association of HCC in low-risk regions[2]. The cirrhosis has a variety of causes but is most often the consequence of chronic alcohol abuse. Other causes including chronic HBV infection and haemochromatosis, as well as so-called 'cryptogenic cirrhosis', play a lesser but nevertheless important role. The risk of HCC supervention is, in fact, similar in male cirrhotics with alcoholic, post-hepatitic and cryptogenic cirrhosis[14,33]; women with cryptogenic cirrhosis are at higher risk than those with other forms of cirrhosis[14].

The presence of cirrhosis (or perhaps chronic active hepatitis) predisposes either directly or indirectly to malignant transformation. Two possible mechanisms for this complication have been postulated. The first is that neoplasia is a direct and inevitable consequence of the hyperplasia of cirrhosis, i.e. that malignant transformation occurs in the cirrhotic liver in the absence of exposure to carcinogens[2]. If this mechanism was universally operative, a parallel geographical distribution between cirrhosis and HCC would be expected. Although this does apply for post-viral macronodular cirrhosis, it does not hold true for alcoholic cirrhosis. The most important determinants of malignant transformation in the cirrhotic liver in low-incidence populations seem to be male sex and increasing age, the latter presumably including, at least to some extent, the duration of the cirrhosis[5,11,34]. The apparently widely varying risk of HCC formation in different aetiological forms of cirrhosis may largely be explained by differences in sex distribution. For example, HCC has rarely been described to develop in patients with primary biliary cirrhosis, but if only male patients are analysed a substantial risk of malignant transformation becomes apparent. The reason why fewer women with alcoholic cirrhosis develop HCC may be that they die from the effects of the initial disease before the tumour has had time to supervene.

The second postulated mechanism for tumorigenesis in the cirrhotic liver is that the presence of cirrhosis renders the individual susceptible to a variety of environmental carcinogens[2]. It may do so by virtue of the increased hepatocyte turnover rate acting as a promoter. Cells in mitosis are more susceptible to DNA alterations by chemicals or other agents. In addition, rapid cell turnover rates interfere with DNA repair processes so that DNA alterations are transmitted to daughter cells and are thus fixed in the progeny. Malignant change is thus favoured by an increase in cell turnover which renders the cell more susceptible to ubiquitous environmental chemical carcinogens. In first-world countries, industrial chemicals would most likely constitute the carcinogens. This effect is independent of the original cause of the cirrhosis. The fact that HCC develops several to many years after alcohol-induced cirrhosis argues against alcohol being carcinogenic as well as cirrhotogenic. In support of this belief is the absence of any experimental evidence that alcohol is carcinogenic. The same argument has been used in connection with HBV-related HCC in low-incidence populations, i.e. that it causes HCC only by virtue of its first causing cirrhosis. However, some patients in low-incidence regions do develop HBV-related HCC in the absence of cirrhosis. Although experimental evidence is available that the cirrhotic liver is predisposed to aflatoxin-induced hepatocarcinogenesis, significant levels of exposure to afla-toxin are unlikely in highly industrialized countries.

In low-risk populations the few patients with HCC in a non-cirrhotic liver are generally younger, more often female, and have a different aetiological spectrum, including a lesser association with persistent HBV infection[11,34,35]. Oral contraceptive steroids and anabolic androgenic steroids have been implicated in this group of patients[36], and the fibrolamellar variant of HCC occurs particularly in this setting.

CONCLUSION

Although cirrhosis and hepatocellular carcinoma frequently co-exist, the precise nature of the relation between these two pathological conditions remains uncertain and a role for cirrhosis in hepatocarcinogenesis has not been proven.

Cirrhosis occurs in a similar proportion of patients with hepatocellular carcinoma in different geographical regions. Despite this, there is mounting evidence that its relation to the tumour differs between populations having a high- and a low-incidence of hepatocellular carcinoma. In high-risk populations in Africa and Asia, the two diseases appear to share a common aetiology, and the likely culprit in the majority of patients is persistent hepatitis-B virus infection. The virus may not only function as an initiator of hepatocarcinogenesis, but may also cause the necro-inflammatory hepatic disease which acts as a promotor of carcinogenesis by increasing the hepatocyte turnover rate.

In populations in which hepatocellular carcinoma is uncommon, cirrhosis precedes the onset of the tumour by several to many years and is itself the major aetiological association of the tumour. Chronic alcohol abuse is the most common cause of the associated cirrhosis in these populations, although all forms of this disease may predispose to the tumour. There is no evidence that alcohol is directly oncogenic. Male sex and increasing age (and presumably duration of cirrhosis) appear to be the major determinants of the risk of malignant transformation in cirrhosis. Whether hepatocellular carcinoma is an inevitable consequence of cirrhosis, or whether cirrhosis renders the hepatocytes susceptible to ubiquitous environmental carcinogens by increasing their turnover rate, remains to be determined.

References

1. Beasley, R. P. and Hwang, L-Y. (1984). Hepatocellular carcinoma and the hepatitis-B virus. *Sem. Liver Dis.*, **4**, 113–21
2. Kew, M. C. and Popper, H. (1984). Relationship between hepatocellular carcinoma and cirrhosis. *Sem. Liver Dis.*, **4**, 136–46
3. Newberne, P. M. (1984). Chemical carcinogenesis: Mycotoxins and other chemicals to which humans are exposed. *Sem. Liver Dis.*, **4**, 122–35
4. Kew, M. C., Dos Santos, H. A. and Sherlock, S. (1971). The diagnosis of primary cancer of the liver. *Br. Med. J.*, **4**, 408–11
5. Johnson, P. J., Krasner, N., Portmann, B., Eddleston, A. L. W. F. and Williams, R. (1978). Hepatocellular carcinoma in Great Britain: influence of age, sex, HBsAg status and aetiology of underlying cirrhosis. *Gut*, **19**, 1022–6
6. Leevy, C. M., Gellene, R. and Ning, M. (1964). Primary liver cancer in cirrhosis of the alcoholic. *Ann. N. Y. Acad. Sci.*, **114**, 1026–40
7. Sung, J. L., Wang, T. H. and Yu, J. Y. (1967). Clinical study of primary carcinoma of the liver in Taiwan. *Amer. J. Dig. Dis.*, **12**, 1036–49
8. Alpert, E., Hutt, M. S. R. and Davidson, C. S. (1969). Primary hepatoma in Uganda. A prospective clinical and epidemiologic study of 46 patients. *Amer. J. Med.*, **46**, 794–802
9. Lai, C. L., Lam, K. C., Wong, K. P., Wu, P. C. and Todd, D. (1981). Clinical features of hepatocellular carcinoma: Review of 211 patients in Hong Kong. *Cancer*, **47**, 2746–55
10. Kew, M. C. and Geddes, E. W. (1982). Hepatocellular carcinoma in rural southern African Blacks. *Medicine*, **61**, 98–108
11. Melia, W. M., Wilkinson, M. L., Portmann, B. C., Johnson, P. J. and Williams, R. (1984). Hepatocellular carcinoma in the non-cirrhotic liver: a comparison with that complicating cirrhosis. *Q. J. Med.*, **33**, 391–400
12. Ihde, D. C., Sherlock, P., Winawer, S. J. and Fortner, J. G. (1974). Clinical manifestations of hepatoma. *Amer. J. Med.*, **56**, 83–91
13. Omata, M., Ashcavai, M., Liew, C-T. and Peters, R. L. (1979). Hepatocellular carcinoma in the USA: Etiologic considerations. *Gastroenterology*, **76**, 279–87
14. Ferenci, P., Dragosics, B., Marosi, L. and Kiss, F. (1984). Relative incidence of primary liver cancer in cirrhosis in Austria. Etiological considerations. *Liver*, **4**, 7–14
15. Okuda, K., Nakashima, T., Sakomoto, K., Ikari, T., Hidaka, H., Kubo, Y., Sakuma, K., Motacki, Y., Okuda, H. and Obata, H. (1982). Hepatocellular carcinoma arising in non-cirrhotic and highly cirrhotic livers. *Cancer*, **49**, 450–5
16. Gibson, J. B., Wu, P. C., Ho, J. C. I. and Lauder, J. J. (1980). HBsAg, hepatocellular carcinoma and cirrhosis in Hong Kong. A necropsy study. *Br. J. Cancer*, **42**, 370–7
17. Kew, M. C., Geddes, E. W. and Bersohn, I. (1974). Hepatitis-B antigen and cirrhosis in Bantu patients with primary liver cancer. *Cancer*, **34**, 539–41
18. Peters, R. L. (1976). Pathology of hepatocellular carcinoma. In Okuda, K. and Peters, R. L. (eds), *Hepatocellular Carcinoma*. pp. 107–68. (New York: John Wiley)
19. Steiner, P. E. (1960). Cancer of the liver and cirrhosis in trans-Saharan Africa and the USA. *Cancer*, **13**, 1085–145
20. Vogel, C. L., Anthony, P. P., Sadikali, F., Barker, L. F. and Peterson, M. R. (1972). Hepatitis associated antigen and antibody in hepatocellular carcinoma: Results of a continuing study. *J. Natl. Cancer Inst.*, **48**, 1583–8
21. Tong, M. J., Sun, S-C., Schaeffer, B. T., Chang, N. K., Lo, K-J. and Peters, R. L. (1971). Hepatitis associated antigen and hepatocellular carcinoma in Taiwan. *Ann. Intern. Med.*, **75**, 687–91

22. Kew, M. C., McKnight, A., Hodkinson, J., Bukofzer, S. and Esser, J. D. (1989). The role of membranous obstruction of the inferior vena cava in the etiology of hepatocellular carcinoma in southern African Blacks. *Hepatology*, **9**, 121–5
23. MacDonald, R. A. (1957). Primary carcinoma of the liver. A clinico-pathologic study of 108 cases. *Arch. Intern. Med.*, **99**, 266–77
24. Purtilo, D. J. and Gottlieb, L. S. (1973). Cirrhosis and hepatoma occurring at Boston City Hospital (1917–1968). *Cancer*, **32**, 458–62
25. Powell, L. W., Mortimer, R. and Harris, O. D. (1971). Cirrhosis of the liver: A comparative study of the four major aetiological groups. *Med. J. Austral.*, **1**, 941–50
26. Higginson, J. (1963). The geographical pathology of primary liver cancer. *Cancer Res.*, **23**, 1624–33
27. Shanmugaratnam, K. (1956). Primary carcinoma of the liver and biliary tract. *Br. J. Cancer*, **10**, 232–46
28. Lee, F. I. (1967). Cirrhosis and hepatoma in alcoholics. *Gut*, **7**, 77–85
29. Prince, A. M., Szmuness, W., Michon, J., Demaille, J., Diebolt, G., Linhard, J., Quenum, C. and Sankali, M. (1975). A case/control study of the association between primary liver cancer and hepatitis B infection in Senegal. *Int. J. Cancer*, **16**, 376–83
30. Kew, M. C. (1984). The possible etiologic role of the hepatitis B virus in hepatocellular carcinoma: Evidence from southern Africa. In Chisari, F. V. (ed.), *Advances in Hepatitis Research*, pp. 203–15. (New York: Masson Publishing).
31. Trichopoulos, D., Tabor, E., Gerety, R. J., Xirouchaki, E., Sparros, L., Munoz, N. and Linsell, C. A. (1982). Hepatitis B and primary hepatocellular carcinoma in a European population. *Lancet*, **2**, 1217–19
32. Gerin, J. L., Tennant, B. C., Popper, H., Tyeryar, F. J. and Purcell, R. H. (1986). The woodchuck model of hepadna virus infection and disease. In Brown, F., Chanock, F. and Lerner, R. (eds), *Vaccines '86: New Approaches to Immunization*, pp. 383–6. (Cold Spring Harbor, New York: Spring Harbor Laboratory).
33. Lehmann, F. G. and Wegner, T. (1979). Etiology of human liver cancer: controlled prospective study in liver cirrhosis. *J. Toxicol. Environ. Health*, **5**, 281–99
34. Zaman, S. N., Melia, W. M., Johnson, R. D., Portmann, B. C., Johnson, P. J. and Williams, R. (1985). Risk factors in development of hepatocellular carcinoma in cirrhosis: Prospective study of 613 patients. *Lancet*, **1**, 1357–9
35. Johnson, P. J., Melia, W. M., Palmer, M. K., Portmann, B. and Williams, R. (1981). Relationship between serum alpha-fetoprotein, cirrhosis and survival in hepatocellular carcinoma. *Br. J. Cancer*, **44**, 502–5
36. Mays, E. T. and Christopherson, W. (1984). Hepatic tumors induced by sex steroids. *Sem. Liver Dis.*, **4**, 147–15

6
Liver cancer incidence and its relation to alcoholic liver cirrhosis in Hungary

K. LAPIS AND Z. SCHAFF

INTRODUCTION

It is well known that — like the United States — most European countries (including Hungary) are regarded as so-called 'low-incidence regions' concerning the incidence of primary hepatocellular carcinoma (PHC). In the last two to three decades, however, in the majority of these countries (including Hungary) profound changes have taken place in the incidence of liver cirrhosis, which is considered to be the most important precursor of liver cancer.

In Hungary, for example, almost parallel with the steep increase of the per capita alcohol consumption (Figure 1), the death rate due to liver cirrhosis has also sharply increased in both sexes. The increase has been more than 400% in males and more than 300% in females during the last 20 years (Figure 2).

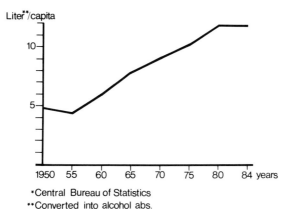

*Central Bureau of Statistics
**Converted into alcohol abs.

Figure 1   Alcohol consumption in Hungary*

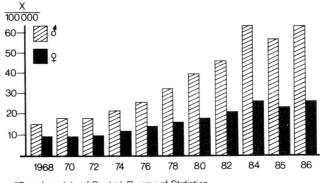

*Based on data of Central Bureau of Statistics

Figure 2 Mortality of cirrhosis in Hungary between 1968 and 1986*

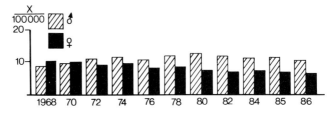

*Based on data of Central Bureau Statistics

Figure 3 Mortality of PHC in Hungary between 1968 and 1986*

Surprisingly — contrary to all expectations — there was no increase reported in the mortality rate owing to PHC in either sex during the same period (Figure 3). This not only failed to meet expectations, but did not concur with our experiences obtained from autopsies either.

Therefore we decided to study how the incidence of PHC in the autopsied cases (over the age of 15 years) has changed during the last 30 years. Altogether 18 557 autopsy protocols — derived from the last 30 years — were reviewed (Table 1). Altogether 1000 but one cases with liver cirrhosis have occurred in this material, which corresponds to 5.3% of the total autopsied

Table 1 Cirrhosis and PHC* in autopsies (1958–84 Budapest, Hungary)

Number of autopsies (over 15 yrs)	18557 (100%)
Total number of cirrhosis	999 (5.3%)
Total number of PHCs	226 (1.2%)
Cirrhosis + PHC	162 (0.9%)

*PHC = primary hepatocellular carcinoma

48

Table 2 Cirrhosis and PHC in autopsies (Budapest, Hungary)

Number of autopsies (over 15 yrs)	1958–67	1968–77	1978–87	1958–87
Total number of autopsies	5105	7477	5975	18557(100%)
Cirrhosis (total)	218 (4.27%)	385 (5.14%)	396 (6.62%)	999(5.3%)
Cirrhosis + PHC	27 (0.52%)	70 (0.93%)	65 (1.08%)	162(0.9%)
PHC (total)	39 (0.76%)	100 (1.33%)	87 (1.45%)	226(1.2%)

PHC = primary hepatocellular carcinoma

cases. If we examine how the proportion of the cirrhotic cases has changed in the three ten-year periods we can register only a slight increase (about 50%) (Table 2). Thus our autopsy findings do not accurately reflect the sharp increase in the mortality rate owing to liver cirrhosis reported by the Central Bureau of Statistics of Hungary. The possible factors which might play a role in this obvious discrepancy will not be discussed, however.

The incidence of PHC in this autopsy material is even more interesting. Out of the 18 557 cases, PHC was seen in 226 cases, i.e. in 1.2% of the autopsied cases (Table 2). The proportion with malignancy in the same material proved to be 1464 cases, that is to say in 24.5% of the autopsied cases some kind of malignant neoplasm has been found. The liver cancer cases totalled 5.94% of all the malignancies found at autopsy (Table 3). When we examined how the proportion of the PHC cases had changed in the three ten-year periods, a 100% increase in the incidence of the PHC was observed up to the end of the third period compared to that seen in the first one (Table 2). This means that while only a slight increase showed up in the incidence of liver cirrhosis, a doubling was seen in the incidence of PHC in the same material. This is most surprising and interesting because there was no increase

Table 3 Occurrence of PHCs in autopsied malignant tumour cases (1975–84, Semmelweis Medical Univ., First Inst. Pathol)

		Percentage in total number of malignant tumours*
Number of cases with malignant tumours	1464	100%
PHC with cirrhosis	65	4.4%
PHC without cirrhosis	22	1.5%
PHC (total)	87	5.94%

PHC = primary hepatocellular carcinoma
*over 15 yrs

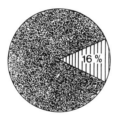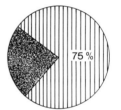

PHC occurred in 16%
of cirrhotic cases (n=396)

75% PHC occurred
in cirrhotic livers

PHC = primary hepatocellular carcinoma

Figure 4 Occurrence of cirrhosis and PHC (autopsies; *n* = 5976, Semmelweis Medical Univ., Budapest, Hungary)

registered in the PHC mortality by the Central Bureau of Statistics while almost a 400% increase was reported in mortality owing to liver cirrhosis.

Out of the 226 PHCs observed in 162 — that is to say in the large majority of the cases — the PHC proved to be associated with liver cirrhosis (Table 2). Analysing this association more closely we have found PHC in more than 16% of the cirrhotic cases and 75% of the PHCs occurring in cirrhotic livers (Figure 4).

Studying this association in the two sexes separately we have found that in males an even larger proportion of the PHCs (exactly 82%) was associated with cirrhosis, with only 18% in females (Table 4). On the other hand, out of the PHCs developed in non-cirrhotic livers, a much larger proportion (40%) occurred in females. Altogether 75% of the PHCs occurred in males.

We have studied the clinical case histories of our cirrhotic and PHC cases. In 13.6% precedent hepatitis, in 24.8% alcoholism was registered in the case histories of cirrhotic patients (Table 5). The incidence of hepatitis was somewhat higher (16.9%) in the PHC cases associated with liver cirrhosis, while alcoholism was registered in a much lower proportion than in the cirrhotic

Table 4 Frequency of PHC in males and females (1958–1977, *n*=12582 autopsies) Budapest, Hungary

	Total	Male	Female
PHC associated with cirrhosis	97 (100%)	80 (82%)	17 (18%)
PHC without cirrhosis	42 (100%)	25 (60%)	17 (40%)
PHC (total)	139 (100%)	105 (75%)	34 (25%)

n = number of cases
PHC = primary hepatocellular carcinoma

Table 5 Case histories of cirrhotic and PHC cases (autopsies, 1975–84) (Semmelweis Medical Univ., First Inst. Pathol., Budapest)

| | Cirrhosis | | Cirrhosis + PHC | | PHC | |
	n	%	n	%	n	%
Hepatitis	45	13.6	11	16.9	0	
Alcohol	82	24.8	8	12.8	3	13.6
Diabetes	83	25.1	8	12.8	2	9.1
No data	121	26.5	38	58.5	17	77.3
Total number of cases	331	100	65	100	22	100

PHC = primary hepatocellular carcinoma

patients. It deserves attention that no precedent hepatitis was registered in any of the patients with PHC occurring in non-cirrhotic livers.

In 50 cirrhotic and in 50 PHC randomly-selected autopsy cases, immuno-histochemical studies were carried out for the detection of viral and certain oncofetal antigens. Out of the 50 PHC cases, 4 proved to be HBsAg and 1 HBcAg positive (Table 6). The HBsAg and HBcAg positivity were only slightly higher in the cirrhotic cases.

The liver biopsy specimens were of course stained with Shikata's orcein staining, but the number of orcein-positive cases proved to be very low. Recently we have carried out subsequent immunohistochemical studies in all of our PHC cases diagnosed in biopsy specimens for the detection of viral antigens.

The proportion of the HBsAg and/or HBcAg positive cases proved to be even much lower than in the autopsy material (Table 7). Several factors may have a role in this finding. It is worth mentioning that the rate of HBV infection in the population of Hungary must be very low, because when screening of blood donors for HBV infection was introduced, <1% of the donors proved to be positive. Another important aspect is the accuracy (or inaccuracy) of the clinical diagnosis of PHC and that of liver cirrhosis in the light of the autopsy findings.

Analysing this problem in our Institute's autopsy material for a ten-year

Table 6 Immunohistochemical localization (PAP, ABC) of viral and oncofetal antigens in autopsies of cirrhotic and PHC cases. (Semmelweis Medical Univ., First Inst. Pathol., Budapest)

| | HBsAg | | HBcAg | | AFP | | CEA | | AAT | | Total | |
	n	%	n	%	n	%	n	%	n	%	n	%
Cirrhosis	5	10	2	4	0	0	0	0	0	0	50	100
PHC	4	8	1	2	20	40	25	50	0	0	50	100

PHC = primary heptocellular carcinoma; PAP = peroxidase antiperoxidase; ABC = avidin-biotin-peroxidase complex; AFP = alpha-fetoprotein; CEA = carcinoembryonic antigen; AAT = alpha 1-antitrypsin

Table 7 Detection of HBV*, CEA*, AFP*, and copper† in liver needle biopsy specimens of PHC cases

Antigens	Number of cases (positive/total)
HBsAg, HBcAg	2/69
Carcinoembryonic antigen	3/24
Alpha-fetoprotein	10/75
Copper	45/91

PHC = primary hepatocellular carcinoma
HBV = hepatitis B virus
HBsAg = hepatitis B virus surface antigen
HBcAg = hepatitis B virus core antigen
CEA = carcinoembryonic antigen
AFP = alpha-fetoprotein

*detected by ABC immunohistochemical method
†detected by orcein and rubeanic acid staining

period we have observed that cirrhosis was found at autopsy in only 61% of cases diagnosed clinically (Table 8). The accuracy of the clinical diagnosis proved to be even worse in the case of PHCs: only one-third of PHCs found at autopsy were diagnosed *in vivo*, and more than two-thirds of the PHCs were not recognized clinically, i.e. the clinical diagnosis in 69% of PHC cases proved to be false negatives. This means that the large majority of liver cancers are not recognized clinically. In light of these data we can understand the striking contradiction existing between the data concerning the mortality rates of cirrhosis and PHC presented at the beginning of this chapter — namely that while a high increase was registered in mortality caused by liver cirrhosis, no increase was reported in the mortality due to liver cancer.

From the data presented from our clinico-pathological studies, the following main conclusions can be drawn:

- There is a striking increase in the mortality rate due to liver cirrhosis, mainly of alcoholic origin, in Hungary in the last 20 years.
- No increase was reported in the mortality rate due to PHC in the same period.
- In large autopsy material however the incidence of PHC doubled during the same period.
- The large majority of the PHCs found at autopsy was not recognized clinically, the ratio of false-negative clinical diagnosis in PHC cases proving to be extremely high (69%).
- 75% of the observed liver cancers occurred in males.
- There was a very close association between cirrhosis and liver cancer: in 16% of cirrhotic cases, PHC was also present; in the majority (75%) of the cases, liver cancer was found in cirrhotic liver.
- This association of PHC with cirrhosis was much more pronounced in males (82%) than in females, in which it was only 18%.

Table 8 Correlation between clinical and pathological diagnosis in cirrhotic and PHC cases (based on autopsies, 1975–84, Budapest, Hungary)

Pathological diagnosis	Clinical diagnosis	
	positive (right)	negative (false)
Cirrhosis	202 (61%)	129 (39%)
Cirrhosis and	42 (64%)	23 (36%)
PHC	20 (31%)	69 (69%)
PHC	7 (32%)	15 (68%)

PHC = primary hepatocellular carcinoma

- Hepatitis was registered only in a small proportion of cirrhotic and PHC cases.
- HBsAg and/or HBcAg positivity were found only in a low proportion (10 and 4, 8 and 2% respectively) in the cirrhotic and PHC cases.
- It seems that the majority of liver cancers observed developed in the cirrhotic livers of alcoholics. The possibility of the role of non-A,non-B hepatitis, however, should also be taken into consideration.

7
Comparative pathobiology of hepatic pre-neoplasia*

P. BANNASCH, H. ENZMANN, H. J. HACKER, E. WEBER AND H. ZERBAN

INTRODUCTION

For a long time, the recognition of prestages of hepatocellular carcinomas in man and experimental animals was predominantly based on histological criteria. Hepatic hyperplasia has been, and in human pathology still is, the favoured candidate for a precancerous lesion[1-12]. A long list of synonyms for this proliferative parenchymal alteration on which complete agreement among pathologists has never been reached reflects the difficulty in interpretation and implies that different pathomorphologic entities might be involved[13]. In addition to cell proliferation, some other cellular alterations associated with hepatic hyperplasia were also noted years ago[2,3,14-18]. However, a detailed analysis of cellular changes in early, intermediate and late stages of hepatocarcinogenesis, which may be morphologically defined as focal hepatic pre-neoplasia, benign nodular neoplasia (adenoma) and malignant neoplasia (carcinoma) was only possible when appropriate animal models were developed and modern cytomorphological, cytochemical, cytogenetic and microbiochemical methods became available[6,19-26]. The bulk of new information still comes from studies in rodent liver treated with various chemical carcinogens, but some comparative investigations in other species including human and non-human primates have been reported[27,28]. Although a particularly large gap exists between the experimental experience in chemical hepatocarcinogenesis and the elucidation of human hepatic pre-neoplasia in cases associated with the hepatitis-B-virus, the recently established animal models of hepadna-virus-induced liver cancer[29-31] and certain strains of transgenic mice prone to develop liver tumours[22,23] should help to bridge this gap rapidly.

---

*Dedicated to Rolf Preussmann on the occasion of his 60th birthday.

Anthony et al.[34] considered liver-cell dysplasia as characterized by hepatocellular enlargement, nuclear atypia and polymorphism to be a premalignant condition in man, but the significance of this lesion has been controversial up to now[7,35-41]. From a review of the literature and observations in more than 200 consecutive autopsy cases of hepatocellular carcinoma, Kojiro and Nakashima[42] concluded that liver-cell dysplasia is a para-neoplastic rather than a pre-neoplastic alteration.

DETECTION AND DEFINITION OF HEPATIC PRE-NEOPLASIA

In their pioneering work on the experimental induction of hepatocellular carcinomas in rats by chemicals, Sasaki and Yoshida[2] noted two types of altered hepatocytes in tumour prestages, namely big clear and small dark cells. However, little attention has been given to these cytological changes in the first instance. Only ten years later, Opie[15] discovered that the dark basophilic staining of the cytoplasm was due to an increase in ribonucleoproteins which have been shown in the meantime to correspond to free or membrane-bound ribosomes[19,43,44]. It took nearly another two decades until a loss of glycogen was cytochemically demonstrated in the basophilic cells[17] and an excessive storage of this polysaccharide (glycogenosis) in the clear cells[45]. At the same time, Gössner and Friedrich-Freksa[46] described a focal reduction in the activity of the microsomal enzyme glucose-6-phosphatase in nitrosamine-treated rat liver. The reduced activity of glucose-6-phosphatase in rat-liver foci has recently been quantified by Fischer et al.[47] A close correlation of this phenomenon with the focal hepatic glycogenosis was frequently but not universally found[48-50]. With microbiochemical methods, Klimek et al.[51] studied the glycogen content in single glycogen storage foci dissected from freeze-dried tissue sections by a laser-beam and were able to show that the lesions contain on an average 100% more glycogen than the normal or the surrounding parenchyma. Some authors emphasized the retention of glycogen in the focal lesions after fasting[52,53]. However, the altered hepatocytes in such foci also store excessive amounts of glycogen in fed animals. Both the excessive storage of glycogen and the decreased glucose-6-phosphatase activity were used as positive or negative 'markers', respectively, for the detection of foci of altered hepatocytes by many workers. In addition, several other enzymatic or functional changes, such as a resistance to exogenously induced haemosiderosis, have been described as positive or negative markers[23,25,54-57].

Although the changes of enzymes involved in the metabolism of drugs or carbohydrates attracted the greatest attention, a detailed knowledge of the morphology of the focal lesions seems to be indispensable if we are to understand the distinct stages of neoplastic development in the liver[19,58]. In conventional paraffin sections stained with H & E, the early emerging glycogenotic lesions appear as clear or acidophilic cell foci (Figure 1a–d). The acidophilia is due to a proliferation of the smooth endoplasmic reticulum. The observations in rat liver treated with chemical carcinogens stimulated studies in man which resulted in the detection of similar hepatocytes[59] now

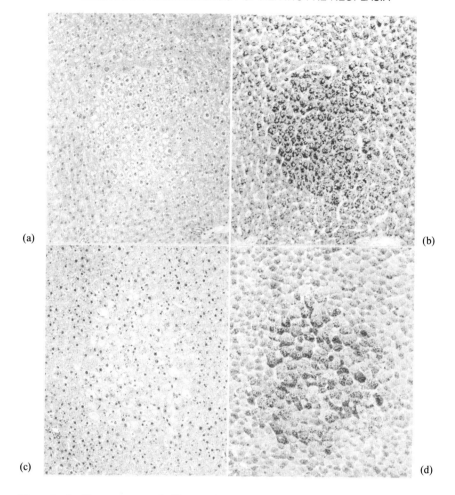

Figure 1a–d Glycogen-storage foci induced in rat liver with N-nitrosomorpholine. (a) Clear-cell focus (H & E, × 90); (b) serial section to (a) showing excessive storage of glycogen in clear cells (Tri-PAS, × 90); (c) clear- and acidophilic-cell focus (H & E, × 90); (d) serial section to (c) showing excessive storage of glycogen in both clear and acidophilic cells (H & E, × 90)

well known as 'ground-glass' cells[60,61]. In contrast to the acidophilic cells of the rat liver, the human ground-glass cells in the lumina of the proliferated smooth endoplasmic reticulum (ER) contain the filamentous hepatitis-B-surface antigen. The ground glass hepatocytes are a morphological feature of the hepatitis-B-virus carrier state in man. Abe and coworkers[31] have just described 'ground-glass' hepatocytes looking exactly like those in man in woodchucks carrying the woodchuck hepatitis virus, and Chisari *et al.*[33] reported typical ground-glass hepatocytes in transgenic mice containing the entire HBV envelope coding region and expressing excessive amounts of the HBV large envelope polypeptide. In both man and experimental animals there is circumstantial evidence of a correlation between the acidophilic cells and hepatocarcinogenesis[19,31,62–65]. In rat liver, all possible transitions lead from the clear and acidophilic cell foci storing glycogen in excess to intermediate and basophilic lesions which are poor in glycogen but rich in ribosomes[19].

On the basis of the cytological criteria outlined, the foci have been classified into clear, acidophilic, intermediate, basophilic and mixed-cell foci. The diagnosis of foci implies that the altered cell populations are perfectly integrated into the architecture of the liver parenchyma and do not show any expansive growth. Hence, at the histological level hepatic *pre-neoplasia may be defined as a phenotypically altered cell population which has no obvious neoplastic nature but has a higher probability of progressing to a benign or malignant neoplasm than the surrounding parenchyma*[56]. This definition includes prestages of benign liver tumours. Thus, 'pre-neoplasia' should be clearly separated from 'pre-cancer', although it is generally accepted that at least in the experimental situation hepatocellular adenomas may be nothing but intermediate stages in the development of carcinomas. What is the evidence for a progression from pre-neoplastic hepatic foci to hepatocellular tumours?

CELL LINEAGES IN HEPATOCARCINOGENESIS

Cholangiolar (oval) cells

The discussion on the cell of origin of hepatocellular carcinomas has been controversial for decades. The old concept[1,66] that, in addition to hepatocytes, poorly differentiated cells deriving from the cholangioles, and designated as oval cells by Farber[67] might be precursors of hepatocytes and hepatoma cells, gained considerable support in recent years from a number of groups[68–78]. However, in detailed autoradiographic studies Tatematsu et al.[79] were not able to provide evidence for a transition from oval cells into hepatocytes or hepatoma cells. In line with earlier reports[80–83], the results of these authors suggested that the majority of oval cells die. The surviving cells undergo so-called 'intestinal metaplasia'[84] or 'cholangiolar mucopolysaccharidosis'[85] and form mucous cholangiofibrotic lesions which have been shown to represent an intermediate stage in the development of cholangiocellular but not hepatocellular tumours[83,86–88]. Among other features, the presence of glucose-6-phosphatase activity in oval cells as demonstrated by cytochemical methods has repeatedly been used as an argument for a transition into cells with a hepatocellular phenotype[73,78,89,90]. However, activity of this enzyme can also be shown by ultrastructural cytochemistry in both many normal bile ductular epithelia and epithelial cells of cholangiofibrotic lesions and cholangiofibromas[91,92]. In the latter case, a strong cytochemical reaction for glucose-6-phosphatase may be combined with a pronounced production of mucus — a feature characteristic of cholangiocellular but not hepatocellular tumours. Another cytochemical marker which can be detected in oval cells as well as hepatoma cells by an immunoreaction is α-fetoprotein[70,73,93–96]. This finding also appeared to support a relationship between these two cell types, but Iwai *et al.*[97] have recently shown that there are consistent differences in the subcellular distribution of α-fetoprotein in oval cells and hepatoma cells.

The most important argument against a crucial role of oval cells in hepato-carcinogenesis is that with low doses of chemical carcinogens, which do not lead to appreciable necrotic changes of the parenchyma, hepatocellular carcinomas develop without any preceding oval-cell proliferation[19]. The same holds true for fibrotic or cirrhotic changes which frequently accompany hepatocarcinogenesis after administration of high doses but are lacking at low dose levels.

Hepatocytes

Rat

In contrast to oval cell proliferation, fibrosis and cirrhosis, the foci of altered hepatocytes appear at all dose levels at which hepatocellular carcinomas develop, and they follow a time–dose relationship which is in principle similar to that of the tumours. In our stop model (which has originally been proposed by Druckrey), we had been treating rats for seven weeks with 80, 120, 160 and 200 mg N-nitrosomorpholine (NNM) per litre of drinking water[98]. Under these conditions, the majority of the foci emerged after withdrawal of the carcinogen as determined by quantitative stereology in H & E stained tissue sections. With increasing doses of NNM, the number of lesions increased considerably, and this was accompanied by an earlier development of mixed and basophilic cell populations. There was no indication of any reversibility of the focal lesions. On the contrary, the foci became larger and acquired phenotypic markers closer to neoplasia independent of further action of the carcinogen. We emphasize, however, that under other experimental conditions, particularly after repeated administration of high doses of one or several hepatocarcinogens, reversible foci and nodules may develop that resemble the persistent lesions in their cytology and cytochemical pattern[25,55,56,99]. Using the increased activity of glucose-6-phosphate dehydrogenase as a marker, we have shown in a Solt/Farber type of experiment that the majority of enzyme-altered foci and nodules induced by this regimen rapidly regress after withdrawal[100]. Similar results have been reported earlier by a number of other groups[56,101]. The significance of the reversion-linked phenotypic instability of focal hepatic lesions induced by carcinogens under extreme conditions is poorly understood. However, this puzzling phenomenon can largely be obviated by appropriate experimental designs, such as the stop experiments mentioned. Small non-persisting foci of altered hepatocytes which apparently disappear due to cellular necrosis after withdrawal of the carcinogen have recently also been observed in stop experiments with NNM[102]. The importance of taking cell death into account in the analysis of hepatocarcinogenesis has been emphasized earlier by Columbano *et al.*[103] and by Bursch *et al.*[104]

The concept of a *precursor–product relationship between foci persisting in stop experiments and hepatocellular adenomas or carcinomas* is substantiated by the observation that the foci of altered hepatocytes and neoplastic hepatic lesions share a number of cytopathological features. Thus, adenomas and occasionally even carcinomas may be predominantly composed of clear or mixed-cell populations resembling those in the focal lesions[19]. The majority of carcinomas consist of cells which are similar to those in glycogen poor, basophilic foci[15,17,105]. From the variety of cytochemical markers for the foci of altered hepatocytes, we particularly studied enzymes related to the alternative pathways of carbohydrate metabolism[51,106–109]. As a rule, the glycogen-storage foci which appear at an early stage show the following histochemical pattern. Whereas the activity of glucose-6-phosphatase and glycogen phosphorylase are reduced, there is a strong increase in the activity of the glucose-6-phosphate dehydrogenase, a key enzyme for the pentose phosphate pathway. A similar metabolic pattern prevails in adenomas and in hepatocellular carcinomas, as has also been shown by biochemical methods in transplantable hepatomas studied in different laboratories, especially in the laboratory of Weber[110] many years ago. Interestingly enough, the same histochemical changes are also demonstrable in one type of expansively growing persistent nodule in cirrhotic livers induced in rats by thioacetamide[109,111] suggesting that this type of nodule is neoplastic rather than hyperplastic. Whether a second type of nodule with a somewhat different enzyme histochemical pattern might be separated from this lesion as a true regenerative hyperplasia remains to be clarified[111].

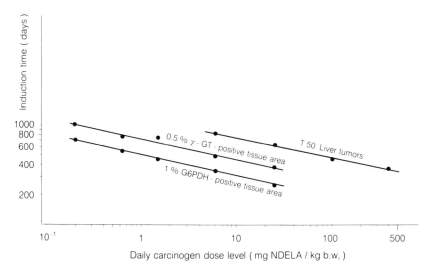

Figure 2 Dose–time response relationship of pre-neoplastic cell areas compared with that of liver tumours. An area density of 1% or 0.05% for glucose-6-phosphate dehydrogenase (G6PDH) and γ-glutamyltransferase (γ-GT), respectively, was taken as a constant parameter of pre-neoplastic alteration. The incidence of 50% lethality from liver tumours served as the parameter for tumour development. Times taken to achieve these effects are plotted against the corresponding dose of N-nitrosodiethanolamine (NDELA). The parallelism of the three lines with the slope indicates an identical dose–time response dependency of G6PDH- and γ-GT-positive areas as was found for tumour development (from ref. 115)

A close *statistical correlation between the enzyme-altered hepatic foci and hepatocellular carcinomas* has been reported from different laboratories[20,112-114]. We have recently studied the correlation between foci showing an increased activity of γ-glutamyltransferase or glucose-6-phosphate dehydrogenase and liver tumours developing after continuous oral administration of N-nitrosodiethanolamine at five different low-dose levels[114,115]. From Figure 2 it is evident that the slope of the lines for the enzyme-altered foci was identical with that of tumour induction. This was true for both enzymatic markers used, though the incidence of the respective lesions differed considerably in absolute terms. The detection of pre-neoplastic lesions allowed an assessment of the carcinogenic risk at dose levels which were much lower than those leading to tumours during the lifespan of the animals. Again, there was no indication of any reversibility of the focal lesions.

From the morphological, cytochemical and morphometric results discussed, we inferred a sequence of cellular changes leading from the clear and acidophilic glycogen-storage foci through intermediate and mixed-cell populations to hepatocellular adenomas and carcinomas. Some authors felt

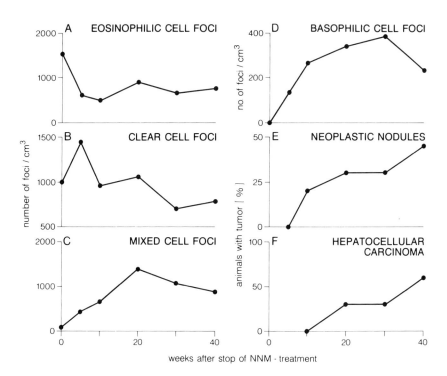

Figure 3 Incidence of focal hepatic lesions at different time points after stopping oral administration of N-nitrosmorpholine in a concentration of 120mg/litre drinking water. (A) Number of eosinophilic cell foci/cm³. (B) Number of clear-cell foci/cm³. (C) Number of mixed cell foci/cm³. (D) Number of basophilic-cell foci/cm³. (E) Percentage of experimental animals with hepatocellular adenomas. (F) Percentage of experimental animals with hepatocellular carcinomas (from ref. 117)

that each of the diverse phenotypes of the focal lesions might represent the result of a specific set of cellular changes and that the foci appearing early do not evolve via progressively more deviated forms to tumours[116]. However, the concept of a sequential phenotypic conversion of altered hepatocytes which we have been pursuing for a number of years, has further been substantiated by studies of the proliferation kinetics and the behaviour of the number and size of the different cell populations emerging during hepatocarcinogenesis. As demonstrated by the incorporation of [³H]-thymidine, the early appearing clear or acidophilic glycogen-storage foci only show a slightly increased cell proliferation[117]. A pronounced and steadily increasing cell proliferation is only linked with the appearance of mixed and basophilic cell populations in foci, nodules and carcinomas. These findings are consistent with the results of morphometric studies of the volume of the different types of foci[118]. When the number of foci was determined from the end of treatment up to 40 weeks after cessation, the total number of all types of foci remained rather constant. However, successive peaks were observed for the glycogen storage, mixed and basophilic cell foci (Figure 3). The increase in number of glycogen-storage foci was due to the additional development of small foci of this phenotype, but the increase in total number of mixed- and basophilic cell foci was correlated with larger lesions of this phenotype. Somewhat later, hepatocellular adenomas and carcinomas developed in a progressive manner. In studies with continuous application of NNM at two different dose levels, namely 6 and 12 mg/kg b.w./day, we observed a basically similar sequence of cellular changes[119]. A comparison of Figures 4 and 5 shows that there was not

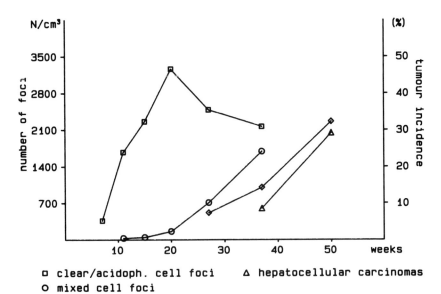

Figure 4 Sequence of pre-neoplastic and neoplastic changes in rat liver after continuous oral administration of 6 mg N-nitrosomorpholine/kg/day.

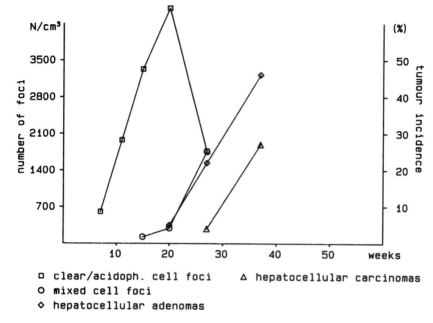

Figure 5 Sequence of pre-neoplastic and neoplastic changes in rat liver after continuous oral administration of 12 mg N-nitrosomorpholine/kg/day.

only an increase in number of the focal lesions but also a higher speed of the sequential cellular changes at the higher dose level, adenomas and carcinomas appearing about 10 weeks earlier than at the low dose level. These results suggest that the phenotypic heterogeneity in pre-neoplastic foci to a large extent reflects different stages in an ordered sequence of cellular changes during hepatocarcinogenesis[118]. It is difficult to reconcile our results with the frequently assumed clonal origin of pre-neoplastic and early neoplastic foci[20,120,121]. The data are more readily compatible with field effects characterized by concurrent alterations in many hepatocytes in large areas of the liver parenchyma[19,122,123].

Although the sequence of cellular changes during hepatocarcinogenesis appears to be rather consistent under controlled experimental conditions, a number of modulating factors may strongly influence the phenotypic pattern and stability of the focal lesions. Some of these modulating factors are the dose and duration of the carcinogenic treatment, the localization of the focal lesions within the liver lobule, the diet and the age, sex and strain of animals[25,26,56,124,125]. A particularly interesting modulation of the phenotype of focal lesions induced in rat liver with NNM has been brought about by additional oral administration of the hormone dehydroepiandrosterone[126] which has earlier been shown to inhibit chemical carcinogenesis in various tissues. Treatment with this hormone results in the relatively frequent appearance of an unusual type of focus staining with both acidophilic and basophilic dyes. We proposed the descriptive term 'amphophilic focus' for this

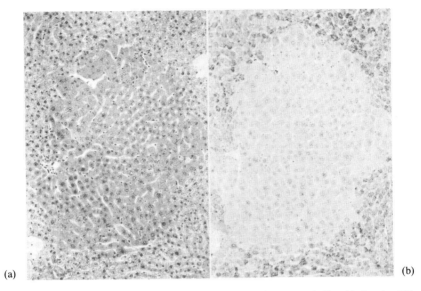

(a)   (b)

Figure 6 Amphophilic focus induced in rat liver with N-nitrosomorpholine (a) Amphophilic focus (H & E, × 90); (b) serial section to (a) showing loss of glycogen (Tri-PAS, × 90)

lesion (Figure 6a, b) which is apparently rich in mitochondria (as shown by a high activity of succinate dehydrogenase) and in peroxisomes (as demonstrated by strong catalase activity). There is evidence that the amphophilic foci, which are always negative for the two frequently used 'marker enzymes' γ-glutamyltransferase[127] and glutathione S-transferase placental form[128] may progress to hepatocellular adenomas and highly-differentiated carcinomas[129].

A different cell lineage leading to hepatic tumours may be represented by the tigroid cell foci which have been explicitly described in rats after oral application of a single dose of aflatoxin[130] and after treatment with chlorocyclohexanes[131] but most probably occur under many other conditions too. These foci are characterized by a pronounced basophilia. However, this basophilia is not present throughout the cytoplasm but organized in a tigroid pattern, due to highly ordered rough endoplasmic reticulum as seen under the electron microscope. Like the amphophilic foci, the tigroid cell foci are negative for γ-glutamyltransferase and the glutathione S-transferase placental form. With respect to the activity of other enzymes, especially that of the glucose-6-phosphate dehydrogenase and the glyceraldehyde-3-phosphate dehydrogenase, the tigroid cell foci resemble the prevalent types of pre-neoplastic hepatic lesions. Even after a single dose of aflatoxin B_1, the tigroid cell foci steadily increased in size and eventually progressed to adenomas which at places showed a tigroid cell pattern[130]. No clear-cut prestages for the tigroid cell foci have been identified so far, but we tentatively assume that they might originate from the large X-cells described earlier[123,132,133]. In this context, it should be mentioned that morphometric studies in extrafocal hepatocytes of NNM-treated rat liver revealed a significant nuclear and cytoplasmic enlargement in many cells, especially in perivenular hepatocytes, persisting up to 40 weeks after the end of treatment[134]. Although the foci of altered hepatocytes are apparently the most typical and the most important features of hepatocarcinogenesis, some participation of the persisting extra-focal changes cannot be ruled out.

Mouse

Foci of altered hepatocytes which show many similarities but also some differences as compared to those of the rat have also been described in other rodents, especially in mice[27,135-137]. Using the single-dose, infant-mouse model developed by Vesselinovitch[138], in which a very clear dose–response for the induction of hepatocarcinogenesis with N-nitrosodiethylamine has been established[139], we observed early focal leisons similar to those produced by single dose of aflatoxin in the rat. There was no obvious glycogenotic prestage[137].

The first lesions which could be identified by histochemical methods were intermediate basophilic, but often also contained considerable amounts of glycogen. Whereas the activity of the glycogen phosphorylase was normal or even somewhat increased, that of the glucose-6-phosphatase was usually decreased as in the majority of rat liver foci. The increased activity of the glucose-6-phosphate dehydrogenase and the glyceraldehyde-3-phosphate dehydrogenase was also comparable to rat liver foci. In hepatocellular adenomas, the enzymatic changes were even more pronounced, and there was frequently an excessive storage of glycogen and fat in large parts of these tumours. As a rule, the transition from adenomas to carcinomas was accompanied by striking additional histochemical changes[140]. The content of glycogen and fat and surprisingly also the activity of the glucose-6-phosphate dehydrogenase were usually reduced. However, the glucose-6-phosphatase activity markedly increased again, and there was a further increase in the activity of the glycolytic enzyme glyceraldehyde-3-phosphate dehydrogenase. In spite of some intriguing discrepancies in the metabolic changes of rat and mouse hepatocytes during carcinogenesis, which are not fully understood at present, a shift from glycogen metabolism towards the pentose phosphate pathway and glycolysis appears to be a common denominator.

In the last few months, we had the opportunity to investigate some livers of transgenic mice which were sent to us for diagnosis by Dr. Paul from Hannover. The mice originated from a colony established by Messing and colleagues[32] who had injected a gene construct composed of the SV40 T antigen gene and metallothionein-human growth hormone fusion gene into fertilized mouse eggs. The offspring carrying the fusion gene developed a high incidence of hepatocellular carcinomas in addition to pancreatic islet cell adenomas and peripheral neuropathies. From the livers of the few transgenic mice which we have studied so far, one case with hepatocellular tumours was particularly remarkable: multiple and multicentric hepatocellular adenomas and carcinomas were associated with prominent clear cell foci storing glycogen in excess. All transitions between clear and basophilic cell populations known from chemically-induced hepatocarcinogenesis were encountered. If these preliminary results can be confirmed, the cellular alterations observed predominantly in chemical hepatocarcinogenesis till now would gain general significance.

Other non-primates

In addition to murine liver, the liver of hamster[141,142], fish[143] and chicken[144] treated with chemical carcinogens has also been analysed for pre-neoplastic lesions. In these species, in principle, the same phenotypic cellular changes were observed in focal hepatic lesions, hepatocellular adenomas and carcinomas as in the respective murine liver lesions.

HEPATIC PRE-NEOPLASIA IN PRIMATES

Monkey

Of particular interest for human pathology are studies of Ruebner et al.[145] on hepatic pre-neoplasia in rhesus monkeys treated with N-nitrosodiethylamine. In accordance with the predominant sequence of cellular changes in rat hepatocarcinogenesis, these investigations revealed an early focal (clear or acidophilic cell) glycogenosis accompanied by a reduction in the activity of glucose-6-phosphatase and proceeding via diverse intermediate stages to basophilic hepatocellular carcinomas poor in glycogen.

Man

There is increasing evidence that the cellular changes during hepatocarcinogenesis in man do not represent an exception to the rules learned from laboratory animals[7,27,62,107,146,147]. Phenotypic alterations of hepatocytes which correspond to those seen in pre-neoplastic hepatic lesions of laboratory animals have been described in human livers by a number of authors[7,148-154]. Of particular interest are the recent observations of Fischer and coworkers[153], who found glycogen storage and enzyme altered foci in women who had taken oral contraceptives over extended periods, and the results of Karhunen and Penttila[154] who detected focal parenchymal lesions composed of clear cells in about 12% of 95 males studied in a consecutive autopsy series in Helsinki. The iron-resistance of such foci in patients suffering from idiopathic haemosiderosis stressed by Hirota et al.[151] is also noteworthy. The predominance of glycogen-rich clear or ground glass cells in many liver-cell adenomas[7,155-157] in focal nodular hepatic hyperplasia[7], in cases of so-called 'adenomatous hepatic hyperplasia'[11], in portions of hepatoblastomas[7,158] and in clear cell carcinomas has been noted by a number of authors[62,159]. According to Wu and colleagues[159], the clear cell variety of hepatocarcinoma may also develop in patients with persistent hepatitis B virus infection. Thung and Gerber[160] described enzymatic changes in a case of so-called nodular 'regenerative' hyperplasia of the liver similar to those known from experimental animals.

An even more interesting aspect of human pathology pertinent to our discussion is the appearance of hepatic tumours increasingly reported in

Table 1 Inborn hepatic glycogenosis and hepatocellular tumours in humans (from ref. 107)

Age (Years)	G-6-Pase Deficiency	Scintigraphy (FD)/ ultrasonogr. (FM)	Hepatic tumours Histopathology	References
0.5	?	—	Carcinoma	Levine et al., 1976
1	+	0	—	Miller et al., 1978
3	+	0	—	Miller et al., 1978
3.5	+	0	—	Howell et al., 1976
3.5	+	—	Adenoma	Berant et al., 1977
4	+	0	—	Miller et al., 1978
5	+	0	—	Miller et al., 1978
6	+	0	—	Miller et al., 1978
6	+	FD	—	Miller et al., 1978
7	—	—	Hepatoma	Fraumeni et al., 1968
7	+	FD	—	Miller et al., 1978
9	+	0	—	Miller et al., 1978
9	+	FD	—	Miller et al., 1978
10.5	+	—	Hepatoma	Mason & Anderson, 1955
11	+	0	—	Grossmann et al., 1981
12	+	0	—	Miller et al., 1978
13	+	0	—	Grossman et al., 1981
14	+	—	Tumour	Bauer, 1964
14	+	—	Carcinoma/Adenomas	Zangeneh et al., 1969
16	—	—	Adenoma	Steim & Zollinger, 1967
16	+	0	—	Miller et al., 1978
16	+	FD	—	Miller et al., 1978
16	+	FM	—	Grossman et al., 1981
19	+	FD	Adenoma	Howell et al., 1976
21	+	FD	—	Howell et al., 1976
21	+	FM	—	Grossman et al., 1981
22	+	FD	—	Miller et al., 1978
22	+	—	Adenoma	Nishio et al., 1981
23	+	—	Hepatoma	Spycher & Gitzelmann, 1971
23	+	FD	Adenoma	Miller et al., 1978
24	+	FD	—	Howell et al., 1976
24	+	FD	Adenoma	Howell et al., 1976
25	+	FD	—	Howell et al., 1976
27	+	FD	—	Howell et al., 1976
27	+	FM	—	Grossman et al., 1981
29	+	FD	Carcinoma	Howell et al., 1976
29	+	FM	—	Grossman et al., 1981
31	+	FD	Carcinoma	Miller et al., 1978
32	—	—	Carcinoma	Maruyama et al., 1962
33	+	FM	Carcinoma	Grossman et al., 1981
36	+	—	Adenoma	Holling, 1963
40	+	—	Adenoma	Holling, 1963

+ G-6-Pase deficiency verified biochemically in the patient or in another member of the respective family
— Not investigated
FD Focal hepatic defect (scintigram)
FM Focal hepatic mass (ultrasonogram)
0 Negative result of scintigraphy or ultrasonography

patients suffering from inborn hepatic glycogenosis, mostly that of the von Gierke type (Table 1). Liver tumours could be detected by scintigrams, sonograms, biopsies or autopsies in many patients with this genetically-fixed disease[107]. Whereas the tumours were relatively rare in the first decade of life, they appeared in all patients who had passed through adolescence. Histologically, both adenomas and carcinomas were diagnosed, and in some cases the clinical course of the disease suggested transformation from adenoma to carcinoma. Since we have collected the data listed in Table 1, we found a number of additional reports[161-165] including a description of two cases of focal nodular hyperplasia in patients with type-I glycogen storage disease[164,166]. Regression of hepatic tumours in type-I glycogen storage disease with dietary therapy has occasionally been observed[167], but it is now generally accepted that this inborn error of metabolism is fraught with an exceedingly high risk to proceed to hepatic tumours after lag periods of about 15 years[163,164,168].

These observations in humans strongly support the hypothesis that the —as yet unknown — molecular changes underlying the hepatocellular glycogenosis induced by carcinogenic agents may be causally related to neoplastic transformation of the hepatocytes[107]. The biochemical data available on carbohydrate metabolism in hepatic prebeoplasia will be discussed in detail by Mayer and colleagues in this volume (see Chapter 28). Our general view is that glucose-6-phosphate, the central metabolite of carbohydrate metabolism, may be transiently accumulated in the pre-neoplastic glycogenotic hepatocytes amongst other metabolites. A cascade of adaptive metabolic changes may be elicited which eventually channels the glucose-6-phosphate towards alternative metabolic pathways, such as the pentose phosphate pathway and glycolysis[169]. An increase in glucose-6-phosphate has in fact recently been found in pre-neoplastic glycogenotic liver cell lines[170] and in rat liver treated with NNM[171].

References

1. Herxheimer, G. (1919). *Schmaus' Grundriß der pathologischen Anatomie*. (Wiesbaden: J. F. Bergmann Verlag)
2. Sasaki, T. and Yoshida, T. (1935). Experimentelle Erzeugung des Leberkarzinoms durch Fütterung mit *o*-Amidoazotoluol. *Virchows Arch.*, **295**, 175–200
3. Reuber, M. D. (1965). Development of preneoplastic and neoplastic lesions of the liver in male rats given 0.025 percent N-2-fluorenyl-diacetamide. *J. Natl. Cancer Inst.*, **34**, 697–724
4. Edmondson, H. A. (1976). Benign epithelial tumors and tumor-like lesions of the liver. In Okuda, K. and Peters, R. L. (eds), *Hepatocellular Carcinoma*. pp. 309–30. (New York: John Wiley)
5. Peters, R. L. (1976). Pathology of hepatocellular carcinoma. In Okuda, K. and Peters, R. L. (eds), *Hepatocellular Carcinoma*. pp. 107–68. (New York, London, Sydney, Toronto: John Wiley)
6. Farber, E. (1973). Hyperplastic liver nodules. *Meth. Cancer Res.*, 7, 345–75
7. Altmann, H. W. (1978). Pathology of human liver tumors. In Remmer, H., Bolt, H. M., Bannasch, P. and Popper, H. (eds), *Primary Liver Tumors*. pp. 53–71. (Lancaster: MTP Press)
8. Stromeyer, F. W. and Ishak, K. G. (1981). Nodular transformation (nodular 'regenerative' hyperplasia) of the liver. A clinicopathologic study of 30 cases. *Human Pathol.*, **12**, 60–71

9. Arakawa, M., Sugihara, S., Kenmochi, K., Kage, M., Nakashima, T., Nakayama, T., Tashiro, S., Hiraoka, T., Suenaga M. and Okuda, K. (1986). Transition from benign adenomatous hyperplasia to hepatocellular carcinoma. *J. Gastroenterol. Hepatol.*, **1**, 3–14

10. Okuda, K. (1986). Early recognition of hepatocellular carcinoma. *Hepatology*, **6**, 729–38

11. Ohta, G. and Nakanuma, Y. (1987). Comparative study of three nodular lesions in cirrhosis. Adenomatoid hyperplasia, adenomatoid hyperplasia with intermediate lesion, and small hepatocellular carcinoma. In Okuda, K. and Ishak, K. G. (eds), *Neoplasms of the Liver*. pp. 177–87. (Tokyo, Berlin, Heidelberg, New York, London, Paris: Springer-Verlag)

12. Furuya, K., Nakamura, M., Yamamoto, Y., Togei, K. and Otsuka, H. (1988). Macroregenerative nodule of the liver. A clinicopathologic study of 345 autopsy cases of chronic liver disease. *Cancer*, **61**, 99–105

13. Weinbren, K. (1984). Precancerous states in the liver. In Carter, R. L. (ed.), *Precancerous States*. pp. 254–77. (London, New York, Toronto: Oxford University Press)

14. Kinosita, R. (1937). Studies on the cancerogenic chemical substances. *Trans. Soc. Path. Jpn.*, **27**, 665–725

15. Opie, E. L. (1946). Mobilisation of basophile substance (ribonucleic acid) in the cytoplasm of liver cells with the production of tumors by butter yellow. *J. Exp. Med.*, **84**, 91–106

16. Firminger, H. J. (1955). Histopathology of carcinogenesis and tumors of the liver in rats. *J. Natl. Cancer Inst.*, **15**, 1427–35

17. Grundmann, E. and Sieburg, H. (1962). Die Histogenese und Cytogenese des Lebercarcinoms der Ratte durch Diäthylnitrosamin im lichtmikroskopischen Bild. *Beitr. path. Anat.*, **126**, 57–90

18. Daoust, R. (1963). Cellular populations and nucleic acid metabolism in rat liver parenchyma during azo dye carcinogenesis. *Canad. Cancer Conf.*, **5**, 225–39

19. Bannasch, P. (1968). The cytoplasm of hepatocytes during carcinogenesis. Electron- and light-microscopical investigations of the nitrosomorpholine-intoxicated rat liver. *Rec. Res. Cancer Res.*, **19**, 1–100

20. Emmelot, P. and Scherer, E. (1980). The first relevant cell stage in rat liver carcinogenesis: a quantitative approach. *Biochim. Biophys. Acta*, **605**, 247–304

21. Pitot, H. C. and Sirica, A. E. (1980). The stages of initiation and promotion in hepatocarcinogenesis. *Biochim. Biophys. Acta*, **605**, 191–215

22. Williams, G. M. (1980). The pathogenesis of rat liver cancer caused by chemical carcinogens. *Biochim. Biophys. Acta*, **605**, 167–89

23. Peraino, C., Richards, W. L. and Stevens, F. J. (1983). Multistage hepatocarcinogenesis. In Slaga, T. J. (ed.), *Mechanisms of Tumor Promotion*, Vol. 1, pp. 1–53. (Boca Raton: CRC Press)

24. Rabes, H. M. (1983). Development and growth of early preneoplastic lesions induced in the liver by chemical carcinogens. *J. Cancer Res. Clin. Oncol.*, **106**, 85–92

25. Moore, M. A. and Kitagawa, T. (1986). Hepatocarcinogenesis in the rat; the effect of the promoters and carcinogens *in vivo* and *in vitro*. *Int. Rev. Cytol.*, **101**, 125–73

26. Préat, V., De Gerlache, D., Lans, M., Taper, H. and Roberfroid, M. (1986). Influence of the nature and the dose of the initiator on the development of premalignant and malignant lesions in rat hepatocarcinogenesis. *Teratogenesis, Carcinogenesis, Mutagenesis*, **6**, 165–72

27. Bannasch, P. (1983). Strain and species differences in the susceptibility to liver tumor induction. *IARC Scientific Publications*, **51**, 9–38

28. Ward, J. M. (1984). Morphology of potential preneoplastic hepatocyte lesions and liver tumors in mice and a comparison with other species. In Popp, J. A. (ed.), *Mouse Liver Neoplasia*. pp. 1–26. (Washington, New York, London: Hemisphere Publishing Corporation)

29. Summers, J., Smolec, J. and Snyder, R. L. (1978). A virus similar to human hepatitis B virus associated with hepatitis and hepatoma in woodchuck. *Proc. Natl. Acad. Sci. USA*, **75**, 4533–7

30. Omata, M., Yokosuka, O., Imazeki, F. and Okuda, K. (1987). Hepadna viruses and hepatocarcinogenesis. In Okuda, K. and Ishak, K. G. (eds), *Neoplasms of the Liver*. pp. 35–45. (Tokyo, Berlin, Heidelberg, New York, London and Paris: Springer-Verlag)

31. Abe, K., Kurata, T. and Shikata, T. (1988). Localization of woodchuck hepatitis virus in the liver. *Hepatology*, **8**, 88–92

32. Messing, A., Chen, H. Y., Palmiter, R. D. and Brinster, R. L. (1985), Peripheral

neuropathies, hepatocellular carcinomas and islet cell adenomas in transgenic mice. *Nature,* **316**, 461–3

33. Chisari, F. V., Filippi, P., Buras, J., McLachlan, A., Popper, H., Pinkert, C. A., Palmiter, R. D. and Brinster, R. L. (1987). Structural and pathological effects of synthesis of hepatitis B virus large envelope polypeptide in transgenic mice. *Proc. Natl. Acad. Sci. USA,* **84**, 6909–13

34. Anthony, P. P., Vogel, C. L. and Barker, L. F. (1973). Liver cell dysplasia: A premalignant condition. *J. Clin. Pathol.,* **26**, 217–23

35. Ruebner, B. H., Michas, C., Kanayama, R. and Bannasch, P. (1976). Sequential hepatic histologic and histochemical changes produced by diethylnitrosamine in the Rhesus monkey. *J. Natl. Cancer Inst.,* **57**, 1261–8

36. Ho, J. C. I., Wu, P.-C. and Mak, T.-K (1981). Liver cell dysplasia in association with hepatocellular carcinoma, cirrhosis and hepatitis B surface antigen in Hong Kong. *Int. J. Cancer,* **28**, 571–4

37. Akagi, G., Furuya, K., Kanamura, A., Chihara, T. and Otsuka, H. (1984). Liver cell dysplasia and hepatitis B surface antigen in liver cirrhosis and hepatocellular carcinoma. *Cancer,* **54**, 315–18

38. Henmi, A., Uchida, T. and Shikata, T. (1985). Karyometric analysis of liver cell dysplasia and hepatocellular carcinoma. Evidence against precancerous nature of liver cell dysplasia. *Cancer,* **55**, 2594–9

39. Cohen, C. and Berson, S. D. (1986). Liver cell dysplasia in normal, cirrhotic and hepatocellular carcinoma patients. *Cancer,* **57**, 1535–8

40. Roncalli, M., Borzio, M., de Biagi, G., Ferrari, A. R., Macchi, R., Tombesi, V. M. and Servida, E. (1986). Liver cell dysplasia in cirrhosis. A serologic and immunohistochemical study. *Cancer,* **57**, 1515–21

41. Pollice, L., Ricco, R., Russo, S., Maiorano, E., Pagniello, G. and Delfino-Pesce, V. (1988). Hepatocellular dysplasia: Immunohistochemical and morphometrical evaluation. *Appl. Pathol.,* **6**, 73–81

42. Kojiro, M. and Nakashima, T. (1987). Pathology of hepatocellular carcinoma. In Okuda, K. and Ishak, K. G. (eds), *Neoplasms of the Liver.* pp. 81–104. (Tokyo, Berlin, Heidelberg, New York, London and Paris: Springer-Verlag)

43. Karasaki, S. (1969). The fine structure of proliferating cells in preneoplastic rat livers during azo-dye carcinogenesis. *J. Cell Biol.,* **40**, 322–35

44. Hirota, N. and Williams, G. M. (1982). Ultrastructural abnormalities in carcinogen-induced hepatocellular altered foci identified by resistance to iron accumulation. *Cancer Res.,* **42**, 2298–309

45. Bannasch, P. and Müller, II. A. (1964). Lichtmikroskopische Untersuchungen über die Wirkung von N-Nitrosomorpholin auf die Leber von Ratte und Maus. *Arzneim. Forsch.,* **14**, 805–14

46. Gössner, W. and Friedrich-Freksa, H. (1964). Histochemische Untersuchungen über die Glucose-6-phosphatase in der Rattenleber während der Cancerisierung durch Nitrosamine. *Z. Naturforsch.,* **19b**, 862–4

47. Fischer, G., Ruschenburg, J., Eigenbrodt, E. and Katz, N. (1987). Decrease in glucokinase and glucose-6-phosphatase and increase in hexokinase in putative preneoplastic lesions of rat liver. *J. Cancer Res. Clin. Oncol.,* **113**, 430–6

48. Friedrich-Freksa, H., Papadopulu, G. and Gössner, W. (1969). Histochemische Untersuchungen der Cancerogenese in der Rattenleber nach zeitlich begrenzter Verabfolgung von Diäthylnitrosamin. *Z. Krebsforsch.,* **72**, 240–53

49. Moulin, M.-C. and Daoust, R. (1971). Glucose-6-phosphatase activity in rat liver parenchyma during azo-dye carcinogenesis. *Int. J. Cancer,* **8**, 81–5

50. Bannasch, P. and Angerer, H. (1974). Glykogen und Glucose-6-phosphatase während der Kanzerisierung der Rattenleber durch N-Nitrosomorpholin. *Arch. Geschwulstforsch.,* **43**, 105–14

51. Klimek, F., Mayer, D. and Bannasch, P. (1984). Biochemical microanalysis of glycogen content and glucose-6-phosphate dehydrogenase activity in focal lesions of rat liver induced by N-nitrosomorpholine. *Carcinogenesis,* **5**, 265–8

52. Farber, E. (1980). The sequential analysis of liver cancer induction. *Biochim. Biophys. Acta,* **605**, 149–66

53. Kaufmann, W. K., MacKenzie, S. A., Rahija, R. J. and Kaufmann, D. G. (1986). Quantitative relationship between initiation of hepatocarcinogenesis and induction of altered cell islands. *J. Cell. Biochem.*, **30**, 1–9

54. Scherer, E. (1984). Neoplastic progression in experimental hepatocarcinogenesis. *Biochem. Biophys. Acta,* **738**, 219–36

55. Goldsworthy, T. L., Hanigan, H. M. and Pitot, H. C. (1986). Models of hepatocarcinogenesis in the rat — Contrasts and comparisons. *CRC Crit. Rev. Toxicol.,* **17**, 61–89

56. Bannasch, P. (1986). Preneoplastic lesions as end points in carcinogenicity testing. I. Hepatic preneoplasia. *Carcinogenesis,* **7**, 689–95

57. Farber, E. and Sarma, D. S. R. (1987). Hepatocarcinogenesis: A dynamic cellular perspective. *Lab. Invest.,* **56**, 4–22

58. Bannasch, P., Zerban, H. and Hacker, H. J. (1985). Foci of altered hepatocytes, rat. In Jones, T. C., Mohr, U. and Hunt, R. D. (eds), *Monographs on Pathology of Laboratory Animals, Digestive System.* pp. 10–30. (Berlin, Heidelberg, New York and Tokyo: Springer-Verlag)

59. Klinge, O. and Bannasch, P. (1968). Zur Vermehrung des glatten endoplasmatischen Retikulum in Hepatocyten menschlicher Leberpunktate. *Verh. Dtsch. Ges. Path.,* **52**, 568–73

60. Hadziyannis, S., Gerber, M. A., Vissoulis, C. and Popper, H. (1973). Cytoplasmic hepatitis B antigen in 'ground-glass' hepatocytes of carriers. *Arch. Pathol.,* **96**, 327–30

61. Popper, H. (1975). The ground glass hepatocyte as a diagnostic hint. *Hum. Pathol.,* **6**, 517–20

62. Bannasch, P. and Klinge, O. (1971). Hepatozelluläre Glykogenose and Hepatombildung beim Menschen. *Virchows Arch. A (Path. Anat.),* **352**, 157–64

63. Nazarewicz, T., Krawczynski, K., Slusarczyk, J. and Nowoslawski, A. (1977). Cellular localization of hepatitis B virus antigens in patients with hepatocellular carcinoma coexisting with liver cirrhosis. *J. Infect. Dis.,* **135**, 298–302

64. Wu, P. C. and Lam, K. C. (1979). Cytoplasmic hepatitis B surface antigen and the ground-glass appearance in hepatocellular carcinoma. *Am. J. Clin. Pathol.,* **71**, 229–34

65. Suzuki, K., Uchida, T., Horiuchi, R. and Shikata, T. (1985). Localization of hepatitis B surface and core antigens in human hepatocellular carcinoma by immunoperoxidase methods. Replication of complete virions of carcinoma cells. *Cancer,* **56**, 321–7

66. Price, J. M., Harmann, J. W., Miller, E. C. and Miller, J. A. (1952). Progressive microscopic alterations in the livers of rats fed the hepatic carcinogens 3'-methyl-4-dimethylaminoazobenzene. *Cancer Res.,* **12**, 192–200

67. Farber, E. (1956). Similarities in the sequence of early histological changes induced in the liver of the rat by ethionine, 2-acetylaminofluorene and 3'-methyl-4-dimethylaminoazobenzene. *Cancer Res.,* **16**, 142–8

68. Inaoka, Y. (1967). Significance of the so-called oval cell proliferation during azo-dye hepatocarcinogenesis. *Gann,* **58**, 355–66

69. Ogawa, K., Minase, T. and Onoé, T. (1974). Demonstration of glucose-6-phosphatase activity in the oval cells in azo-dye carcinogenesis. *Cancer Res.,* **34**, 3379–86

70. Dempo, K., Chisaka, N., Yoshida, Y., Kaneko, A. and Onoe, T. (1975). Immunofluorescent study of 3'-methyl-4-dimethylaminoazobenzene carcinogenesis. *Cancer Res.* **35**, 1282–7

71. Shinozuka, H., Lombardi, B., Sell, S. and Immarino, R. M. (1978). Early histological and functional alterations of ethionine liver carcinogenesis in rats fed a choline-deficient diet. *Cancer Res.,* **38**, 1092–8

72. Sell, S., Osborn, K. and Leffert, H. L. (1981). Autoradiography of 'oval cells' appearing rapidly in the livers of rats fed N-2-fluorenylacetamide in a choline devoid diet. *Carcinogenesis,* **2**, 7–14

73. Yaswen, P., Hayner, N. T. and Fausto, N. (1984). Isolation of oval cells by centrifugal elutriation and comparison with other cell types purified from normal and preneoplastic livers. *Cancer Res.,* **44**, 324–31

74. Yaswen, P., Goyette, M., Shank, P. R. and Fausto, N. (1985). Expression of *c-ki-ras, c-Ha-ras* and *c-myc* genes in specific cell types during hepatocarcinogenesis. *Mol. Cell Biol.,* **5**, 780–6

75. Germain, L., Goyette, R. and Marceau, N. (1985). Differential cytokeratin and α-

fetoprotein expression in morphologically distinct epithelial cells emerging at the early stage of rat hepatocarcinogenesis. *Cancer Res.,* **45**, 673–81

76. Evarts, R. P., Nagy, P., Marsden, E. and Thorgeirsson, S. S. (1987). A precursor–product relationship exists between oval cells and hepatocytes in rat liver. *Carcinogenesis,* **8**, 1737–40

77. Tsao, M. S. and Grisham, J. W. (1987). Hepatocarcinomas, cholangiocarcinomas and hepatoblastomas produced by chemically transformed cultured rat liver epithelial cells. *Am. J. Pathol.,* **127**, 168–81

78. Plenat, F., Braun, L. and Fausto, N. (1988). Demonstration of glucose-6-phosphatase and peroxisomal catalase activity by ultrastructural cytochemistry in oval cells from livers of carcinogen-treated rats. *Am. J. Pathol.,* **130**, 91–102

79. Tatematsu, M., Ho, R. H., Kaku, T., Ekem, J. K. and Farber, E. (1984). Studies on the proliferation and fate of oval cells in the liver of rats treated with 2-acetylaminofluorene and partial hepatectomy. *Am. J. Pathol.,* **114**, 418–30

80. Hutterer, F., Rubin, E., Singer, E. J. and Popper, H. (1961). Quantitative relation of cell proliferation and fibrogenesis in the liver. *Cancer Res.,* **21**, 206–15

81. Grisham, J. W. and Porta, E. A. (1964). Origin and fate of proliferated hepatic ductal cells in the rat; electron microscopic and autoradiographic studies. *Exp. Mol. Pathol.,* 3, 242–61

82. Rubin, E. (1964). The origin and fate of proliferated bile ductular cells. *Exp. Mol. Pathol.,* 3, 279–86

83. Bannasch, P. and Massner, B. (1976). Histogenese und Cytogenese von Cholangiofibromen und Cholangiocarcinomen bei Nitrosomorpholin-vergifteten Ratten. *Z. Krebsforsch.,* **87**, 239–55

84. Terao, K. and Nakano, M. (1974). Cholangiofibrosis induced by short-term feeding of 3-methyl-4-(dimethylamino)azobenzene: an electron microscopic observation. *Gann,* **65**, 249–60

85. Bannasch, P. and Reiss, W. (1971). Histogenese und Cytogenese cholangiocellulärer Tumoren bei Nitrosomorpholin-vergifteten Ratten. Zugleich ein Beitrag zur Morphogenese der Cystenleber. *Z. Krebsforsch.,* **76**, 193–215

86. Tatematsu, M., Kaku, T., Medline, A. and Farber, E. (1985). Intestinal metaplasia as a common option of oval cells in relation to cholangio-fibrosis in liver of rats exposed to 2-acetylaminofluorene. *Lab. Invest.,* **52**, 354–62

87. Moore, M. A., Fukushima, S., Ichihara, A., Sato, K. and Ito, N. (1986). Intestinal metaplasia and altered enzyme expression in propylnitrosamine-induced Syrian hamster cholangiocellular and gall-bladder lesions. *Virchows Arch. B (Cell Pathol.),* **51**, 29–38

88. Thamavit, W., Kongkanuntn, R., Tiwawech, D. and Moore, M. A. (1987). Level of *Opisthorchis* infestation and carcinogen dose-dependence of cholangiocarcinoma induction in Syrian golden hamsters. *Virchows Arch. B (Cell Pathol.),* **54**, 52–8

89. Ogawa, K., Minase, T. and Onoe, T. (1974). Demonstration of glucose-6-phosphatase activity in the oval cells of rat liver and the significance of the oval cells in azo dye carcinogenesis. *Cancer Res.,* **34**, 3379–86

90. Sirica, A. E. and Cihla, H. P. (1984). Isolation and partial characterization of oval and hyperplastic bile ductular cell enriched populations from the livers of carcinogen and noncarcinogen-treated rats. *Cancer Res.,* **44**, 3454–66

91. Benner, U., Hacker, H. J. and Bannasch, P. (1979). Electron microscopical demonstration of glucose-6-phosphatase in native cryostat sections fixed with glutaraldehyde through semipermeable membranes. *Histochemistry,* **65**, 41–7

92. Bannasch, P., Benner, U., Hacker, H. J., Klimek, F., Mayer, D., Moore, M. and Zerban, H. (1981). Cytochemical and biochemical microanalysis of carcinogenesis. *Histochem. J.,* **13**, 799–820

93. Kitagawa, T., Yokochi, T. and Sugano, H. (1972). α-Fetoprotein and hepatocarcinogenesis in rats fed 3-methyl-4-dimethyl-aminoazobenzene or N-2-fluorenylacetamide. *Int. J. Cancer,* **10**, 368–81

94. Okita, K., Gruenstein, M., Klaiber, M. and Farber, E. (1974). Localization of α-fetoprotein by immunofluorescence in hyperplastic nodules during hepatocarcinogenesis induced by 2-acetylaminofluorene. *Cancer Res.,* **34**, 2758–63

95. Sell, S., Nichols, M. and Becker, F. F. (1974). Hepatocyte proliferation and α_1-fetoprotein in pregnant, neonatal and partially hepatectomized rats. *Cancer Res.,* **34**, 865–71

96. Kuhlmann, W. D. (1978). Localization of alpha₁-fetoprotein and DNA-synthesis in liver cell populations during experimental hepatocarcinogenesis in rats. *Int. J. Cancer*, **21**, 368–80

97. Iwai, M., Kashiwadani, M., Takino, T. and Ibata, Y. (1988). Demonstration by light and ultrastructural immunoperoxidase study of α-fetoprotein-positive non-hepatoma cells and hepatoma cells during 3′-methyl-4-dimethylaminoazobenzene hepatocarcinogenesis. *Virchows Arch. B (Cell Pathol.)*, **55**, 117–23

98. Moore, M. A., Mayer, D. and Bannasch, P. (1982). The dose-dependence and sequential appearance of putative preneoplastic populations induced in the rat liver by stop experiments with N-nitrosomorpholine. *Carcinogenesis*, **3**, 1429–36

99. Farber, E. (1984). Precancerous steps in carcinogenesis. Their physiological adaptive nature. *Biochim. Biophys. Acta*, **738**, 171–80

100. Moore, M. A., Hacker, H. J. and Bannasch, P. (1983). Phenotypic instability in focal and nodular lesions induced in a short term system in the rat liver. *Carcinogenesis*, **4**, 595–603

101. Farber, E. (1982). The biology of carcinogen-induced hepatocyte nodules and related liver lesions in the rat. *Toxicol. Pathol.*, **10**, 197–205

102. Enzmann, H. and Bannasch, P. (1988). Non-persisting early foci of altered hepatocytes induced in rats by N-nitrosomorpholine. *J. Cancer Res. Clin. Oncol.*, **114**, 30–4

103. Columbano, A., Ledda-Columbano, G. M., Rao, P. M., Rajalakshmi, S. and Sarma, D. S. R. (1984). Occurrence of cell death (apoptosis) in preneoplastic and neoplastic liver cells: A sequential study. *Am. J. Pathol.*, **116**, 441–6

104. Bursch, W., Lauer, B., Timmermann-Trosiener, T., Barthel, G., Schuppler, J. and Schulte-Hermann, R. (1984). Controlled cell death (apoptosis) of normal and putative preneoplastic cells in rat liver following withdrawal of tumor promoters. *Carcinogenesis*, **5**, 453–8

105. Daoust, R. and Calamai, R. (1971). Hyperbasophilic foci as sites of neoplastic transformation in hepatic parenchyma. *Cancer Res.*, **31**, 1290–96

106. Hacker, H. J., Moore, M. A., Mayer, D., and Bannasch, P. (1982). Correlative histochemistry of some enzymes of carbohydrates metabolism in preneoplastic and neoplastic lesions in the rat liver. *Carcinogenesis*, **3**, 1265–72

107. Bannasch, P., Hacker, H. J., Klimek, F. and Mayer, D. (1984). Hepatocellular glycogenosis and related pattern of enzymatic changes during hepatocarcinogenesis. *Adv. Enzyme Regul.*, **22**, 97–121

108. Seelmann-Eggebert, G., Mayer, D., Mecke, D. and Bannasch, P. (1987). Expression and regulation of glycogen phosphorylase in preneoplastic and neoplastic hepatic lesions in rats. *Virchows Arch. B. (Cell Pathol.)*, **53**, 44–51

109. Klimek, F., Moore, M. A., Schneider, E. and Bannasch, P. (1988). Histochemical and microbiochemical demonstration of reduced pyruvate kinase activity in thioacetamide-induced neoplastic nodules of rat liver. *Histochemistry*, **90**, 37–42

110. Weber, G. (1977). Enzymology of cancer cells. Parts 1 and 2. *N. Engl. J. Med.*, **296**, 486–93, 541–51

111. Bannasch, P. and Zerban, H. (1987). Modulation of hepatocellular phenotype and proliferation in liver cirrhosis. In Boyer, J. L. and Bianchi, L. (eds), *Liver Cirrhosis*. pp. 27–38. (Lancaster: MTP Press)

112. Kunz, W., Schaude, G., Schwarz, M. and Tennekes, H. (1982). Quantitative aspects of drug-mediated tumour promotion in liver and its toxicological implications. In Hecker, E., Fusenig, N. E., Kunz, W., Marks, F. and Thielmann, M. W. (eds), *Carcinogenesis – A Comprehensive Survey*, Vol. 7, pp. 111–25. (New York: Raven Press)

113. Goldsworthy, T. L. and Pitot, H. C. (1985). The quantitative analysis and stability of histochemical markers of altered hepatic foci in rat liver following initiation by diethylnitrosamine administration and promotion with phenobarbital. *Carcinogenesis*, **6**, 1261–9

114. Zerban, H., Preussmann, R. and Bannasch, P. (1988). Dose-time –relationship of the development of preneoplastic liver lesions induced in rats with low doses of N-nitrosodiethanolamine. *Carcinogenesis*, **9**, 607–10

115. Zerban, H., Preussmann, R. and Bannasch, P. (1988). Quantitative morphometric comparison between the expression of two different 'marker enzymes' in preneoplastic liver lesions induced in rats with low doses of N-nitrosodiethanolamine. *Cancer Lett.*, **43**, 99–104

116. Peraino, C., Staffeldt, E. F., Carnes, B. A., Ludeman, V. A., Blomquist, J. A. and

Vesselinovitch, S. D. (1984). Characterization of histochemically detectable altered hepatocyte foci and their relationship to hepatic tumorigenesis in rats treated once with diethylnitrosamine or benzo(a)pyrene within one day after birth. *Cancer Res.*, **44**, 3340–7

117. Zerban, H., Rabes, H. M. and Bannasch, P. (1985). Kinetics of cell proliferation during hepatocarcinogenesis. *Eur. J. Cancer Clin. Oncol.*, **21**, 1424

118. Enzmann, H. and Bannasch, P. (1987). Potential significance of phenotypic heterogeneity of focal lesions at different stages in hepatocarcinogenesis. *Carcinogenesis*, **8**, 1607–12

119. Weber, E. and Bannasch, P. (1988). Dose-dependence of preneoplastic lesion phenotype in N-nitrosomorphine-induced hepatocarcinogenesis. *Falk Symposium No. 51, Liver Cell Carcinoma*, 43

120. Rabes, H. M., Bücher, T., Hartmann, A., Linke I. and Dünnwald, M. (1982). Clonal growth of carcinogen-induced enzyme-deficient preneoplastic cell populations in mouse liver. *Cancer Res.*, **42**, 3220–7

121. Weinberg, W. C. and Iannaccone, P. M. (1988). Clonality of preneoplastic liver lesions: Histological analysis in chimeric rats. *J. Cell Sci.*, **89**, 423–31

122. Willis, R. A. (1953). *Pathology of Tumors*, 2nd edn (London: Butterworths)

123. Bannasch, P., Mayer, D. and Hacker, H. J. (1980). Hepatocellular glycogenosis and hepatocarcinogenesis. *Biochim. Biophys. Acta*, **605**, 217–45

124. de Gerlache, J., Lans, M., Taper, H., Préat, V. and Roberfroid, M. (1982). Promotion of the chemically initiated hepatocarcinogenesis. In Sorsa, M. and Vainio, H. (eds), *Mutagens in our Environment*. pp. 35–46. (New York: Alan R. Liss, Inc.)

125. Ohlhauser, D., Enzmann, H., Dettler, T. and Bannasch, P. (1988). Response of early preneoplastic liver lesions to fructose. *Falk Symposium No. 51, Liver Cell Carcinoma*, 47

126. Weber, E., Moore, M. A. and Bannasch, P. (1988). Enzyme histochemical and morphological phenotype of amphophilic foci and amphophilic/tigroid cell adenomas in rat liver after combined treatment with dehydroepiandrosterone and N-nitrosomorpholine. *Carcinogenesis*, **9**, 1049–54

127. Hanigan, M. H. and Pitot, H. C. (1985). Gamma-glutamyl transpeptidase — its role in hepatocarcinogenesis. *Carcinogenesis*, **6**, 165–72

128. Tatematsu, M., Mera, Y., Inoue, T., Satoh, K. and Ito, N. (1988). Stable phenotypic expression of γ-glutamyltransferase in rat liver preneoplastic and neoplastic lesions. *Carcinogenesis*, **9**, 215–20

129. Weber, E., Moore, M. A. and Bannasch, P. (1988). Phenotypic modulation of hepatocarcinogenesis and reduction in N-nitrosomorpholine-induced hemangiosarcoma and adrenal lesion development in Sprague–Dawley rats by dehydroepiandrosterone. *Carcinogenesis*, **9**, 1191–5

130. Bannasch, P., Benner, U., Enzmann, H. and Hacker, H. J. (1985). Tigroid cell foci and neoplastic nodules in the liver of rats treated with a single dose of aflatoxin β_1. *Carcinogenesis*, **6**, 1641–8

131. Schröter, C., Parzefall, W., Schröter, H. and Schulte-Hermann, R. (1987). Dose–response studies on the effects of a α-, ß- and γ-hexachlorocyclohexane on putative preneoplastic foci, monooxygenases, and growth in rat liver. *Cancer Res.*, **47**, 80–8

132. Bannasch, P., Papenburg, J. and Ross, W. (1972). Cytomorphologische und morphometrische Studien der Hepatocarcinogenese. I. Reversible und irreversible Veränderungen am Cytoplasma der Leberparenchymzellen bei Nitrosomorpholin-vergifteten Ratten. *Z. Krebsforsch.*, **77**, 108–33

133. Wanson, J.-C., Bernaert, D., Penasse, W., Mosselmans, R. and Bannasch P. (1980). Separation in distinct subpopulations by elutriation of liver cells following exposure of rats to N-nitrosomorpholine. *Cancer Res.*, **40**, 459–71

134. Enzmann, H. and Bannasch, P. (1987). Morphometric studies of alterations of extrafocal hepatocytes of rat liver treated with N-nitrosomorpholine. *Virchows Arch. B (Cell Pathol.)*, **53**, 218–26

135. Goldfarb, S., Pugh, T. D., Koen, H. and He, Y.-Z. (1983). Preneoplastic and neoplastic progression during hepatocarcinogenesis in mice injected with diethylnitrosamine in infancy. *Environ. Health Perspect.*, **50**, 149–61

136. Ward, J. M. (1984). Morphology of potential preneoplastic hepatocyte lesions and liver tumors in mice and a comparison with other species. In Popp, J. A. (ed.), *Mouse Liver Neoplasia*. pp. 1–26. (Washington: Hemisphere Publishing Corporation)

137. Vesselinovitch, S. D., Hacker, H. J. and Bannasch, P. (1985). Histochemical characterization of focal hepatic lesions induced by single diethylnitrosamine treatment in infant mice. *Cancer Res.,* **45**, 2774–80

138. Vesselovitch, S. D. (1980). Infant mouse as a sensitive system for carcinogenicity in N-nitroso compounds. *IARC Scientific Publications,* **31**, 645–55

139. Vesselinovitch, S. D. and Mihailovich, N. (1983). Kinetics of diethylnitrosamine hepatocarcinogenesis in the infant mouse. *Cancer Res.,* **43**, 4253–9

140. Hacker, H. J., Mtiro, H., Bannasch, P. and Vesselinovitch, S. D. (1988). Histochemical pattern of hepatocellular adenomas and carcinomas induced in mice by single dose of diethylnitrosamine. *Falk Symposium No. 51, Liver Cell Carcinoma*

141. Stenbäck, F., Mori, H., Furuya, K. and Williams, G. M. (196). Pathogenesis of dimethylnitrosamine-induced hepatocellular cancer in hamster liver and lack of enhancement by phenobarbital. *J. Natl. Cancer Inst.,* **76**, 327–33

142. Thamavit, W., Ngamying, M., Boonpucknavig, V., Boonpucknavig, S. and Moore, M. A. (1987). Enhancement of DEN-induced hepatocellular nodule development by *Opisthorchis viverrini* infection in Syrian golden hamsters. *Carcinogenesis,* **8**, 1351–3

143. Couch, J. A. and Courtney, L. A. (1987). N-nitrosodiethylamine-induced hepatocarcinogenesis in estuarine sheephead minnow (*Cyprinodon variegatus*): Neoplasms and related lesions compared with mammalian lesions. *J. Natl. Cancer Inst.,* **79**, 297–321

144. Brunn, H., Schmidt, E., Reinacher, M., Manz, D. and Eigenbrodt, E. (1987). Histology and histochemistry of the liver of chickens after DEN-induced hepatocarcinogenesis and ingestion of low chlorinated biphenyls. *Arch. Toxicol.,* **60**, 337–42

145. Ruebner, B. H., Michas, C., Kanayama, R. and Bannasch, P. (1976). Sequential hepatic histogenic and histochemical changes produced by diethylnitrosamine in the Rhesus monkey. *J. Natl. Cancer Inst.,* **57**, 1261–8

146. Balázs, M. (1976). Lichtmikroskopische Untersuchungen in einem Fall von primärem Leberkarzinom in Säuglingsalter. *Zbl. allg. Path.,* **120**, 3–13

147. Pitot, H. C. (1988). Hepatic neoplasia: Chemical induction. In Arias, J. M., Jacoby, W. B., Popper, H., Schachter, D. and Shafritz, D. A. (eds), *The Liver. Biology and Pathobiology.* pp. 1125–46. (New York: Raven Press)

148. Shapiro, P., Ikeda, R. M., Ruebner, B. H., Connors, M. H., Halsted, C. C. and Abildgaard, C. F. (1977). Multiple hepatic tumors and peliosis hepatis in Fanconi's anemia treated with androgens. *Am. J. Dis. Child.,* **131**, 1104–6

149. Cain, H. (1978). Liver cell carcinoma in infancy and childhood. In Remmer, H., Bolt, H., Bannasch, P. and Popper, H. (eds), *Primary Liver Tumors.* pp. 73–85. (Lancaster: MTP Press)

150. Heine, W. D. (1981). Experimentelle und menschliche hepatozelluläre Lebertumoren und ihre Vorstufen — histologische enzymhistochemische und zellkinetische Charakteristika. In Zelder, O., Röher, H. D., Fischer, M. and Bode, J. Ch. (eds), *Experimentelle und klinische Hepatologie.* pp. 13–24. (Stuttgart, New York: F. K. Schattauer Verlag)

151. Hirota, N., Hamazaki, M. and Williams, G. M. (1982). Resistance to iron accumulation and presence of hepatitis B surface antigen in preneoplastic and neoplastic lesions in human hemochromatic livers. *Hepato-Gastroenterol.,* **29**, 49–51

152. Mori, H., Tanaka, T., Sugie, S., Takahashi, M. and Williams, G. (1982). DNA content of liver cell nuclei of N-2-fluorenylacetamide-induced altered foci and neoplasms in rats and human hyperplastic foci. *J. Natl. Cancer Inst.,* **69**, 1277–82

153. Fischer, G., Hartmann, H., Droese, M., Schauer, A. and Bock, K. W. (1986). Histochemical and immunohistochemical detection of putative preneoplastic liver foci in woman after long-term use of oral contraceptives. *Virchows Arch. B (Cell Pathol.),* **50**, 321–37

154. Karhunen, P. J. and Penttilä, A. (1987). Preneoplastic lesions of human liver. *Hepato-Gastroenterol.,* **34**, 10–15

155. Popper, H., Maltoni, C., Selikoff, I. J., Squire, R. A. and Thomas, L. B. (1977). Comparison of neoplastic hepatic lesions in man and experimental animals. In Hiatt, H. H., Watson, J. D. and Winsten, J. A. (eds), *Origin of Human Cancer, Book C, Human Risk Assessment, Cold Spring Harbor Conferences on Cell Proliferation,* Vol. 4. pp. 1359–82. (Cold Spring Harbor)

156. Wheeler, D. A., Edmondson, H. A. and Reynolds, T. B. (1986). Spontaneous liver cell

adenoma in children. *Am. J. Clin. Pathol.,* **85**, 6–12

157. Goodman, Z. D. (1987). Benign tumors of the liver. In Okuda, K. and Ishak, K. G. (eds), *Neoplasms of the Liver.* pp. 105–25. (Tokyo, Berlin, Heidelberg, New York, London and Paris: Springer-Verlag)

158. Stocker, J. T. and Ishak, K. G. (1987). Hepatoblastoma. In Okuda, K. and Ishak, K. G. (eds), *Neoplasms of the Liver.* pp. 127–36. (Tokyo, Berlin, Heidelberg, New York, London and Paris: Springer-Verlag)

159. Wu, P. C., Lai, C. L., Lam, K. C., Lok, A. S. F. and Lin, H. J. (1983). Clear cell carcinoma of liver. An ultrastructural study. *Cancer,* **52**, 504–7

160. Thung, S. and Gerber, M. (1981). Enzyme pattern and marker antigens in nodular 'regenerative' hyperplasia of the liver. *Cancer,* **47**, 1796–9

161. Biondetti, P. R., Fiore, D. and Muzzio, P. C. (1980). Computerized tomography of the liver in von Gierke's disease. *J. Comput. Assist. Tomogr.,* **4**, 685–6

162. Bowerman, R. A., Samuels, B. I. and Siver, M. T. (1983). Ultrasonographic features of hepatic adenomas in type I glycogen storage disease. *J. Ultrasound Med.,* **2**, 51–4

163. Coire, C. I., Qizilbash, A. H. and Castelli, M. F. (1987). Hepatic adenomata in type Ia glycogen storage disease. *Arch. Pathol. Lab. Med.,* **111**, 166–9

164. Limmer, J., Fleig, W. E., Leupold, D., Bittner, R., Ditschuneit, H. and Beger, H. -G. (1988). Hepatocellular carcinoma in type I glycogen storage disease. *Hepatology,* **8**, 531–7

165. Poe, R. and Snover, D. C. (1988). Adenomas in glycogen storage disease type 1. Two cases with unusual histologic features. *Am. J. Surg. Pathol.,* **12**, 477–83

166. Pizzo, C. J. (1980). Type I glycogen storage disease with focal nodular hyperplasia of the liver and vasoconstrictive pulmonary hypertension. *Pediatrics,* **65**, 341–3

167. Parker, P., Burr, J., Slonim, A., Gishan, F. K. and Greene, H. (1981). Regression of hepatic adenomas in type Ia glycogen storage disease with dietary therapy. *Gastroenterology,* **81**, 534–6

168. Howell, R. R., Stevenson, R. E., Ben-Menachem, Y., Phyliky, R. L. and Berry, D. H. (1976). Hepatic adenomata with type 1 glycogen-storage disease. *J. Am. Med. Assoc.,* **236**, 1481–4

169. Bannasch, P. (1988). Phenotypic cellular changes as indicators of stages during neoplastic development. In Iversen, O. H. (ed.), *Theories of Carcinogenesis.* pp. 231–49. (Washington: Hemisphere Publishing Corporation)

170. Mayer, D. (1988). Regulation of carbohydrate metabolism in a glycogen storing liver cell line. In Roberfroid, M. B. and Préat, V. (eds), *Experimental Hepatocarcinogenesis.* pp. 283–96. (New York, London: Plenum Press)

171. Enzmann, H., Dettler, T., Ohlhauser, D. and Bannasch, P. (1988). Elevation of glucose-6-phosphate in early stages of hepatocarcinogenesis induced in rats by N-nitrosomorpholine. *Horm. Metabol. Res.,* **20**, 128–9.

Section 2
Hepadna viruses and hepatocarcinogenesis

8
Unravelling the life cycle of hepatitis B viruses

H. -J. SCHLICHT, A. ESSER, R. BARTENSCHLAGER, P. GALLE,
C. KUHN, M. NASSAL, M. NIEPMANN, G. RADZIWILL AND
H. SCHALLER

INTRODUCTION

The hepatitis B viruses, also called hepadnaviruses, represent a small group of primarily hepatotropic enveloped DNA viruses with a simple morphology (Figure 1). The most important member of this virus family is the human hepatitis B virus (HBV) which is the causative agent of a severe form of hepatitis. However, other than man, HBV is only infectious for chimpanzees, and therefore several hepadnaviruses which infect animals more amenable to experimental studies have been isolated and characterized. To date, three such viruses which either infect ducks (DHBV), woodchucks (WHV), or ground

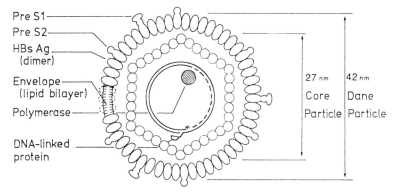

Figure 1 Schematic representation of the hepatitis B virus particle (Dane particle). In the case of HBV, the viral envelope contains three different surface proteins which are referred to as the HBsAg (S protein), the pre-S1 and the pre-S2 protein. The core particle is formed by 180 identical subunits of core protein. It contains the viral polymerase and the genome which consists of a partially double-stranded DNA molecule to which a protein is covalently linked

79

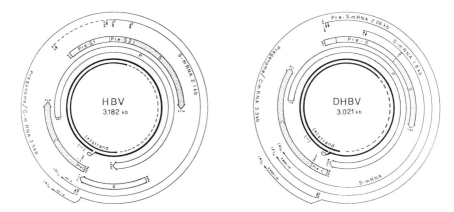

Figure 2 Genetical, physical, and transcriptional map of the HBV and DHBV genomes. The inner circles represent the two DNA strands of the viral genome. The gap within the plus strand is dotted. The viral genes which encode the surface proteins (pre-S/S gene), the core protein (C gene), the polymerase (P gene), and the X-protein (X gene, absent in DHBV) are depicted as arrows. The outer lines represent the viral transcripts. The mRNA starting upstream from the HBV pre-S1 region is partially dotted since to date this mRNA has only been detected in tissue culture

squirrels (GSHV) have been examined in detail[1,2]. In our laboratory we have chosen the avian hepadnavirus DHBV to develop an animal model system for HBV since this virus allows the systematic investigation of virus mutants *in vivo*. In addition, since DHBV is the member of the hepatitis B virus family most distantly related to HBV, a comparative study of both viruses should allow insight into the principles of hepadnaviral gene expression.

Characteristic of all hepatitis B viruses is a small compact genome with extensively overlapping reading frames and a unique replication strategy which includes reverse transcription of a RNA pregenome[3]. The organization of the HBV and DHBV genomes is shown in Figure 2. The C-gene encodes the core-protein. It overlaps at its 3' end with the P-gene, whose proposed gene product shares significant homologies with certain retroviral reverse transcriptases[4] and which is therefore believed to encode the viral polymerase. The preS/S-gene, which completely overlaps with the P-gene, encodes the surface proteins. The only gross difference between both genomes is that the X-gene, whose gene product can enhance viral gene expression[5,6], is absent in DHBV.

In this chapter we discuss recent work mainly from our laboratory dealing with the tissue and species specificity of the hepadnaviruses, the expression strategy of the viral core and polymerase gene, and the viral replication strategy. As will become clear by the discussion of these data, there are now powerful systems available which allow the study of all aspects of hepatitis B virus biology at the molecular level.

HOW TO GROW HEPATITIS B VIRUS IN CULTURED CELLS

Two especially prominent features of all hepadnaviruses are their very narrow host range and their pronounced tissue tropism which restricts virus replication almost exclusively to hepatocytes. Until recently, the latter property was a major obstacle to the study of hepadnaviral gene expression, since even after transfection of cloned viral DNA into cultured cells only a small fraction of the viral proteins (that is the major surface proteins) were expressed. A clue to the reason for this finding came initially from the analysis of the viral mRNAs in infected liver tissue. As shown in Figure 2, there are basically two types of mRNAs transcribed from the viral genomes. The small mRNAs of about 2 kb encode the major surface proteins. The long mRNA of about 3.5 kb, which has more than genome length, initiates upstream from the core gene. This RNA, however, not only codes for protein (i.e. the core protein), but in addition is also the template for a new viral genome generated by reverse transcription (see below). Since no core protein could be detected in cells after transfection with viral DNA, it appeared most likely that expression of the long mRNA was controlled by regulatory elements which were only active in differentiated liver cells. That this assumption was indeed correct has now been proven by several independent experimental findings.

Firstly, and most importantly, the search for a permanent cell line competent for hepatitis B virus replication resulted in the description of two exceptionally well-differentiated human hepatoma cell lines, HepG2 and HUH-7, which produce complete virus particles upon transfection with cloned viral DNA[7-11]. Secondly, systematic studies employing endogenously or experimentally DHBV infected primary duck hepatocytes showed that the loss of the differentiated state during prolonged cell culture is paralleled by a drastic reduction in core protein synthesis and virus replication (Galle *et al.*, submitted for publication). These findings are consistent with the view that cellular factors that are only present in differentiated hepatocytes are required for expression of the 3.5 kb RNA, and that these factors are usually lost very quickly after the cells have been withdrawn from their natural environment. To date, however, almost nothing is known about these factors, and information about the viral target sequences is scarce and at least partially controversial[12-14]. That these liver-cell factors might be of general importance for the expression of liver-specific genes is suggested by the finding that the HepG2 and HUH-7 cell lines are also competent for the replication of the duck hepatitis B virus, the hepadnavirus most distantly related to the HBV[15,16]. Thus, it appears that hepadnaviral gene expression is essentially dependent on a highly-conserved regulatory mechanism that controls gene expression in hepatocytes across the species barrier. In addition, the transfection data imply that the strict species specificity of the hepadnaviruses is due to an early step of the infectious cycle, most likely a requirement for the binding of the virus to a still undefined species-specific host-cell receptor.

Direct proof that expression of the long viral RNA is indeed the only liver cell-specific event after entrance of the viral genome was then obtained through experiments carried out with HBV genomes in which the tissue-specific viral promoter had been replaced by an ubiquitously active promoter. With these constructs, it was not only possible to express all known viral gene products but even complete HBV particles in the human HeLa cell line[17] as well as in mouse fibroblasts (H. J. Schlicht, unpublished). Thus, molecular analysis of the hepadnaviral genome has now enabled us to construct a variety of cell lines which can continuously produce all viral gene products.

THE HBeAg ENIGMA

The principal viral protein forming the viral nucleocapsid is called the core protein or, in case of the human hepatitis B virus, the core antigen (HBcAg), and is encoded by the viral C (or core) gene. This protein aggregates readily into viral cores, even when expressed in bacterial cells, with 180 copies forming a viral capsid. Though remarkable, this behaviour is not especially surprising since it is the function of a capsid protein to form a protective protein shell around the viral nucleic acid. A more peculiar finding was that significant amounts of a non-particulate core-gene encoded polypeptide could also be detected in the serum of HBV-infected individuals. This protein, which was called 'e'-antigen or HBeAg, was first distinguished from the HBcAg serologically with the help of antisera which reacted either with the HBcAg or the HBeAg[18]. Later experiments then showed that treatment with proteases or certain detergents could convert 'c'-antigenicity into 'e'-antigenicity[19]. Moreover, the biochemical characterization of both proteins showed that a C-terminal sequence present in the HBcAg is removed during generation of the HBeAg[20]. Thus, it was initially assumed that the HBeAg represents a degradation product of the full-length core protein that is released into circulation by lysed liver cells.

This view was first challenged by the finding that a short coding sequence located immediately upstream from the C-gene (the so-called pre-C region; see Figures 2 and 3) appeared to be essential for e-antigen generation[21]. Analysis of serum samples taken from ducks infected with the duck hepatitis B virus then revealed that C-terminally truncated non-particulate core proteins are also generated during DHBV infection[22]. The bulk of these proteins, however, is glycosylated, and therefore cannot be produced by core-protein degradation but rather must be actively secreted by the virus-infected cells (in the case of the human virus the HBeAg cannot be glycosylated since it does not contain a glycosylation site). A detailed mutational analysis of both, the HBV[17] and the DHBV[22] core genes then resulted in the elucidation of an exceptional expression mechanism which leads to the production of two different core-gene products from one gene.

As is outlined in Figure 3, there are two translation initiation codons located at the 5'-end of the C gene. The coding sequence between these initiation codons is referred to as the pre-C region. If this region is interrupted by a stop codon or if the pre-C ATG is deleted, production of the secretory core gene product is abolished[17,22]. As could be shown by further experiments, the pre-C peptide functions as a signal sequence which mediates HBeAg secretion[23,24]. However, only a fraction of the core-gene encoded proteins

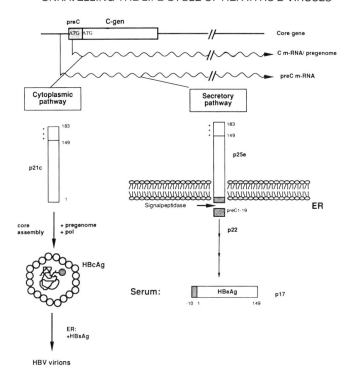

Figure 3 Schematic representation of the two different biosynthetic pathways which are entered by the hepatitis-B virus core gene products. The pre-C region, which is confined by the pre-C and the C-ATG, is shaded. Two different mRNAs which encode either the cytoplasmic or the secretory core-gene product (HBcAg or HBeAg, respectively) are depicted as wavy lines. The cytoplasmic form (HBcAg; p21c) assembles into core particles, thereby encapsidating the viral pregenome and polymerase. Budding takes place at the endoplasmic reticulum (ER). A pre-C/C protein with a molecular mass of about 25 kD (p25e), encoded by the longer mRNA, enters the secretory pathway and eventually results in the formation of the HBeAg (p17). During this process, most of the pre-C sequence (19 of 29 amino acids) as well as the strongly basic C-terminus (amino acids 150–183) are cleaved from the p25e precursor

contains this signal sequence since most of the long viral mRNA molecules start between the pre-C and the C-ATG[48] (Figure 2). Consequently, translation of these mRNAs results in a core-gene product lacking the pre-C sequence. These protein molecules remain within the cell where they aggregate to form core particles. A minor fraction of the RNA molecules, however, must start upstream from the pre-C region. These slightly longer mRNAs then code for a pre-C/C protein which, because of the attached signal sequence, enters the secretory pathway where it is subjected to certain processing steps and is finally released from the cell. Thus, there is no precursor–product relationship between the HBcAg and the HBeAg. Instead, these proteins represent the end products of a rarely encountered gene-expression strategy which leads to the production of two different proteins from one gene via the optional usage of a signal sequence.

Why do hepatitis B viruses produce a secretory core protein? Since this feature is conserved between the most distantly-related hepadnaviruses, HBV and DHBV, production of a secretory core-gene product should be beneficial for the hepatitis B viruses in general. But to date, the nature of this benefit is obscure. That e-antigen production is not essential for the establishment of a hepadnavirus infection could be demonstrated in the DHBV system. For these studies, a DHBV mutant was constructed in which the pre-C region was interrupted by a stop codon and which therefore was defective with respect to e-antigen synthesis. Intrahepatic injection of the mutated viral DNA into ducklings resulted in a productive infection in the absence of e-antigen synthesis[22]. Injection of serum samples taken from these animals into ducklings again resulted in an e-antigen negative DHBV infection, proving that virus particles generated in the absence of pre-C expression are infectious and that the inability to synthesize e-antigen can be transmitted as a stable trait. The finding that production of infectious virus is not necessarily coupled with e-antigen synthesis is of general importance in clinical diagnosis since the HBeAg is considered as a marker indicating virus production[25,26]. The reliability of this marker, however, has been challenged by the finding that in several sera negative for both, HBeAg and anti-HBeAg, viral DNA has been detected[27,28]. It will be interesting to see whether such cases are due to infection with an HBV pre-C mutant.

HEPADNAVIRAL REVERSE TRANSCRIPTION: VARIATIONS ON A THEME

Though hepadnaviruses contain a DNA-genome, they do not multiply their genetic information by semi-conservative replication, but rather by reverse transcription[4]. This exceptional replication strategy has only been found in one other DNA virus family, the caulimoviruses of plants[29]. As with all viruses, the hepadnavirus life cycle (outlined in Figure 4) begins with the entry of a virus particle into a host cell, a process which most likely requires the binding of one of the viral surface proteins to a species-specific cell receptor. After uncoating, the viral genome is transported into the nucleus. However, before this genome can be used as a template for mRNA synthesis, it must be subjected to several repair reactions. This is necessary because the hepadnaviral genome consists of an only partially double stranded DNA molecule (figures 1 and 2). Moreover, at the 5' end of the minus strand, a protein is covalently bound, which most likely functions as the primer for reverse transcription of the pregenomic RNA$_{30-32}$. Upon entry of a viral genome into a new host cell, the genome-linked protein is removed from the minus-strand, the plus strand is completed, and a superhelical covalently closed circular (CCC)–DNA is formed from which the viral mRNAs are transcribed.

Whereas the short transcripts function as normal mRNAs, the large transcript is not only translated but serves also as a template for synthesis of a new viral genome. This process is believed to start with the encapsidation of this RNA into a viral core particle (Figure 4). DNA synthesis is most likely primed by the protein which is later found covalently bound to the 5' end of

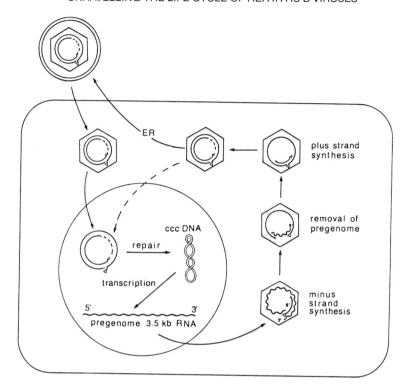

Figure 4 Proposed replication pathway of the hepatitis B viruses. Details are given in the text

the virion-minus strand DNA. During reverse transcription, the RNA template is degraded. A small fragment from the 5' end, however, remains intact and serves as a primer for plus-strand synthesis[33]. As mentioned above, virus budding usually occurs before plus-strand synthesis has been completed.

During the past few years, much effort has been undertaken to characterize the two proteins which are essential for reverse transcription: the protein primer and the reverse transcriptase. However, so far all attempts to isolate these proteins from liver tissue, purified virus, or core particles have failed (unpublished data from our laboratory). With respect to these studies, it was especially puzzling that no proteins co-purifying with core particles could be detected by protein staining. That the polymerase is virally encoded was strongly suggested by the fact that the proposed P-gene product shares homologies with certain retroviral reverse transcriptases[4]. However, attempts to detect P-gene-encoded proteins with a multitude of different P-protein-specific antisera were also unsuccessful (unpublished data from our laboratory). With the establishment of the new tissue culture systems, we therefore decided to study P-gene expression by mutational analysis. For this purpose, mutations were introduced into the P-gene and the respective constructs transfected into HepG2 cells. After two days, core particles were isolated from cell lysates by immunoprecipitation and used to perform an endogenous polymerase reaction. This reaction is based on the fact that the core-associated polymerase incorporates nucleotides into the incomplete viral genome when core or virus particles are incubated with deoxynucleotide triphosphates under suitable conditions[34]. Thus, with this experimental system it is possible to assay polymerase expression without the need to identify the polymerase protein itself. This analysis, done in parallel with DHBV and HBV, first provided strong evidence that the P-gene indeed encodes the viral polymerase[35,36]. Moreover, it could be demonstrated that the regions within the proposed P-gene product that exhibit homology to retroviral reverse transcriptases are indeed of functional significance since even single amino acid exchanges within these regions abolished polymerase activity[36].

We then used this experimental system to examine in detail how hepadnaviral reverse transcriptase is expressed. As has been discussed, nothing is known about the protein(s) encoded by the P-gene. The only hint at a possible mode of P-gene expression came from the analysis of tissue samples obtained from HBV-positive human liver tumours, in which occasionally proteins were detected which appeared to be generated by fusion of core and polymerase sequences[37]. This finding suggested that hepadnaviral reverse transcriptase might be synthesized by the same biosynthetic pathway utilized by retroviruses and retrotransposons, i.e. via the production of C/Pol fusion protein intermediates[38-40].

If the genomes of different retroviruses or retrotransposons are compared, a characteristic overlap between the 3' end of the core gene and the 5' end of the P-gene can be found in most cases[41]. The significance of this genomic arrangement became evident only recently when the molecular details of the biosynthetic pathway leading to polymerase production were elucidated for several retroviruses[38-40,42]. These studies showed that the retroviral polymerase is synthesized via a core–polymerase (gag/Pol) fusion protein intermediate which is proteolytically processed after incorporation into nascent core particles. Most interestingly, these fusion proteins were not due to spliced mRNAs but rather, in most cases, were generated by ribosomal frameshifting which occurred in the gag/Pol overlap region. Conceptually, this biosynthetic pathway which primarily leads to the production of an enzymatically inactive precursor which, because of its core portion, co-assembles into nascent core particles, was especially intelligible since it provided an explanation as to how random reverse transcription of cellular RNAs can be avoided in retrovirus-infected cells. Though not experimentally proven, it is assumed that such a process should be harmful for the cells, and therefore would be incompatible with the continuous virus production generally observed in retrovirus-infected cells.

Since hepadnaviruses also contain the characteristic C/Pol overlap region (Figure 2) and also cause no obvious cell damage, it appeared very likely that the mechanism of polymerase production would be the same as for retroviruses. However, the analysis of DHBV and HBV P-gene expression unambiguously showed that hepadnaviruses have evolved a unique strategy for polymerase synthesis which clearly distinguishes this virus family from the retroviruses[35,36]. As is outlined in Figure 5, hepadnaviral reverse transcriptase is not synthesized via a core–polymerase fusion protein, as is the case for retroviruses, but rather as an authentic P-gene product. Synthesis of this protein most likely starts by internal initiation within the long 3.5 kb mRNA which also encodes the core protein and serves as the template for reverse transcription. The resulting P protein appears to consist of two domains separated by a spacer region which is largely dispensable for polymerase function. Whereas the reverse transcriptase (RT) and the RNaseH activity are located in the C–terminal domain, the N-terminal domain represents the protein that acts as a primer for reverse transcription[36,43]. Upon binding of this multifunctional P-protein to the pregenomic RNA, reverse transcription is initiated. Whether elongation of the DNA-strand indeed requires cleavage of the P-protein, as is shown in Figure 5, is under investigation. In fact, recent data from our laboratory rather suggest that the P-protein is not cleaved[43].

What are the consequences of an expression strategy that does not require the formation of a core–polymerase fusion protein intermediate? Does this mean that hepadnavirus-infected cells contain free reverse transcriptase which could also use cellular RNAs as a template? For certain retroviruses it has been shown that cellular RNAs can be packaged quite efficiently into viral capsids, especially in the absence of specific viral RNA[44]. These RNAs can then be reverse transcribed and the resulting DNA copies can integrate into the genome of a new host cell where they may even be expressed[45]. For this reason it can be assumed that retroviral reverse transcriptase would very rapidly disturb the cellular metabolism by altering the gene dosage of many genes, if it were not efficiently packaged into virus particles. As has been discussed, in the case of retroviruses this process is facilitated by the fact that the polymerase precursors can co-assemble into nascent core particles because of their core portion. How can this problem be solved in the case of hepadnaviral reverse transcriptases which is not synthesized via a core–polymerase fusion protein intermediate? As outlined in Figure 5, hepadnaviral reverse transcriptase appears to be synthesized as a multidomain protein containing its own primer. Although the sequence(s) recognized by this primer are unknown, mapping of the 5′ end of the minus strand indicates that priming occurs within a DR sequence present in the terminally redundant part of the pre-genomic RNA[31,43,46–48]. Thus, it might be the specificity of the priming event that prevents the reverse transcription of cellular RNAs.

This situation, however, could be quite different if aberrant polymerase products are produced. As has been noted, large amounts of proteins consisting of core and polymerase sequences have been detected in several HBV-induced tumours[37]. Considering the results of the experiments discussed here, it is now clear that these proteins do not represent regular viral gene products but most likely have been expressed from re-arranged viral genomes. However, since these proteins contain an altered N-terminal domain, and therefore lack the correct primer, it can be speculated that such P-gene products are more promiscuous with respect to the templates that they can reverse transcribe. If so, expression of aberrant P-gene products could be one factor leading to the transformation of HBV-infected cells.

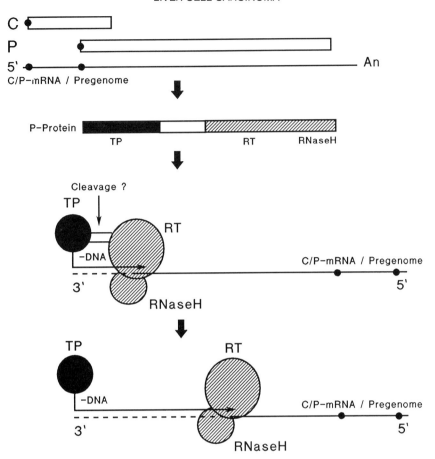

Figure 5 Expression strategy of the hepadnaviral P-gene and a model for initiation of reverse transcription. The bars in the upper part of the figure represent the viral C and P gene. The respective translation initiation codons are shown as dark dots. Internal initiation within the long C/P-mRNA gives rise to a P protein consisting of two domains which are connected by a spacer sequence. The N-terminal domain (black) represents the protein primer used for initiation of reverse transcription which remains covalently bound to the DNA minus-strand (here referred to as terminal protein, TP). The C-terminal domain (hatched) contains the reverse-transcriptase (RT) and RNaseH activity. Upon binding of the P-protein to the pre-genomic RNA, reverse transcription is initiated. Whether elongation of the DNA-strand indeed requires cleavage of the P-protein, as is shown in the figure, or can proceed without this process, is under investigation

PERSPECTIVES

As demonstrated by the data summarized in this chapter, there are now powerful experimental systems available which allow the analysis of all aspects of hepadnaviral gene functions on the molecular level. Thus, it should be possible in the near future to gain much deeper insight into the mechanisms by which liver disease can be caused by hepatitis B viruses. With this knowledge, it might then also be possible to develop specific drugs that interfere with the viral life cycle. With several hundred million chronically HBV-infected individuals worldwide, the need for specific therapies is evident.

Acknowledgements

We thank N. Schek for critical reading of the manuscript. Work performed in this laboratory was supported by the Deutsche Forschungsgemeinschaft, SFB 229, the Bundesministerium für Forschung und Technologie, BCT 0381-5, and the Fonds der Chemischen Industrie.

References

1. Ganem, D. and Varmus, H. (1987). The molecular biology of the hepatitis B viruses. *Ann. Rev. Biochem.,* **56**, 651–93
2. Summers, J. (1981). Three recently described animal virus models for human hepatitis B virus. *Hepatology,* **1**, 179–83.
3. Summers, J. and Mason, W. (1982) Replication of the genome of a hepatitis B-like virus by reverse transcription of an RNA intermediate. *Cell,* **29**, 403–15.
4. Toh, H., Hayashida, H. and Miyata, T. (1983). Sequence homology between retroviral reverse transcriptase and putative polymerases of hepatitis B virus and cauliflower mosaic virus. *Nature (London),* **305**, 827–9.
5. Twu, J. S. and Schloemer, R. H. (1987). Transcriptional transactivating function of hepatitis B virus. *J. Virol.,* **61**, 3448–53.
6. Spandau, D. and Lee, C. (1988). Trans-activation of viral enhancers by the hepatitis B virus X protein. *J. Virol.,* **62**, 427–34
7. Sureau, C., Roup-Lemonne, J., Mullins, J. and Essex, M. (1986). Production of hepatitis B virus by a differentiated human hepatoma cell line after transfection with cloned circular HBV DNA. *Cell,* **47**, 37–47
8. Chang, C., Jeng, K., Hu, C., Lo, S., Su, T., Ting, L., Chou, C., Han, S., Pfaff, E., Salfeld, J. and Schaller, H. (1987). Production of hepatitis B virus *in vitro* by transient expression of cloned HBV DNA in a hepatoma cell line. *EMBO J.,* **6**, 675–80
9. Tsurimoto, T., Fujiyama, A. and Matsubara, K. (1987) Stable expression and replication of heptaitis B virus genome in an integrated state in a human hepatoma cell line transfected with the cloned viral DNA. *Proc. Natl. Acad. Sci USA,* **84**, 444–7
10. Acs, G., Sells, M., Purcell, R., Price, P., Engle, R., Shapiro, M. and Popper, H. (1987). Hepatitis B virus produced by transfected Hep G2 cells causes hepatitis in chimpanzees. *Proc. Natl. Acad. Sci. USA,* **84**, 4641–4
11. Yaginuma, K., Shirakata, Y., Kobayashi, M. and Koike, K. (1987). Hepatitis B virus (HBV) particles are produced in a cell culture system by transient expression of transfected HBV DNA. *Proc. Natl. Acad. Sci. USA,* **84**, 2678–82
12. Shaul, Y., Rutter, W. and Laub, O. (1985) A human hepatitis B viral enhancer element. *EMBO J.,* **4**, 427–30
13. Shaul, Y. and Ben-Levy, R. (1987) Multiple nuclear proteins in liver cells are bound to hepatitis B virus enhancer element and its upstream sequences. *EMBO J.,* **6**, 1913–20
14. Vannice, J. L. and Levinson, A. D. (1988). Properties of the human hepatitis B virus enhancer: position effects and cell-type nonspecificity. *J. Virol.,* **62**, 1305–13
15. Galle, P., Schlicht, H. J., Fischer, M. and Schaller, H. (1988). Production of infectious duck hepatitis B virus in a human hepatoma cell line. *J. Virol.,* **62**, 1736–40
16. Pugh, J. C., Yaginuma, K., Koike, K. and Summers, J. (1988). Duck hepatitis B virus (DHBV) particles produced by transient expression of DHBV DNA in a human hepatoma cell line are infectious *in vitro. J. Virol.,* **62**, 3513–16

17. Junker, M., Galle, P. and Schaller, H. (1987). Expression and replication of the hepatitis B virus genome under foreign promoter control. *Nucl. Acids Res.*, **15**, 10117–32

18. Magnius, L. O. and Espmark, J. A. (1972). New specificities in Australia antigen positive sera distinct from the Le Bouvier determinants. *J. Immunol.*, **109**, 1017–21

19. MacKay, P., Lees, J. and Murray, K. (1981) The conversion of hepatitis B core antigen synthesized in E. coli into e antigen. *J. Med. Virol.*, **8**, 237–43

20. Takahashi, K., Machida, A., Funatsu, G., Nomura, M., Usuda, S., Aoyagi, S., Tachibana, K., Miyamoto, H., Imai, M., Nakamura, T., Miyakawa, Y. and Mayumi, M. (1983). Immunochemical structure of hepatitis B e-antigen in the serum. *J. Immunol.*, **130**, 2903–7

21. Ou, J., Laub, O. and Rutter, W. (1986). Hepatitis B virus gene function: The precore region targets the core antigen to cellular membranes and causes the secretion of the e antigen. *Proc. Natl. Acad. Sci. USA*, **83**, 1578–82

22. Schlicht, H. J., Salfeld, J. and Schaller, H. (1987). The pre-C region of the duck hepatitis B virus is essential for synthesis and secretion of processed core proteins but not for virus formation. *J. Virol.*, **61**, 3701–9

23. Bruss, V. and Gerlich, W. (1988). Formation of transmembraneous hepatitis B e-antigen by cotranslational *in vitro* processing of the viral precore protein. *Virology*, **163**, 268–75

24. Garcia, P. D., Ou, J. H., Rutter, W. J. and Walter, P. (1988). Targeting of the hepatitis B virus precore protein to the endoplasmic reticulum membrane: after signal peptide cleavage translocation can be aborted and the product released into the cytoplasm. *J. Cell Biol.*, **106**, 1093–2004

25. Weller, I. V. D., Fowler, M. J. F., Monjardino, J. and Thomas, H. C. (1982). The detection of HBV DNA in serum by molecular hybridization: A more sensitive method for the detection of complete HBV particles. *J. Med. Virol.*, **9**, 273–80

26. Liebermann, H. M., La Brecque, D. R., Kew, M. C., Hadziyannis, S. J. and Shafritz, D. A. (1983). Detection of hepatitis B virus DNA directly in human serum by a simplified molecular hybridization test: comparison to HBeAg/anti-HBe status in HBsAg carriers. *Hepatology*, **3**, 285–91

27. Harrison, T. J., Bal, V., Wheeler, E. G., Meacock, T. J., Harrison, J. F. and Zuckerman, A. J. (1985). Hepatitis B virus DNA and e antigen in serum from blood donors in the United Kingdom positive for hepatitis B surface antigen. *Brit. Med. J.*, **290**, 663–4

28. Krogsgard, K., Kryger, P., Aldershville, J., Andersson, P., Brechot, C. and the Copenhagen Hepatitis Acute Programme (1985). Hepatitis B virus DNA in serum from patients with acute hepatitis B. *Hepatology*, **5**, 10–13

29. Hohn, T., Hohn, B. and Pfeiffer, P. (1985). Reverse transcription in CaMV. *Trends Biochem. Sci.*, **5**, 205–9

30. Gerlich, W. and Robinson, W. (1980). Hepatitis B virus contains protein covalently attached to the 5′-terminus of its complete DNA strand. *Cell*, **21**, 801–9

31. Molnar-Kimber, K., Summers, J., Taylor, J. and Mason, W. (1983). Protein covalently bound to minus-strand DNA intermediates of duck hepatitis B virus. *J. Virol.*, **45**, 165–72

32. Bosch, V., Bartenschlager, R., Radziwill, G. and Schaller, H. (1988) The duck hepatitis B virus P-gene codes for protein strongly associated with the 5′-end of the viral minus DNA strand *Virology*, **166**, 475–85

33. Lien, J., Aldrich, C. and Mason, W. (1986). Evidence that a capped oligoribonucleotide is the primer for duck hepatitis B virus plus strand DNA synthesis. *J. Virol.*, **57**, 229–36

34. Kaplan, P., Greenman, R., Gerin, J., Purcell, R. and Robinson, W. (1973). DNA polymerase associated with human hepatitis B antigen. *J. Virol.*, **12**, 995–1005

35. Schlicht, H. J., Radziwill, G. and Schaller, H. (1989) Synthesis and encapsidation of the duck hepatitis B virus reverse transcriptase does not require the formation of core/polymerase fusion proteins. *Cell* 56, 85–92

36. Radziwill, G. (1989). PhD thesis, University of Heidelberg

37. Will, H., Salfeld, J., Pfaff, E., Manso, C., Theilmann, L. and Schaller, H. (1986). Putative reverse transcriptase intermediates of human hepatitis B virus in primary liver carcinomas. *Science*, **231**, 594–6

38. Jacks, T. and Varmus, H. (1985). Expression of the Rous sarcoma virus *pol* gene by ribosomal frame shifting. *Science*, **230**, 1237–42

39. Jacks, T., Townsley, K., Varmus, H. and Majors, J. (1987). Two efficient ribosomal frameshifting events are required for synthesis of mouse mammary tumor virus *gag*-related polyproteins. *Proc. Natl. Acad. Sci. USA*, **84**, 4298–302

40. Jacks, T., Power, M. D., Masiarz, F. R., Luciw, P. A., Barr, P. J. and Varmus, H. (1988). Characterization of ribosomal frameshifting in HIV-I *gag-pol* expression. *Nature*, **331**, 280–3

41. Hull, R. and Covey, S. (1986). Genome organization and expression of reverse transcribing elements: variations and a theme. *J. Gen. Virol.*, **67**, 1751–8

42. Weiss, R., Teich, N., Varmus, H. and Coffin, J. (eds). (1982). *RNA Tumor Viruses.* (New York: CSH Press)

43. Bartenschlager, R. and Schaller, H. (1988) The aminoterminal domain of the hepadnaviral P-gene encodes the terminal protein (genome linked protein) believed to prime reverse transcription. *EMBO J.* 7, 4185–92

44. Embretson, J. and Temin, H. (1987) Lack of competition results in efficient packaging of heterologous murine retroviral RNAs and the reticuloendotheliosis virus encapsidation-minus RNAs by the reticuloendotheliosis virus helper cell line. *J. Virol.*, **61**, 2675–83

45. Linial, M. (1987) Creation of a processed pseudogene by retroviral infection. *Cell,* **49**, 93–102

46. Lien, J. Petcu, D., Aldrich, C. and Mason, W. (1987) Initiation and termination of duck hepatitis-B virus DNA synthesis during virus maturation. *J. Virol.*, **61**, 3832–40

47. Seeger, C., Ganem, D. and Varmus, H. E. (1986) Biochemical and genetic evidence for the hepatitis B virus replication strategy. *Science*, **232**, 477–484

48. Will, H., Reiser, W., Weimer, T., Pfaff, E., Büscher, M., Sprengel, R., Cattaneo, R. and Schaller, H. (1987) Replication strategy of human hepatitis B virus. *J. Virol,* **61**, 904–911

9
Viral DNA integration, chromosome aberrations and growth factor activation in hepatocellular carcinomas of hepadna virus carriers

C. E. ROGLER, O. HINO, D. YANG AND D. A. SHAFRITZ

PATHWAY OF VIRAL DNA IN HEPATOCYTES

One of the earliest events following penetration and uncoating of hepadna viruses is conversion of the viral DNA into a covalently closed circular (CCC) molecule[1] (Figure 1). The CCC DNA accumulates in the nucleus and is believed to serve as the template for synthesis of viral RNAs, including pre-genome RNA and mRNAs encoding viral proteins. The pre-genome RNAs are packaged into particles with viral core protein in the cytoplasm and reverse transcription occurs, leading to production of a full-length viral DNA minus-strand[2]. Plus-strand DNA synthesis begins approximately 250 bp (base pairs) from the 5' end of the minus-strand, and is primed by an RNA oligonucleotide from the 5' end of the RNA pre-genome[3]. After plus-strand DNA synthesis reaches the 5' end of the minus-DNA strand it 'jumps the gap' to the 3' end of the minus-DNA strand resulting in circularization of the minus-strand DNA. For reasons which are unclear, virions are formed and secreted before plus-strand DNA synthesis is completed and therefore, DNA molecules in virions are open circular and contain a single-strand region. Completion of the viral DNA plus-strand is the first event after the virus infects a permissive host cell (Figure 1). Transcription and translation of viral genes proceeds in an unidirectional fashion utilizing all three translational reading frames due to the overlap of viral genes (Figure 2A; see ref. 4 for a full description).

It should be emphasized that in contrast to RNA-containing retroviruses, in hepadna viruses, reverse transcription occurs during viral assembly rather than viral disassembly. The work of Tuttleman *et al.*[5], also supports a model in which DNA molecules in core particles are recycled into the nucleus where they are converted to the CCC form. This recycling mechanism is believed to provide a continuous source of viral DNA for replication of the virus. Unlike retroviruses, integration of

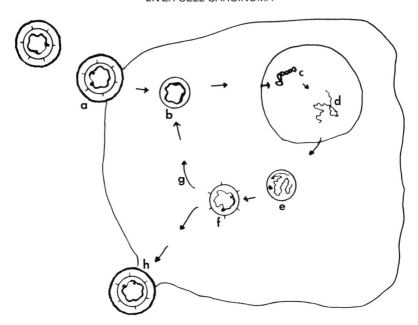

Figure 1 Schematic diagrams of the pathway of hepadna viral nucleic acids involved in hepadna virus replication (viral mRNAs are not included in the illustration). (a) Viral attachment. (b) Penetration of hepatocyte, completion of plus-strand DNA. (c) Conversion of viral DNA to the CCC form in nucleus. (d) Transcription of pre-genomic RNA. (e) Packaging of pre-genome RNA in viral core particles. (f) Reverse transcription in core particles, generation of minus-strand viral DNA and open circular molecules after plus-strand synthesis. (g) Recycling of some viral core particles to the nucleus where they provide a source of CCC DNA. (h) Viral maturation and excretion (Diagram by J. Tuttleman)

viral DNA is not required for the hepadna virus replication cycle. However, hepadna virus integration does occur during persistent infection[6]. Recent studies also suggest that the integration process may be augmented during a state of persistent infection in which viral DNA replication continues but there is a block in the virus assembly/secretion mechanism[7].

VIRAL DNA INTEGRATION AND HEPATOCELLULAR CARCINOMA

The association of hepatocellular carcinoma (HCC) with long-term persistent HBV infection in humans was recognized soon after discovery of the virus[8]. Prospective studies of HBV carriers have shown that HBV carriers have a 200-fold greater risk of HCC than uninfected individuals from the same population. Males are more prone to develop persistent infection and male HBV carriers have greater than 40% lifetime risk of HCC[8]. Persistent infection with each of the animal hepadna viruses, woodchuck hepatitis virus (WHV), ground squirrel hepatitis virus (GSHV) and duck hepatitis B virus (DHBV) also leads to HCC in the respective hosts. The association of persist-

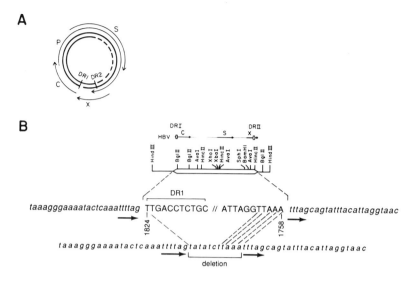

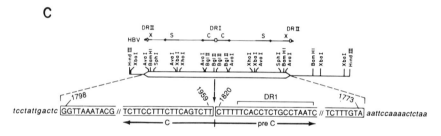

Figure 2 Examples of a linear HBV integration with one viral–cell junction at the DR1 sequence and the second viral cell junction at a site of 5-bp homology with cellular DNA and a second integration containing inverted duplication of integrated HBV sequences at a chromosome trans-location. (A) Genetic map of HBV including the virion open-circular DNA structure (solid circular line) with a single-stranded region (dashed line). Arrangement of genes for the viral core protein (C), surface antigen (S), polymerase (P) and X gene shown with arrows to show the direction of transcription. The position of the 11 base-pair directly-repeated sequences (DR1 and DR2), and plus-strands, respectively, are shown on the viral map at the termini of the viral minus- and plus-strands, respectively. (B) Example of a prototype linear HBV integration[23]. Lines: (1) genetic map of the integrated HBV sequences; (2) restriction endonuclease map of the integrated HBV sequences. The DNA sequences of the left and right viral–cell junctions are shown below the restriction map. The DNA sequence of normal cellular DNA at the HBV integration site along with the 5–11 bp deletion are shown on the bottom line. HBV DNA sequences are in capitals and cellular DNA in lower case. The region of homology between HBV DNA and cellular DNA at the right viral–cell junction is noted by dashed lines. The solid arrows under the sequence indicated a 5-bp directly repeated cellular DNA sequence at the integration site. (C) Inverted HBV integration at the site of a chromosome translocation t(17, 18) (q21, q11). Top two lines: Genetic map of inverted HBV sequences and restriction endonuclease map of the integrated HBV. Bottom line: DNA sequence at the left and right viral–cell junctions and the HBV DNA inversion point. Nucleotide 1820 of HBV at this inversion point is the 3′ end of the HBV DNA-minus strand. Nucleotide numbers are in reference to the unique EcoR 1 site in the HBV genome

ent infection with HCC is the strongest in woodchucks, which show nearly a 100% lifetime risk. While primary HCCs are the predominant tumour which arise in woodchucks, rare cholangiocarcinomas have also been reported[9,10].

The initial discovery that HCCs arising in WHV and HBV carriers contain clonal viral DNA integrations raised interest in the potential role of integrations in hepatic oncogenesis[11,12]. In HBV carriers, integrated DNA is usually the sole form of viral DNA remaining in tumour tissue[11], whereas in woodchucks, episomal WHV DNA is present in some tumours, in addition to clonal integrations[12]. Initially, it was hoped that by cloning the integrations from HCCs it would be possible to identify cellular genes which function, in association with viral DNA, as hepatic oncogenes. The first integrations to be cloned were from two woodchuck hepatomas, each of which contained only a single WHV DNA integration[13]. Unique cellular DNA sequences flanking the WHV integration were used to screen a large panel of woodchuck HCCs for a common cellular integration site, but none was found (unpublished data). Subsequent cloning of additional HBV, WHV and DHBV DNA integrations from HCCs has confirmed the initial observation that viral integrations do not occur at a common site in HCCs. Therefore, it is now generally accepted that insertional mutagenesis of a specific cellular gene is not the predominant mechanism by which hepadna virus integrations function in hepatic oncogenesis.

In a few cases, hepadna virus integrations adjacent to genes involved in cellular growth control have been reported[14,15]. Cases in which WHV DNA integration is in or near the *c myc* gene[14] and one case in which HBV is integrated in a cellular gene with homology to the *v-erb-A* and steroid receptor genes[15] have been reported. The mechanism by which these integrations alter the transcription of these respective genes and modify the function of the viral proteins leading to tumorigenesis has not yet been clarified.

Sequencing of viral integrations and restriction mapping of cellular integration sites have provided clues as to how such integrations occur and the mechanism(s) by which integrated viral sequences function in oncogenesis. Two general groups of integrations, those with linear integrated sequences and those with rearranged viral DNA sequences, have been described (Figure 2). The linear integrations show a strong preference to have one viral–cell junction within, or immediately adjacent to, one of two 11 base-pair directly-repeated sequences in the viral genome, designated DR1 and DR2 (Figure 2)[16,17]. The DR1 sequence is the site of initiation of minus-strand DNA synthesis and is present in the unique triple-strand structure in virion DNA[4]. The other viral–cell junction of linear integrations apparently occurs at random positions in viral DNA. Short homologies of 2–5 base pairs between viral and cellular DNA are common but not essential at the second viral–cell junction. The integration described in Figure 2B may be considered a proto-type linear integration which exhibits both of the above characteristics.

Since the DR sequences are 'hot spots' for viral integration, these sequences were examined for homology with cleavage sites for cellular enzymes known to be important in DNA recombination and repair mechanisms. Topoisomerase I (Topo I) has been shown *in vitro* to specifically cleave integrated SV40 DNA at sites in which the virus is spontaneously excised *in vivo* in somatic cell hybrids[18]. Similar preferred Topo I cleavage sites were observed in the DR sequences of hepadna viruses and a recent report[19] has shown that Topo I specifically cleaves WHV virion DNA at two places in the immediate vicinity of the DR sequences. Work is currently in progress to identify the exact Topo I cleavage sites and compare them to known integration sites in viral DNA. Since Topo I can link heterologous DNAs at cleavage sites, a possible role of Topo I in viral integration is suspected. Double-stranded viral DNA cleaved at the DR1 site or single-stranded replicative intermediates could function as substrates for Topo I mediated integration. Since not all rearrangement sites are in the DR sequences or at Topo I cleavage sites, this represents only one of several mechanisms involved in generating integration and rearrangements of viral DNA.

The most common rearrangements of viral sequences in integrations are inverted duplications accompanied by deletion of viral sequences between the inversion[20]. Direct duplications or short deletions are also common[20]. Rearrangements of viral DNA are usually accompanied by rearrangement of flanking cellular DNA. The first clearly characterized rearrangement of cellular DNA at an HBV integration site was a large deletion (≥ 13 kbp) which occurred[21] at chromosome 11p13. Inverted duplication of HBV and cellular sequences has also been reported in a HBV clone from a Japanese patient[22]. Another integration contained an inverted duplication of HBV sequences in which the inversion served as the focal point for a chromosome 17q22:18q11 translocation[23]. Interestingly, one of the HBV sequences at the viral DNA inversion point was immediately adjacent to the DR1 sequence, at the exact position of the 3' end of virion minus-strand DNA and a preferred Topo I cleavage site (Figure 2C). When the inverted duplication of HBV DNA from this clone was introduced into transgenic mice, the HBV sequences were rearranged in the mice at a high frequency[24]. Whether this instability is a specific property of the inverted HBV sequences or is common to any inverted duplication of foreign DNA in transgenic mice, has yet to be determined. Several additional HBV integrations, cloned from HCCs, have been localized to chromosome translocations, each on a different chromosome[20].

In summary, initial studies on the role of HBV integrations in HCC have focused primarily on their potential to activate cellular oncogenes. These experiments have, instead, demonstrated that the location of HBV integrations in tumours is not specific for any oncogene and occurs on many chromosomes. In addition, in cases where the cellular genome has been mapped, major rearrangements of cellular DNA have often been observed. Reports which have compared viral DNA integrations in primary tumours to the integrations present in cell lines established from these tumours have shown that deletion and rearrangement of integrations can occur during the establishment of cell lines[25]. These post-integration rearrangements are also quite likely to occur during chronic active hepatitis as a consequence of continuous cellular regeneration. The occurrence of integrations which have linear viral sequences versus those with varying degrees of rearrangement fits a general model in which post-integration rearrangements are derived from integrations which initially have a specific linear structure.

The above model is consistent with results obtained from sequencing of five integrations from the liver and tumours of two young Japanese children[17]. The common features of these integrations were: (1) that they were all composed of linear viral DNA sequences without internal rearrangements and (2) that one viral–cell junction was in or adjacent to the DR1 sequence in four of the cases. One explanation for these results, in the context of the above model, is that the relatively short period of chronic infection in the children (relative to the 20–40 year carrier state before HCC usually occurs in humans) did not provide sufficient cell generations for rearrangement of viral integrations to occur.

Three consequences of post-integration rearrangements which are significant with regard to cancer are:

(1) That such rearrangements, whether they involve excision, transposition or translocation of viral and/or cellular DNA, result in the gradual accumulation of mutations in the cellular genome. Accumulation of mutations will invariably cause a cell to become predisposed to malignant transformation or may directly cause a mutation which results in transformation.

(2) That they may cause cellular DNA mutations which are no longer linked to viral DNA. This was clearly the case for the viral integration which was characterized at a chromosome translocation[23] (Figure 2C) in which the reciprocal chromosome arm (18q11-centromere) contained a deletion of cellular DNA and no detectable viral DNA. Thus, it is clear that in addition to the translocation, viral DNA integration can generate chromosome aberrations by a 'hit and run' mechanism.

(3) That the integration site in a tumour is not necessarily the cellular site at which the integration originated or caused a mutation predisposing the cell to malignant transformation. The apparent random distribution of HBV and WHV DNA integration sites in HCCs is consistent with this conclusion. Furthermore, only a few selected integrations would be expected to be associated with genes known to participate in oncogenesis. Experiments to trace the 'footprints' (sites of excision) of integrations in the genome and possibly work backwards to identify cellular DNA rearrangements which are no longer associated with viral DNA, but are common to many HCCs, are in progress. This may lead to the identification of common cellular mutation sites in HCCs.

In light of the complications associated with utilizing HBV integrations to study genes and chromosomes involved in HCC, additional methods which are not dependent on cloning viral integrations have been applied to this problem. These methods, described below, can detect chromosome defects which have relevance to mechanisms of cancer involving the loss of tumour suppressor genes.

POSSIBLE ROLE OF RECESSIVE ONCOGENES (TUMOUR SUPPRESSOR GENES) IN HCC

Since it has become clear that dominant oncogenes present only a partial picture of tumorigenesis mechanisms *in vivo*, the recessive oncogene hypothesis, originally proposed by Knudson and Strong[26], has attracted considerable attention. According to this hypothesis, a cell must lose, or otherwise inactivate, both copies of a recessive oncogene (another term for which is 'tumour suppressor gene') before cancer can develop. This hypothesis has gained strong experimental support through the study of genetic tumours, such as Wilms' tumor[26,27] and retinoblastoma[28]. In these tumours, an individual who inherits a chromosome in which one copy of the 'tumour suppressor gene' has been inactivated will be predisposed to cancer because inactivation of the second allele for this tumour suppressor gene will result in complete loss of function of both genes. Tumours arise at high rates in individuals who inherit chromosomes which predisposes them to the tumorigenic consequences of the a 'second' hit. Tumour suppressor genes have been localized on chromosome sites 11p13 in the case of Wilms' tumour[27,29], and 13q14 in the case of retinoblastoma[28].

One molecular test of the Knudson hypothesis, which has been successfully applied to Wilms' tumours[30-33] and retinoblastoma[28], is that tumour tissues should exhibit the specific loss of alleles (or loss of heterozygosity) in regions of chromosomes in which tumour suppressor genes reside. Restriction fragment length polymorphisms (RFLPs) are normal variations in DNA sequence in the human population. Using probes for genes which exhibit RFLPs, it is possible to distinguish between the maternal or paternal copies of a gene, and to detect the specific losses of one allele of a gene in tumour tissues. The only requirement of this analysis is that the initial normal tissues must be heterozygous for the RFLP to detect loss of one of the alleles in tumour tissues.

Since HCC is a solid tumour of epithelial origin, as are Wilms' tumours and retinoblastoma, HCCs from HBV carriers have been examined to determine if they also exhibit specific chromosome losses particularly associated with chromosomes containing tumour suppressor genes, using the loss of RFLPs as the genetic marker. Normal and HCC tumour tissues were screened with polymorphic gene probes from 20 chromosomes using Southern blotting. This study revealed a high frequency of loss of alleles from chromosomes 11p (45%) and 13q (50%) in tumour DNAs[34]. Nine of fourteen tumours exhibited the loss of one allele from either chromosome 11p, 13q or in some cases both 11p and 13q, as opposed to random losses on other chromosomes. By analyzing tumour DNAs with probes spanning the region of chromosome 11p15 to 11p13, it was possible to localize deletions to either the distal end of 11p or internally at 11p13 (Figure 3). The data are consistent with previous reports for Wilms' tumour in which some deletions were limited to the 11p15 region and others were localized to 11p13[30-33]. Both chromosomes 13q and 11p are believed to contain tumour suppressor genes. In the HCCs examined, deletions occurred in 13q, 11p or both 11p and 13q, raising the possibility that the tumour suppressor genes on these chromosomes may affect a common third site. Specifically, loss of alleles at 11p and/or 13q may serve to remove suppressor genes which then allows expression of a recessive oncogene located elsewhere in the genome.

In each of the HCCs studied, the deletion of an allele for a gene resulted in a hemizygous condition in which the remaining allele of that gene was not

Chromosome 11p

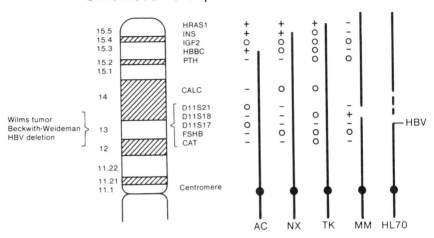

Figure 3 Diagram of deletions in chromosome 11p which caused loss of heterozygosity of genes, on chromosome 11p in primary hepatocellular carcinomas from five HBV carriers. *Left:* Diagram of chromosome 11p with chromosome bands numbered. The location of the tumour suppressor gene involved in Wilms' tumour is denoted to the left and the gene probes used for restriction fragment length polymorphism (RFLP) analysis of tumour DNA are noted to the right of the banded chromosome diagram. *Right:* Stick diagrams illustrating the results of RFLP analysis using chromosome 11p gene probes. Deletions of chromosome 11p are noted by a shorter stick diagram or a break in the line. The RFLP results for each probe are presented to the left of each stick diagram for chromosome 11p. The code for interpretation of RFLP results is as follows: (+) Normal DNA was heterozygous for this locus and tumour DNA was hemizygous meaning there was a deletion of one allele (O) Normal DNA was homozygous at the locus and no conclusion was possible (–). Normal DNA was heterozygous and tumour DNA was also heterozygous (no deletion at this locus.)

re-duplicated in the tumour. In this respect the HCC data contrast those of Wilms' tumour and retinoblastoma in which the predominant mechanism involves re-duplication of the remaining allele to establish a homozygous condition of the mutant allele[28,30–33]. In embroyonal tumours there is probably a strong selection against monosomy and therefore loss of chromosomes by mitotic non-dysjunction is accompanied by re-duplication of the remaining chromosome. In adult tumours, it is likely that the action of a 'hit and run' carcinogenic agent, such as an HBV integration, would result in deletions of chromosome segments without the need to re-duplicate the remaining chromosomal counterpart.

TRANSCRIPTIONAL ACTIVATION OF INSULIN-LIKE GROWTH FACTOR II IN HCC

One aspect of the tumour suppressor theory is that loss of the suppressor gene should allow expression of a recessive cellular oncogene. In addition to the

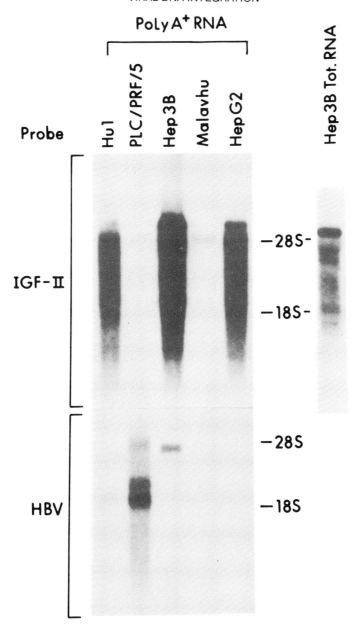

Figure 4 Northern blot of poly A⁺ RNA from five HCC cell lines hybridized with human insulin-like growth factor II cDNA probe (upper panel) or HBV probes (lower panel). The dark smear in the IGF-II panel is due to multiple transcripts of the IGF-II gene. Hybridization of total Hep3B RNA to the IGF-II probe is shown to the right of the main blot and reveals specific IGF-II transcripts. Cell lines Hu1, PlC/PRF/5 and Hep 3B contain integrated HBV DNA and HBV RNA was detected in these lines when the same blot was hybridized with HBV probe (lower panel)

Wilms' tumour gene at chromosome 11p13, several other genes involved in endocrine and autocrine control of growth are located on chromosome 11p including c-H-Ras, Insulin, Insulin-like growth factor II (IGF-II), and parathyroid hormone at 11p15 and follicle stimulating hormone, and calcitonin in the 11p13 region. Since IGF-II is a fetal growth factor highly expressed in liver[35,36], its expression was studied in human HCC cell lines. Three out of five HCC cell lines examined contained high levels of IGF-II RNA, and the IGF-II RNAs were characteristic of transcripts present in fetal human liver (Figure 4). Studies of primary human HCCs have shown a fetal liver pattern of IGF-II RNA in most cases[37]. Since IGF-II is a fetal growth factor, it might be expected to come under the control of suppressor genes whose function is to maintain the adult program of differentiation in hepatocytes. Expression of alpha-fetoprotein in HCCs is another example of a 'fetal' gene which is de-repressed in most HCCs.

Studies of IGF-II transcription in woodchucks have shown that IGF-II RNA is also highly elevated in most woodchuck HCCs[38]. A series of IGF-II transcripts were identified in woodchuck HCCs which were not detectable in normal liver (Figure 5). By analogy with the rat IGF-II gene, several of these RNAs are probably initiated from a promoter which is inactive in adult tissue and is active in fetal rat liver[39]. *In situ* hybridization has demonstrated early cancer nodules with high levels of IGF-II RNA (Figure 6) and pre-cancerous nodules also contain high levels of IGF-II RNA[38]. IGF-II activation, therefore, occurs at an early stage in cancer development. A two- or three-fold

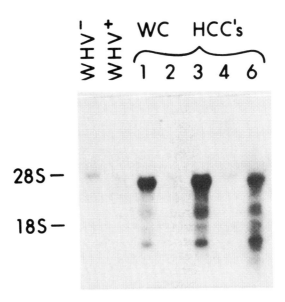

Figure 5 Northern blot of total cellular RNA (7 ng/lane) from woodchuck liver and HCCs hybridized with prepro-human IGF-II cDNA probe. The blot was exposed 16 hours at $-70°$C: WHV, normal uninfected woodchuck liver RNA; WHV$^+$, liver RNA from chronically infected woodchuck. WC HCCs, RNA from five primary woodchuck HCCs. Three HCCs were strongly positive for IGF-II (1, 3, 6) and two were negative (2, 4)

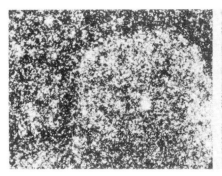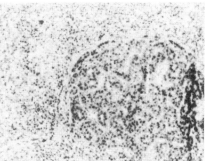

Figure 6 *In situ* hybridization of an early cancer nodule with a [³⁵S]-human IGF-II cDNA probe. *Left:* Dark field illumination illustrating specific hybridization (bright spots) to the tumour module. *Right:* Bright field illumination of the same section illustrating histological charcteristics of an early differentiated HCC

elevation of serum IGF-II levels was also detected in woodchucks with chronic active hepatitis in the pre-cancerous stages[38]. The biological activity of IGF-II in liver has not been directly determined, however, since IGF-II is expressed in fetal liver and is a potent mitogen in cell culture[40], it is likely that it performs either autocrine or paracrine functions to stimulate regeneration of liver cells during chronic hepatitis. It is, therefore, not unreasonable that IGF-II may remain active in tumours which develop from cells in which the gene is activated.

MODEL FOR TUMORIGENESIS IN WHV CARRIERS

A schematic representation of the series of events in the progression from initial WHV infection in woodchucks to HCC is presented in Figure 7. The model proposes that once WHV persistent infection is established, portal hepatitis (PH) ensues and several pathological reactions occur on a self-perpetuating basis. These include (1) death and regeneration of hepatocytes, (2) inflammatory reaction primarily limited to the portal tracts and (3) mild proliferation of bile ducts (Figure 7, line 2). As the disease progresses to chronic active hepatitis (CAH), involvement of the rest of the hepatic lobule becomes evident (lobular hepatitis) (Figure 7, line 3). The inflammatory reaction, composed primarily of lymphocytes with some macrophages and plasma cells, spills over the limiting plate and initiates a disruption of the lobular architecture. Clusters of dysplastic nodules arise in the liver at this pre-cancer stage. As a result of de-repression of specific cellular gene expression, IGF-II transcription is activated and elevated IGF-II is also detected in the serum of woodchucks with CAH before cancer develops. In addition, WHV DNA Integrations can be cloned from infected liver cells at this stage[6].

Within the cellular milieu maintained by CAH, hepatocellular carcinomas develop with distinct phenotypic and biochemical characteristics (Figure 7, line 4), some of which include IGF-II activation and others which do not. The role of

103

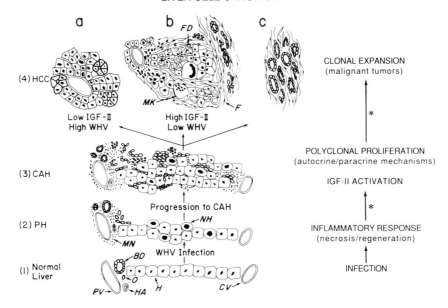

Figure 7 Diagram of the pathological changes in woodchuck livers during the progression from initial persistent WHV infection through malignant HCCs. (See text for full explanation.) *Left panel: line 1*, normal liver cell profile; *line 2*, PH, portal hepatitis during early persistent infection; *line 3*, CAH, progression to chronic active hepatitis; *line 4*, HCC, fully malignant HCCs exhibiting heterogeneous gene expression. High IGF-II means high level of IGF-II RNA in HCC tissue. High WHV means high level of WHV RNA in tumour tissue. *Right panel:* Several factors important in the development of HCC at different stages of disease.*Places in the progression to HCC where viral integration may function by mechanisms discussed in text

the virus in this process includes maintenance of a selective pressure for regeneration and generation of chromosome aberrations which accumulate and predispose the cell to malignant transformation. Whether the virus plays a direct role in IGF-II activation or whether the activation is a consequence of proliferation of 'liver stem cells' is a matter for further investigation. In any event, it is clear that polyclonal expansion during chronic active hepatitis generates a population of cells in the pre-cancerous liver (regenerative nodules) which represent the first step to cancer. Mutational events within these cells eventually lead to transformation of a single cell and its clonal expansion to a fully malignant HCC.

References

1. Mason, W. S., Halpern, M. S., England, J. M., Seal, G., Egan, J., Coates, L., Aldrich, C. and Summers, J. (1983). Experimental transmission of duck hepatitis B virus. *Virology*, **131**, 575–84
2. Summers, J. and Mason, W. S. (1982). Replication of the genome of a hepatitis B-like virus by reverse transcription of an RNA intermediate. *Cell*, **29**, 403–15

3. Lien, J. M., Aldrich, C. E. and Mason, W. S. (1986). Evidence that a capped oligoribonucleotide is the primer for duck Hepatitis B Virus plus-strand DNA synthesis. *J. Virol.,* **57**, 229–36

4. Ganem, D. and Varmus, H. E. (1987). The molecular biology of the hepatitis B virus. *Ann. Rev. Biochem.,* **56**, 651–93

5. Tuttleman, J. S., Pourcel, C. and Summers, J. (1986). Formation of the pool of covalently closed circular viral DNA in hepadnavirus infected cells. *Cell,* **47**, 451–60

6. Rogler, C. E. and Summers, J. (1984). Cloning and structural analysis of integrated woodchuck hepatitis virus sequences from a chronically infected liver. *J. Virol.,* **50**, 832–7

7. Raimondo, G., Burk, R. D., Lieberman, H. M., Muschel, J., Hadziyannis, S. J., Will, H., Kew, M. C., Dusheiko, J. M. and Shafritz, D. A. (1988). Interrupted replication of hepatitis B virus in liver tissue of HBsAg carriers with hepatocellular carcinoma. *Virology,* **165**, in press.

8. Beasley, R. P., Hwang, L. Y., Lin, C. C. and Chien, C. S. (1981). Hepatocellular carcinoma and hepatitis B virus. *Lancet,* **3**, 1129–33

9. Summers, J., Smolec, J. M. and Snyder, R. (1978). A virus similar to human hepatitis B virus associated with hepatitis and hepatomas in woodchucks. *Proc. Natl. Acad. Sci. USA,* **75**, 4533–7

10. Snyder, R. L. and Summers, J. (1980). Woodchuck hepatitis virus and hepatocellular carcinoma from viruses in naturally occurring cancers. In Essex, M., Todaro, G. and Zur Hausen, H. (eds), *Cold Spring Harbor Conference of Cell Proliferation,* Vol. 7, pp. 447–57

11. Shafritz, D. A., Shouval, D., Sherman, H. I., Hadziyannis, S. J. and Kew, M. C. (1981). Integration of hepatitis B virus DNA into the genome of liver cells in chronic liver disease and hepatocellular carcinoma. *New Engl. J. Med.,* **305**, 1067–73

12. Summers, J., Smolec, J. M., Werner, B. G., Kelly, T. G., Jr., Tyler, G. V. and Snyder, R. L. (1980). Hepatitis B virus and woodchuck hepatitis virus are members of a novel class of DNA viruses in viruses in naturally occurring cancers. In Essex, M., Todaro, G. and Zur Hausen, H. (eds), *Cold Spring Harbor Conference on Cell Proliferation,* Vol. 7, 459–70

13. Ogston, C. W., Jonak, G. J., Rogler, C. E., Astrin, S. M. and Summers, J. (1982). Cloning and structural analysis of integrated woodchuck hepatitis virus sequences from hepatocellular carcinomas of woodchucks. *Cell,* **29**, 385–94

14. Moroy, T., Marchio, A., Etiemble, J., Trepo, C., Tiollais, P. and Buendia, M. A. (1986). Rearrangement and enhanced expression of *c-myc* in hepatocellular carcinoma of hepatitis virus infected woodchucks. *Nature,* **324**, 276–80

15. Dejean, A., Bougueleret, L., Grzeschik, K. H. and Tiollas, P. (1986). Hepatitis B virus DNA integration in a sequence homologous to *v-erb-A* and steroid receptor genes in a hepatocellular carcinoma. *Nature,* **322**, 70–2

16. Dejean, A., Sonigo, P., Wain-Hobson, S. and Trollais, P. (1984). Specific hepatitis B virus integration in hepatocellular carcinoma DNA through an all base-pair direct repeat. *Proc. Natl. Acad. Sci. USA,* **81**, 5350–4

17. Yaginuma, K., Kobayashi, H., Kobayashi, M., Morishima, T., Matsuyama, K. and Koike, K. (1987). Multiple integration sites of hepatitis B virus DNA in hepatocellular carcinoma and chronic active hepatitis tissues from children. *J. Virol.,* **61**, 1808–13

18. Bullock, P., Champoux, J. J. and Botchan, M. (1985). Association of crossover points with Topoisomerase I cleavage sites: A model for nonhomologous recombination. *Science,* **230**, 954–8

19. Wang, H. P. and Rogler, C. E. (1987). Evidence for topoisomerase I cutting of WHV virion DNA in the cohesive overlap region. Presented at Cold Spring Harbor Hepatitis B Viruses Meeting, September 28–October 1. Abstr. p. 121

20. Nagaya, T., Nakamura, T., Tokino, T., Tsurimoto, M., Mayumi, T., Kamino, K., Yamamura, K. and Matsubara, K. (1987). The mode of hepatitis B virus DNA integration in chromosomes of human hepatocellular carcinoma. *Genes and Devel.,* **1**, 773–82

21. Rogler, C. E., Sherman, M., Su, C. Y., Shafritz, D. A., Summers, J., Shows, T. B., Henderson, A. and Kew, M. (1985). Deletion in chromosome 11p associated with a hepatitis B integration site in hepatocellular carcinoma. *Science,* **230**, 319–22

22. Mizusawa, H., Taira, M., Yaginuma, K., Kobayashi, H., Yoshida, E. and Koike, K. (1985). Inversely repeating integrated hepatitis B virus DNA and cellular flanking sequences in the human hepatoma-derived cell line huSP. *Proc. Natl. Acad. Sci. USA,* **82**, 208–12

23. Hino, O., Shows, T. B. and Rogler, C. E. (1986). Hepatitis B virus integration site in hepatocellular carcinoma at chromosome 17; 18 translocation. *Proc. Natl. Acad. Sci. USA*, **83**, 8338–42

24. Hino, O., Nomura, K., Ohtahe, K., Kitagawa, T., Sugano, H., Kimura, S., Yokoyamo, M. and Katsuki, M. (1986). Rearrangement of integrated HBV DNA in descendants of transgenic mice. *Proc. Jap. Acad. Ser. B*, **62**, 1–4

25. Unora, M., Kobayashi, K., Fukuoka, K., Matsushita, F., Morimoto, H., Oshima, T., Kameko, S., Hattori, N., Murakami, S. and Yoshikawa, H. (1985). Establishment of a cell line from a woodchuck hepatocellular carcinoma. *Hepatology*, **6**, 1106–11

26. Knudson, A. G. and Strong, I. C. (1972) Mutation and cancer: A model for Wilms' tumor of the kidney. *J. Natl. Cancer Inst.*, **48**, 313–24

27. Francke, U. and Riccardi, V. M. (1979). Aniridia–Wilms' tumor association: evidence for specific deletion of 11p13. *Cytogenet. Cell Genet.*, **23**, 185–92

28. Cavenee, W. K., Dryja, T. P., Phillips, R. A., Benedict, W. F., Godbout, R., Gallie, B. O., Murphree, A. L., Strong, L. C. and White, R. L. (1983). Expression of recessive alleles by chromosomal mechanisms in retinoblastoma. *Nature*, **305**, 779–84

29. Glaser, T. G., Lewis, W. H., Bruns, G. A. P., Watkins, P. C., Rogler, C. E., Shows, T. B., Powers, V. E., Willard, H. F., Goguen, J. M., Simola, K. O. J. and Housman, D. E. (1986). The ß-subunit of follicle stimulating hormone is deleted in patients in aniridia and Wilms' tumor, allowing a further definition of the WAGR locus. *Nature*, **321**, 882–7

30. Koufos, A., Hansen, M. F., Lampkin, B. C., Workman, M. L., Copeland, N. G., Jenkins, N. A. and Cavenees, W. K. (1984). Loss of alleles at loci on human chromosome 11 during genesis of Wilms' tumor. *Nature*, **309**, 170–2

31. Orkin, S. H., Goldman, D. S. and Sallan, S. E. (1984). Development of homozygosity for chromosome 11p markers in Wilms' tumor. *Nature*, **309**, 172–4

32. Reeve, A. E., Housiaux, P. J. and Gardner, R. J. M. (1984). Loss of Harvey ras allele in sporadic Wilms' tumor. *Nature*, **309**, 174–6

33. Fearon, E. R., Vogelstein, B. and Feinberg, A. P. (1984). Somatic deletion and duplication of genes on chromosome 11 in Wilms' tumors. *Nature*, **309**, 176–8

34. Wang, H. P. and Rogler, C. E. (1988). Deletions in chromosomearms 11p and 13q in primary hepatocellular carcinomas. *Cytogenet. Cell Genet.*, **48**, 72–8

35. Soares, M. B., Ishii, D. N. and Efstratiadis, A. (1985). Developmental and tissue-specific expression of a family of transcripts related to rat insulin-like growth factor II mRNA. *Nucl. Acids Res.*, **14**, 1119–34

36. Frunzio, R., Chiarotti, L., Brown, A., Graham, D. E., Rechler, M. W. and Bruni, C. B. (1986). Structure and expression of the rat insulin-like growth factor II (rIGF-II) gene. *J. Biol. Chem.*, **261**, 17138–49

37. Cariani, E., Lasserre, C., Seurin, D., Hamelin, B., Kemeny, F., Franco, D., Czech, M. P., Ullrich, A. and Brechot, C. (1988). Differential expression of insulin-like growth factor II mRNA in human primary liver cancers, benign liver tumors and liver cirrhosis. *Cancer Res.*, **48**, 6844–9

38. Fu, X. X., Su, C. Y., Lee, Y., Hintz, R., Biempica, L., Snyder, R. and Rogler, C. E. (1988). Insulin-like growth factor II expression and oval cell proliferation associated with hepatocarcinogenesis in woodchuck hepatitis virus carriers. *J. Virol.*, **62**, 3422–30

39. Soares, M. B., Turken, A., Ishii, D., Mills, L., Epeskopou, V., Cotter, S., Zeitlin, S. and Efstratiadis, A. (1986). Rat insulin-like growth factor II gene, a single gene with two promoters expressing a multitranscript family. *J. Mol. Biol.*, **192**, 737–53

40. Dulak, N. C. and Temin, H. M. (1973). Multiplication-stimulating activity for chicken embryo fibroblasts from rat liver cell conditioned medium. A family of small polypeptides. *J. Cell Physiol.*, **82**, 161–70

10
Hepatitis B virus (HBV) DNA as a marker of HBV infection

E. NAKAJIMA, V. THIERS, D. LARZUL, P. TIOLLAIS AND
CH. BRECHOT

INTRODUCTION

The cloning of hepatitis B virus (HBV) DNA has provided a tool for the detection of viral DNA in serum and tissues of HBV carriers. This chapter will focus on the use of HBV DNA as a diagnostic test for HBV infection.

Two different groups of patients will be analysed according to the presence or absence of detectable serum HBsAg with a standard radioimmunoassay (RIA) (Abbott Laboratory).

HBsAg-POSITIVE PATIENTS

For HBsAg-positive patients, the detection of viral surface antigen indicates the presence of HBV; the problem is then to determine the presence or absence of viral multiplication and thus the level of infection in the serum. We have compared the HBeAg and serum HBV DNA status in 140 HBV chronic carriers with chronic active hepatitis (with associated cirrhosis or not): viral multiplication was not detected in about 20% of HBeAg-positive patients with chronic active hepatitis (CAH) with or without cirrhosis. Furthermore, HBV multiplication was also identified in 20% of HBsAg-positive, HBeAg-negative subjects. A similar result (with no association between HBeAg status and HBV multiplication) has also been observed at the acute stage of infection, i.e. acute fulminant and non-fulminant hepatitis.

Therefore the detection of HBV DNA is now recognized as the best marker for HBV multiplication. It should be used for selection of patients to be treated with antiviral therapy (such as interferon and adenine arabinoside) and for assessment of their efficacy.

The prevalence of anti-HBe positive, serum HBV DNA-positive, chronic HBV carriers is variable according to geographical area; indeed rates up to

40–50% have been reported in Asia and Greece, as compared to 10–20% observed in northern Europe.

HBV DNA SEQUENCES IN THE LIVER AND SERUM OF HBsAg-NEGATIVE PATIENTS WITH CHRONIC LIVER DISEASE: PATHOGENIC AND EPIDEMIOLOGICAL IMPLICATIONS

Viral DNA has been detected in liver cells of most patients we have investigated with HBsAg-negative hepatocellular carcinoma (HCC) and associated cirrhosis. The findings led to the suggestion that even in low and intermediate endemic areas the relationship between chronic HBV infection and HCC might also hold true; however, the effect of the virus in the development of these liver cancers and of HBsAg-positive tumours occurring in high endemic areas might obviously differ. In addition, in alcoholics it appeared that those without HCC had a much lower rate (about 10%) of HBV DNA positivity; therefore it was hypothesized that the presence of HBV DNA in the liver of these subjects might delineate a population at high risk of HCC. More recently evidence has also been obtained, although at a lower frequency, for the presence of HBV DNA in some patients with haemochromatosis and HCC. By contrast, our preliminary study of HCC without associated cirrhosis indicates that HBV DNA seems to be much less frequently identified in this situation (work is in progress). Thus, interactions between HBV infection, cirrhosis, iron excess and/or alcohol would be involved in the pathogenesis of HBsAg-negative hepatocellular carcinoma. That HBV DNA sequences can be detected in liver samples from HBsAg-negative subjects has now been shown by other groups and this has been further supported by the cloning of HBV DNA from a tumour, from a tumour-derived cell line and from the liver of an HBsAg-negative subject with CAH. In addition, HBsAg determinants were also identified in the serum of some HBsAg-negative subjects when RIA was performed with some monoclonal anti-HBs (M-RIA).

Although the liver DNA restriction patterns observed in HBsAg-negative patients are often suggestive of integration or of free monomeric HBV DNA, in some of these patients DNA replicative forms can be identified. Furthermore, that viral multiplication might occur was evidenced by the detection of HBV DNA sequences in some HBsAg-negative sera; in our experience such DNA sequences were identified in the serum of about 10% of patients with HBsAg-negative CAH or alcoholic liver disease, including even subjects without any conventional HBV marker. The detection of such viral DNA sequences was also reported by Wands et al.[3] in sera from HBsAg-negative patients as well as chimpanzees inoculated with a 'non-A, non-B' strain. Recently we were able to show the specificity of these results by injection into chimpanzees of HBV DNA and M-RIA-positive sera obtained from two HBsAg-negative alcoholic subjects (one with HCC). Transmission of the viral particles was obtained, even in some anti-HBs-positive animals; the HBsAg determinants were detectable with M-RIA (but not with P-RIA) in the serum of the chimpanzees, while HBV DNA sequences were detected in their liver samples.

However, although it now seems clear that HBV DNA can be found in HBsAg-negative liver samples, the exact frequency of these findings is still debated. For example, in subjects with CAH, Figus *et al.* reported in Italy a very high rate of positivity: 16 of 19 HBsAg-negative cases including 4 without HBV markers, whereas Harrison *et al.* and Fowler *et al.* showed far less positive results. In France we found a rate of 59% of HBV DNA-positive liver samples. In patients with HCC, different results were obtained in Japan, where Hino *et al.* described only 4 positive samples out of 62 cases, whereas Koike *et al.* reported 5 positive and 4 'ambiguous' results from 12 subjects.

Thus some discrepancies appear in the results and interpretations presented by different groups; this may reflect technical problems, as might be expected from any laborious procedure, as well as geographical variation in the HBV endemic rate. To be able to compare different studies aimed at detecting HBV DNA in liver samples where a limited percentage of cells may contain HBV DNA, various conditions are required. The sensitivity of the assay is of the order of 1–10 pg of HBV DNA marker; this sensitivity, however, may vary in the same laboratory according to the efficiency of hybridization, and remains hard to estimate accurately even when several assays are conducted for each sample. In addition, the possible heterogeneity of HBV DNA localization (in particular in HCC) is also an important consideration. On the other hand, it is now well known that false-positive results might be due to plasmids or, in general, to bacterial DNA contaminating the liver DNA (even when the probe is carefully prepared). Such bacterial DNA, often present in autopsy but also in surgical or needle-biopsy samples, may reflect either a true liver bacterial proliferation or a laboratory contamination. This stresses the need for systematic control experiments. Furthermore, the choice of the restriction enzymes is also an important and underestimated problem. Different results might, for example, be obtained if only Hind-III or Eco-RI digestion are performed: the former may yield positive results only if free HBV is present or if clonal proliferation of the infected cells occurs whereas the latter may show internal HBV bands even in the case (frequently observed in non-cirrhotic tissue) of integration at several sites or concatemeric organization. Furthermore, HBV DNA rearrangements due to HBV variations may change the restriction sites and further complicate such analysis.

Thus, altogether, it is possible that the reported data may point out differences in the prevalence of HBsAg-negative HBV DNA-positive cases in various geographical areas. However, it also clearly appears that exchange of DNA samples between different laboratories is needed before reaching any definitive conclusion. Finally, it is clear that, with the procedures usually described, no hybridization occurs between HBV and normal cellular DNA. In addition, studies such as those of anti-HBs-positive cases either with normal liver histology, in alcoholics without HCC, or of resolved acute hepatitis (unpublished data) showed that simple exposure to HBV does not always imply further detection of HBV DNA in liver samples. Obviously, however, the prevalence of asymptomatic carriers of HBV DNA will also have to be determined in each geographical area to clarify the implications of HBV DNA detection.

The dissociation between the usual HBV serology and HBV DNA or the M-RIA assay is likely to reflect variations in HBV expression. This would include different (and not exclusive) possibilities. For many anti-HBc and anti-HBs-positive patients, HBsAg might be 'hidden' in immune complexes, the viral particles being only identified by the M-RIA and hybridization tests. In addition, restricted HBV gene expression in the infected hepatocytes can be due either to lower transcription or to modification in the assembly and/or exportation of viral particles; this would account for the immunohistochemical detection of HBsAg in the liver of some of the HBsAg-negative HBV DNA-positive subjects. Variations in the number of viral particles secreted might occur in some HBV infections or be related to some treatments, as suggested in children treated with chemotherapy; furthermore, this might also hold true in alcoholic liver disease, since inhibition of protein secretion by alcohol has been well demonstrated.

Additional explanations are needed, however, when anti-HBc and anti-HBs are not detected in the serum while HBV DNA and HBsAg determinants are present. A low or non-response to both HBsAg and HBcAg might occur in some patients, but this may also reflect heterogeneity of the viral antigens. Indeed, the development of monoclonal antibody assays for several viruses such as influenza, measles, rabies, and more recently HBV clearly demonstrated such variations of the viral antigenic determinants. Modifications in the viral genomes would then account for the negative results obtained with conventional tests and the absence of cross-protection between two different HBV strains. In view of this, an intriguing observation was obtained from the nucleotide sequence of different integrated HBV DNA in the single Alexander cell line; indeed, the results suggested that several infections with different HBV subtype occurred in the HBsAg-positive subject whose tumour was used to establish this cell line.

Such data could well imply that a fraction of the so-called 'non-A, non-B' infections might be related to HBV infection either with a low level of viral antigen expression or with viral genomic variations; however, the precise incidence of such HBV variants in different populations as well as their definitive characterization remains to be elucidated.

The polymerase chain reaction (PCR) assay allows specific amplification of a short DNA sequence located between two primers, the sequences of which are complementary to both strands of the DNA analysed. We have synthesized primers specific for the S, pre-S, C and X regions of the viral genome. After 30–40 cycles of amplification, the viral DNA has been identified by spot test and Southern blot with an oligonucleotide probe located between the two primers.

CONCLUSIONS

For HBsAg-positive patients, HBV DNA detection in the serum is possible with PCR. The sensitivity is markedly enhanced and would reach 100 particles/ml.

For HBsAg-negative patients with chronic liver diseases, the PCR test allows ready identification of viral DNA. In addition, it has recently been possible to clone these short amplified DNA sequences. This approach will allow a first characterization of these 'HBV-related' viruses.

Development and standardization of the PCR assay should allow generation of new diagnostic tests, probably using non-radioactive probes. These tests should allow identification of viral DNA in serum, liver and mononuclear blood cells.

References

1. Bréchot, C., Hadchouel, M., Scotto, J. *et al.* (1981). State of hepatitis B virus DNA in hepatocytes of patients with hepatitis B surface antigen-positive and negative liver diseases. *Proc. Natl. Acad. Sci. USA*, **78**, 3906–10
2. Pasquinelli, C., Lauré, F., Chatenoud, L. *et al.* (1986). Hepatitis B virus DNA in mononuclear blood cells: a frequent event in hepatitis B surface antigen positive and negative patients with acute and chronic liver disease. *J. Hepatol.*, **3**, 95–103
3. Wands, J., Fujita, Y. K., Isselbacher, J., Degott, C., Schellekens, H., Dazza, M. C., Tiollais, P. and Bréchot, C. (1986). Identification and transmission of hepatitis B virus related variants. *Proc. Natl. Acad. Sci. USA*, **83**, 6608–12
4. Larzul, D., Thiers, V., Couroucé, A. M., Bréchot, C. and Guesdon, J. L. (1987). Non-radioactive hepatitis B virus DNA probe for detection of HBV-DNA in serum. *J. Hepatol.*, **5**, 199–204
5. Thiers, V., Fujita, Y. K., Takahashi, H., Schellekens, H., de Reus, A., Driss, F., Degott, C., Isselbacher, K., Tiollais, P., Wands, J. and Bréchot, C. (1988) Hepatitis B virus DNA sequences in the serum of HBsAg negative patients with chronic liver diseases: transmission of viral particles to chimpanzees in viral hepatitis and liver disease. In Zuckerman, A. J. (ed.) 553–57. (New York: Alan R. Liss Inc.)

11
Trans-acting factors regulating the replication and malignant transformation of hepatitis B virus

G. ACS, S. KARPEN, R. BANERJEE, M. A. SELLS, G. VAJTA, P. PRICE, M. SUNG, G. LENGYEL AND M. SHVARTSMAN

At the last Falk conference entitled *Modulation of Liver Cell Expression*, we described a new cell line derived from Hep G_2 cells transfected with HBV DNA. The cells of this line contain integrated and episomal HBV DNA, synthesize all the viral antigens, replicative intermediates and secrete mature surface antigen and viral particles into the medium which morphologically are indistinguishable from those found in the serum of infected patients[1].

Our data reported herein show that the *in vitro* produced virus is also infectious *in vivo*. In collaboration with Dr Purcell's group[2], chimpanzees were inoculated intravenously with approximately 9×10^8 and 3.6×10^8 virus particles. About 3 weeks after the inoculation, both HB_s and HB_c antigens were detected in the serum followed by the appearance of the respective antibodies. Simultaneously, the enzyme levels characteristic for hepatic microinflammation were found to be elevated. The liver biopsies revealed, as judged by the late Dr Popper, characteristic lesions in the parenchyma and portal tracts. The restriction map pattern of the viral DNA produced in the chimpanzees is identical to the cloned DNA. Thus, HBV DNA transfected Hep G_2 cells can support the replication of HBV which in turn produces hepatitis in chimpanzees.

The permanent, virus-producing cell lines described by us and simultaneously by two other groups of investigators[3,4] have, however, two shortcomings: (1) the parent cells capable of supporting viral replication are tumorigenic by themselves; and (2) the *in vitro* produced virus, similarly to Dane particles, isolated from infected patients, is infectious in chimpanzees but is not infectious on cultured Hep G_2 cells. Nevertheless, we obtained circumstantial evidence regarding the oncogenic potential of HBV and characterized liver-specific transacting factors binding to regulatory sequences on the HBV genome which might be responsible for the liver tropism of the virus.

In collaboration with Dr Paronetto, we have injected 0.5×10^6 HBV-producing-cells subcutaneously into nude mice; within 2 weeks, large tumours were formed in all the mice. Simultaneously, HB_s antigen and viral particles were found in the serum. By injecting the virus-producing cells into the spleen of nude mice, xenografts were found in the liver and HB_s, HB_c antigens as well as virus were present in the serum. Thus, by injecting the HBV DNA transfected cells into nude mice, we obtained an animal model where HBV production can be monitored and modulated.

Although there is some evidence for HBV replication in non-liver tissue[5,6], the principal site of clinical pathology is the liver. The finding that Hep G_2 cells derived from a hepatoblastoma are capable of supporting viral replication made it feasible to search for specific trans-acting factors in these cells which are capable of binding to regulatory elements present in the HBV genome. For this purpose, we constructed a plasmid containing the enhancer elements[7] of HBV DNA and the core promoter to which the bacterial chloramphenicol acetyltransferase (CAT) gene is ligated. This plasmid was transfected into a variety of cell lines such as Hep G_2, virus-producing Hep G_2, monkey kidney CV-1, mouse and rat fibroblasts. CAT expression was observed only in Hep G_2 and in the virus-producing Hep G_2 cells indicating that titratable, specific, trans-acting factors are responsible for the tissue-specific expression of this plasmid. This was further proven by the findings that co-transfection of this plasmid with either enhancer or core promoter sequences strongly inhibited the expression of the CAT gene. In order to characterize these tissue-specific trans-acting factors and localize their target site within the regulatory elements, we performed gel electrophoretic mobility shift assays using Hep G_2 nuclear extract and ^{32}P labelled fragments of the enhancer and core promoter region. The mobility of both DNA sequences on a non-denaturing agarose gel was retarded if they were pre-incubated with the nuclear extracts. The factors responsible for binding to these two regulatory regions are distinct since unlabelled enhancer sequences compete in the binding of the factors to the radiolabelled enhancer sequences but do not affect the binding to the radiolabelled core sequences. Vice versa, the non-labelled core sequences compete only with the binding to the radiolabelled core sequences and not to the enhancer sequences. At least two factors bind to the enhancer sequences; one is heat labile and the other heat stable. Only one factor binds to the core promoter. By methylation interference asssays[8], we mapped the regions to which these trans-acting factors bind. Both encompass a relatively short segment and both contain palindromic sequences. Analogous, but not identical, results were obtained by others regarding the enhancer binding protein using DNAse-1 protection analyses[9,10].

DNA of various members of the papovavirus, adenovirus, and herpes virus families are capable of augmenting the expression of CAT gene linked to the long terminal repeats (LTR) of the human immunodeficiency virus, HIV[11]. We investigated the expression of HIV-promoted CAT gene in Hep G_2 and HBV-producing Hep G_2 cells and found that liver trans-acting factors recognize regulatory sequences in the HIV LTR. In cells producing HBV, the expression of the factors is modulated. Namely, the HIV-directed CAT gene is less effectively expressed in the HBV-producing cells than in the parent Hep

G_2 cells. The modulating activity can be counteracted by the TAT gene product of HIV whose target is the TAR region of HIV. A strong sequence homology was found between the TAR region and the enhancer region of HBV. We are investigating whether one of the above described liver-specific trans-acting factors binding to the enhancer is also capable of binding to the TAR region and thereby modulating the expression of HIV promoted transcripts.

References

1. Sells, M. A., Chen, M.-L. and Acs, G. (1987). Production of hepatitis B virus particles in Hep G_2 cells transfected with cloned hepatitis B virus DNA. *Proc. Natl. Acad. Sci. USA,* **84**, 1005–9
2. Acs, G., Sells, M. A., Purcell, R. H., Price, P., Engle, R., Shapiro, M. and Popper, H. (1987). Hepatitis B virus produced by transfected Hep G_2 cells causes hepatitis in chimpanzees. *Proc. Natl. Acad. Sci. USA,* **84**, 4641–4
3. Sureau, C., Romet-Lemonne, J-L., Mullins, J. I. and Essex, M. (1986). Production of hepatitis B virus by a differentiated human hepatoma cell line after transfection with cloned circular HBV DNA. *Cell,* **47**, 37–47
4. Tsurimoto, T., Fujuyama, A. and Matsubara, K. (1987). Stable expression and replication of hepatitis B virus genome in an integrated state in a human hepatoma cell line transfected with the cloned viral DNA. *Proc. Natl. Acad. Sci. USA,* **84**, 444–8
5. Lie-Injo, L. E., Balasegaram, M., Lopez, C. G. and Herrera, A. R. (1983). Hepatitis B virus DNA in liver and white blood cells of patients with hepatoma. *DNA,* **2**, 301–8
6. Elfassi, E., Romet-Lemonne, J.-L., Essex, M., McLane, M. F. and Haseltine, W. (1984). Evidence of extra chromosomal forms of hepatitis B viral DNA in a bone marrow culture obtained from a patient recently infected with hepatitis B virus. *Proc. Natl. Acad. Sci. USA,* **81**, 3526–8
7. Shaul, Y., Rutter, W. J. and Laub, O. (1985). A human hepatitis B viral enhancer element. *EMBO J.,* **4**, 427–30
8. Gilman, M. Z., Wilson, R. N. and Weinberg, R. A. (1986). Multiple protein-binding sites in the 5'-flanking region regulates *c-fos* expression. *Mol. Cell. Biol.,* **6**, 4305–16
9. Jameel, S. and Siddiqui, A. (1987). The HBV enhancer and trans-acting factors. In Robinson, W., Koike, K. and Will, H. (eds). *Hepadna Viruses.* pp. 65–76. (New York: Alan R. Liss, Inc.)
10. Shaul, Y. and Ben-Levy, R. (1987). Multiple nuclear proteins in liver cells are bound to hepatitis B virus enhancer element and its upstream sequence. *EMBO J.,* **6**, 1913–20
11. Gendelman, H. E., Phelps, W., Feigenbaum, L., Ostrove, J. M., Adachi, A., Howley, P. M., Khoury, G., Ginsberg, H. S. and Martin, M. A. (1986). Trans-activation of the human immunodeficiency virus long terminal repeat sequence by DNA viruses. *Proc. Natl. Acad. Sci. USA,* **83**, 9759–63

12
Transactivation by HBV X gene product

R. KOSHY, P. ZAHM, M. WOLLERSHEIM AND P. H. HOFSCHNEIDER

INTRODUCTION

Hepatitis B virus (HBV) is the aetiological agent in the development of primary liver cancer in many areas of the world[1]. The molecular mechanisms of HBV-mediated cell transformation are not understood. Studies to date have failed to identify common viral integration sites in tumour cell chromosomes or to provide a basis for a common *cis*-acting virus function in tumorigenesis. The elucidation[2] of the replicative strategy of HBV (hepadnaviruses) involving a viral reverse transcriptase (hitherto a distinctive feature of retroviruses) has stimulated further comparisons between HBV and retroviruses. A physical map of the HBV genome is shown in Figure 1. Such studies have revealed analogies in the organization of genes on their respective genomes[3]. The X open reading frame (ORF) of HBV is one of four viral genes and the only one without a known function. This gene occupies a position corresponding to the *tat* gene of human T lymphotropic viruses (HTLV) which encodes a transactivating function necessary for virus replication[4] and is also suggested to be a factor in T-lymphocyte transformation[5]. These reasons encouraged us to investigate the X ORF of HBV for transactivational activity.

X GENE STIMULATION OF PSV2 CAT

Plasmid constructs consisting of the X ORF and varying upstream regions were tested for the ability to stimulate the expression of the chloramphenicol acetyltransferase gene (CAT) from the SV40 early promoter (pSV2cat) following cotransfection of X test DNA and pSV2cat DNA into cells of human liver origin (CCL13). The amount of acetylation of ^{14}C labelled chloramphenicol in lysates of transfected cells provided the measure of stimulation of CAT expression.

The results of these experiments are depicted in Figure 2. In these initial constructs the promoters of the pre-S and S genes were used for the

117

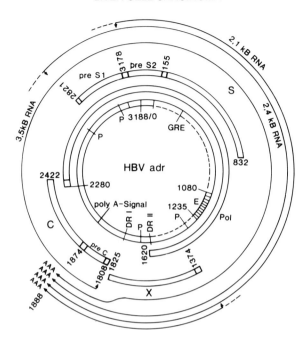

☐ AUG – Startcodon

Figure 1 Physical map of the HBV genome. The basic diagram of the genome is taken from Tiollais *et al.* 1985[8]. Updating modifications and details of regulatory sequences and transcription of the X region are added. The reading frames of the HBV genes are shown by broad arrows and are referred to as S for surface, C for core, P for polymerase proteins, and X, which is discussed in this chapter. The thin arrows correspond to the major transcripts which have different start sites but terminate at a common sequence

expression of the X gene. The plasmids used were as follows: Plasmid pHBV 2836 consisted of a 2.3-kb BglII-BglII fragment of HBV DNA which consisted of the pre-S and S genes and their promoters as well as the X ORF and the downstream termination sequences. This contiguous fragment of DNA also had the HBV enhancer element[6,7] at map position 1000–1200. This plasmid very efficiently stimulated CAT expression (ca. 50-fold). Since there was a possibility that the enhancer could have been responsible for the observed effect plasmid pHBV 2836 Δ Nco/Xho was constructed in which the enhancer was deleted. This plasmid stimulated CAT expression to a similar degree as pHBV 2836 indicating that the enhancer was not the reason for the activity. Furthermore, the enhancer appeared not to influence the level of expression in these experiments in which the X transcripts arose from the S or pre-S promoters. When the region 5′ to the X ORF was removed, as in pHBV 824, thereby rendering it promoterless, there was no stimulation of CAT expression in transfected cells. The expression of transcripts was investigated by Northern blot analyses of RNA isolated from cells transfected with the

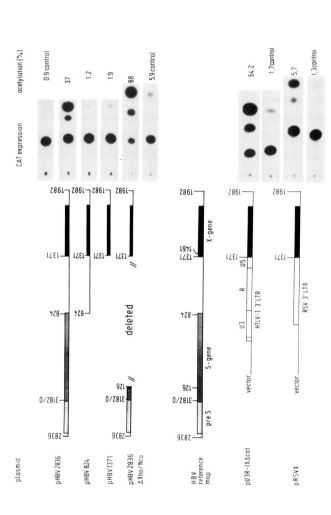

Figure 2 HBV-plasmid constructs and CAT expression in CCL13 cells. Levels of transactivation in CCL13 cells by cloned subgenomic HBV fragments containing the X region. HBV plasmids with names and the genome positions of the cloned HBV DNA are depicted. A physical map of the relevant genome sequences is given for reference. On the right side CAT expression from pSV2cat in the presence of the respective test plasmids is shown. A 10-fold molar excess of the co-transfected test plasmids over pSV2cat was used in experiments with HBV promoters. For pU3R-IXΔcat and pRSVX the molar ratios of test and indicator plasmids were 1:1 and 4:1 respectively. Optimum molar ratios were experimentally determined. The CAT assays of representative controls were with pSV2cat alone (for pU3R-IXΔcat and pRSVX) and with the test plasmid pMLΔBS (Not to scale.)

119

plasmids described. X-specific transcripts were made in cells transfected with pHBV 2836 and pHBV 2836Δ Nco/Xho whereas no RNA was seen in cells transfected with pHBV 824 which was devoid of a promoter (Figure 3). Thus it was clear from these results that pSV2cat stimulation was a function of X gene expression.

IDENTIFICATION OF X GENE PROMOTER

In naturally-infected hepatocytes the major viral RNA transcripts are 2.3 kb and 3.5 kb in size arising from the S promoter and the C promoter, respectively (for a review see Tiollais *et al.,* 1985)[8], which may also give rise to X protein. However, in cells transfected with viral DNA smaller transcripts have been seen[9], which suggested the presence of another promoter

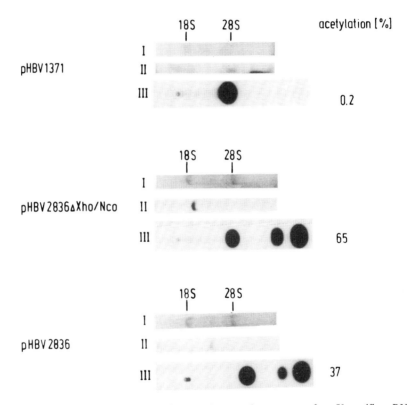

Figure 3 Transactivation of pSV2cat is dependent on the presence of an X-specific mRNA. Northern analyses of total RNA (II) and CAT activity (III) of extracts from CCL13 cells transfected with pSV2cat and test plasmids pHBV1371 (molar ratio 1:10), pHBV2836ΔXho/Nco and pHBV2836 are shown. Methylene blue staining of the filters (I) indicates comparable amounts of total RNA in each case. The percentage of ^{14}C labelled chloramphenicol acetylated is also given. The value for pHBV2836ΔXho/Nco is taken from an independent experiment than that depicted in Figure 2

immediately upstream of the X ORF. We have investigated this by means of a plasmid construct consisting of a AccI-NcoI fragment of HBV (nucleotides 824–1374) containing the putative X promoter and the HBV enhancer cloned upstream of the CAT gene in a promoterless vector (pCAT3M). Clones were obtained with the HBV fragment in both orientation (pHBVXcat+ and pHBVXcat–) with respect to the CAT gene. Plasmids with the HBV DNA in the same orientation as the CAT gene efficiently expressed the CAT gene in transfected cells whereas no expression was seen when the HBV DNA was in an inverted orientation (Figure 4). This strongly suggests the presence of a promoter within the fragment of HBV DNA used. X transcripts of about 0.8 kb are abundantly expressed in transfected cells (e.g. see Fig. 7c). Assuming poly (A) residues of about 0.2 kb, the promoter lies within 100 bases of the X start site. These results corroborate other recently presented evidence[10] on the existence of this promoter.

REQUIREMENT FOR X PROTEIN

In two additional constructs, pU3R-IXΔ cat and pRSVX, the X ORF was placed under the control of heterologous promoters, namely, the human T lymphotropic virus 1 (HTLV-1) long terminal repeat (LTR) and the Rous

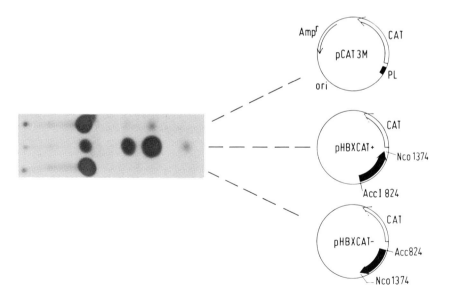

Figure 4 Evidence for a promoter upstream to the X gene. A fragment of HBV DNA (AccI-NcoI, nucleotides 824–1376) was inserted into the BglII site of vector pCAT3M after Klenow I + treatment of vector and insert DNA. pHBXcat+ has the HBV DNA in the correct orientation with respect to the CAT gene. pHBXcat– has the HBV segment in the wrong orientation. In transfected CCL13 cells, the CAT gene is expressed only when the HBV fragment is in the correct orientation

sarcoma virus (RSV) LTR, respectively. These plasmids were also able to stimulate pSV2cat expression very efficiently (Figure 2). In order to prove unequivocally that a protein product of the X ORF is required for the stimulatory activity frame-shift mutations were introduced into plasmids pRSVX and pU3R-IX Δcat by Bam HI cleavage of the plasmid in the unique site within the X gene, filling in the cohesive ends so generated with T₄ DNA polymerase and religating the newly created blunt ends using T₄ DNA ligase. This procedure introduced four bases into the sequences thus shifting the reading frame by one base. The frame-shifted plasmids pRSVXfs and pU3R-IXΔcatfs in each case failed to provide stimulatory activity (Figure 2), even though Northern analyses showed that the RNA expression was comparable to that obtained with the wild-type plasmids. The RNA analyses using pU3R-IXΔcat and its frame-shifted version pU3R-IX Δcatfs are presented in Figure 5. These experiments confirmed that the stimulatory activity provided by the HBV X gene was dependent on the expression of a functional protein.

STIMULATION OF CAT EXPRESSION IS TRANSCRIPTIONAL

RNA isolated from cells transfected with the various plasmids were analysed by hybridisation of Northern blots with a CAT-specific probe. The levels of

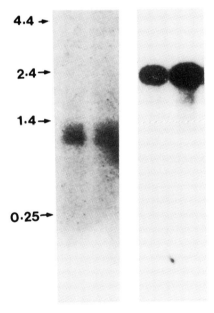

Figure 5 Transcription of X-specific RNA in cells transfected with plasmid DNA bearing a frame-shift mutation in the X coding sequences. Poly(A) selected RNA from CCL13 cells transfected respectively with equal amounts of the frame-shifted plasmid, pU3R-IXfsΔcat (left lane) and with the wild-type plasmid pU3R-IXΔcat (right lane) were analysed. The panel on the left shows hybridization to an X probe and the panel to the right shows the same filter strip-washed and re-hybridized to a ß-actin probe

CAT RNA were elevated in cells transfected with plasmids that stimulated CAT activity, i.e. pGEMHBV2 (which consists of two head-to-tail copies of the HBV genome in the vector pGEM), pHBV2836, and pHBV2836Δ Nco/Xho, as compared to the very minimal expression of the same transcripts in cells transfected with vector plasmid alone (Figure 6). Re-probing the same filter with ß-actin (not shown) and methylene blue staining showed that similar amounts of total RNA were present in different lanes (Figure 6, compare lanes, a, b and d). The results of this experiment as well as the frame-shift experiment described above demonstrate that the stimulation of CAT expression by the X product is by stimulation of transcription.

STIMULATION BY X PROTEIN IS IN *TRANS*

The observation discussed above strongly suggested that the X product is a transfunctioning protein. In order to unequivocally demonstrate this, we obtained clones of cells in which the X gene is stably integrated into the cellular chromosomes. HepG2 hepatoblastoma cells were co-transfected with plasmids pAG2HBV, containing two head-to-tail copies of the HBV genome

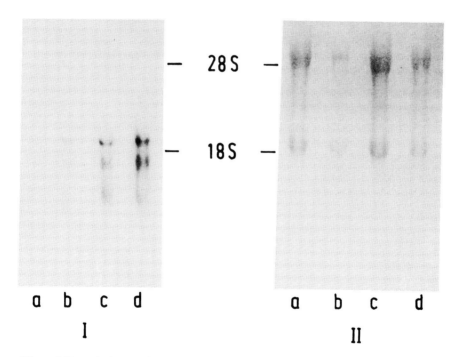

Figure 6 Transcriptional activation of pSV2cat by different HBV plasmids. (I) Northern-blot hybridization of CAT RNA in CCL13 cells transfected with pSV2cat and a 10-fold molar excess of the test plasmids pMLΔBS (a), pGEMHBV2 (b), pHBV2836 (c) and pHBV2836ΔXho/Nco (d). The probe was nick translated HindIII-BamHI CAT fragment from pSV2cat. (II) Methylene blue stain of the same filter as in (I)

and pAG60 which encodes resistance to the drug G418. Resistant clones of cells were isolated after selection of the transfected cultures with G418. Clones containing HBV DNA were identified by hybridization of cellular DNA with HBV probe and radioimmunoassay of culture medium for secreted hepatitis B surface antigen. X-protein mediated transactivation was studied in several such cell clones after transfection of pSV2cat DNA. Parental HepG2 cells lacking HBV DNA were used as a control in these experiments. The results of such experiments with a representative clone 15/1 are shown in Figure 7. Southern blot analyses show that intact viral DNA is integrated in the cellular DNA (Figure 7 A). X mRNA is abundantly expressed in these cells (Figure 7 C). The size of the RNA is consistent with expression from the X promoter. As seen in Figure 7B, CAT expression is stimulated 15-fold in 15/1 cells but

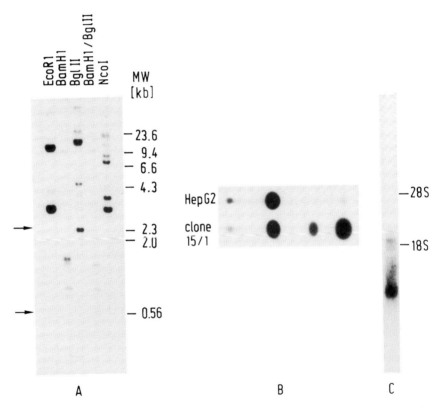

Figure 7 Analyses of HepG2 clone 15/1 cells. **A**: Southern blot of 15/1 cellular DNA digested with the indicated enzymes and hybridized with an HBV probe. The 2.3-kb Bgl II fragment and the 0.58 kb BamH I/Bgl II fragment of HBV (arrows) indicate intact X sequences integrated in the cellular DNA. **B**: Transient CAT expression in parental HepG2 and 15/1 cells transfected pSV2cat DNA. In HepG2 the acetylation was 3.4% and in clone 15/2 it was 45.4% **C**: Northern blot of Poly(A) selected RNA of 15/1 cells hybridized with an HBV probe indicating the abundant expression of X transcripts of about 800 nucleotides, derived from integrated HBV DNA

absent in HepG2 cells. These experiments establish that the stimulatory potential of the X protein is in *trans*.

EFFECT OF X ON DIFFERENT PROMOTERS

In order to test the specificity of the transactivation response of different promoters to the X protein, plasmids were constructed, as described[11] in which the CAT gene was placed under the control of various eukaryotic viral promoters, viz., the herpes simplex virus I thymidine kinase promoter (pBLcat2), the Rous sarcoma virus LTR (pRSV-LTRcat), the mouse mammary tumour virus LTR (pMMTV-LTRcat), and the human T lymphotropic virus I LTR (pHTLV-LTRcat). A general ability of the X product to stimulate CAT expression was demonstrated (Figure 8) although the MMTV LTR was not stimulated to any significant extent. In that case, the experiment was performed in the absence of dexamethasone in order to dissociate the possible stimulatory effect of the X protein from that which would be conferred by hormones. Thus, even though the effect of the X protein is not a very specific one there seems to be some degree of preference. Only one cellular promoter, the human metallothionein promoter (MTIIA), so far

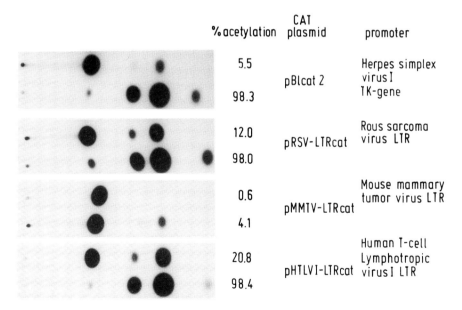

% acetylation	CAT plasmid	promoter
5.5	pBlcat 2	Herpes simplex virus I TK-gene
98.3		
12.0	pRSV-LTRcat	Rous sarcoma virus LTR
98.0		
0.6	pMMTV-LTRcat	Mouse mammary tumor virus LTR
4.1		
20.8	pHTLVI-LTRcat	Human T-cell Lymphotropic virus I LTR
98.4		

Figure 8 Transactivation of different eukaryotic promoters by pBV2836 or pHBV1982. Stimulation of transient CAT expression from the indicated promoters by HBV DNA is presented. The control assays were done with cells transfected with the same molar amounts of pMLΔBS. Transactivating test plasmid was pHBV2836 and in the case of pBLcat2, the transactivating plasmid was pHBV1982 (containing the Bgl II-BglII HBV DNA fragment from position 2836 to 1982 in the opposite orientation as pHBV2836)

tested was also comparatively only poorly stimulated (less than 3-fold, data not shown). These results raise the possibility that in infected cells particular cellular genes may be activated or stimulated. It is very likely that alterations in gene expression contribute to pathogenesis and, as discussed below, may have implications in tumorigenesis.

X PRODUCT STIMULATES ITS OWN EXPRESSION

The observation that a variety of viral enhancer/promoter elements are stimulated by the X protein suggests that the effect of the protein may be via the enhancer rather than directly on the promoter and further that the X protein does not bind directly to the DNA but more likely to other cellular proteins. This speculation is consistent with the observation that the X protein has been localized by immunofluorescence to the cytoplasm[12]. The possible binding of the X protein to cellular cytoplasmic protein(s) may activate it and cause limited amounts of such complexes to be transported to the nucleus where it functions as a transcriptional transactivator. The temporal and regulated expression of the X protein in infected cells is not understood, partly because purified X protein and antibodies to it are not yet available. However, the studies to date (for a review see Ganem and Varmus, 1987)[13] indicate that the expression of this gene is well controlled. We studied the effect of the X protein on the HBV enhancer and X promoter. Plasmid pHBVXcat, described above, comprising the CAT gene under the control of the HBV enhancer and X promoter when transfected into CCL13 cells at low concentrations (i.e. 1 μg/100 mm plate) did not lead to CAT expression. However, when this plasmid was co-transfected with another plasmid pU1.4 (see Figure 11 for a description of this plasmid) expressing the X gene, there was stimulation of CAT expression (Figure 9), indicating that the X product has a positive feedback on its own expression. This effect has been determined to occur via the enhancer as shown by the use of constructs in which the enhancer was deleted (see Figure 11 and discussion below).

CELLULAR FACTORS IN TRANSACTIVATION

As discussed above, the action of the X protein may be in concert with cellular proteins. These considerations and the fact that infection with HBV is tissue and species tropic led us to examine the properties of the X protein in cells of different species, the experiments described thus far having been done in human liver derived CCL13 cells. A variety of cells were used including HeLa (human), Fisher rat fibroblasts, CV-I (monkey), Vero (monkey), GL2/2 (feline), BHK (hamster) and NIH 3T3 (mouse). The results of some of the experiments are shown in Figure 10. It was clear that the best stimulation of CAT expression occurred in human liver cells. However, HeLa cells which are of human non-liver origin were also good expressers of the function. Fisher rat cells permitted CAT stimulation to a much lower extent and then only at higher amounts of DNA transfection. The experiments with mouse,

plasmid   coplasmid

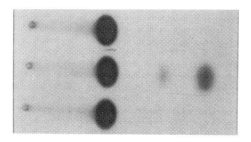

pHBXCAT + ——————

pHBXCAT + pU 1.4

pHBXCAT + pUC 19

Figure 9 The X product transactivates the X promoter. Plasmid pHBXcat (described in Figure 4) was transfected into CCL13 cells at a concentration too low for it to be expressed (1 µg/plate). Co-transfection with an X expressing plasmid, pU1-4 (see Figure 11) resulted in CAT expression. Co-transfection with vector pUC19 did not have any effect

hamster and cat cells confirmed these trends thus suggesting that there are cellular factors required for optimum transactivation and that these factors though similar in function are phylogenetically diverged.

INTEGRATED HBV DNA FROM TUMOURS RETAINS TRANSACTIVATIONAL POTENTIAL

The possibility of a HBV transactivating function being important in hepato-carcinogenesis has been suggested[14]. Therefore, having determined that such a function is indeed encoded by HBV DNA, we wanted to study this property in integrated HBV DNA. For this purpose, integrated viral DNA along with cellular flanking sequences were isolated by molecular cloning from cells of a primary hepatocellular carcinoma containing two integrated copies of HBV DNA. Restriction mapping of the cloned DNA (Figure 11) shows that there are 2.1 kb of viral DNA with 12.6 kb of cellular DNA adjacent to it. The viral DNA present on the clone comprises only the surface (S) gene and most of the X gene. The core (C) gene and the pre-surface (pre-S) gene are deleted, as is the S promoter. Sequence analyses (not shown) reveal that the last 28 nucleotides of the X ORF are deleted. This cloned DNA, pU1.4, was tested in CCL13 cells and found to be extremely efficient in stimulating expression of cotransfected pSV2cat (Figure 11). Because of the presence of a large amount of cellular sequences on the clone, it was necessary to reduce the tested DNA by progressive deletions in order to be sure that the stimulatory activity was a function of the X sequences and to exclude any contributory effect of the cellular DNA. The plasmids thus produced were tested for their stimulatory capacity (Figure 11). The results clearly indicate that a considerable part of the cellular DNA can be removed (pU4.31) without diminution of the activity. A deletion of part of the X sequences (pU4.31ΔX) results in total loss of activity. Removal of sequences upstream of the X gene, i.e. enhancer and promoter (pU4.31 Bam-Eco) also renders the construct inactive. Plasmid

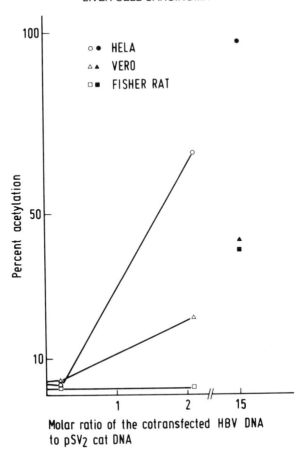

Figure 10 Transactivation of pSV2cat by pHBV2AG60 and pKKHBs34 in cells of different species. Stimulation of transient CAT expression from pSV2cat by pHBV2AG60 (○, △, □) and pKKHBs34 (●, ▲, ■), is shown for each cell line used

pU4.31 Acc-Eco which retains a small region upstream of the X ORF but which is missing the enhancer and promoter shows a much diminished activity. Plasmid pU4.31 Sph-Eco containing the promoter but missing the enhancer is less active than the original. Thus, it can be concluded that the stimulatory activity of the plasmid pU4.31 is encoded by the X sequences. Furthermore, the enhancer is necessary for optimum expression of the X gene.

EXPRESSION OF FUSION X-CELLULAR RNA TRANSCRIPT

The process of integration, as seen in plasmid pU4.31, led to the deletion of the last 28 bases of the X gene as well as the 3′ flanking sequences normally

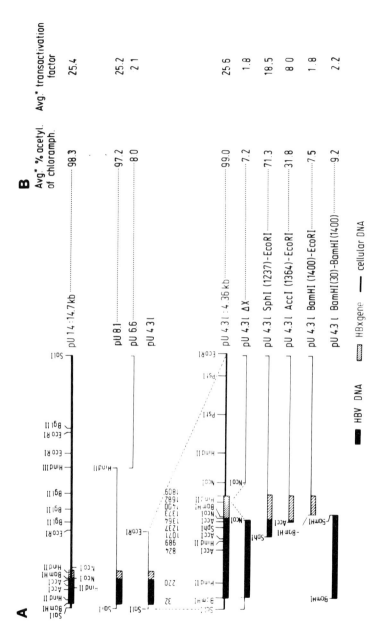

Figure 11 Restriction map of integrated HBV DNA clone pU1.4 and its deletion derivatives. The extents of deletions are indicated and the stimulatory activities obtained upon transfection into CCL13 cells are presented to the right of each construct.

required for production of viral mRNA. Therefore, in order to generate a functional X message, transcription would have to proceed through adjacent cellular DNA and terminate at a cellular polyadenylylation site. We have examined RNA isolated from CCL13 cells transfected ith PU4.31 DNA. . An unexpectedly long X transcript of about 10 kb is produced (Figure 12). The failure of this transcript to hybridize to a probe derived from S sequences indicates that it could only have arisen from the X promoter, which means that the transcript contained up to 9 kb of cellular RNA. Nucleotide sequence analyses (not shown) indicated that there is a fused open-reading frame between the viral X gene and at least 228 bases of cellular DNA, indicating that a fusion protein is possible. While there is no direct evidence for the

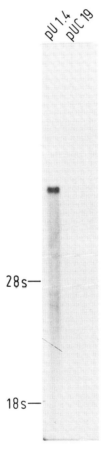

Figure 12 Fusion mRNA consisting of X and cellular domains. Plasmid pU1.4 DNA was transfected into CCL13 cells. RNA was isolated 48 h after transfection, and analysed by Northern blotting. An X-specific probe was used for hybridization. There was no signal when the filter was strip-washed and hybridized to an S-specific probe (data not shown). Cells transfected with pUC 19 vector DNA did not produce RNA hybridizing to the X probe. Ribosomal 28S and 18S RNA were used as size markers.

synthesis of such a protein, the results of the transactivation experiments strongly suggest that it is made. Lack of tissue from the original tumour precludes any effort to determine whether such a product was actually made *in vivo*. Future experiments with other tumours will provide important information on this question.

The experiments described in this report and Wollersheim *et al.* (Ref. 11 in a paper submitted for publication) thus establish that the hepatitis B virus produces a protein with the ability to stimulate gene expression by a *trans* mechanism. This product which is encoded within the X gene of HBV increases the level of transcription of the activated gene. A frame-shift mutation in the X coding sequence abolishes the activity. In transfection experiments a promoter lying upstream of the X ORF is efficient in transcription of the gene, although this particular promoter has not yet been shown to be active in naturally-infected cells. A number of viral enhancer–promoters tested show that the activity of the X product is rather broad, even though in certain cases there was little activity under the experimental conditions used. This indicates that the X protein may function indirectly by interacting with cellular proteins rather than directly with DNA. Experiments using a variety of cell lines strongly suggested the existence of cellular factors which influence the function of the X protein. The results indicate phylogenetically closer related species to be more supportive of X function, thus encouraging the speculation that X gene function may have some role in determining the tropism of the virus.

The observation that various enhancer–promoters are activated by the X product also might suggest that the effect is exerted at the level of the enhancer. The efficient expression of the X gene itself is dependent on the presence of the enhancer. This view is supported by the fact that when the enhancer is deleted as in plasmid pU4.3 Sph-Eco, the level of activity is considerably reduced (Figure 11). Similar conclusions have been recently reported by other investigators[15]. In addition to the X promoter[10], the surface[16] and core[6,17], promoters have also been shown to be influenced by the HBV enhancer. The product of the X gene in turn has a positive effect on the enhancer (Figure 9). Thus, there could be a mechanism by which all the viral genes can be regulated by the X-gene product via the enhancer. This possibility must be considered in attempting to define the viral function(s) of the X gene. It may well be that in the absence of a functional X product viral gene expression and virus replication are diminished. Recent experiments with frame-shift mutation of the X gene led to the conclusion that the X gene was not necessary for the replication of HBV[18]. However, the system used in those studies was among the first ever established for HBV replication and, as such, perhaps not sensitive enough to monitor X gene modulation of virus replication. Moreover, the conservation of the gene in mammalian hepadnaviruses[19], and the effects of its product on viral promoters would argue for an essential role. In the integrated HBV sequences from a tumour, described above, the X gene was functional in transactivation despite the deletion of 28 bases at its 3′ end. This raises the possibility that a truncated X gene could give rise to a functional product(s). This would also be consistent with the results of Yaginuma *et al.*[18] in whose experiments the frame-shift mutation was introduced in the 3′ portion of the X gene.

Whatever the viral function of the X gene, the ability of its product to transactivate gene expression may have important implications in HBV-induced liver diseases, particularly hepatocellular carcinoma. The need to consider the possible importance of transactivation in tumour development is also underscored by the lack of evidence for a common HBV cis-mediated role. The observation that the X function of integrated HBV in tumours is conserved in a number of cases studied (this report and unpublished observations) adds substance to this speculation. HBV-X sequences are frequently present in tumour cells even when other HBV genes are not[19,20]. Because integration often involves DNA sequences in the X region[20] the gene is often truncated and this leads to the expression of fusion transcripts of X-cellular composition and which as a consequence have altered properties[21]. The significance of such products for transformation is being investigated. In HTLV-related human T-cell leukaemias, the HTLV I transactivator gene is shown to be able to activate the promoter of the gene encoding interleukin-2 receptor (IL $2R\alpha$)[5,22]. Since IL $2R\alpha$ is specifically expressed in infected cells and is strongly implicated in T-lymphocyte transformation, there is good reason for considering transactivation to be very important to the process of viral transformation. Analogous mechanisms might be envisioned in HBV-related hepatocarcinogenesis. It is important to identify cellular genes involved in transformation and to study their possible activation by hepatitis B virus.

Acknowledgements

We are grateful to Drs. P. Gruss, B. Howard, R. Miksicek, R. Renkawitz, H. Schaller and H. Will for kind gifts of plasmids. We thank Elisabeth Bürgelt, Sabine Hankel and Antje Klem-Andres for excellent technical assistance. The contributions of Ute Debelka to this work are also acknowledged. This study was supported by funds from the Deutsche Stiftung für Krebsforschung.

Note added in proof

Since the submission of this paper, the work of Wollersheim et al. has been published; Oncogene, 3, 545–52 (1988).

References

1. Beasley, R. P. (1982). Hepatitis B virus as the etiologic agent in hepatocellular carcinoma —epidemiologic considerations. Hepatology, 2, 21–6
2. Summers, J. and Mason, W. S. (1982). Replication of the genome of a hepatitis B-like virus by reverse transcriptase of an RNA intermediate. Cell, 29, 403–15
3. Miller, R. H. and Robinson, W. S. (1986). Common evolutionary origin of hepatitis B virus and retroviruses. Proc. Natl. Acad. Sci. USA, 83, 2531–5
4. Wong-Staal, F. and Gallo, R. C. (1985). Human T-lymphotropic retroviruses. Nature, 317, 395–403

5. Cross, S. L., Feinberg, M., Wolf, J. B., Holbrook, N. J., Wong-Staal, F. and Leonard, W. J. (1987). Regulation of the human interleukin-2-receptor alpha-chain promoter: Activation of a nonfunctional promoter by the transactivator gene of HTVL-1. *Cell*, **49**, 47–56

6. Shaul, Y., Rutter, W. J. and Lamb, O. (1985). A human hepatitis B viral enhancer element. *EMBO Journal*, **4**, 427–30

7. Tognoni, A., Cattaneo, R., Serfling, E. and Schaffner, W. (1985). A novel expression selection approach allows precise mapping of the hepatitis B virus enhancer. *Nucl. Acids Res.*, **13**, 7457–72

8. Tiollais, P., Pourcel, C. and Dejean, A. (1985). The hepatitis B virus. *Nature*, **317**, 489–95

9. Gough, N. M. (1983). Core and E antigen synthesis in rodent cells transformed with hepatitis B virus DNA is associated with greater than genome length viral messenger RNAs. *J. Mol. Biol.*, **165**, 683–99

10. Treinin, M. and Laub, O. (1987). Identification of a promoter element located upstream from the hepatitis B virus X gene. *Mol. Cell Biol.*, **7**, 545–8

11. Zahm, P., Hofschneider, P. H. and Koshy, R. (1988). The HBV X-ORF encodes a transactivator: A potential factor in viral hepatocarcinogenesis. *Oncogene*, **3**, 169–77

12. Siddiqui, A., Jameel, S. and Mapoles, J. (1987). Expression of hepatitis B virus X gene in mammalian cells. *Proc. Natl. Acad. Sci. USA*, **84**, 2513–17

13. Ganem, D. and Varmus, H. E. (1987). The molecular biology of the hepatitis B virus. *Ann. Rev. Biochem.*, **56**, 651–93

14. Koshy, R. (1987). Integrated hepatitis B virus genomes in human primary liver cancer: A consideration of molecular mechanisms of oncogenesis. In Hofschneider, P. H. and Munk, K. (eds) Viruses in human tumors, *Contr. Oncol.*, Vol. **24**, pp. 97–112

15. Spandau, F. D. and Lee, C-H. (1988). Transactivation of viral enhancers by the hepatitis B virus X protein. *J. Virol.*, **62**, 427–34

16. Chang, H. K., Chou, C. K., Chang, C., Su, T. S., Hu, C. P., Yoshida, M. and Ting, L. P. (1987). The enhancer sequence of human hepatitis B virus can enhance the activity of its surface gene promoter. *Nucl. Acids Res.*, **15**, 2261–8

17. Roosinck, M. J., Jameel, S., Loukin, S. H. and Siddiqui, A. (1986). Expression of hepatitis B viral core region in mammalian cells. *Mol. Cell Biol.*, **6**, 1393–1400

18. Yaginuma, K., Shirakata, Y., Kobayashi, M. and Koike, K. (1987). Hepatitis B virus (HBV) particles are produced in a cell culture system by transient expression of transfected HBV DNA. *Proc. Natl. Acad. Sci. USA*, **84**, 2678–82

19. Kodama, K., Ogasawara, N., Yoshikama, H. and Murakami, S. (1985). Nucleotide sequence of a cloned woodchuck hepatitis virus genome: Evolutionary relationship between hepadnaviruses. *J. Virol.*, **56**, 978–86

20. Nagaya, T., Nakamura, T., Tokino, T., Tsurimoto, T., Imai, M., Mayumi, T., Kamino, K., Yamamura, K. and Matsubara, K (1987). The mode of hepatitis B virus DNA integration in chromosomes of human hepatocellular carcinoma. *Genes and Development*, **1**, 773–82

21. Freytag von Loringhoven, A., Koch, S., Hofschneider, P. H. and Koshy, R. (1985). Co-transcribed 3' host sequences augment expression of integrated hepatitis B virus DNA. *EMBO Journal*, **4**, 249–55

13
Is there a direct genetic role for hepatitis B virus in oncogenesis?

G. M. DUSHEIKO

The major antecendent factors preceding the development of hepatocellular carcinoma (HCC) are chronic hepatitis B virus (HBV) infection, cirrhosis, and exposure to chemical carcinogens. The majority of cases of HCC worldwide are associated with chronic HBV infection, but the role of HBV in hepatocarcinogenesis is incompletely understood[1]. Chronic phasic necro-inflammation associated with hepatitis B virus (HBV) infection may induce regeneration and eventually malignant transformation. However, HBV may of itself exert direct genetic effects during long-standing infection which may play a role in the pathogenesis of HCC.

HBV virus integrations are accumulated during chronic infection, but the functional significance of these integrations is unknown[2]. They may be inconsequential, or actually play a central role in carcinogenesis[3-5]. The fact that the HBV virus is a retrovirus-like agent[6] argues for its oncogenic potential, but we must reconcile the knowledge that:

1. HCC usually develops several decades after the original infection, and after viral integrations can be detected by molecular hybridization during the phase of chronic infection.
2. A common unique integration has not been isolated in man.
3. The hepatitis B virus lacks a known oncogene.
4. The tumour develops in only a minority of patients with chronic HBV infection.

HBV integration undoubtedly plays an initiating role; integration of HBV genomes in host hepatocytes confers a selective growth advantage to affected cells, as viral nucleocapsid antigens (HBcAg and HBeAg)[7] are not expressed in these hepatocytes, and they are consequently protected from the host immune response. However, can a further direct genetic effect be considered?

In some cases, insertional mutagenesis may play a role. There are recent reports of the production of a new cellular gene containing a HBV integration and coding for a retinoic acid–DNA binding receptor gene[8,9]. The characterization of this fusion gene is interesting but the functional significance of such a novel gene is unknown. Deletions and translocations induced by HBV integration may lead to loss of cellular alleles, and in particular loss of tumour-suppressor genes[10]. In the woodchuck *c-myc* amplification associated with woodchuck HBV integration has been reported[11].

Are these chromosomal aberrations the important ones? Are these aberrations one of two, three or many required for malignant transformation? The dispersal of HBV DNA within the genome as a result of the chromosomal instability conferred by HBV integrations, and the resulting translocations may be critical genetic factors, but we have not yet explained the sequence of events, and the cascade of genetic effects may not be the same in all tumours. These events may indeed be difficult to track, since the human genome comprises four gigabases (1 gigabase is 4×10^9 bases) with at least 100 000 genes. Only 2% of the human genome is composed of genes and the remainder contains repetitive sequences whose function is unknown. We lack the critical evidence incriminating the insertion of 3200 bases of HBV virus that may be of critical importance.

Several regions of the hepatitis B virus genome have been shown to possess promoter or gene regulatory function. More precise genetic information is emerging, however. An enhancer region of the hepatitis B virus genome has been identified as an important controlling element of the C and S gene promoters[12,13]. The HBV enhancer shows some tissue specificity and since enhancers may activate native and heterologous genes relatively independently of orientation with respect to the coding region, may conceivably activate cellular genes.

If HBV virus integrates anywhere in the cell, for it to play a direct genetic role, it must be capable of activating cellular genes at a distance. This mechanism is termed 'transactivation'. The X gene of HBV and the *tat* gene of HTLV I are positioned identically with respect to their genome organization[14]. The *tat* gene plays a key role in HTLV I viral replication, and also interacts with specific target sequences, notably the enhancers located in the long terminal repeats of this virus[15]. The *tat* gene is probably essential for viral regulation and also may play a key role in the transforming effect of the virus[16]. Recent evidence has suggested that the X gene of HBV is a transactivating factor for viral enhancers (Figure 1), and that the X gene encodes a protein having the ability to stimulate transcription[18]. Such a transactivating protein may stimulate heterologous cellular enhancers and indeed serve as a modulator of gene expression. Chapter 12 by Koshy *et al.* provides further elegant experimental evidence that the X gene may function as a transactivator.

These new developments take advantage of powerful new methodology including computer modelling, and rapid methods of sequencing, as well as transfection cell systems, which will greatly expedite our understanding of any direct genetic role that HBV may play in hepatocarcinogenesis. Although we are a long way from understanding this role, it is possible that the verification of a transactivating function of the X gene may have implications that are immediately applicable, such as the recognition of cellular neo-

Trans-activating role x gene?

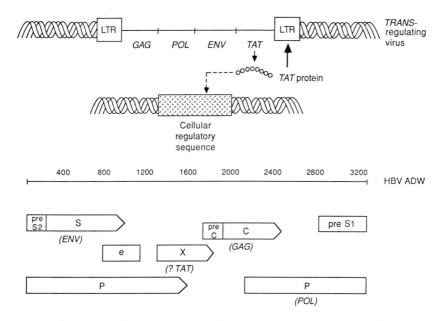

Figure 1 Comparison of the genome organization of a *trans*-regulating retrovirus (upper sequence) and HBV (lower sequence)

differentiation associated with expression of X gene in patients with chronic hepatitis; such evidence may facilitate the screening of hepatitis B virus carriers who may be at risk for hepatocellular carcinoma. Finally, the recognition that X gene may play a transactivating role may also lead to more rational antiviral therapy for hepatitis B carriers.

References

1. Beasley, R. P. and Hwang L-Y. (1984). Epidemiology of hepatocellular carcinoma. In Vyas, G. N., Dinstag, J. L. and Hoofnagle, J. H. (eds) *Viral Hepatitis and Liver Disease*. pp. 209–24. (New York: Grune & Stratton Orlando)
2. Brechot, C., Hadchouel, N., Scotto, J. *et al.* (1981). Detection of hepatitis B virus DNA in liver and serum: a direct appraisal of the carrier state. *Lancet,* **2**, 765–8
3. Tiollais, P., Pourcel, C. and Dejean, A. (1985). Hepatitis B virus. *Nature,* **317**, 489–95
4. Alexander, J. J., Bey, E., Geddes, E. W. *et al.* (1976). Establishment of a continuously growing cell line from a primary carcinoma of the liver. *S. Afr. Med. J.,* **50**, 2124–8
5. Brechot, C., Pourcel, C., Louise, A. *et al.* (1980). Presence of integrated hepatitis B virus DNA sequences in cellular DNA of human hepatocellular carcinoma. *Nature,* **286**, 533–5
6. Bishop, J. M. (1983). Cellular oncogenes and retroviruses. *Annu. Rev. Biochem.,* **52**, 301–54
7. Chen, J-Y., Harrison, T. J., Lee, C-Siu *et al.* (1988). Detection of hepatitis B virus DNA in hepatocellular carcinoma: analysis by hybridization with sub-genomic DNA fragments. *Hepatology,* **8**, 518–23

8. Dejean, A., Bougueleret, L., Grzeschik, K. H. *et al.* (1986). Hepatitis B virus DNA integration in a sequence homologous to *v-erb-A* and steroid receptor genes in a hepatocellular carcinoma. *Nature,* **322**, 70–2

9. Benbrook, D., Lernhardt, E. and Pfahl, M. (1988). A new retinoic acid receptor identified from a hepatocellular carcinoma. *Nature,* **333**, 669–72

10. Hino, O., Shows, T. B. and Rogler, C. E. (1986). Hepatitis B virus integration site in hepatocellular carcinoma at chromosome 17;18 translocation. *Proc. Natl. Acad. Sci. USA,* **83**, 8338–42

11. Moroy, T., Marchio, A., Etiemble, J. *et al.* (1986). Rearrangement and enhanced expression of *c-myc* in hepatocellular carcinoma of hepatitis virus in infected woodchucks. *Nature,* **324**, 276–9

12. Shaul, Y., Rutter, W. J. and Laub, O. (1985). A human hepatitis B viral enhancer element. *EMBO J.,* **4**, 427–30

13. Siddiqui, A., Jameel, S. and Mapoles, J. (1986). Transcriptional control elements of HBsAg gene. *Proc. Natl. Acad. Sci. USA,* **83**, 566–70

14. Miller, R. H. and Robinson, W. S. (1986). Common evolutionary origin of hepatitis B virus and retroviruses. *Proc. Natl. Acad. Sci. USA,* **83**, 2531–5

15. Arya, F. K., Guo, C., Josephs, S. F. and Wong-Staal, F. (1985). Transactivator gene of human T-lymphotropic virus type III (HTLV-III). *Science,* **229**, 69–73

16. Chen, I. S. Y., Flamon, J. D., Rosenblatt, N. P. *et al.* (1985). The X gene is essential for HTLV replication. *Science,* **229**, 54–8

17. Spandau, D. F. and Lee, C-H. (1988). Transactivation of viral enhancers by the hepatitis B virus X protein. *J. Virol.,* **62**, 427–34

18. Twu, J-S. and Schloemer, R. H. (1987). Transcriptional transactivating function of hepatitis B virus. *J. Virol.,* **61**, 3448–53

14
Structure, expression, and potential oncogenicity of hepatitis B virus proteins

W. H. GERLICH, K. -H. HEERMANN, V. BRUSS, M. HÖHNE,
B. KRONE, S. SCHAEFER AND M. SEIFER

INTRODUCTION

Hepatitis B virus (HBV) of man belongs to the hepadnavirus family. As with the other mammalian viruses of this family, HBV encodes four open-reading frames (orf) in its DNA-minus strand: C for core (or capsid) proteins, S for surface (or envelope) proteins, P for polymerase, and X for a small protein of unknown function[1]. This chapter will focus on the structure, function, and expression of S and C proteins and present preliminary findings on oncogenesis *in vitro* by HBV.

SURFACE PROTEINS

Nomenclature

The circular genome of hepadnaviruses is one of the smallest among all viruses. The encoding capacity of its ca. 3200 bases is, however, extremely economically used. One example of this is the S-orf. It is situated completely within the larger P-orf. Moreover, it encodes not only one, but three, proteins. It does so by using three functional initiation codons for protein translation (AUG) but only one stop codon. Thus, three co-terminal proteins of different size are derived from the S-orf (see Figure 1).

Originally only the smallest protein was discovered as the major component of hepatitis B surface antigen (HBsAg) particles in the blood of virus carriers[2]. In SDS gel electrophoresis this protein had an apparent molecular weight of 22 to 26 kilodaltons (kDa). It occurs also in a form[2] which contains a complex glycan linked to its Asn-146. We refer to this protein as P24^s and GP27^s or SHBs for small HBsAg protein but the terms

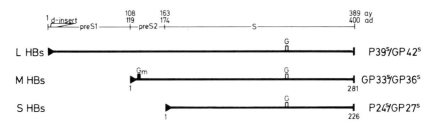

Figure 1 Organization and products of the open reading frame for the surface proteins (S-orf). Gy, N-linked glycoside; Gm, mannose-rich glycoside. The numbers refer to the codons or amino acids respectively; 'ay' and 'ad' refer to the HBsAg subtypes.

P25[s] and GP28[s] are also used. The gene[2] encoding SHBs was named gene S and the 5' proximal part of the S-orf region preS because its function was not known at this time[3].

In 1982, two further protein bands were detected in purified HBsAg particles from the blood of HBV carriers which were named[4] GP33[s] and GP36[s]. These proteins[5,6] are co-terminal with SHBs; they have an amino terminal extension which is encoded by the preS2 segment[3,7-10]. A mannose-rich glycan is linked to Asn-4 of GP33[s] and GP36[s]. The only difference between GP33[s] and GP36[s] is that GP36[s] has a complex glycan[5] linked at the same site as GP27[s]. We suggest middle HBsAg proteins as a name for these proteins.

The blood of chronic HBV carriers contains three types of virus-derived particles: 22-nm HBsAg particles, filamentous HBsAg particles, and the virions themselves. The 22-nm particles are the most abundant and usually reach titers[11] up to 10^{14}/ml serum or typically 10–500 μg HBsAg proteins/ml. The filaments are less abundant (<1 μg/ml) and the virions are least abundant (<100 ng/ml). By gel electrophoretic analysis of filaments and virions two further proteins P39[s] and GP42[s] became visible[12], which were later shown to be encoded by the complete S-orf[13-16]. We refer to these proteins as large HBsAg protiens (LHBs).

The gene of LHBs is evidently identical with the S-orf (except the few codons upstream of the first AUG). We suggest designating the genes of the three HBs proteins as *lhbs, mhbs* and *shbs*. The three initiation codons of *lhbs* divide it into three functional segments. In agreement with previous nomenclature[1], we suggest the terms preS1 for the segment present only in *lhbs*, preS2 for the segment present in *mhbs* also, and S for the carboxy-terminal part in *mhbs* or *lhbs*. The corresponding protein domains are Pre-S1, PreS2 and S. The numbering of the codons or amino acids depends on the subtype of HBsAg. Most 'd'-subtypes have an insertion of 11 amino acids after the two first amino acids of PreS1[17]. Thus, the length of *lhbs* is 389 codons for subtypes 'y' and 400 for most subtypes 'd'. For better comparability some authors use the same number for subtypes 'd' and 'y', with codon 3 to 13 being absent in 'y'. The length of *mhbs* and *shbs* is identical for all subtypes.

The small HBsAg protein (SHBs)

Physical properties

The small HBsAg protein is the major component of all three HBV-associated particles in the blood of virus carriers. In natural HBsAg particles, ca. 40% of the SHBs are glycosylated but glycosylation seems not to be essential for morphogenesis, secretion, or conformation of the protein. SHBs from many transfected cell cultures contains much less glycoside but still forms authentic 22-nm particles. The particles contain approximately 25% lipid derived from the ER membrane[18]. This is different to most viral envelopes where the lipid is derived from the plasma membrane and where its proportion is much higher. Thus, HBsAg 22-nm particles have a higher density than most enveloped viruses; they band at 35% (w/w) sucrose or 1.20 g/cm^3 in CsCl solution. The SHBs protein is extremely hydrophobic, especially a sequence between amino acids 81 and 99 and the whole carboxy-terminal region beyond amino acid 148. A typical property of SHBs in all mammalian hepadnaviruses is the high content of Trp and the low content of Tyr. Thus SHBs has a very high specific UV absorbance at 280 nm of 4.2 per g/litre and a distinct Trp-specific peak at 291 nm[11]. SHBs is extremely resistant to proteases, heat, and chaotropic substances, but very sensitive to ionic detergents and reduction.

Antigenicity

A region between amino acids 120 and 148 has been shown to be surface exposed and to be antigenic. The major B-cell epitopes of this more hydrophilic region are conformational and highly dependent on disulphide bonds. In fact the region contains 7 cysteines which are intra-molecularly cross-linked. Cys-121, 124, and 221 are probably involved in inter-molecular cross-linking[19].

Immunization of laboratory animals or human vaccinees with 22-nm particles does not lead to well-detectable levels of SHBs sequence-specific antibodies while conformational antibody titres are usually very high after relatively small doses of HBsAg[13]. An exchange of Arg-122 (d) to Lys (y) has been shown to generate one major subtype-specific epitope but there are certainly other subtype-specific epitopes with other exchanges being involved[20]. The antigenic part of the S domain contains more subtype-specific nucleotides and amino acid exchanges than the other parts of SHBs.

Several peptides of the region were able to induce antibodies to natural HBsAg particles (antiHBs) and some of them induced also partial protection in chimpanzees which had been immunized with them[21]. A cyclic peptide was found to be more immunogenic than the corresponding linear peptide[22]. However, not only intra-molecular conformation but also inter-molecular assembly seems to confer antigenicity. A HBV-neutralizing monoclonal antibody RF6 was found to react with dimers or polymers of SHBs, but not with monomeric SHBs[23]. Thus, the prospect of using SHBs partial peptides as vaccine components instead of whole HBsAg particles is not very promising.

However, a T-cell epitope has been defined at partial peptide amino acid 4–33 which is more efficiently presented by denatured or fragmented SHBs than by native particles[24].

Biosynthesis of HBsAg 22-nm particles

The other parts of SHBs are either buried in the lipid layer or face toward the internal side of the particles. SHBs contains an amino-terminal signal peptide for insertion into the endoplasmic reticulum (ER) and an additional internal translocation signal at amino acids 81 to 98. In spite of being highly hydrophobic the carboxy-terminal part does not induce translocation to the ER by itself. The polypeptide chain of SHBs spans at least twice[25] but probably four or more times the lipid layer[19]. Glycosylation of GP27[s] is co-translational. After completed protein synthesis, SHBs molecules are attracted to each other by unknown forces and extrude as particles to the lumen of the ER. Secretion of the particles is much less rapid as for typical secretory proteins and requires 24 h[26]. All mammalian cells are able to form and secrete HBsAg particles. Insect cells synthesize SHBs particles very efficiently under the control of baculovirus vectors[27], but the secretion of the particles may be even more sluggish than in mammalian cells[28]. Yeast cells synthesize non-glycosylated SHBs efficiently, but particle formation is incomplete or only induced *in vitro* after extraction[23,29]. *E. coli* does not synthesize complete SHBs efficiently and assembly of particles does not occur at all.

The middle protein (MHBs)

Discovery and biochemical properties of MHBs

MHBs was definitively described only in 1982 although SDS gel electrophoresis had been applied to HBsAg particles since 1970. One reason for this was the weak staining of all HBs proteins by Coomassie Blue and the inability to distinguish the MHBs protein band from impurities. A second reason was that the proportion of MHBs to SHBs is highly variable in different human carriers of HBsAg. Highly viraemic carriers have not only more HBsAg (typically 100 μg/ml) than low viraemic carriers (typically 10 μg/ml) but they have also more MHBs. Although exact figures are not available, staining intensities suggest that HBsAg from viraemic carriers contains 5–10% MHBs (molar ratio) while low viraemic carriers contain 1–3% MHBs. Thus, the appearance of MHBs in gels was a variable and partially irreproducible finding. A third reason was the use of proteases for purification of HBsAg by many investigators. Since the major protein SHBs was very resistant against all kinds of proteases, the loss of a minor component was not noted. The most widely-used hepatitis B vaccine made from human viraemic plasma was in fact treated with pepsin. Other plasma-derived vaccines were not treated with protease but for safety reasons they were made from low viraemic plasma. Thus, they had a variable and always very low content of MHBs.

Unambiguous detection of MHBs in highly-purified HBsAg became initially possible by silver staining of SDS gels. All three HBs proteins are more intensely stained by silver than most other proteins. In an independent approach MHBs was discovered by Machida *et al.* by its ability to bind polymerized human serum albumin (pHSA). A very efficient way of detection is the immunoblot using antisera against natural HBsAg particles[13]. In contrast to antibodies against S epitopes, the preS2 epitopes are mostly (or completely) sequential[15]. Thus, the MHBs may be selectively stained by poly-valent antiserum against natural HBsAg in spite of being a minor component. The relationship between MHBs and SHBs was shown by partial proteolysis[5]. Some tryptic fragments of MHBs and SHBs were identical, while other fragments were consistent with the hypothesis that MHBs contained (in addition to SHBs) an amino-terminal extension of glycosylated preS2. The overall amino acid composition of MHBs and SHBs was very similar. Machida *et al.* showed in addition that the three carboxy-terminal amino acids of MHBs and SHBs were identical[6]. They also found the amino-terminal amino acid of MHBs to be methionine. In our experience the amino end of MHBs is difficult or impossible to detect by Edman degradation (K. -H. Heermann, unpublished observation). The presence of the preS2 sequence in MHBs was proved by Machida *et al.* by analysing the amino acid composition of its amino-terminal CNBr fragment[7]. Neurath *et al.* showed further that a preS2-specific peptide antiserum stained MHBs but not SHBs[8].

The presence of N-linked mannose-rich glycans in MHBs was shown by digestion of HBsAg particles with endoglycosidase H^4. This enzyme converts $GP36^s$ to a $GP33^s$ and $GP33^s$ to a $P30^s$ while $GP27^s$ is resistant. Endoglyco-sidase F which also cleaves complex N-linked glycans[13] converted $GP36^s$ and $GP33^s$ to $P30^s$ and $GP27^s$ to $P24^s$. A non-glycosylated P30-MHBs protein has not yet been found in natural HBsAg particles. The glycan always seems to be located at Asn-4 of preS2. The mannose-rich glycan contains terminal sialic acid, because the size of $GP33/36^s$ is slightly but significantly reduced by digestion with neuraminidase[4]. Asn-146 of the S domain is less frequently glycosylated in MHBs than in SHBs. In MHBs containing HBsAg particles from mammalian cell culture, this site is often completely unoccupied, e.g. in a new vaccine derived from Chinese hamster ovary cells[30]. The addition of sialic acid to this glycan is possibly a secondary event because mannose-rich glycans are usually secreted without terminal sialic acid. Glycoprotein with-out terminal sialic acid should theoretically be trapped by the liver-specific asialoglycoprotein receptor and finally be released again with terminal sialic acid. The conservation of the glycosylation signal Asn–X–Ser or Thr in the otherwise barely homologous preS2 domains of all mammalian HBVs suggests a functional role for the glycan which is, however, not yet understood.

Trypsin cleaves the PreS2 domain in natural HBsAg particles rapidly at arginines 16 and/or 18. Thus, this site is well exposed at the surface of the particles. Digestion of preS2-rich HBsAg particles with trypsin increases the reactivity with SHBs-specific antibodies[13]. These data suggest that the preS2 domain covers the external sites of the S domain in MHBs. Particles con-taining only MHBs would probably not expose the complete S antigenicity.

Biosynthesis of MHBs

The HBV genome contains an efficient promoter within the preS1 gene segment[31]. This promoter lacks the so-called TATA box. It is similar to the Simian virus 40 late (SV40L) promoter and resembles the promoters of many constitutively expressed 'house-keeping genes'. Mammalian cells indeed express MHBs and SHBs in an unregulated way if HBV genomes or sufficient parts of it are transfected to them. The TATA box adjusts the RNA polymerase to initiate transcription at a defined site downstream. In the absence of a TATA box, several initiation sites may be used. In the case of the SV40L-like promoter, a part of the mRNA initiates at a site upstream of the preS2 segment and a part downstream[32]. Thus, this promoter governs the expression of both MHBs and SHBs protein. It is not yet clear which factors determine the variable ratio between *mhbs* and *shbs* expression *in vivo*. In the absence of heterologous regulatory sequences, production of SHBs is always more efficient and the HBsAg particles contain less than 10% MHBs. Even if pure *mhbs* RNA is translated *in vitro* some SHBs is formed[33]. Apparently, the AUG of preS2 is not flanked by the optimal bases and may occasionally be ignored at the initiation of translation.

The amino-terminal region of PreS2 may possibly not function as translocation signal to the ER. Its complete glycosylation shows, however, that it is translocated to the lumen of the ER. The translocation itself is apparently induced by the first signal sequence within the S domain. The appearance of additional S antigenicity after removal of the PreS2 domain (see above) suggests that at least the folding and transmembranous configuration of MHBs beyond amino acid 100 of S is similar to that of SHBs. MHBs is also cross-linked by disulphide bonds with itself and/or SHBs because very little SHBs or MHBs is visible in gel electrophoresis without prior reduction[4].

Albumin binding by PreS2

The interaction of HBsAg with 'polymerized' human serum albumin has been known since the early seventies. Initially misunderstood as 'anti-albumin', it became clear that HBsAg was able to aggregate albumin-coated erythrocytes. The interaction between HBsAg and albumin is species-specific so that human and chimpanzee albumin are reactive while serum albumins from other species are inactive[6]. Since liver cells were also found to bind 'polymerized' albumin, the idea came up that the albumin receptor would adsorb HBV via albumin to the liver cell. This hypothesis is consistent with the narrow host range of HBV, its organ tropism and with the fact that viraemic carriers had more albumin receptors than low viraemic carriers. A problem of this theory is the fact that only glutaraldehyde-treated albumin binds efficiently to HBsAg[34]. Glutaraldehyde causes cross-linking or 'polymerization' of albumin and consequently it was suggested that the binding was specific for polymerized human serum albumin (pHSA). It turned out, however, that other agents for cross-linking of albumin including ageing were ineffective in generating binding capacity for PreS2. On the other hand, glutaraldehyde-treated monomeric albumin is able to bind to PreS2 in protein blots[35]. We suggest that not the *polymerization* but a *modification* of albumin generates strong binding to PreS2[36]. Most assay systems are, however, designed in a way that polymerization may further increase the binding. The dependence of the albumin binding on glutaraldehyde raises serious doubts about the biological significance of this *in vitro* phenomenon. A further argument against its significance is the fact that with the woodchuck HBV no such phenomenon is observed[37].

Nevertheless, albumin binding also occurs *in vivo* in the absence of artificial chemicals. HSA has for long been identified as a component of purified HBsAg particles from human plasma. Only recently it was shown that the HSA is not only a contaminant but that it co-purifies with HBsAg particles in gel chromatography and density-gradient centrifugation[35]. In CsCl, HSA is partially dissociated from HBsAg. Unmodified HSA either in purified form or in normal human serum binds to CsCl-purified HBsAg as can be shown by a slight increase of size and density[35]. The binding depends on the presence of PreS2 because pretreatment with trypsin abolishes the binding of albumin and anti-PreS2-specific monoclonal antibodies inhibit the binding (B. Krone, unpublished observations). The binding of natural albumin can also be inhibited by pHSA and vice versa. It has also been noted that SHBs may bind albumin at its physiological concentrations of ca. 40 mg/ml[38], but binding to PreS2 occurs at albumin concentrations below 1 mg/ml. The exact site of HSA binding within the PreS2 domain is now known. The binding of HSA is inhibited by a set of three non-overlapping sequential epitopes (B. Krone, unpublished observations) represented by three antibodies (Q19/10 [ref. 36] or F124, F376 [ref. 43] and E21/14, K.-H. Heermann, unpublished observations).

The HSA which bound to PreS2 was in our experience monomeric although the serum from which the HBsAg was isolated[35,36] contained some natural pHSA. Possibly, an unknown cofactor induces both binding to HBV and at another site to the hepatocyte membrane. The very low binding capacity of HSA in normal human serum for ca. 10 nM PreS2/litre suggests[36] that only a modified HSA can bind to PreS2. Using a PreS2-specific antibody Q19/10, most HBsAg carriers with $< 10 \mu g$ HBsAg/ml were unreactive in an ELISA, while carriers with higher concentrations gave a positive reaction for PreS2 antigen[36]. When the unreactive HBsAg was analysed by immunoblot the same antibody detected MHBs in them. Viraemic carriers usually have high concentrations of HBsAg and a higher proportion of MHBs, and this allows for the presence of free PreS2 domains in their serum. The low viraemic carrier (who is usually anti-HBe positive) contains MHBs in connection with HSA. This explains the often noted correlation of free pHSA receptors with viraemia.

The biological significance of the HSA binding remains unsolved. The original suggestion of a pHSA linker between HBV and hepatocyte membranes can be confirmed *in vitro* but the PreS1 domain seems to be far more important for the binding to hepatocytes (A. Pontisso, pers. commun.) Moreover, there is no evidence that a natural pHSA which binds to HBV occurs *in vivo*.

The importance of the PreS2 domain and also of HSA binding is, however, documented by the protective immunity induced by PreS2 peptides. Antisera to peptide 1-25 are able to neutralize 3000 infectious doses of HBV in chimpanzees[39]. Even more significantly, peptide 14-32 coupled to the hapten carrier keyhole limpet haemocyanin (KLH) induces direct protection by immunization[49]. Possibly, this protection is mediated merely by agglutination. It may, however, also indicate neutralization of an essential biological function.

Besides an ill-defined role in binding of HBsAg to hepatocytes, an important side effect of the HSA binding may be masking of the immunodominant B-cell recognition site. The binding is, however, not strong enough to prevent humoral immunity to PreS2 after recovery of a hepatitis B infection. There is neither confirmed evidence for an immunosuppressive effect of the PreS2 domain nor for induction of autoimmunity to albumin[41] both of which have been suggested as major pathogenic mechanisms in acute and chronic hepatitis B[42]. Several studies[43,44] reported early appearance of anti-PreS2 after acute hepatitis B and its absence in chronic carriers of HBV irrespective of the clinical state. Recipients of a recombinant PreS2-containing hepatitis B vaccine developed high titres of anti-S, anti-PreS2 antibodies but no evidence of liver damage, or of antibodies against albumin[30]. On the other hand, it remains to be shown if the PreS2 containing vaccine is indeed more immunogenic and/or more protective than conventional SHBs vaccines from yeast or mammalian cells.

The large HBsAg protein (LHBs)

Discovery and biochemical properties

The large HBsAg protein was the last discovered HBsAg protein because it is least abundant in the blood of virus carriers. However, as noted before, it forms a major part of the virion envelope and of the HBsAg filaments. The relationship of P39^s and GP42^s to SHBs and MHBs was first recognized by staining with anti-S and anti-PreS2-specific antibodies. The size of P39^s was consistent with a non-glycosylated translation product of the whole S-orf. Digestion with the Glu-specific V8 protease generated an expected 18-kDa Pre-S fragment. This fragment reacted with an HBV-specific monoclonal antibody (MA18/7) which did not bind to MHBs or SHBs[13]. The absence of N-linked glycan in P39^s or in the 18-kDa PreS fragment derived from P39^s and GP42^s showed that the PreS2 domain in LHBs was indeed not glycosylated. GP42^s contains, however, a N-linked glycan which can be removed[13] by endoglycosidase F. Although its position has not been experimentally studied, it is very likely that it is linked to Asn-146 of the S domain as with the other HBs proteins. The proportion of GP42^s to P39^s is higher[13] than that of GP36^s to GP33^s and of GP27^s to P29^s. The GP42^s band stains in fact usually stronger than the P39^s band when purified virions of HBsAg filaments are analyzed by gel electrophoresis. The mechanism of how the whole PreS sequence increases glycosylation of Asn-146 while the PreS2 sequence alone decreases it, is unknown. Even more astonishing is the fact that Asn-4 of PreS2 is completely glycosylated in MHBs and completely free in LHBs. The example of the HBs proteins shows that N-glycosylation is highly dependent on the amino-terminal sequences in a growing peptide chain.

The identity of the amino-terminal sequence in LHBs with the PreS1 sequence was suggested by the observation that LHBs from subtype 'ad' virions was ca. 1 kDa larger than that from subtype 'ay' carriers. This difference was not found for MHBs and SHBs. DNA sequence data had already shown that the PreS1 domain from subtype 'ad' had an insertion[17] of 11 codons between position 2 and 13. This conclusion was confirmed by the fact that the LHBs-specific antibody MA18/7 bound to 13 kDa preS1 encoded protein expressed in *E. coli*[45]. MA18/7 bound also to a fusion protein containing PreS amino acids 28–136 provided by J. Sninsky[14] (K.-H. Heermann, unpublished observations). Later, Neurath *et al.*[15] and Takahashi *et al.*[16] provided further structural evidence by staining LHBs with PreS1-specific peptide antisera.

Native virions and filaments reacted strongly with MA18/7. This suggested that the epitope of MA18/7 was accessible at the surface of these particles[13]. Digestion of virions or filaments with the Arg-specific protease clostripain cleaves LHBs very rapidly to a P32^s and GP35^s probably at Arg-101 (K.-H. Heermann, unpublished observations). Trypsin cleaves LHBs of subtype 'ay' also very well but LHBs of subtype 'ad' is relatively resistant. This is due to a subtype-specific exchange from a neighbouring Asn to Asp which prevents trypsin activity[47]. Furthermore, the arginines in the PreS2 domain which are accessible in MHBs cannot be cleaved in LHBs without prior cleavage of the PreS1 domain[46]. This suggests that the PreS1 domain masks the PreS2 domains in LHBs. It appears also that the PreS2 domain of LHBs does not contribute to the albumin binding capacity of virions[47] whereas denatured LHBs binds pHSA *in vitro* as well as MHBs does. The masking of the PreS2 and S domains by PreS1 is furthermore recognized by the impossibility to surface label the tyrosines in PreS2 or S which are accessible in MHBs or SHBs (W. H. Gerlich, unpublished observations). It is, however, not clear if PreS2 and S are *merely* covered by PreS1 or if they have a completely different folding in LHBs.

The PreS1 domain does not contain cysteines or large hydrophobic sequences. Thus, it is expected to be resistant against reduction or detergents. PreS1 antigen is indeed easily detectable by ELISA in reduced and alkylated HBsAg[46]. However, much anti-PreS reactivity is lost when fully denatured LHBs is used in immunoblots[46]. This finding suggests the presence of dominant conformational epitopes in the PreS1 domain. A detergent-sensitive element in the PreS1 domain may be myristic acid (a C_{14} fatty acid) which is bound as an amide to Gly-2 of the PreS1 sequence. Persing *et al.*[48] detected this interesting post-translational modification by adding radioactive myristic acid to cell cultures which produced LHBs after transfection. The radiolabel was found together with LHBs. Myristylation occurs at an amino-terminal peptide sequence Met–Gly which is conserved in PreS domains of all hepadnaviruses. Myristylation causes membrane insertion of proteins which might be otherwise located in the cytoplasm. It is very likely that the myristic acid inserts the amino end of PreS1 into the lipid layer of the virion envelope.

Biosynthesis of LHBs

Upstream of the LHBs gene is a promoter with a TATA box from which a 2.4-kb mRNA can be transcribed[32]. This mRNA can be translated to LHBs. It is a minor species in livers from acutely or chronically HBV-infected animals, like chimpanzees, woodchuck and ground squirrels. The preS specific mRNA is more abundant in HBV-infected ducks[49]. Expression of the 2.4-kb mRNA was shown first in the hepatoma cell line PLC/PRF/5. But even in this cell line it is also a minor transcript compared to the 2.1-kb mRNA[32]. Transcription in this cell line comes most likely from an HBV DNA insert which was cloned as plasmid pAI 10.7. Transfection of this plasmid to a mouse fibroblast cell line resulted in very efficient transcription of 2.1-kb mRNA and synthesis of PreS2 containing 22-nm HBsAg particles, but the 2.4-kb mRNA and PreS1 antigen were not expressed[50]. The same plasmid yielded a very good expression of all three HBs proteins after transfection into HeLa cells[51]. It is possible to grow these transfected tumour cells as solid tumour cells in nude mice. Growth of the PLC/PRF/5 cells in nude mice resulted in secretion of HBsAg to the serum of the mice. The tumours contain all three HBs proteins. Growth of the HeLa cells which had been transfected with PAI 10.7 did not lead to secretion of HBsAg. However, the tumour contained much LHBs as the only HBs protein. When the tumour cells were explanted to cell culture, secretion of LBsAg started again. These findings showed that the ratio of LHBs to the smaller HBs proteins was highly dependent on the nature of the cell and of its growth conditions. *In vivo* growth apparently favoured expression of *lhbs* and certain tumour cells also supported the expression of *lhbs*[52].

Expression of LHBs in HBV carriers is not yet fully understood. Viraemic carriers have more LHBs in form of virions and filaments in their blood than low viraemic carriers. The intrahepatic distribution of LHBs, as shown by immunofluorescence using monoclonal antibody MA 18/7, follows in viraemic carriers closely that of MHBs and of total HBs[53]. In low viraemic carriers the pattern is more complicated. They certainly have less LHBs in the serum but they have often much LHBs in the liver. This becomes most apparent by enzyme immunohistology (H. Dienes, pers. commun; H. C. Hsu, pers. commun.) but it has also been found by immunofluorescence[54]. It appears that in viraemic carriers, LHBs is usually exported by an excess of SHBs. Low viraemic carriers seem to have two types of HBV-positive cells. One type produces SHBs but very little LHBs and they secrete 22-nm HBsAg particles. In the other cell type, much more LHBs is produced and this prevents secretion. These cells resemble probably the well-known ground-glass cells of 'healthy' HBsAg carriers, and may present a milder form of the storage phenomenon found in the LHBs over-producing transgenic mice (see below).

The different expression of the *hbs* genes in hepatocytes may be caused by a different state of differentiation. Another explanation is the integration of HBV DNA in the host genome. Integrated HBV DNA is often incomplete. Those cells which harbour the *shbs* gene without *lhbs* would probably secrete SHBs at a moderate level. Cells where *lhbs* is integrated next to positive cellular regulation elements may over-express LHBs in relation to SHBs and MHBs[55].

Mouse fibroblasts[50,56] (LTK) and mouse hepatocytes[57] (line FMH 202, M. Höhne and S. Schaefer, unpublished observations) did not support much *lhbs* expression after transfection, but a transfected human hepatoma cell line[58] (Hep G 2.2.15) did. This points to the importance of species-specific factor(s) in the regulation of *lhbs*. Recently, a negative transcriptional factor was identified which binds to sequences within the preS1 segment and inhibits *lhbs* expression[59]. This factor seems to be inactive or absent in HeLa cells and in HepG2 cells. The growth phase may possibly also regulate the expression of *lhbs*.

The expression of *lhbs* can of course be forced by linkage to heterologous promoters and enhancers. Using SV40 vectors[60], retroviral vectors[61] or Vaccinia vectors[62] a strong expression of LHBs was obtained in the absence of MHBs or SHBs. These systems showed in agreement with the transfected Hela cells[52] that LHBs by itself cannot be secreted. Titration of mRNAs for LHBs, MHBs and SHBs in micro-injected oocytes showed an excess of LHBs inhibited secretion of SHBs as well[63]. *lhbs* coupled to the very strong albumin promoter or inducible metallothionein promoter was used to generate transgenic mice. These mice did not secrete HBsAg but they stored large amounts of LHBs in the ER[64]. The lumen of the ER was filled with very long filaments which were otherwise morphologically similar to the shorter filaments in the serum of virus carrier (see Chapter 16).

The analysis of HBsAg particles in serum suggests that a small proportion of LHBs ($<3\%$) does not visibly alter the morphology of spherical particles, a moderate proportion (10–20%) generates filaments, while particles containing $>20\%$ are not secreted. Combination of LHBs-rich (10–20%) HBsAg with virion core particles leads evidently to the secretion of virions. It is not proven that a high LHBs content is required for the maturation of virions. LHBs is, however, the morphogenetic factor for the filaments. The transfected Hela cells screte both 22-nm particles and filaments[52]. These filaments are as rich in LHBs as the particles in serum while the 22-nm particles are almost devoid of LHBs[56]. Treatment of filaments with trypsin not only degrades LHBs but it also leads to disintegration of the filaments into clusters of 20-nm particles (K.-H. Heermann, unpublished observations).

Binding of PreS1 to hepatocytes

This was first shown by Neurath in a seminal paper[65]. PreS1-rich HBsAg particles were immobilized on an affinity column and various cells passed through this column. The human hepatoma cell Hep G2 was bound specifically while liver cells of other species or human cells from other organ specificity were not bound. Although this assay system was relatively artificial, it reproduced the organ- and species-specificity of human HBV. The binding could be inhibited by PreS1 peptides between sequence 27 and 47 (subtype 'd') and by antibodies to them. Pontisso *et al.* isolated sinusoidal hepatocyte membranes from human liver. They showed that LHBs expressed in transfected yeast bound to these membranes. Binding could be inhibited by the

PreS1 specific antibody MA18/7 (Pontisso *et al.*, pers. commun.). This antibody binds highly efficiently to a PreS1 peptide 12–47 (P. Coursaget, pers. commun.). MA18/7 binds to all HBsAg subtypes[66]. In the corresponding peptide only amino acids 40–47 do not show subtype-specific exchanges. Since hepatocyte binding is probably not subtype-specified either, it appears likely that sequence 40–47 contributes to the hepatocyte binding. Virions and filaments from human serum bind also to hepatocyte membranes and their binding can also be inhibited by MA18/7 (P. Pontisso, pers. commun.)

The hepatocyte receptor sequence is not an immuno-dominant site. Only few convalescents contain antibodies which inhibit MA18/7 binding to Pre-S1. However, good responders to plasma-derived vaccines (anti-HBs titre >10000 IU/litre) usually contain antibodies which compete with MA18/7 for PreS1 (R. Deepen, unpublished observations). Such antibodies could be considered as anti-receptor antibodies. Noteworthy, the pepsin-treated plasma-derived vaccine also induced such antibodies.

CORE PROTEINS

Nomenclature

Most isolates of hepadnavirus genomes contain a C-orf with two functional initiation codons. We suggest designating the product of the whole C-orf as 'HBe protein' because it is processed *in vivo* to HBeAg. The smaller protein may be named 'HBc protein' because it forms the core particle and the HBc antigen associated with it[67] (see Figure 2). If characterization by size is required, a superscript 'e' such as P25^e or a 'c' such as P22^c is recommended. This is especially useful for the HBe proteins because they occur due to post-translational clipping and modification in several different sizes between 16 and 25 kDa (see Figure 2). The corresponding genes would be *hbe* and *hbc*. The small DNA segment between the first and the second initiation codon has already been termed 'preC' and the *hbc* gene is also referred[17] to as 'gene C'. Several authors use the superscript 'preC' for the HBe proteins (such as P25^{prec}).

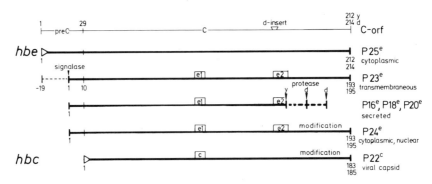

Figure 2 Organization and products of the open reading frame for the core proteins (C-orf). e1, e2, and c refer to antigen determinants; 'y' and 'd' to subtype-specific proteolytic sites.

The HBc and HBe *proteins* should not be confused with HBc and HBe antigens. Both proteins contain a major antigenic site between codon 70 and 90 of *hbc*. This site displays HBcAg (c in Figure 2) as a component of natural core particles and the HBeAg-el determinant (e1 in Figure 2) after disturbance of the native core particles structure (H. Schaller, pers. commun.). HBe protein does not usually fold to HBc antigenicity and always displays the HBe1 determinant. The second antigenic site of HBeAg, e2, is hidden within native core particles; under natural conditions HBeAg is derived from *hbe* and HBcAg from *hbc*.

HBV genome isolates of HBsAg subtype 'adw' have an insertion of two codons at position 151 of *hbc*. The carboxy-terminal clipping is, moreover, different in the various HBV subtypes (H. Schaller, pers. commun.).

The HBc protein

P22^c is the major component of the virion capsid which encloses the viral DNA genome. The capsids are usually referred to as virion 'cores' because they are enveloped by the three HBs proteins[68]. Core particles without envelope are found in the nuclei of infected hepatocytes[69]. Before the advent of gene technology it was very difficult to obtain sufficient amounts of HBcAg for biochemical or diagnostic studies. It had to be extracted either from large volumes of infected blood or from the livers of deceased immunodeficient HBV carriers. The identity of natural P22^c with the *hbc* gene product was confirmed by carboxy-terminal sequencing and the relative amino acid composition[70]. However, amino-terminal sequencing was not achieved. Only expression of the *hbe* and *hbc* in mammalian[71] or bacterial cells[72] using comparable plasmid constructs made clear that *hbc* encoded P22^c.

Packaging of viral RNA

HBc protein packages during the viral life cycle the pre-genomic RNA (which is its own mRNA) and the viral polymerase precursor (see Chapter 8). The RNA pre-genome is only later converted to the viral DNA pre-genome by the viral reverse transcriptase[73]. Recent observations from our laboratory (V. Bruss, in preparation) suggest that the packaging of the pre-genome results from a specific interaction between HBc protein and its mRNA. P22^c can be easily expressed by all vector/host systems, e.g. in *E. coli* using a small expression plasmid[67,72]. Purified core particles from *E. coli* contain a tightly-bound nucleic acid which co-migrates in agarose gel electrophoresis with core particles. This nucleic acid is resistant to nucleases. After extraction with SDS/phenol, the nucleic acid can be digested with RNase but not with DNase. Thus, even in the presence of large amounts of HBcAg encoding plasmid DNA, RNA is preferably packaged by the core protein. The HBc protein has, moreover, a clear preference for its own mRNA. The mRNA for ß-lactamase, which is expressed in similar amounts by the same plasmid, is barely detectable within the core particles (V. Bruss, unpublished observations).

P25[e] expressed in *E. coli* has, in contrast to P22[c], a higher affinity to DNA than to RNA[72]. P22[c] also binds DNA, but this was detected only after SDS gel electrophoresis and blotting[74]. This probably non-specific binding is due to the arginine-rich carboxy-terminal domain of P22[c]. Removal of the arginine-rich domain by trypsin abolishes the ability to bind nucleic acid in immunoblots (M. Melegari, unpublished observations). Hepadnavirus-infected ground squirrels express both HBe and HBc proteins, but only the mRNA for HBc protein (i.e. the CmRNA) is packaged within the core particles[75,76]. This, and the above-mentioned results in *E. coli*, suggest that the HBc protein but not the HBe protein has a specific affinity to its own mRNA. A too-long 5′ terrminal extension upstream of *hbc* blocks packaging while 3′ terminal extension beyond *hbc* up to the natural (supergenomic) length is tolerated but not required. According to the current model of hepadnaviral genome replication, a polymerase precursor including a protein primer should have an affinity for the 3′ end of the pre-genome and, thus, also become packaged within the core particle.

It appears unlikely that P22c would non-specifically package cellular RNA, e.g. mRNA of oncogenes *and* the polymerase precursor. If such an event did occur (e.g. after non-homologous recombination), it would theoretically contribute to viral oncogenesis. However, in hepadnaviruses there is no experimental evidence for this mechanism, which often occurs with retroviruses.

Post-translational modification

Core particles of all hepadnaviridae contain an endogenous protein kinase, i.e. an enzyme that transfers phosphate from a nucleotide triphosphate to HBc protein. The enzyme co-purifies with core particles and transfers $^{32}PO_4$ from γ^{32} ATP to Ser[77] or to a lesser extent to Thr[78]. The *in vitro* bound $^{32}PO_4$ is protected against alkaline phosphatase unless the core particles are lysed by SDS[77]. Core particles with low density contain more endogenous protein kinase activity than dense core particles which also contain endogenous DNA polymerase[77,79]. Partial proteolysis of human core particles with clostripain or V8 protease cleaves P22[c] around amino acid 80 or around amino acid 130[80]. Only the former cleavage generates ^{32}P-labelled fragments after endogenous protein kinase labelling. However, these fragments were HBeAg negative. The latter cleavage fragments were HBeAg positive but ^{32}P negative. Thus, the ^{32}P label was added to carboxy-terminal sites beyond amino acid 130. This domain contains several serines next to two basic amino acids which would serve as phosphate-acceptor site. Two-dimensional separation of peptides after complete trypsin digestion showed that the ^{32}P-labelled phosphopeptides were conserved in human and ground squirrel HBc proteins[78]. Since the only homology between the two proteins is found in the carboxy-terminal domain, it is evident that *in vitro* phosphorylation occurs at this site[81]. P22[c] expressed in *E. coli* does not exhibit autophosphorylation (V. Bruss, unpublished observations). Thus, an enzyme is required for this modification. The origin of this enzyme is not known. Some authors have observed that the enzyme is able to phosphorylate exogenous substrates like casein[79]. On the other hand, the endogenous phosphorylation site seems to be internal[77]. Recent evidence (O. Laub, pers. commun.) suggests that there are two protein kinase activities associated with core particles, one being externally bound, and another being an integral part of the capsid.

Although the protein kinase phosphorylates only serine or threonine as endogenous substrates, it cannot be ruled that tyrosine or even other substrates could be phosphorylated if they were available in the endogenous labelling reaction. In view of the specificity of other kinases, this is not very likely to occur.

The phosphorylation of the carboxy-terminal domain may have an effect on its interaction with nucleic acids, but there is no direct evidence for this. P22^c isolated from virions has very little effect and P22^c from human liver nuclei had no detectable binding capacity for RNA *in vitro* (V. Bruss, in preparation). Since P22^c from *E. coli* bound RNA, we conclude that the carboxy-terminal domain is modified in the natural host of HBV. The most obvious modification would be phosphorylation. However, treatment with alkaline phosphatase did not restore the RNA binding. Apparently another, or a subsequent, modification of this domain occurs *in vivo*. Such a possible modification would be ADP ribosylation. This possibility cannot be ruled out. However, phosphodiester bonds are apparently not present in the modification because treatment with phosphodiesterase did not restore RNA binding (V. Bruss, in preparation). It has still to be elucidated whether [^{32}P] phosphate, present through *in vitro* phosphorylation, remains resistant to alkaline phosphatase even after lysis of the core particles[77]. This would suggest that a part of this ill-understood modification is indeed nucleotidetriphosphate-dependent and that it also occurs *in vitro* within purified core particles.

Antigenicity and immunogenicity

The most amazing property of the core particle is its extreme immunogenicity. Antibodies against HBcAg (anti-HBc) are the first to appear during acute infection. Their titre is usually very high and they persist longer than other HBV antibodies[82]. Chronic carriers of HBV usually have the highest titres of antiHBc. This suggests that anti-HBc is not protective and not able to terminate infection. It has even been suggested that large doses of anti-HBc prevent efficient immune elimination by an HBc-specific T-cell cytotoxicity[83].

The first humoral immune response against HBcAg is via IgM antibodies which reach very high titres in acute hepatitis B virus infection. Chronic carriers with liver disease have often moderate fluctuating titres of IgM antiHBc while naturally immune persons or healthy HBsAg carriers are usually IgM anti-HBc negative[84]. Detectable IgM anti-HBc has also been found with increased frequency in patients with HBsAg-positive liver carcinoma[85].

Total anti-HBc is the most universal marker for previous or ongoing HBV infection but the current inhibition assays produce, unfortunately, 0.5–1.5% non-specifically positive results in normal populations (A. Uy, pers.

commun.). These false-positive results are usually close to the detection limit and further characterized by the absence of other HBV markers. The significance of IgM anti-HBc is hampered by the lack of a standardized assay. Only quantitative assays will enable distinction between acute and chronic hepatitis B.

The high immunogenicity depends on the quaternary structure of P22[c] in the core particles. HBcAg induces, in native form, anti-HBc independent of T-helper cells[86]. Other epitopes linked to core particles also acquire this high B-cell immunogenicity. Core particles have been used successfully as carriers for a neutralizing FMDV epitope[87]. P22[c] which has been truncated carboxy-terminally by recombinant DNA techniques, still assembles core particles which now, however, display HBeAg. This particulate HBeAg is also a very effective B-cell immunogen (Milich *et al.,* pers. commun.). Besides the immunodominant B-cell epitope, P22[c] has also highly active T-cell epitopes. These T-cell epitopes are required for a humoral immune response against soluble HBe protein[86] and for the enhancement of the anti-HBs response against complete HBV[88].

A cellular immune response against HBcAg and/or HBeAg was suggested some time ago[89] as a major pathogenic mechanism in chronic hepatitis B. Both core-particle-specific T-helper/inducer and T-suppressor/killer cells have been identified[90]. It has to be kept in mind that HBcAg must be presented as degraded partial peptides by monocytes or B-cells in the T-cell assays. If HBcAg is considered strictly as conformational antigen, the target antigen for the T cell may more properly be described as HBeAg. However, both antigens are defined at the antibody level and not at the T-cell level.

THE HBe PROTEIN

The nature of HBeAg was not known for a long time, and even today its function is not well understood. Magnius and Espmark[61] detected it in 1972 as the third antigen antibody system of HBV. HBeAg is usually detectable in those HBV carriers who have a high blood virus titre and who transmit the infection in even very small volumes of blood, such as sharing needles in the case of drug abusers. Anti-HBe is present in most carriers who have no detectable virions in blood and who usually transmit the infection only in very large volumes of blood (like transfusion) or not at all. These observations suggest that HBeAg may have a function in the development and maintenance of massive viraemia, or that immunity against HBeAg has some effect on virus production. However, it cannot be excluded that both HBeAg and anti-HBe are unnecessary side products of viral replication and that the prognostically favourable seroconversion from HBeAg to anti-HBe reflects no more than a general decrease in viral expression.

Origin of HBeAg

Genetic analysis of all known hepadnaviruses suggests that there is a subtle function of HBeAg in the survival of this virus family during evolution. All hepadnaviruses have a short preC segment which has the characteristics of a signal peptide for translocation to the ER. In the case of human[92–94] and duck HBV[95] it has been experimentally shown that the PreC sequence may cause translocation of HBe protein, and that it may be cleaved contranslationally by the signal peptidase. Expression of the *hbe* gene in mammalian cells or *in vitro* translation systems generates P25[e]. A part of the nascent P25[e] is translocated and processed to P23[e] by removal of the 19 amino-terminal amino acids[96]. The preC sequence is not in complete agreement with the minimal requirements of a typical signal sequence and, thus, a part of P25[e] remains unprocessed[94]. The processed P23[e] remains transiently in a transmembrane position. It appears that the accumulation of basic amino acids in the carboxy-terminal part prevents complete translocation to the lumen of the ER[94]. The transmembranous P23[e] may follow two different pathways: one part may return to the cytoplasm and becomes modified[93] to a P24[e]. Another part becomes clipped at the beginning of, or within, the carboxy-terminal domain and is secreted from HBV-transfected cells as P16[e] in the case of HBV subtype 'ayw' and 'adr'[70] or as P18[e] and P20[e] with subtype 'adw'. HBeAg purified from serum has been found as 16-kDa protein clipped at Val-149[56]. Immunoblot analysis of HBeAg from a HBV carrier subtype 'adw' showed a P20[e] and a P18[e] (E. Zyzik, unpublished observations). P20[e] and P18[e] both from human serum or transfected cell media were converted to a P16[e] by trypsin. Denatured P22[c] was converted in control experiments by trypsin[56,94] to a slightly smaller P15[e]. This suggests that the HBeAg in serum originates indeed from the *hbe* gene and not from degraded P22[c].

Potential functions of HBe proteins

The variable patterns of processing and of intracellular distribution suggest that the HBe proteins may exert several functions. The function which is certainly not taken by the HBe protein is that of a precursor for the major core protein. Thus, the designation 'precore protein' is better not used.

P23[e] as a potential transmembrane protein could theoretically have a function in virus maturation. Its carboxy-terminal domain remains in the cytoplasm and could fix the HBV pre-genome at the ER. Assembly of P22[c] to core particles around this pre-genome would generate ER-bound core particles which would eventually acquire an envelope and become complete virions[94]. Virions from human serum contain a small amount of a 23-kDa protein which binds anti-HBe in immunoblots. Core particles isolated from human hepatocellular nuclei do not contain such a protein consistent with a direct migration from cytoplasm to nucleus (K.-H. Heermann, unpublished observations). These data suggest that the P23[e] may be involved in the formation of secrete virions. Transfection of ducks with a preC-deficient mutant yields, however, viable virus *in vivo*[95,97]. The mutant virus did, however, not produce HBeAg. Transfection of human cells with preC-deficient human HBV also yielded secreted virions, but no HBeAg[98]. Possibly, several ways of interaction between core particles and HBs protein allow for the formation of viable virus.

The occurrence of secreted HBe protein may, possibly, interfere with the T-cell immune response. As pointed out above, HBV-producing cells would probably contain core peptides which may be presented by MHC class I or II molecules to T cells. Circulating HBe protein as an immunological homologue of denatured HBe protein might compete with the presented peptide for the T-cell receptor. This speculation is consistent with the clinical experience that loss of HBeAg in chronic HBV carriers is often associated with activation of liver disease.

Unprocessed $P25^e$ or cytoplasmic $P23^e$ seems to have an affinity to the nucleus (J. Ou, pers. commun.). Although no function of this $P25^e$ in the nucleus in known, it is noteworthy that transfection of mouse fibroblasts with functional *hbe/c* gene but not with defect ones, inhibits induction of the ß-interferon synthesis[99]. While the constructs used by Twu *et al.* would theoretically allow expression of both HBe and HBc protein, our experience with transfected mouse cells suggests that HBe proteins are far more efficiently expressed[56]. HBe-specific immunofluorescence of HBe-producing mouse cells showed, besides a strong cytoplasmic and a membranous staining, small dots within the nucleus (M. Seifer, unpublished observations). It is known that HBV replication is sensitive against interferon and that chronic HBV carriers have reduced levels of interferon. Thus, HBe protein may interfere with the host's defence.

REPLICATION OF HBV DNA IN MAMMALIAN CELLS

Transfection of human hepatoma cells, like HepG2 or Huh7, by dimerized HBV genomes has recently allowed *in vitro* production of complete HBV (see for example Chapter 11). We studied the expression of dimerized HBV genomes in mouse fibroblasts[56]. Since it had been reported that the HBV enhancer was liver-specific[100] we introduced into the transfected DNA an additional SV40 enhancer which acts ubiquitously. Many stable clones which expressed HBV proteins were obtained. The clones contained HBV typical mRNAs for SHBs and MHBs of 2.1 kb and for HBe/c proteins of 3.6 kb. Expression of LHBs was low and detectable only by a sensitive PreS1 specific ELISA. $P22^c$ was also barely detectable, but $P24^e$, $P23^e$, and $P20^e$ were readily found by immunoblot in the cells and in the supernatants. The data suggest that most of the 3.6-kb mRNA started upstream of the preC sequence and encoded HBe protein. As mentioned previously only *hbc* mRNA but not *hbe* mRNA is packaged within the virions.

Nevertheless, extra-chromosomal HBV DNA was detectable within the cells and in the pellets of the culture media. The DNA consisted of 3.2-kbp and heterogeneous smaller molecules. The 3.2-kbp molecule was probably not circular. It banded in density gradients like virions. In contrast to virion DNA, this DNA was not completely protected against degradation by added DNase. This suggested that it was associated with HBs and HBe proteins but that it was not packaged within a closed particle. During extraction with phenol, the HBV DNA partitioned in the phenol phase, unless it was first digested with protease. The HBV DNA was apparently synthesized by the mode of HBV and not by cellular enzymes. This involves reverse transcription by the viral reverse transcriptase beginning at a protein primer[73]. The resulting DNA is covalently linked to protein[101]. The secreted virus-like particles also contained an endogenous DNA polymerase as is the case for authentic virions. Thus, the cells were able to perform several essential steps of HBV genome replication like synthesis of the reverse transcriptase, of the protein primer, and of a RNA template. The failure to form authentic virions was probably due to the under-expression of $P22^c$ and of LHBs.

MALIGNANT TRANSFORMATION OF HEPATOCYTES

We wanted to study if mouse hepatocytes would express the HBV genome in a more appropriate way than mouse fibroblasts. The target cells[57] were the fetal mouse hepatocytes cell line FMH 202. This cell line was derived from transgenic mice which carried SV40 TAg under the control of the metallo-thionein promoter. The presence of SV40 TAg caused constitutive expression of c-myc and allowed, probably, the establishment of this immortalized cell line. The cell line was, however, non-malignant in that it did not grow in soft agar or in nude mice. It was also fully differentiated and required liver-specific growth factors (M. Höhne, unpublished observations). These cells were co-transfected with the dimerized HBV genome and with a neomycin resistance gene, both under the control of the SV40 enhancer. Many resistant clones were obtained and many of them secreted HBsAg and HBeAg. All of the clones which had been analysed further secreted HBV DNA in the form as described above for the transfected mouse fibroblasts. SHBs, MHBs and HBe protein were well expressed but HBc or LHBs were still deficient. There was, however, a strong expression of an X-specific 0.9-kb RNA which was not seen in the fibroblasts.

Surprisingly, most of the HBV expressing clones showed an altered morphology and a more rapid growth to a higher density. All these clones grew in soft agar and three of four clones grew as tumours in nude mice. Some of the nine evaluated tumours had the histology of trabecular hepatomas with the typical sinusoid-like spaces; other tumours grew as solid infiltrating cell masses (I. Fiebig, pers. commun.) Most clones showed in cell culture constitutive expression of c-fos which was not seen in the parent cell.

An important difference between the tumour growth in cell culture and in vivo (nude mouse) was methylation of HBV DNA. The clones expressed in cell culture 3.6-kb and 2.1-kb mRNAs of HBV before and after growth as nude mouse tumour, but in the nude mouse expression was very low. This observation resembles the findings in transgenic mice which carried and expressed HBV genes. Transformation of explanted hepatocytes from these mice with SV40 resulted in a shut-off of HBsAg synthesis[102]. Expression of the X mRNA was variable. In one clone no decrease of X mRNA was found in vivo; in another clone the 0.9 kb mRNA was suppressed in vivo as the other viral mRNAs, but a new large mRNA appeared which hybridized to an X probe. This was probably a read-through from X to cellular sequences. The transformed FMH 202 cells reflected apparently a typical property of human HBV-associated hepatomas which also rarely express HBsAg or HBe/cAg.

Another interesting feature of the system is the occurrence of HBV gene amplification and rearrangements. In Southern blots, all HBV-expressing clones had an individual pattern of which one showed alterations in the nude mouse tumour and further alterations in the explanted tumours. This suggests that the initial integration occurred at variable sites and that the pattern of integration was not stable *in vivo*. Numerous rearrangements of viral and cellular sequences are a typical property of human HBV-positive hepatomas.

Our data suggest that HBV may directly induce malignant transformation with high efficiency if a pre-transformed hepatocyte (like FMH 202) is hit. One could argue that the process of transfection itself induces malignancy in the cell. A control transfection of the resistance gene in the same vector did, however, not alter cell morphology or growth behaviour.

Although the mechanism of malignant transformation has not yet been studied in our system, the preliminary data suggest that expression of the X protein may induce this process. X protein is probably expressed in very low amounts during acute or chronic infection, because its mRNA is very difficult to detect. However, fragments of HBV DNA are frequently integrated in such a way that X mRNA could be very well expressed while other HBV genes would be absent, truncated, or inactive. Expression of X mRNA has been found in human hepatomas[103]. X-protein is known to be a non-specific activator of transcription which acts on many enhancers including the HBV enhancer (see Chapter 12). Activation of *c-myc* by the X protein has been demonstrated (K. Koike *et al.* and M. Levrero *et al.*, pers. commun.). Although this is not of importance in our system, it is consistent with the assumption that it may activate oncogenes.

Malignant transformation by the X protein is still not a well-established fact or theory. The relatively rare finding of X protein in natural HBV-associated hepatomas, and the frequent detection of insertional mutagenesis of oncogenes and anti-oncogenes (see Chapter 9) by HBV does, however, not rule out an important function of X protein in natural oncogenesis. Our data suggest that transformation by X protein (if it is indeed the transforming agent in our system) may start a series of rearrangements which may result in secondary, even more malignant, events.

Acknowledgements

We acknowledge the personal communications by the many colleagues mentioned in text. Work from our laboratory was supported by DFG grant Ge 345/7–3. We are indebted to the head of our department, R. Thomssen, for his support and to U. Goldmann and R. Hobein for technical assistance.

References

1. Tiollais, P., Pourcel, C. and Dejean, A. (1985). The hepatitis B virus. *Nature,* **317**, 489–95

2. Peterson, D. L., Nath, N. and Gavilanes, F. (1982). Structure of hepatitis B surface antigen. *J. Biol. Chem.*, **257**, 10414–20
3. Tiollais, P., Charnay, P. and Vyas, G. N. (1981). Biology of hepatitis B virus. *Science,* **213**, 406–11
4. Stibbe, W. and Gerlich, W. H. (1982). Variable protein composition of hepatitis B surface antigen from different donors. *Virology*, **123**, 436–42
5. Stibbe, W. and Gerlich, W. H. (1983). Structural relationships between minor and major proteins of hepatitis B surface antigen. *J. Virol.*, **46**, 626–8
6. Machida, A., Koshimoto, S., Ohnuma, H. *et al.* (1983). A hepatitis B surface antigen polypeptide (P31) with the receptor for polymerized human as well as chimpanzee albumins. *Gastroenterology*, **85**, 268–74
7. Machida, A., Kishimoto, S., Ohnuma, H., Miyamoto, H., Baba, K., Itoh, Y. *et al.* (1984). A polypeptide containing 55 amino acid residues coded by the pre-S region of hepatitis B virus deoxyribonucleic acid bears the receptor for polymerized human as well as chimpanzee albumins. *Gastroenterology*, **86**, 910–18
8. Neurath, A. R., Kent, S. B. H. and Strick, N. (1984). Location and chemical synthesis of a pre-S gene coded immunodominant epitope of hepatitis B virus. *Science,* **224**, 392–5
9. Michel, M.-L., Pontisso, P., Sobczak, E., Malpièce, Y. and Streeck, R. E. (1984). Synthesis in animal cells of hepatitis B surface antigen particles carrying a receptor for polymerized human serum albumin. *Proc. Natl. Acad. Sci. USA*, **81**, 7708–12
10. Persing, D. H., Varmus, H. E. and Ganem, D. (1985). A frameshift mutation in the pre-S region of the human hepatitis B virus genome allows production of surface antigen particles but eliminates binding to polymerized albumin. *Proc. Natl. Acad. Sci. USA*, **82**, 3440–4
11. Gerlich, W. and Thomssen, R. (1975). Standardized detection of hepatitis B surface antigen: determination of its serum concentration in weight units per volume. *Devel. Biol. Standard.,* **30**, 78–87
12. Stibbe, W. and Gerlich, W. H. (1983). Characterization of pre-S gene products in hepatitis B surface antigen. *Devel. Biol. Standard.,* **54**, 33–43
13. Heermann, K.-H., Goldmann, U., Schwartz, W., Seyffarth, T., Baumgarten, H. and Gerlich, W. H. (1984). Large surface proteins of hepatitis B virus containing the pre-S sequence. *J. Virol.,* **52**, 396–402
14. Wong, D. T., Nath, N. and Sninsky, J. J. (1985). Identification of hepatitis B virus polypeptides encoded by the entire of pre-S open reading frame. *J. Virol.,* **55**, 223–31
15. Neurath, A. R., Kent, S. B. H., Strick, N., Taylor, P. and Stevens, C. E. (1985). Hepatitis B virus contains pre-S gene-encoded domains. *Nature*, **315**, 154–6
16. Takahashi, K., Kishimoto, S., Ohnuma, H., Machida, A., Takai, E., Tsuda, F., Miyamoto, H., Tanaka, T., Matsushita, K., Oda, K., Miyakawa, Y. and Mayumi, M. (1986). Polypeptides coded for by the receptor for polymerized human serum albumin: Expression on hepatitis B particles produced in the HBeAg or anti-HBe phase of hepatitis B virus infection. *J. Immunol.*, **136**, 3467–72
17. Tiollais, P., Dejean, A., Brechot, C., Michel, M. L., Sonigo, P. and Wain-Hobson, S. (1981). Structure of hepatitis B virus DNA. In Vyas, G. N., Dienstag, J. L. and Hoofnagle, J. H. (eds) *Viral Hepatitis and Liver Disease*, pp. 57–70. (Orlando: Grune & Stratton)
18. Gavilanes, F., Gonzalez-Ros, J. M. and Peterson, D. L. (1982). Structure of hepatitis B surface antigen. *J. Biol. Chem.,* **257**, 7770–7
19. Guerrero, E., Gavilanes, F. and Peterson, D. L. (1988). Model for the protein arrangement in HBsAg particles based on physical and chemical studies. In Zuckerman, A. J. (ed.) *Viral Hepatitis and Liver Disease*, pp. 606–13. (New York: Alan R. Liss)
20. Peterson, D. L., Paul, D. A., Lam, J., Tribley, J. J. E. and Achord, D. T. (1984). Antigenic structure of hepatitis B surface antigen: identification of the 'd' subtype determinant by chemical modification and use of monoclonal antibodies. *J. Immunol.,* **132**, 920–7
21. Neurath, A. R., Kent, S. B. H., Strick, N. and Parker, K. (1988). Delineation of contiguous determinants essential for biological functions of the pre-S sequence of the hepatitis B virus envelope protein: its antigenicity, immunogenicity and cell-receptor recognition. *Ann. Inst. Pasteur/Virol.,* **139**, 13–38
22. Howard, C. R., Stirk, H. J., Brown, S. E. and Steward, M. W. (1988). Towards the development of synthetic hepatitis B vaccines. In Zuckerman, A. J. (ed.) *Viral Hepatitis and Liver Disease*, pp. 1094–101. (New York: Alan R. Liss)

23. Hauser, P., Thomas, H. C., Waters, J., Simoen, E., Voet, P., De Wilde, M., Stephenne, J. and Pétre, J. (1988). Induction of neutralizing antibodies in chimpanzees and humans by a recombinant yeast-derived hepatitis B surface antigen particle. In Zuckerman, A. J. (ed.) *Viral Hepatitis and Liver Disease*, pp. 1031–7. (New York: Alan R. Liss)

24. Celis, E., Ou, D. and Otvos, L. (1988). Identification of a major antigenic determinant of hepatitis B surface antigen for human T cells by means of synthetic peptides. In Zuckerman, A. J. (ed.) *Viral Hepatitis and Liver Disease*, pp. 650–5. (New York: Alan R. Liss)

25. Eble, B. E., Lingappa, V. R. and Ganem, D. (1986). Hepatitis B surface antigen: An unusual secreted protein initially synthesized as a transmembrane polypeptide. *Mol. Cell. Biol.*, **6**, 1454–62

26. Patzer, E. J., Nakamura, G. R., Simonsen, C. C., Levinson, A. D. and Brands, R. (1986). Intracellular assembly and packaging of hepatitis B surface antigen particles occur in the endoplasmic reticulum. *J. Virol.*, **58**, 884–92

27. Cochran, M. A., Ericson, B. L., Knell, J. D. and Smith, G. E. (1987). Use of baculovirus recombinants as a general method for the production of subunit vaccines. In Chanock, R. M., Lerner, R. A., Brown, R. and Ginsberg, H. (eds) *Vaccines 87*, pp. 384–8. (Cold Spring Harbor Laboratory)

28. Lanford, R. E., Kennedy, R. C., Dreesman, G. R., Eichberg, J. W., Notvall, L., Luckow, V. A. and Summers, M. D. (1988). Expression of hepatitis B virus surface and core antigens using a baculovirus expression vector. In Zuckerman, A. J. (ed.) *Viral Hepatitis and Liver Disease*, pp. 372–8. (New York: Alan R. Liss)

29. Wampler, D. E., Lehman, E. D., Boger, J., McAleer, W. J. and Scolnick, E. M. (1985). Multiple chemical forms of hepatitis B surface antigen produced in yeast. *Proc. Natl. Acad. Sci. USA*, **82**, 6830–4

30. Adamowicz, Ph., Tron, F., Vinas, R., Mevelec, M. N., Diaz, I., Couroucé, A. M., Mazert, M. C., Lagarde, D. and Girard, M. (1988). Hepatitis B vaccine containing the S and pre S-2 antigens produced in Chinese hamster ovary cells. In Zuckerman, A. J. (ed.) *Viral Hepatitis and Liver Disease*, pp. 1087–90. (New York: Alan R. Liss)

31. Cattaneo, R., Will, H., Hernandez, N. and Schaller, H. (1983). Signals regulating hepatitis B surface antigen transcription. *Nature*, **305**, 336–8

32. Ou, J.-H. and Rutter, W. S. (1985). Hybrid hepatitis B virus–host transcripts in a human hepatoma cell. *Proc. Natl. Acad. Sci. USA*, **82**, 83–7

33. Ou, J. H. and Rutter, W. J., (1987). Regulation of secretion of the hepatitis B virus major surface antigen by the preS-1 protein. *J. Virol.*, **61**, 782–6

34. Yu, M. W., Finlayson, J. S. and Shih, J. W.-K. (1985). Interaction between various polymerized human albumins and hepatitis B surface antigen. *J. Virol.*, **55**, 736–43

35. Lenz, A. (1987). Bindung von nativem Humanalbumin an die Prä.S2 Domäne des Hepatitis B Virus. Dissertation (Göttingen)

36. Heermann, K.-H., Waldeck, F. and Gerlich, W. H. (1988). Interaction between native human serum and the preS2 domain of hepatitis B virus surface antigen. In Zuckerman, A. J. (ed.) *Viral Hepatitis and Liver Disease*, pp. 697–700. (New York: Alan R. Liss)

37. Pohl, C., Cote, P., Purcell, R. and Gerin, J. (1986). Failure to detect polyalbumin-binding sites on the woodchuck hepatitis virus surface antigen: Implications for the pathogenesis of hepatitis B virus in humans. *J. Virol.*, **60**, 943–9

38. Ishihara, K., Waters, J. A., Pignatelli, M. and Thomas, H. C. (1987). Characterization of the polymerized and monomeric human serum albumin binding site in hepatitis B surface antigen *J. Med. Virol.*, **21**, 89–95

39. Neurath, A. R., Kent, S. B. H., Parker, K., Prince, A. M., Strick, N., Brotman, B. and Sproul, P. (1986). Antibodies to a synthetic peptide from the pre-S 120–145 region of the hepatitis B virus envelope are virus-neutralizing. *Vaccine*, **4**, 35–7

40. Itoh, Y., Takyi, E., Ohnuma, H., Kitajima, K., Tsuda, F., Machida, A., Mishiro, S. and Nakamura, T. (1986). A synthetic peptide vaccine involving the product of the pre-S(2) region of hepatitis B virus DNA: protective efficacy in chimpanzees. *Proc. Natl. Acad. Sci. USA*, **83**, 9174–8

41. Alberti, A., Cavalletto, D., Pontisso, P., Chemello, L., Tagariello, G. and Belussi, F. (1988). Antibody response to pre-S2 and hepatitis B virus induced liver damage. *Lancet*, **1**, 1421–4

42. Hellström, U., Sylvan, S., Kuhns, M. and Sarin, V. (1986). Absence of pre-S2 antibodies in natural hepatitis B virus infection. *Lancet* **2**, 889–93

43. Budkowska, A., Dubreuil, P., Capel, F. and Pillot, J. (1986). Hepatitis B virus pre-S gene-encoded antigenic specificity and anti-pre-S antibody: Relationship between anti-pre-S response and recovery. *Hepatology,* **6**, 360–8

44. Alberti, A., Pontisso, P., Schiavon, E. *et al.* (1984). An antibody which precipitated Dane particles in acute hepatitis type B: relation to receptor sites which bind polymerized human serum albumin on virus particles. *Hepatology,* **4**, 220–6

45. Uy, A. (1984). Expression der Prä-Core und der Prä-S Sequenz aus dem Hepatitis B Virus Genom in *Escherichia coli* und immunologische Charakterisierung der Produkte. Dissertation (Göttingen)

46. Heermann, K.-H., Kruse, F., Seifer, M. and Gerlich, W. H. (1987). Immunogenicity of the gene S and pre-S domains in hepatitis B virions and HBsAg filaments. *Intervirology,* **28**, 14–25

47. Quiroga, J. A., Mora, I., Carreno, V., Herreras, M. I., Porres, J. C. and Gerlich, W. H. (1987). Inhibition of albumin binding to hepatitis B virions by monoclonal antibody to the pre-S2 domain of the viral envelope. *Digestion,* **38**, 212–20

48. Persing, D. H., Varmus, H. E. and Ganem, D. (1987). The pre-S1 protein of hepatitis B virus is acylated at its amino terminus with myristic acid. *J. Virol.,* **61**, 1672–7

49. Marion, P. L. (1988). Use of animal models to study hepatitis B virus. *Prog. Med. Virol.,* **35**, 43–75

50. Freytag von Loringhoven, A., Koch, S., Hofschneider, P. H. and Koshy, R. (1985). Co-transcribed 3' host sequences augment expression of integrated hepatitis B virus DNA. *EMBO J.,* **4**, 249–55

51. Marquardt, O., Heermann, K.-H., Seifer, M. and Gerlich, W. H. (1987). Cell type specific expression of pre-S1 antigen and secretion of hepatitis B surface antigen. *Postgrad. Med. J.,* **63**, 41–50

52. Marquardt, O., Heermann, K.-H., Seifer, M. and Gerlich, W. H. (1987). Cell specific expression of pre S1 antigen and secretion of hepatitis B virus surface antigen. *Arch. Virol.,* **96**, 249–56

53. Thung, S. N., Gerber, M. A., Kasambalides, E. J., Gilja, B. K., Keh, W. and Gerlich, W. H. (1986). Demonstration of pre-S polypeptides of hepatitis B virus in infected livers. *Hepatology,* **6**, 1315–18

54. Hadziyannis, S. J. (1983). Use of a monoclonal antibody in the detection of HBsAg in the liver by immunofluorescence. *Devel. Biol. Standard.,* **55**, 517–21

55. Dienes, H. P., Bianchi, L., Gerlich, W. and Hess, G. (1988). Different patterns of HBsAg and pre-S antigens in liver biopsies from healthy carriers. In Zuckerman, A. J. (ed.) *Viral Hepatitis and Liver Disease*, pp. 290–1. (New York: Alan R. Liss)

56. Seifer, M. (1987). Expression und Replikation des Hepatitis B Virus-Genoms in transfizierten animalen Zellen. Dissertation (Göttingen)

57. Paul, D., Höhne, M. Pinkert, C., Piasecki, A., Ummelmann, E. and Brinster, R. L. (1988). Immortalized differentiated hepatocyte lines derived from transgenic mice harboring SV40 T-antigen genes. *Exp. Cell Res.,* **175**, 354–62

58. Sells, M. A., Chen, M.-L. and Acs, G. (1987). Production of hepatitis B virus particles in HepG2 cells transfected with cloned hepatitis B virus DNA. *Proc. Natl. Acad. Sci. USA,* **84**, 1005–9

59. De-Medina, T., Faktor, O. and Shaul, Y. (1988) The S promoter of hepatitis B virus is regulated by positive and negative elements. *Mol. Cell. Biol.,* **8**, 2449–55

60. Persing, D. H., Varmus, H. E. and Ganem, D. (1986). Inhibition of secretion of hepatitis B surface antigen by a related presurface polypeptide. *Science,* **234**, 1388–91

61. McLachlan, A., Milich, D. R., Raney, A. K., Riggs, M. G., Hughes, J. L., Sorge, J. and Chisari, F. V. (1988). Expression of hepatitis B virus surface and core antigens: Influences of pre-S and precore sequences. *J. Virol.,* **61**, 683–92

62. Moss, B., Smith, G. L., Gerin, J. L. *et al.* (1984). Live recombinant Vaccinia virus protects chimpanzees against hepatitis B. *Nature,* **311**, 67–9

63. Standring, D. N., Ou, J. and Rutter, W. J. (1986). Assembly of viral particles in *Xenopus* oocytes: Presurface antigens regulate secretion of the hepatitis B viral surface envelope particle. *Proc. Natl. Acad. Sci. USA,* **83**, 9338–42

64. Filippi, P., Buras, J., McLachlan, A., Popper, H., Pinkert, C. A., Palmiter, R. D., Brinster, R. L. and Chisari, F. V. (1988). Overproduction of the hepatitis B virus large envelope polypeptide causes filament storage, ground-glass-cell formation, hepatocellular injury, and

nodular hyperplasia in transgenic mice. In Zuckerman, A. J. (ed.) *Viral Hepatitis and Liver Disease*, pp. 632–40. (New York: Alan R. Liss)

65. Neurath, A. R., Kent, S. B. H., Strick, N. and Parker, K. (1986). Identification and chemical synthesis of a host cell receptor binding site on hepatitis B virus. *Cell, 46*, 429–36

66. Seyffarth, T. (1986). Die Bedeutung der Prä-S1-Domäne in der Hülle des Hepatitis B virus. Dissertation (Göttingen)

67. Stahl, S., MacKay, P., Magazin, M., Bruce, S. A. and Murray, K. (1982). Hepatitis B virus core antigen: Synthesis in *Escherichia coli* and application in diagnosis. *Proc. Natl. Acad. Sci. USA, 79*, 1606–10

68. Almeida, G. D., Rubenstein, D. and Stott, E. D. (1971). New antigen–antibody system in Australia-antigen positive hepatitis. *Lancet, 2*, 1225–7

69. Gerety, R. J., Hoofnagle, J. A. and Barker, L. F. (1974). Humoral and cell-mediated immune responses to two hepatitis B virus antigens in guinea pigs. *J. Immunol., 113*, 1223–9

70. Takahashi, K., Machida, A., Funatsu, G., Nomura, M., Usuda, S., Aoyagi, S., Tachibana, K., Miyamoto, H., Imai, M., Nakamura, T., Miyakawa, Y. and Mayumi, M. (1983). Immunochemical structure of hepatitis B e antigen in the serum. *J. Immunol., 130*, 2903–7

71. Ou, J., Laub, O. and Rutter, W. J. (1986). Hepatitis B virus gene function: The precore targets the core antigen to cellular membranes and causes the secretion of the e antigen. *Proc. Natl. Acad. Sci. USA, 83*, 1578–82

72. Uy, A., Bruß, V., Gerlich, W. H., Köchel, H. G. and Thomssen, R. (1986). Precore sequence of hepatitis B virus inducing e antigen and membrane association of the viral core protein. *Virology, 155*, 86–96

73. Summers, J. and Mason, W. S. (1982). Replication of the genome of a hepatitis B-like virus by reverse transcription of an RNA intermediate. *Cell, 29*, 403–15

74. Petit, M. A. and Pillot, J. (1985). HBc and HBe antigenicity and DNA binding activity of major core protein P22 in hepatitis B virus core particles isolated from the cytoplasm of human liver cell. *J. Virol., 53*, 543–51

75. Enders, G. H., Ganem, D. and Varmus, H. E. (1987). 5'-terminal sequences influence the segregation of ground squirrel hepatitis virus RNAs into polyribosomes and viral core particles. *J. Virol., 61*, 35–41

76. Seeger, C., Ganem, D. and Varmus, H. E. (1986). Biochemical and genetic evidence for the hepatitis B virus replication strategy. *Science, 232*, 447–83

77. Gerlich, W. H., Goldmann, U., Müller, R., Stibbe, W. and Wolff, W. (1982). Specificity and localization of the hepatitis B virus associated protein kinase. *J. Virol., 42*, 761–6

78. Feitelson, M. A., Marion, P. L. and Robinson, W. S. (1982). Core particles of hepatitis B virus and ground squirrel hepatitis virus. *J. Virol., 43*, 687–96

79. Hantz, O., Fourel, I., Buendia, B., Baginski, I. and Trepo, C. 1988. Specificity of the woodchuck hepatitis virus-associated protein kinase. In Zuckerman, A. J. (ed.) *Viral Hepatitis and Liver Disease*, pp. 471–5. (New York: Alan R. Liss)

80. Baumgarten, U. (1983). Kartierung des HBeAg-Epitops im Core-Protein des Hepatitis B virus. Dissertation (Göttingen)

81. Argos, P. and Fuller, S. D. (1988). A model for the hepatitis B virus core protein: prediction of antigenic sites and relationship to RNA virus capsid proteins. *EMBO J., 7*, 819–24

82. Hoofnagle, J. H., Gerety, R. J. and Barker, L. F. (1973). Antibody to hepatitis-B-virus core in man. *Lancet, 2*, 869–73

83. Thomas, H. C. (1988). Treatment of hepatitis B viral infection. In Zuckerman, A. J. (ed.) *Viral Hepatitis and Liver Disease*, pp. 817–22. (New York: Alan R. Liss)

84. Gerlich, W. H., Uy, A., Lambrecht, F. and Thomssen, R. (1986). Cutoff levels of immunoglobulin M antibody against viral core antigen for differentiation of acute, chronic, and past hepatitis B virus infections. *J. Clin. Microbiol., 24*, 288–93

85. Roggendorf, M., Hwang, L. Y., Beasley, R., Chen, P.-H., Chen, T.-C., Lo, K.-R. and Deinhardt, F. (1987). Anti-HBc IgM in cases of hepatocellular carcinoma and cirrhosis in Taiwan. *J. Hepatol., 5*, 268–73

86. Milich, D. R. and McLachlan, A. (1986). The nucleocapsid of hepatitis B virus is both a T-cell-independent and a T-cell-dependent antigen. *Science, 234*, 1398–401

87. Clarke, B. E., Newton, S. E., Carroll, A. R., Francis, M. J., Appleyard, G., Syred, A. D., Highfield, P. E., Rowlands, D. J. and Brown F. (1987). Improved immunogenicity of a peptide epitope after fusion to hepatitis B core protein. *Nature, 330*, 381–4

88. Milich, D. R., McLachlan, A., Thornton, G. B. and Hughes, J. L. (1987). Antibody production to the nucleocapsid and envelope of the hepatitis B virus primed by a single synthetic T cell site. *Nature,* **239,** 547–9

89. Mondelli, M. U., Mieli-Vergani, G., Alberti, A., Vergani, D., Portmann, B., Eddleston, A. L. W. F. and Williams, R. (1982). Specificity of T lymphocyte cytotoxicity to autologous hepatocytes in chronic hepatitis B virus infection: evidence that T cells are directed against HBV core antigen expressed on hepatocytes. *J. Immunol.,* **129,** 2773–8

90. Ferrari, C., Penna, A., Mondelli, M. U., Fiaccadori, F and Chisari, F. V. (1988). Intrahepatic, HBcAg specific regulatory T-cell networks in chronic active hepatitis B. In Zuckerman, A. J. (ed.) *Viral Hepatitis and Liver Disease,* pp. 641–4. (New York: Alan R. Liss)

91. Magnius, L. O. and Espmark, J. A. (1972). New specificities in Australia antigen positive sera distinct from the Le Bouviert determinants. *J. Immunol.,* **109,** 1017–21

92. Weimer, T., Salfeld, J. and Will, H. (1987). Expression of the hepatitis B virus core gene *in vitro* and *in vivo. J. Virol.,* **61,** 3109–13

93. Garcia, P. D., Ou, J. H., Rutter, W. J. and Walter, P. (1988). Targeting of hepatitis B virus precore protein to the endoplasmatic reticulum membrane after signal peptide cleavage translocation can be aborted and the product released into the cytoplasm. *J. Cell. Biol.* **106,** 1093–1104

94. Bruss, V. and Gerlich, W. H. (1988). Formation of transmembranous hepatitis B e antigen by cotranslational *in vitro* processing of the viral precore protein. *Virology,* **163,** 268–75

95. Schlicht, H. J., Salfeld, J. and Schaller, H. (1987). The duck hepatitis B virus pre-C region encodes a signal sequence which is essential for synthesis and secretion of processed core proteins but not for virus formation. *J. Virol.,* **61,** 3701–9

96. Standring, D. N., Ou, J.-H. and Rutter, W. J. (1987). Expression of hepatitis B viral antigens in *Xenopus* oocytes. In Robinson, W., Koike, K. and Will, H. (eds) *Hepadna Viruses,* pp. 117–27. (New York: A. Liss)

97. Chang, C., Enders, G., Sprengel, R., Peters, N., Varmus, H. E. and Ganem, D. (1987). Expression of the precore region of an avian hepatitis B virus is not required for viral replication. *J. Virol.,* **61,** 3322–5

98. Junker, M., Galler, P. and Schaller, H. (1987). Expression and replication of the hepatitis B virus genome under foreign promoter control. *Nucl. Acids Res.,* **15,** 10117–32

99. Twu, J.-S., Lee, C.-H. and Schloemer, R. H. (1987). Interaction between hepatitis B virus and human beta-interferon. In Robinson, W., Koike, K. and Will, H. (eds) *Hepadna Viruses,* pp. 47–63. (New York: Alan R. Liss)

100. Shaul, Y., Rutter, W. J. and Laub, O. (1985). A human hepatitis B viral enhancer element. *EMBO J.,* **4,** 427–30

101. Gerlich, W. and Robinson, W. S. (1980). Hepatitis B virus contains protein attached to the 5′ terminus of its complete DNA strand. *Cell,* **21,** 801–9

102. Paul, D., Farza, H., Höhne, M. and Pourcel, C. (1988). Production of hepatitis B virus surface antigen in normal and immortalized transgenic mouse hepatocytes. In Zuckerman, A. J. (ed.) *Viral Hepatitis and Liver Disease,* pp. 379–80. (New York: Alan R. Liss)

103. Wollersheim, M. and Hofschneider, P. H. (1988). Transactivation by a product of the X gene of hepatitis B virus. In Zuckerman, A. J. (ed.) *Viral Hepatitis and Liver Disease,* pp. 334–40. (New York: Alan R. Liss)

15
The hepatitis B virus large envelope polypeptide can cause liver cell injury and multifocal nodular hyperplasia in transgenic mice

F. V. CHISARI

The hepatitis B virus (HBV) is a circular, double-stranded hepatotropic DNA virus that causes self-limited (acute) or prolonged (chronic) infection and hepatocellular injury (reviewed in ref. 1). HBV replicates by reverse transcription of an RNA intermediate and it may integrate into the host chromosomes after prolonged infection. Integration is random with respect to the host genome and it is associated with the development of primary hepatocellular carcinoma (PHC) after several decades of chronic infection with attendant active liver disease.

The mechanisms responsible for hepatocellular injury and malignant transformation are not known although considerable circumstantial evidence suggests that a cellular immune response to HBV encoded antigens expressed at the liver cell membrane is involved in hepatocytolysis. The virus does not contain an acutely transforming oncogene and does not appear to activate a common cellular proto-oncogene so its role in PHC is not well defined and it probably represents one of a series of events that lead to malignant transformation.

In an effort to understand the pathogenesis of HBV infection we have developed a transgenic mouse system in which each of the HBV genes can be expressed in the liver in the presence and absence of an HBV specific immune response. In this way it is possible to determine the extent to which HBV gene products are directly hepatocytotoxic and the role played by the immune response in the development of liver cell injury and PHC.

A subgenomic fragment of HBV which contains all the coding information necessary to produce the three envelope polypeptides containing HBsAg was cloned into liver-specific vectors containing either the zinc-inducible mouse metallothionein promoter or the strongly constitutively expressed mouse albumin promoter[2-4]. These recombinants were injected into the male pronuclei of unicellular mouse embryos; neonates that contained the microinjected HBV DNA and expressed the HBsAg were selected for breeding and subsequent analysis.

Production of the three envelope polypeptides during conventional HBV infection is transcriptionally regulated[1]. Three, in-frame translational start codons define the amino-termini of envelope polypeptides that share a common carboxy-terminus. The smallest polypeptide (P24) is most abundant (therefore designated 'major') and contains the family of determinants recognizes HBsAg, the major structural protein of the viral envelope. The middle polypeptide (P34) contains the entire major polypeptide plus an additional 55 N-terminal amino acids containing the preS(2) region that may be involved in virus–cell interactions. The large polypeptide (P39) contains the entire middle polypeptide plus an additional 108 N-terminal amino acids containing the preS(1) region. To date no specific function has been identified for this polypeptide but it is known to be relatively enriched in the envelope of the complete infectious HBV 'Dane' particle and the subviral filamentous forms, and to be absent from the subviral spherical forms[5,6] which constitute the vast majority of HBsAg particles in the blood of infected patients. Thus the large envelope polypeptide is associated with unique viral structures that appear in the circulation at relatively low concentrations.

The constructs used in our studies were designed such that synthesis of the major envelope polypeptide is driven by a viral promoter located within the pre-S region, while production of the large envelope polypeptide is controlled by the exogenous metallothionein or albumin promoter–enhancer elements. Secretion of 22-nm diameter subviral HBsAg particles by the transgenic hepatocyte is influenced by the relative intracellular abundance of each of the HBV envelope polypeptides of which the particles are composed[3]. Specifically, whereas the major envelope polypeptide (P25) and the middle envelope polypeptide (P34) form spherical particles within the endoplasmic reticulum that are rapidly transported to the Golgi apparatus and efficiently secreted by the cell, the large envelope polypeptide (P39) forms long filaments that become entrapped within the smooth endoplasmic reticulum. Since all of the envelope polypeptides form mixed aggregates with one another within the ER membrane[7-9], over-production of P39 can also entrap P34 and P25 within the cell, presumably due to structural constraints it imposes on particle formation when it is present in excess. Under these conditions the envelope polypeptides progressively accumulate and the hepatocytes assume the appearance of 'ground-glass' cells[4] often seen in the human HBsAg carrier state. Eventually intracellular envelope polypeptide levels can be reached that impair hepatocyte viability leading to acidophilic degeneration, Councilman-like body formation, feathery degeneration, and single-cell necrosis[4]. These changes occur in the absence of a humoral or cellular immune response to the HBV envelope antigens since the transgenic mice are immunologically tolerant to these polypeptides which are recognized as self[3]. The hepatocellular changes are reflected in elevated serum alanine aminotransferase levels and they become progressively more severe as a function of time. Injury is accompanied by Kupffer cell hyperplasia, focal inflammatory cell infiltration and hepatocellular pleomorphism characterized by cytomegaly, enlarged hyper-chromatic nuclei, bizarre multinucleate hepatocytes and abnormal mitoses indicative of active hepatocellular regeneration. These events evolve over a period of approximately 14 months and are only seen in the transgenic lineages that accumulate the highest concentrations of HBV envelope polypeptides within the liver. Ultimately, the regenerative process can become extreme producing a massively enlarged liver containing multiple grossly evident hyperplastic nodules (nodular regenerative hyperplasia). Nodular regnerative hyperplasia is considered a premalignant condition[10]. Other trans-genic lineages that do not over-produce the large envelope polypeptide have histologically normal livers throughout their entire lifespan and die of unrelated causes at 24–30 months of age.

We conclude that hepatocellular over-production of the large envelope polypeptide generates a long filamentous HBsAg particle that becomes en-trapped within the endoplasmic reticulum and cannot be secreted by the cell. 'Ground glass' hepatocytes are formed early in this process. Eventually, intra-cellular HBsAg concentrations are reached that interfere with cellular homeo-statis. As the hepatocytes die the liver displays many of the cytological and histological changes characteristic of viral hepatitis. Thus, it is formally possible for liver cell injury to occur as a direct consequence of HBV gene expression and for injury to initiate a regenerative hyperplastic response by surviving hepatocytes. The extent to which this process occurs during HBV infection in man and the degree to which it is superimposed upon a cytolytic, HBV-specific, immune response are currently under investigation in our laboratory.

Acknowledgements

I thank Pierre Filippi, Carl Pinkert, Richard Palmiter and Ralph Brinster for collaboration in the production and analysis of transgenic mice. I thank Janette Sanders for manuscript preparation. This research was supported by NIH grants CA40489, CA38635, AI20001, AI20720, HD17321, HD0912 and HD07155 and by a North Atlantic Treaty Organization grant for Inter-national Collaboration (675/84). This is publication number 5372BCR from the Department of Basic and Clinical Research, Research Institute of Scripps Clinic, La Jolla, California.

References

1. Tiollais, P., Pourcel, C. and Dejean, A. (1985). The hepatitis B virus. *Nature*, **317**, 489–95
2. Chisari, F. V., Filippi, P., McLachlan, A., Milich, D. R., Riggs, M., Lee, S., Palmiter, R. D., Pinkert, C. A. and Brinster, R. L. (1986). Expression of hepatitis B virus large envelope polypeptide inhibits hepatitis B surface antigen secretion in transgenic mice. *J. Virol.*, **60**, 880–7
3. Chisari, F. V., Pinkert, C. A., Milich, D. R., Filippi, P., McLachlan, A., Palmiter, R. D. and Brinster, R. L. (1985). A transgenic mouse model of the chronic hepatitis B surface antigen carrier state. *Science*, **230**, 1157–60

4. Chisari, F. V., Filippi, P., Buras, J., McLachlan, A., Popper, H., Pinkert, C. A., Palmiter, R. D. and Brinster, R. L. (1987). Structural and pathological effects of synthesis of hepatitis B virus large envelope polypeptide in transgenic mice. *Proc. Natl. Acad. Sci. USA*, **84**, 6909–13

5. Heermann, K. H., Goldmann, U., Schwartz, W., Seyffarth, T., Baumgarten, H. and Gerlich, W. H. (1984). Large surface proteins of hepatitis B virus containing the pre-s sequence. *J. Virol.*, **52**, 396–402

6. Takahashi, K., Kishimoto, S., Ohnuma, H., Machida, A., Takai, E., Tsuda, F., Miyamoto, H., Tanaka, T., Matsushita, K., Oda, K., Miyakawa, Y. and Mayumi, M. (1986). Polypeptides coded for by the region pre-s and gene s of hepatitis B virus DNA with the receptor for polymerized human serum albumin: Expression on the hepatitis B particles produced in the HBeAg or anti-HBe phase of hepatitis B virus infection. *J. Immunol.*, **136**, 3467–72

7. Eble, B. E., Lingappa, V. R. and Ganem, D. (1986). Hepatitis B surface antigen: an unusual secreted protein initially synthesized as a transmembrane polypeptide. *Mol. Cell. Biol.*, **6**, 1454–63

8. Patzer, E. J., Nakamura, G. R., Simonsen, C. C. and Levinson, A. D. (1984). Intracellular assembly and packaging of hepatitis B surface antigen particles occur in the endoplasmic reticulum. *J. Virol.*, **58**, 884–92

9. Patzer, E. J., Nakamura, G. R. and Yaffe, A. (1984). Intracellular transport and secretion of hepatitis B surface antigen in mamalian cells. *J. Virol.*, **51**, 346–53

10. Edmondson, H. A. (1958). Tumor-like lesions. *Tumors of the Liver and Intrahepatic Bile Ducts*, pp. 191–2. (Washington, DC: Armed Forces Institute of Pathology)

16
Hepatitis B virus in non-hepatocytes

H. E. BLUM, E. WALTER, K. TEUBNER, W.-B. OFFENSPERGER, S. S. OFFENSPERGER AND W. GEROK

INTRODUCTION

Infection with hepatitis B virus (HBV) is endemic throughout much of the world. Viral infection is associated with a wide spectrum of clinical presentations, ranging from the healthy carrier state to acute or fulminant hepatitis, to chronic hepatitis and liver cirrhosis. Further, chronic HBV infection is clearly involved in the development of hepatocellular carcinoma (HCC), worldwide a leading cause of death from cancer[1,2].

The structural and biological characteristics of HBV and the related viruses of the woodchuck[3] (WHV), the ground squirrel[4] (GSHV), the tree squirrel[5] (TSHV) and the Pekin duck[6] (DHBV) have been discussed in several recent reviews[7-9]. On the basis of their similar structural and biological properties, these viruses have been classified as hepatotropic DNA viruses (hepadnaviruses). The two cardinal biological features of hepadnavirus infection are species specificity and hepatotropism. While hepadnavirus infections have been considered strictly hepatotropic for many years, recent evidence suggests that HBV and the related viruses can exist in cells other than hepatocytes, i.e. in non-hepatocytes. In the following we will review four aspects of HBV in non-hepatocytes: (1) the type of non-hepatocytes (cells, tissues, organs) in which HBV has been detected (HBV standing for all hepadnaviruses); (2) the structure of viral nucleic acids in non-hepatocytes; (3) the correlation between the presence of HBV in non-hepatocytes and HBV serology or liver disease; (4) the significance of HBV in non-hepatocytes.

HBV-INFECTED NON-HEPATOCYTES

The host range of HBV and the related viruses is very narrow. In permissive hosts, viral antigens and nucleic acids are found primarily in liver cells. Recently, hepadnaviruses have also been detected, however, in cells other than hepatocytes (Table 1): in bile-duct epithelial cells[10-12] and endothelial

Table 1 HBV in non-hepatocytes

- Non-hepatocytes in liver
  Bile-duct epithelial cells
  Endothelial cells
- Pancreas
- Adrenal cortex
- Kidney
- Skin
- Kaposi sarcoma
- Spermatozoa
- Placenta
- Macrophages
- Spleen
- Bone marrow cells
- Peripheral white blood cells

cells[10] in the liver, in pancreas[6,11-17], in adrenal cortex[15], in kidney[11,12,14,16,18,19], in skin[14], in spleen[12,16-18,26], in bone marrow cells[27-29] and in various peripheral white blood cells[23,30-44]. These data are summarized in Table 2.

By immunohistochemical analyses, in DHBV-infected ducks DHBsAg has been identified in liver cells and in bile-duct epithelial cells (Figure 1), in

Table 2 HBV DNA, RNA and antigens in non-hepatocytes

Cells/Tissues	DNA	RNA	Antigen(s)	References
Non-hepatocytes in liver	+			10, 12
			+	11
Pancreas			+	6, 13, 15
	+	+	+	11
	+			14, 16, 17
	+		+	12
Adrenal cortex			+	15
Kidney	+			14, 16, 18, 19
	+	+	+	11
	+		+	12
Skin	+			14
Kaposi sarcoma	+			20
Spermatozoa	+			21–24
Placenta	+			19
Macrophages			+	25
Spleen	+			12, 16–18, 26
Bone-marrow cells	+		+	27
	+			28
			+	29
Peripheral white blood cells	+			23, 30, 32–36, 38–43
			+	31
	+	+		37
		+		44

LIVER

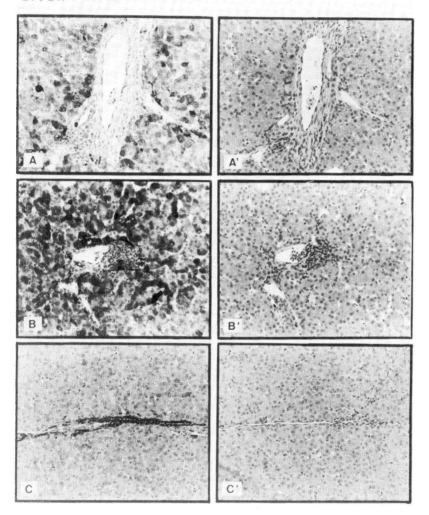

Figure 1   Detection of DHBsAg in the liver of DHBV-infected ducks, (A) and (B) hepatocytes and bile-duct epithelial cells, (C) bile-duct epithelial cells stained with antiDHBs antibodies, (A′–C′) same fields stained with pre-immune serum

pancreas and in kidney (Figure 2). By *in situ* hybridization viral DNA could be detected in liver cells and spleen from a patient with HBsAg- and HBeAg-positive chronic active hepatitis B (Figure 3); further in liver cells and pancreas from DHBV-infected ducks (Figure 4). These examples clearly demonstrate that HBV can exist outside hepatocytes, i.e. in non-hepatocytes in the liver, in pancreas, adrenal cortex, kidney, skin, Kaposi sarcoma, spermatozoa, placenta, macrophages, spleen, bone-marrow cells and a variety of peripheral white cells.

PANCREAS

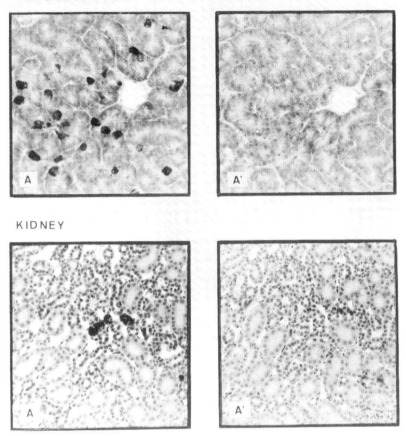

KIDNEY

Figure 2 Innumohistochemical detection of DHBsAg in pancreas (top) and kidney (bottom) of DHBV-infected ducks. Staining with anti DHBs antibodies (A) and pre-immune serum (A')

STRUCTURE OF VIRAL NUCLEIC ACIDS IN NON-HEPATOCYTES

Structure of viral DNA

The structure of hepadnaviral DNA species has been analyzed by agarose gel electrophoresis and Southern blot hybridization. Southern blot analyses of DNA extracted from HBV-infected liver tissue demonstrated that HBV DNA in hepatocytes can exist in two different states: (1) as free, extrachromosomal actively replicating, monomeric or oligomeric viral DNA (Figure 5A); and (2) as DNA sequences covalently integrated into the cellular genome (Figure 5B). The hybridization pattern in a patient with active viral replication is characterized by the presence of large amounts of free, extrachromosomal low-molecular-weight nascent DNA molecules (Figure 5A). These species were

LIVER   SPLEEN

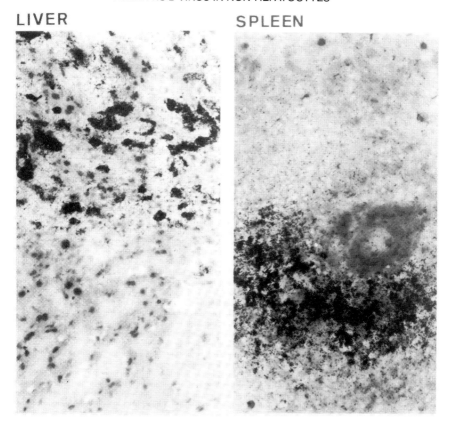

Figure 3 Detection of HBV DNA by *in situ* hybridization in liver (left) and spleen (right) from a patient with HBsAg- and HBeAg-positive chronic active hepatitis

shown to be predominantly single-stranded and of minus-strand polarity, demonstrating the asymmetric replication of the hepadnavirus genome[45-50]. By contrast, in a hepatocellular carcinoma (HCC) from a patient serologically positive for anti-HBc IgG and anti-HBs HBV DNA was found to be predominantly integrated into the host cell genome, frequently detectable as DNA species larger than 3.2 kbp after digestion with restriction endonucleases (Figure 5B), due to flanking host cellular sequences.

Southern blot analyses have also been applied to study the presence and state of viral DNA in non-hepatocytes. Detailed structural analyses have been performed in cells of hematopoietic origin. The data published to date are summarized in Table 3. In principle, all viral DNA species described in hepadnavirus-infected liver tissues have also been detected in cells of hematopoietic origin: low-molecular-weight replicative intermediates (ri), linear monomeric (lm), open circular (oc), covalently-closed circular (ccc) and oligomeric (oligo) HBV DNA species. Further, in some studies integrated viral DNA has been described[32,33,35-37,40,42]; the distinction between extra-

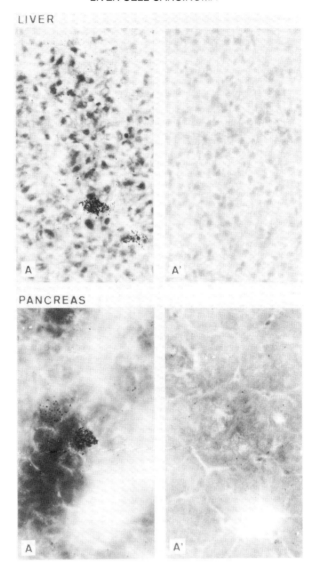

Figure 4 Detection of DHBV DNA by *in situ* hybridization in liver and pancreas. (A) DHBV-infected duck, (A') uninfected duck

chromosomal, high-molecular-weight oligomeric and truly integrated viral DNA species appears rather tenuous, however, in most studies. In any event, it is obvious from the data (Table 3) that in the majority of the studies of cells of hematopoietic origin, novel free, extrachromosomal, higher-molecular-weight oligomeric forms of HBV DNA are found; these nucleic acid species have rarely been detected in infected liver cells and are unknown in serum.

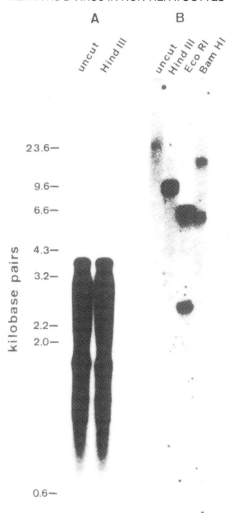

Figure 5 Detection of HBV DNA by Southern blot hybridization in the liver from a patient with HBsAg- and HBeAg-positive chronic active hepatitis (A) and in the hepatocellular carcinoma from a patient serologically positive for anti-HBc IgG and anti-HBs (B). Restriction enzymes are indicated at the top

The level of HBV DNA in peripheral blood lymphocytes (PBL) of chimpanzees was only 0.1 to 0.3 HBV genome equivalent per cell[37], i.e. 10–30-fold less than that observed for HBV in human PBL[30,32,35]. In both chimpanzees and woodchucks the level of viral DNA in PBL was approximately 100-fold less than that observed in hepatocytes[37].

Table 3 Structure of HBV DNA in cells of hematopoietic origin

Cell type	Free*					Integrated	References
	ri	lm	oc	ccc	oligo		
Lymphoblastoid cells			+	+			28
White blood cells					+		30
Mononuclear cells		+			+	(+)	32
White blood cells	(+)		+	+		+	33
Polymorphonuclear cells		+				+	34
Lymphocytes		+				(+)	35
Mononuclear cells	+	+				+	36
Lymphocytes		(+)			+	(+)	37
Monocytes	+				+		38
Mononuclear cells	+				+		39
Mononuclear cells		+			+	(+)	40
White blood cells		+	+	+	+		41
White blood cells		+					23
T cells					+	(+)	42

*ri = replicative intermediates; lm = linear monomeric forms; oc = open-circular forms; ccc = covalently-closed circular forms; oligo = high-molecular-weight oligomeric forms

Structure of viral RNA

The structure of hepadnaviral RNA species has been analyzed by agarose gel electrophoresis and Northern blot hybridization[7-9,51,52]. Northern blot analyses of RNA extracted from the liver of HBV-infected individuals and animals identified three major RNA species: (1) 3.5-kb genomic mRNA species, containing the full complement of the genetic information and serving as replication templates; (2) 2.1-kb subgenomic mRNA species for the pre-S2 and S proteins (middle and major proteins); (3) 2.4-kb subgenomic mRNA species for the expression of the pre-S1, pre-S2 and S proteins (large, middle and major proteins).

Northern blot analyses have also been applied to the study of the structure of viral transcripts in PLB of HBV-infected chimpanzees and WHV-infected woodchucks[37]: HBV RNA in the chimpanzee PBL existed primarily as 7.5-kb species; in some RNA samples, a 3.8-kb species was also observed. Interestingly, the migration pattern of HBV RNA in chimpanzee PBL differed from that observed in the liver of infected animals. WHV RNA isolated from the PBL of two chronic carrier woodchucks was present primarily as 4.3-, 3.8- and 2.3-kb species, similar to that observed in the animals' hepatocytes (Table 4). The level of viral RNA in the PBL of both chimpanzees and woodchucks was approximately 30-fold less than that observed in hepatocytes of these

Table 4 Structure of HBV/WHV RNA species in cells of hematopoietic origin

Cell type	RNA species	Reference
Lymphocytes	HBV: 3.8, 7.5 kb WHV: 2.3, 3.8 kb	37

animals[37]. Very importantly, this study for the first time demonstrates that viral DNA in non-hepatocytes can be transcriptionally active. By *in situ* hybridization, viral RNA has recently also been detected in mononuclear cells from HBsAg-positive and -negative individuals[44].

Table 5 Correlation between HBV in cells of hematopoietic origin and HBV serology

HBV serology		% HBV DNA/RNA positive (n)	References
Group I: HBsAg+, HBeAg+		66 (06)	32
		44 (25)	33
		100 (03) HIV +	39
		100 (05) HIV −	39
		40 (10)	41
		66 (12)	23
		58 (17)	44
	Average	56 (75)	
Group II: HBsAg+, anti-HBe+		62 (08)	32
		5 (22)	33
		66 (03)	34
		100 (02) HIV +	39
		33 (09) HIV −	39
		44 (18)	44
	Average	32 (60)	
Group III: HBsAg−, anti-HBs+		0 (03)	33
		100 (02) HIV +	35
		100 (10) HIV +	39
		33 (10) HIV −	39
		33 (03)	44
	Average	25 (16)	
Group IV: HBV marker negative		100 (01) HIV +	39
		0 (12) HIV −	39
		0 (11)	41
		100 (02)	44
	Average	8 (25)	

CORRELATION BETWEEN HBV IN NON-HEPATOCYTES AND HBV SEROLOGY OR LIVER DISEASE

The presence of HBV DNA or RNA in cells of hematopoietic origin has been correlated with the prevalence of serological markers of HBV infection and the type of disease. These data are of particular interest for our understanding of the epidemiological and clinical aspects of HBV in non-hepatocytes.

HBV in non-hepatocytes and HBV serology

In several clinical studies, the presence of HBV DNA or RNA in cells of hematopoietic origin has been correlated with the prevalence of serological markers of HBV infection. Four serological groups have been analyzed (Table 5): in group I, i.e. in patients with serological evidence for active viral replication (HBsAg- and HBeAg-positive) the frequency of HBV DNA or RNA in peripheral white blood cells was 56% (excluding HIV-positive patients). By comparison, in group II, i.e. in patients serologically positive for HBsAg and anti-HBe, the frequency was 32%. Most remarkably, however, in group III, i.e. in individuals serologically immune to HBV infection and in group IV, i.e. in patients negative for all markers of HBV infection, 25% and 8% of patients, respectively, had viral DNA or RNA in their peripheral white blood cells. Very interestingly, in all four groups all the HIV-positive patients appear to carry HBV in their mononuclear cells (Table 5).

HBV in non-hepatocytes and liver disease

In several clinico-pathological studies, the presence of HBV DNA or RNA in cells of hematopoietic origin has been correlated with the type of associated liver diseases. Five different groups of liver diseases have been analyzed (Table 6): asymptomatic patients, patients with acute hepatitis, patients with chronic persistent hepatitis (CPH), patients with chronic active hepatitis (CAH) and patients with hepatocellular carcinoma (HCC). The highest frequency of HBV DNA or RNA in peripheral white blood cells (excluding HBsAg-negative patient) was found in patients with acute hepatitis B (77%), CPH (75%) and CAH (60%). By comparison, only 39% of asymptomatic HBV carriers and 27% of patients with HCC had HBV DNA or RNA in their mononuclear cells.

SUMMARY AND PERSPECTIVES

HBV has been detected in non-hepatocytes, including bile-duct epithelial cells and endothelial cells in the liver, pancreas, adrenal cortex, skin, Kaposi sarcoma, spermatozoa, placenta, macrophages, spleen, bone-marrow cells and various peripheral white blood cells (Tables 1 and 2).

The viral DNA and RNA species in cells of hematopoietic origin have been

Table 6 Correlation between HBV in cells of hematopoietic origin and liver disease

Liver disease		% HBV DNA/RNA positive (n)	References
I. Asymptomatic			
		66 (06)	32
		33 (06)	40
		33 (12)	41
		33 (12)	44
	Average	39 (36)	
II. Acute hepatitis			
		100 (08) HBsAg +	40
		60 (03) HBsAg –	40
		40 (05)	41
	Average	77 (13)	
III. CPH			
		66 (06)	23
		80 (10)	44
	Average	75 (16)	
IV. CAH			
		57 (07)	32
		86 (21) HBsAg +	40
		33 (15) HBsAg –	40
		33 (15)	41
		71 (07)	23
		40 (10)	44
	Average	60 (32)	
V. Hepatocellular carcinoma			
		18 (11)	30
		66 (03) HBsAg +	40
		31 (16) HBsAg –	40
		27 (15)	41
	Average	27 (29)	

characterized in great detail (Tables 3 and 4). HBV DNA and RNA species found in these non-hepatocytes frequently differ in structure from the pattern seen in infected hepatocytes. Further, viral DNA and RNA species in these cells are present in significantly lower copy number than in productively infected liver cells[30,32,35,37].

The presence of HBV in non-hepatocytes is a frequent event (Tables 5 and 6): in some studies, in up to 100% of patients HBV DNA or RNA is found in cells of hematopoietic origin. The presence of HBV in non-hepatocytes correlates with HBV serology and the type of liver disease. The highest frequency is found in patients with serological evidence for viral replication (HBsAg- and HBeAg-positive) and in patients with histologic evidence for viral hepatitis, i.e. in patients with acute hepatitis B, CPH or CAH. Further, all HIV-positive patients appear to carry HBV in their peripheral white blood cells, irrespective of their HBV serology.

Despite possible artefacts in some studies (non-specific method of detection of viral antigens or nucleic acids; cross-reaction or cross-hybridization of antibodies or probes with cellular constituents induced by HBV infection, HIV infection or others; 'contamination' of cellular or tissue preparations with HBV from serum; adhesion or adsorption of HBV to cell membranes; phago- or endocytosis of extracellular HBV), several lines of evidence demonstrate the true existence of HBV in non-hepatocytes: (1) Dane-like particles have been detected in the culture medium of lymphoblastoid cells from the bone marrow of a patient with HBV infection[27]; (2) viral RNA and antigens have been detected in peripheral white blood cells, indicating that viral genes are transcriptionally active in these cells (Tables 3 and 4); (3) the structure of viral DNA and RNA in peripheral white blood cells is frequently different from the forms detected in serum or hepatocytes (Tables 3 and 4).

The biological significance of HBV in non-hepatocytes remains largely undefined. The findings mentioned above demonstrate, however, that HBV and its related animal viruses are not strictly hepatotropic and that the tissue tropism of these viruses is broader than once thought: obviously, non-hepatocytes are permissive for all aspects of the life cycle of HBV, including attachment of the virus to the cell surface, internalization of the virus, viral replication[45-50] and integration as well as expression of viral genes[51,52]. One can speculate that non-hepatocytes are the initial site of viral infection and/or the site of viral persistence and the reservoir for (re-)infection of hepatocytes, even in the face of the host's immune response (Table 5). Finally, one can hypothesize that viral infection of non-hepatocytes may have direct biological consequences and may be involved in the pathogenesis of disease, such as AIDS-related complex, AIDS, aplastic anemia, agranulocytosis, pancytopenia, polyarthritis nodosa, glomerulonephritis and possibly others.

To firmly establish the HBV specificity and the genetic identity of HBV in hepatocytes and non-hepatocytes, the fine structure of viral DNA in non-hepatocytes should be determined by molecular cloning and nucleotide sequence analyses. For these analyses, it would be extremely helpful to have non-hepatocytes in culture, stably carrying the viral genome and expressing viral genes. In such a cell line, e.g. lymphoblastoid cells, lymphocytes or Kupffer cells, one could study: (1) the biology of HBV in non-hepatocytes; (2) the impact of HBV infection on host cellular functions; and (3) the effect of antiviral therapy on the biology of HBV in non-hepatocytes, possibly an important aspect for the long-term success of therapeutic strategies.

Acknowledgements

We thank Ms. P. Kary and Ms. C. Zeschnigk for expert technical assistance. The experimental studies were supported by a grant from the Deutsche Forschungsgemeinschaft (SFB154 Project A2) and a Hermann-and-Lilly-Schilling professorship from the Stifterverband fuer die Deutsche Wissenschaft to H. E. Blum.

References

1. Okuda, K. and Mackay, I. (eds.) (1982). *Hepatocellular Carcinoma*. Technical Report Series, Vol. 74 (Geneva: International Union against Cancer)
2. Blum, H. E., Gerok, W., Tong, M. J. and Vyas, G. N. (1986). Hepatitis B virus infection and hepatocellular carcinoma. *IM (International Medicine for the Specialist)*, 7, 195–211
3. Summers, J., Smolec, J. and Snyder, R. (1978). A virus similar to human hepatitis B virus associated with hepatitis and hepatoma in woodchucks. *Proc. Natl. Acad. Sci. USA*, 75, 4533–7
4. Marion, P. L., Oshiro, L. S., Regnery, D. C., Scullard, G. A. and Robinson, W. S. (1980). A virus in Beechy ground squirrel that is related to hepatitis B virus of humans. *Proc. Natl. Acad. Sci. USA*, 77, 2941–5
5. Feitelson, M. A., Millman, I. and Blumberg, B. S. (1986). Tree squirrel hepatitis B virus: Antigenic and structural characterization. *Proc. Natl. Acad. Sci. USA*, 83, 2994–7
6. Mason, W. S., Seal, G. and Summers, J. (1980). Virus of Pekin ducks with structural and biological relatedness to human hepatitis B virus. *J. Virol.*, 36, 829–36
7. Tiollais, P., Pourcel, C. and Dejean, A. (1985). The hepatitis B virus. *Nature*, 317, 489–95
8. Standring, D. N. and Rutter, W. J. (1986). The molecular analysis of hepatitis B virus. *Prog. Liver Dis.*, 8, 311–33
9. Ganem, D. and Varmus, H. E. (1987). The molecular biology of the hepatitis viruses. *Annu. Rev. Biochem.*, 56, 651–93
10. Blum, H. E., Stowring, L., Figus, A., Montgomery, C. K., Haase, A. T. and Vyas, G. N. (1983). Detection of hepatitis B virus DNA in hepatocytes, bile duct epithelium, and vascular elements by *in situ* hybridization. *Proc. Natl. Acad. Sci. USA*, 80, 6685–8
11. Halpern, M. S., England, J. M., Deery, D. T., Petcu, D. J., Mason, W. S. and Molnar-Kimber, K. L. (1983). Viral nucleic acid synthesis and antigen accumulation in pancreas and kidney of Pekin ducks infected with duck hepatitis B virus. *Proc. Natl. Acad. Sci. USA*, 80, 4865–9
12. Freiman, J. S., Jilbert, A. R., Dixon, R. J., Holmes, M., Gowans, E. J., Burrell, C. J., Wills, E. J. and Cossart, Y. E. (1988). Experimental duck hepatitis B virus infection: Pathology and evolution of hepatic and extrahepatic infection. *Hepatology*, 8, 507–13
13. Shimoda, T., Shikata, T., Karasawa, T., Tsukagoshi, S., Yoshimura, M. and Sakurai, I. (1981). Light microscopic localization of hepatitis B virus antigens in the human pancreas. Possibility of multiplication of hepatitis B virus in the human pancreas. *Gastroenterology*, 81, 998–1005
14. Dejean, A., Lugassy, C., Zafrani, S., Tiollais, P. and Brechot, C. (1984). Detection of hepatitis B virus DNA in pancreas, kidney and skin of two human carriers of the virus. *J. Gen. Virol.*, 65, 651–5
15. Halpern, M. S., Egan, J., Mason, W. S. and England, J. M. (1984). Viral antigen in endocrine cells of the pancreatic islets and adrenal cortex of Pekin ducks infected with duck hepatitis B virus. *Virus Res.*, 1, 213–23
16. Tagawa, M., Omata, M., Yokosuka, O., Uchiumi, K., Imazeki, F. and Okuda, K. (1985). Early events in duck hepatitis B virus infection. Sequential appearance of viral deoxyribonucleic acid in the liver, pancreas, kidney and spleen. *Gastroenterology*, 89, 1224–9
17. Jilbert, A. R., Freiman, J. S., Gowans, E. J., Holmes, M., Cossart, Y. E. and Burell, C. J. (1987). Duck hepatitis B virus DNA in liver, spleen and pancreas: Analysis by *in situ* and Southern blot hybridization. *Virology*, 158, 330–8
18. Ganem, D., Weiser, B., Barchuck, A., Brown, R. J. and Varmus, H. E. (1982). Biological characterization of acute infection with ground squirrel virus. *J. Virol.*, 44, 366–73
19. Naumova, A. K., Favorov, M. O., Keteladze, E. S., Nosikov, V. V. and Kisselev, L. L. (1985). Nucleotide sequences in human chromosomal DNA from nonhepatic tissues homologous to the hepatitis B virus genome. *Gene*, 35, 19–25
20. Siddiqui, A. (1983). Hepatitis B virus DNA in Kaposi sacroma. *Proc. Natl. Acad. Sci. USA*, 80, 4861–4
21. Karayiannis, P., Novick, D. M., Lok, A. S. F., Fowler, M. J. F., Monjardino, J. and Thomas, H. C. (1985). Hepatitis B virus DNA in saliva, urine, and seminal fluid of carriers of hepatitis Be antigen. *Br. Med. J.*, 290, 1853–5
22. Hadchouel, M., Scotto, J., Huret, C., Molinie, C., Villa, E., Degos, Q. and Brechot, C.

(1985). Presence of HBV in spermatozoa. A possible vertical transmission via the germ line. *J. Med. Virol.,* **16**, 61–6

23. Davison, F., Alexander, G. J. M., Trowbridge, R., Fagan, E. A. and Williams, R. (1987). Detection of hepatitis B virus DNA in spermatozoa, urine, saliva and leucocytes of chronic HBsAg carriers. *J. Hepatol.,* **4**, 37–44

24. Jenison, S. A., Lemon, S. M., Baker, L. N. and Newbold, J. E. (1987). Quantitative analysis of hepatitis B virus DNA in saliva and semen of chronically infected homosexual men. *J. Infect. Dis.,* **156**, 299–307

25. Milovanovic, M. V., Zivanovic-Marinkovic, V., Nanusevic, N. and Stankovic, D. (1987). Hepatitis B virus in tissue culture systems. I. Serial propagation of virus in human macrophages. *Intervirology,* **27**, 1–8

26. Blum, H. E. and Vyas, G. N. (1983). Hepatitis B virus in non-hepatocytes. *Lancet,* **2**, 920, (Letter to the Editor)

27. Romet-Lemonne, J. -L., Frances-McLane, M., Elfassi, E., Haseltine, W. A., Azocar, J. and Essex, M. (1983). Hepatitis B virus infection in cultured human lymphoblastoid cells. *Science,* **221**, 667–9

28. Elfassi, E., Romet-Lemonne, J. -L., Essex, M., Frances-McLane, M. and Haseltine, W. A. (1984). Evidence of extrachromosomal forms of hepatitis B viral DNA in a bone marrow culture obtained from a patient recently infected with hepatitis B virus. *Proc. Natl. Acad. Sci. USA,* **81**, 3526–8

29. Zeldis, J. B., Mugishima, H., Steinberg, H. N., Nir, E. and Gale, R. P. (1986). *In vitro* hepatitis B virus infection of human bone marrow cells. *J. Clin. Invest.,* **78**, 411–17

30. Lie-Injo, L. E., Balasegaram, M., Lopez, C. G. and Herrera, A. R. (1983). Hepatitis B virus DNA in liver and white blood cells of patients with hepatoma. *DNA,* **2**, 301–8

31. Ding, J. L. and Oon, C. J. (1984). Detection of HBeAg in the lymphocytes of sero-HBeAg negative patients with chronic hepatitis B and primary hepatocellular carcinoma. *Cytobios,* **39**, 29–33

32. Pontisso, P., Poon, M. C., Tiollais, P. and Brechot, C. (1987). Detection of hepatitis B virus DNA in mononuclear blood cells. *Br. J. Med.,* **288**, 1563–6

3 Gu, J.-R., Chen, Y.-C., Jiang, H.-Q., Zhang, Y.-L., Wu, S.-M., Jiang, W.-L. and Jian, J. J. (1985). State of hepatitis B virus DNA in leucocytes of hepatitis B patients. *J. Med. Virol.,* **17**, 73–81

34. Hoar, D. I., Bowen, T., Matheson, D. and Poon, M. C. (1985). Hepatitis B virus DNA is enriched in polymorphonuclear cells. *Blood,* **66**, 1251–3

35. Laure, E., Zagury, D., Saimot, A. G., Gallo, R. C., Hahn, B. H. and Brechot, C. (1985). Hepatitis B virus DNA sequences in lymphoid cells from patients with AIDS and AIDS-related complex *Science,* **229**, 561–3

36. Morichika, S., Hada, H., Arima, T., Togawa, K., Watanabe, M. and Nagashima, H. (1985). Hepatitis B virus DNA replication in peripheral blood mononuclear cells. *Lancet,* **2**, 1431. (Letter to the Editor)

37. Korba, B. E., Wells, F., Tennant, B. C., Yoakum, G. H., Purcell, R. H. and Gerin, J. L. (1986). Hepadnavirus infection of peripheral blood lymphocytes *in vivo:* Woodchuck and chimpanzee models of viral hepatitis. *J. Virol.,* **58**, 1–8

38. Yoffe, B., Noonan, C. A., Melnick, J. L. and Hollinger, F. B. (1986). Hepatitis B virus DNA in mononuclear cells and analysis of cell subsets for the presence of replicative intermediates of viral DNA. *J. Infect. Dis.,* **153**, 471–7

39. Noonan, C. A., Yoffe, B., Mansell, P. W. A., Melnick, J. L. and Hollinger, F. B. (1986). Extrachromosomal sequences of hepatitis B virus DNA in peripheral blood mononuclear cells of acquired immune deficiency syndrome patients. *Proc. Natl. Acad. Sci. USA.,* **8**, 5698–702

40. Pasquinelli, C., Laure, F., Chatenoud, L., Beaurain, G., Gazengel, C., Bismuth, H., Degos, F., Tiollais, P., Bach, J. F. and Brechot, C. (1986). Hepatitis B virus DNA in mononuclear blood cells. A frequent event in hepatitis B surface antigen-positive and -negative patients with acute and chronic liver disease. *J. Hepatol.,* **3**, 95–103

41. Shen, H.-D., Choo, K.-B., Lee, S.-D., Tsai, Y.-T. and Han, S.-H. (1986). Hepatitis B virus DNA in leucocytes of patients with hepatitis B virus-associated liver diseases. *J. Med. Virol.,* **18**, 201–11

42. Laure, F., Chantenoud, L., Pasquinelli, C., Gazengel, C., Beaurain, G., Torchet, M. -F., Zagury, D., Bach, J. F. and Brechot, C. (1987). Frequent lymphocyte infection by hepatitis

B virus in haemophiliacs. *Br. J. Haematol.,* **65**, 181–5
43. Shen, H.-D., Choo, K.-B., Wu, T.-C. and Han, S.-H. (1987). Hepatitis B virus infection of cord blood leucocytes. *J. Med. Virol.,* **22**, 211–16
44. Hadchouel, M., Pasquinelli, C., Fournier, J. G., Hugon, R. N., Scotto, J., Bernard, O. and Brechot, C. (1988). Detection of mononuclear cells expressing hepatitis B virus in peripheral blood from HBsAg positive and negative patients by *in situ* hybridisation. *J. Med. Virol.,* **24**, 27–32
45. Summers, J. and Mason, W. S. (1982). Replication of the genome of a hepatitis B-like virus by reverse transcription of an RNA intermediate. *Cell,* **29**, 403–15
46. Miller, R. H., Tran, C.-T. and Robinson, W. S. (1984). Hepatitis B virus particles of plasma and liver contain viral DNA–RNA hybrid molecules. *Virology,* **139**, 53–63
47. Miller, R. H., Marion, P. L. and Robinson, W. S. (1984). Hepatitis B viral DNA–RNA hybrid molecules in particles from infected liver are converted to viral DNA molecules during an endogenous DNA polymerase reaction. *Virology,* **139**, 64–72
48. Blum, H. E., Haase, A. T., Harris, J. D., Walker, D. and Vyas, G. N. (1984). Asymmetric replication of hepatitis B virus DNA in human liver: Demonstration of cytoplasmic minus-strand DNA by blot analyses and *in situ* hybridization. *Virology,* **139**, 87–96
49. Seeger, C., Ganem, D. and Varmus, H. E. (1986). Biochemical and genetic evidence for the hepatitis B virus replication strategy. *Science,* **232**, 477–84
50. Will, H., Reiser, W., Weimer, T., Pfaff, E., Büscher, M., Sprengel, R., Cattaneo, R. and Schaller, H. (1987). Replication strategy of human hepatitis B virus. *J. Virol.,* **61**, 904–11
51. Catteneo, R., Will, H. and Schaller, H. (1984). Hepatitis B virus transcription in the infected liver. *EMBO J.,* **3**, 2191–6
52. Enders, G., Ganem, D. and Varmus, H. E. (1985). Mapping the major transcripts of ground squirrel hepatitis virus: The presumptive template for reverse transcriptase is terminally redundant. *Cell,* **42**, 297–308

Section 3
Chemicals and hepato carcinogenesis

17
Experimental induction of hepatocellular carcinoma by chemical carcinogens

G. N. WOGAN AND G. McMAHON

INTRODUCTION

Several hundreds of chemicals have been shown to have carcinogenic activity in experimental animals, and the literature is replete with examples of organic compounds representing many chemical classes that produce liver cell carcinomas or other liver tumours when administered to animals under appropriate conditions. In a large proportion of these investigations, the carcinogens were used as model compounds in experiments dealing with one or another facet of the carcinogenesis process. Useful as such information may be in contributing to improved understanding of underlying mechanisms, it has not greatly enhanced elucidation of the aetiologic factors for primary hepatocellular carcinomas in man, because most of the model compounds that have been used would probably never be encountered by human populations. However, with the recent discovery of oncogenes and mechanisms for their activation, including mutations or other DNA sequence changes of the type caused by chemical carcinogens in experimental systems, the technical capability has evolved to determine whether similar molecular and cellular changes exist in human tumours. Direct comparison of experimentally-induced cancers with those appearing in humans may therefore reveal much additional information concerning the possible role of chemical carcinogens in the aetiology of human cancer risk.

The number of known synthetic carcinogens is now large and the list is continuously expanding as additional chemicals are tested for carcinogenic activity. Classes of synthetic chemical carcinogens include the large group of polycyclic aromatic hydrocarbons, aromatic amines, azo compounds, alkylating agents, lactones, N-nitroso compounds, metals, and many other specific chemical structures. On the basis of available evidence, there seems to be no strong reason to invoke most of these carcinogens as possible aetiologic agents for primary hepatocellular carcinoma, with the exceptions of nitrosamines, certain chlorinated hydrocarbons, and specific compounds such as ethanol and urethan which impact human populations in a variety of ways.

In addition to the above carcinogens, which are androgenic in origin, a number of very potent carcinogens of natural origin have also been characterized, and the possibility that certain of them may be aetiologic factors for human disease has been extensively discussed. Those compounds in this group that induce primary liver cancer in animals include aflatoxins and certain other mycotoxins, pyrrolizidine alkaloids, cycasin, and several other constituents of edible plants. Most are encountered by man as a consequence of their presence in food or beverages. In some circumstances, carcinogenic agents are either present as normal constituents of plants or plant products used as foods, herbal medicines or teas.

The geographic pathology of human liver cancer suggests the involvement of environmental factors, including infection with the hepatitis B virus. In this respect, liver cell cancer represents a generic problem that exemplifies the most difficult aspects of environmental carcinogenesis. The number of possible carcinogens that might constitute the total carcinogenic burden for the liver is potentially very large. In many instances, the carcinogens themselves or precursors capable of forming them are widely distributed in the environment. Both factors create a large potential for exposure, which is probably long-term, low-level in character, characteristics that make it extremely difficult to establish cause and effect relationships. For these reasons, in making assessments of public health risk represented by carcinogens, heavy reliance must be placed upon evidence of carcinogenicity in experimental animals coupled with estimates of the extent to which human populations are exposed to specific carcinogens.

On the basis of the various chemical carcinogens known to induce liver cell cancer in animals, the strongest evidence for involvement in human liver cancer exists for the aflatoxins. Others that might be involved include: sterigmatocystin and perhaps other mycotoxins; certain pyrrolizidine alkaloids; cycasin and related glycosides; carcinogenic nitrosamines and nitrosamides formed through the interaction of nitrite and nitrosatable substrates in the environment; the components of alcoholic beverages such as ethanol and urethan. It is impossible to assess with any certainty the importance of other known synthetic carcinogens, such as the chlorinated hydrocarbons, even though some of them are widely distributed at low levels in the environment. Although many other experimental carcinogens are known to exist, there seems no reason to implicate them as aetiologic agents for the human disease in the absence of further evidence.

Aflatoxins

The carcinogenic properties of the aflatoxins have been very extensively studied, and much information has been produced concerning various aspects of their mechanisms of action, occurrence in foods, and their possible involvement as human cancer risk factors. A fairly recent comprehensive review is that of Busby and Wogan[1], in which is summarized detailed information concerning many aspects of the field. In the context of the present discussion, several attributes of the aflatoxins relevant to human primary hepatocellular carcinoma are of particular interest. Aflatoxins, especially aflatoxin B_1 (AFB$_1$), are so frequently encountered in some constituents of human diets as to be virtually unavoidable contaminants, usually at levels of a few parts per billion or less. An extensive amount of data has been generated associating elevated exposure of such agents to human populations with elevated incidence of primary hepatocellular carcinoma. Studies of metabolism of AFB$_1$ have revealed that the compound is activated to its electrophilic DNA binding form, through an epoxidation pathway that is identical in human cells and in experimental systems that respond to its biological effects. Furthermore, activation and DNA binding produces identical DNA adduct profiles, with the N^7-position of guanine representing the only site of adduct formation, in experimental animals and humans. AFB$_1$ is a potent mutagen for cells (including those of human origin) in culture, and is also a powerful carcinogen for the liver of many experimental animals, including sub-human primates.

Taken together, this evidence strongly suggests that humans consuming diets contaminated with aflatoxins may be at elevated risk for their carcinogenic and other genotoxic effects, in particular for liver cancer. For these reasons, our group has had a long-standing interest in pursuing lines of investigation that may elucidate further the significance of aflatoxins as environmental carcinogens. We have recently been investigating the role of oncogene activation in aflatoxin-induced liver cancer in rodents.

EXPERIMENTAL APPROACHES

Animal models of hepatocarcinogensis have provided important information with regard to the metabolism of co-carcinogens and interaction of carcinogens with the DNA molecule. Since much is known regarding the metabolism and binding of chemical carcinogens to DNA, we sought to correlate whether exposure of an animal to a known hepatocarcinogen, aflatoxin B$_1$, would result in the mutagenic activation of oncogenes. Since most of the past work has been performed in rats, our inclination was to attempt to identify oncogenes in AFB$_1$-induced rat liver tumours. However, the detection of oncogenes in rat liver tumours derived by treatment of other carcinogenic chemicals has been elusive. Specifically, no oncogenes have been identified in spontaneous or chemically-induced rat liver tumours. In contrast, c-Ha-*ras* oncogenes have been identified in some spontaneous[2] and chemically-induced liver tumours from the B6C3F1 mouse[3]. The reason for this apparent discrepancy is unclear at this time. Nonetheless, we sought to determine whether rat liver tumours induced by exposure of the animal to AFB$_1$ would result in the appearance of transforming genes.

As we have described previously[4], male Fischer rats were administered AFB$_1$ in multiple intraperitoneal injections for 2 months. All of the treated animals developed hepatocellular carcinomas within 16 months. In contrast, none of the control animals developed any evidence of aberrant liver histopathology. The schemes used to detect oncogenes involved DNA-mediated transfer into NIH3T3 mouse fibroblasts using calcium phosphate co-precipitation followed by selection for transformed fibroblasts. The first approach to identify oncogenes utilized DNA transfection of genomic DNA isolated from the primary liver tumour into mouse fibroblasts followed by selection of transformed foci. The second approach utilized the co-transfection of liver tumour DNA with a plasmid containing a selectable growth marker[5]. Use of this latter method resulted in a population of G418-resistant fibroblast clones which could be pooled and injected subcutaneously into athymic Nu–Nu mice. In this case, tumour formation indicated the presence of a rat oncogene. Using both the focus formation and Nu–Nu assay, we were able to identify biologically-active oncogenes which were stable and effective in transforming NIH3T3 cells in subsequent transfections. Southern blot analysis of the transformant DNA led to the identification of these oncogenes as those of the c-Ki-*ras* gene family in 4/10 (40%) liver tumours assayed by these methods.

The research of others strongly suggested that the activation of c-*ras* proto-oncogenes to oncogenic forms may be due to single-base mutations which result in single amino acid substitutions in the p21 protein. Moreover, it has been shown that the predominant sites for such subtle genetic changes occur in regions which include codon 12 or 61 of the gene[6]. In addition, bacterial mutagenesis studies with AFB$_1$ suggested[7] that the AFB$_1$-induced mutations occur predominantly at G–C base pairs resulting in both G–C to T–A base transversions (89%) and G–C to A–T base transitions (6%). For these reasons, we chose to analyse the first exon of the rat c-Ki-*ras* gene which has been shown to contain codon 12 including two potential G–C base pairs which may be mutated by AFB$_1$ exposure. To accomplish this, we employed selective hybridization of synthetic oligonucleotides to identify particular mutated alleles resulting in amino acid substitutions at codon 12. Using this technique, mutant homoduplexes between the radiolabelled oligonucleotide and the mutated oncogene DNA would be stable whereas heteroduplexes containing the mutant oligonucleotide would be unstable and melt at elevated temperature. Analysis of the transformants hybridized to particular mutant oligomers indicated the presence of activating mutations in codon 12 resulting in TGT (Cys), GAT (Asp), and GTT (Val) codons. In these cases, different mutated alleles were present in transformants from individual AFB$_1$-induced liver tumours. Importantly, the mutations in all the oncogenes resided at G–C base pairs and resulted in both G–C to T–A (3/4) and G–C to A–T (1/4) base changes. Such mutations are very consistent with the nature of AFB$_1$-induced mutations detected in bacterial mutation assays. Consequently, our results strongly indicated that the genetic changes in the liver oncogenes may have been a direct consequence of AFB$_1$–DNA interaction.

The analysis of such genetic changes in the oncogenes relied upon the stable transfer of the mutated gene into NIH3T3 cells followed by appropriate selection of the transformed fibroblast. We felt that since the transfection procedure relied upon a rare recombinant many genetic changes in this gene region may be missed. Consequently, the fortuitous mutant alleles we have scored may under-represent the full spectrum of genes containing somatic mutations in the liver tumour cell. In addition, we hypothesized that some mutated oncogenes may not transform fibroblasts efficiently but may have

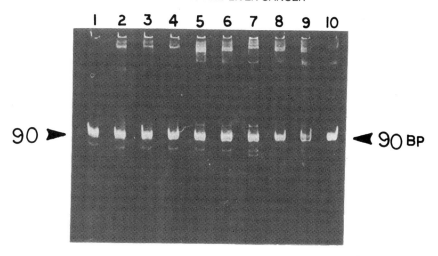

Figure 1 Analysis of PCR DNA product derived from AFB₁-induced rat hepatocellular carcinomas. PCR DNA was derived from the first exon of the rat c-Ki-*ras* gene using synthetic oligonucleotide primers spanning codons 1–35. The PCR reactions contained *Taq* polymerase and were performed for 40 cycles. The DNA product was analysed by electrophoresis in a native 10% polyacrylamide gel, stained with ethidium bromide, and photographed. The photograph indicates independent rat liver tumour samples (1–10) and the resultant 90-bp DNA bands.

more relevance in hepatocarcinogenesis. To confirm the presence of these oncogenic mutations in the liver and to identify novel mutated alleles in this gene region, we employed the polymerase chain reaction (PCR) DNA amplification method[8]. This methodology utilizes sequential annealing of gene-specific oligonucleotide primers followed by extension with polymerase to enzymatically amplify specific gene regions in eukaryotic DNA. We have employed the PCR method for the first exon of the rat c-Ki-*ras* gene from codons 1–35 as we have described previously[9]. Initial studies using the Klenow fragment of *E. coli* DNA polymerase resulted in PCR DNA of multiple forms resulting from mispriming of oligonucleotide (amplimers) at non-specific sites in the rat DNA. The recent use of the thermostable DNA polymerase, isolated from *T. aquaticus (Taq* polymerase), results in a more specific amplification of the c-Ki-*ras* gene (Fig. 1). We have since shown that the mutation frequency present in the PCR DNA reflects the mutation frequency in the original template suggesting its application to estimates of the mutant allele distribution in the primary tumour DNA. To quantitate the mutation frequency and to detect novel mutant alleles we have employed several methodologies. They include (i) allele-specific oligonucleotide hybridization (ASO), (ii) direct DNA sequencing of PCR, DNA, and (iii) cloning and sequencing of PCR product into M13 phage. As we have described, the ASO procedure utilizes selective hybridization of synthetic oligomers specific for particular mutated alleles. This method has been described for the detection of oncogene mutations by Verlaan-de Vries *et al.*[10]. We have applied this approach to determine mutations in NIH3T3 transformant DNA containing a single mutation. The second, direct DNA sequencing, approach has the advantage of not restricting the analysis to specific nucleotide domains, as in the case of ASO. In general, this approach relies upon the annealing of radiolabelled oligomer to PCR DNA followed by polymerase extension in the presence of dideoxy-nucleotide triphosphates. For our purposes, we have routinely radiolabelled either of the two amplimers from the PCR reaction using polynucleotide kinase in the presence of $[^{32}P]$ATP. However, this method is not effective for mutated alleles which are at low frequency in the tumour DNA preparation since wild-type DNA sequences are predominant.

Sine we wished to analyse the gene region in detail, we cloned and sequenced PCR DNA product derived from the AFB_1-induced rat liver tumours. As shown in Fig. 2, amplimers for the PCR reaction included a gene-specific primer binding region and a restriction site linker domain. After sequential primer-directed DNA amplification, a PCR product was generated which contained a DNA region bound by the gene-specific primer binding

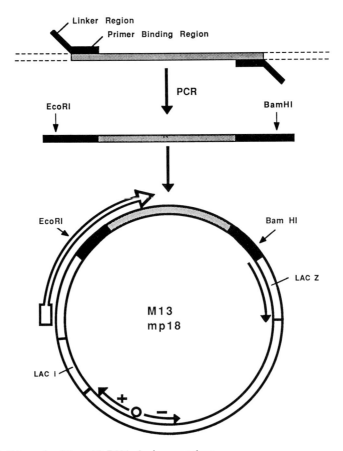

Figure 2 Schematic of the PCR DNA cloning procedure.

regions with additional DNA segments containing novel restriction enzyme cutting sites. Restriction of the PCR DNA results in cohesive ends which are easily cloned into M13 bacteriophage. The resultant recombinants are then sequenced using conventional methods.

A compilation of some of the mutated alleles derived from AFB$_1$-induced liver tumours is illustrated in Fig. 3. It is important to note that multiple mutated alleles have been derived from individual liver tumour DNA preparations. In all cases, one such allele from each tumour DNA correlates with codon 12 mutation determined in the transformation assays. However, additional alleles have been detected which were not scored in the transformation assays. For instance, one allele contained multiple mutations resulting in three amino acid substitutions for which two of them resided in codons 13 and 14. Another mutated allele from a different tumour DNA, resulted in a single amino acid substitution in codon 14. Analysis of hundreds of phage derived from *Taq*-amplified PCR DNA of control rat livers did not indicate the presence of any mutations. Therefore, the clustering of amino acid substitutions in the 12–14 codon region of the genes derived from primary liver tumours suggests that such a region in the protein may have an important role in the formation of the neoplasia. Importantly, this methodology enables us to estimate the relative allele distribution for a given tumour DNA preparation. As predicted, the oncogene alleles scored by either focus formation or the tumorigenicity assay represented a subset of the mutated genes present in the original template. In addition, it appears that the frequencies of the genetic changes indicated by oncogene identification are an underestimate of the AFB$_1$-induced mutational spectrum present in this gene region.

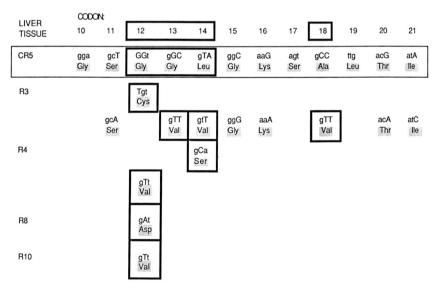

Figure 3 Summary of mutations and amino acid substitutions in c-Ki-*ras* genes derived from AFB$_1$-induced rat liver tumours. Upper case letters refer to mutated nucleotides. Amino acid substitutions are indicated by those codons outlined in bold lines.

DISCUSSION

Since the mutations we have scored are somatic, the presence of mutations implicates oncogenic *c-ras* proteins in the mechanism underlying chemically-induced hepatocarcinogenesis. However, the temporal and/or causal role of oncogenic c-*ras* proteins in the cancer process is undefined. In addition, our findings of different oncogenic mutations and the apparent absence of onco-genes in some tumour DNA preparations suggest that alternate oncogenic proteins may replace, augment, or complement the mutant c-*ras* gene products in liver neoplasia. For instance, other investigators have shown that oncogenic c-Ha-*ras* protein alone is generally incapable of transforming primary rat fibroblasts. However, the simultaneous presence of the mutant c-*ras* protein and an additional nuclear oncogene of the c-*myc* class of oncogenic products is sufficient to bring about transformation[11]. It is of interest in this context that we have found elevated levels of c-*myc* mRNA in rat livers during dosing with AFB_1. In addition, we have noted a 10–20-fold elevation of c-*myc* mRNA in AFB_1-induced primary liver tumours. We can therefore conjecture that the presence of increased c-*myc* protein may signal cell proliferative events during compensatory regeneration, which could in turn cooperate with chemically-induced c-*ras* oncoproteins to transform the hepatocyte. This hypothesis is strengthened by findings relating elevation of c-*myc* mRNA in livers of rats following partial hepatectomy[12]. It can further be postulated that the cell-proliferative events may, alternatively, be signalled by agents which could include chemical promoters, cell regeneration, or hepatitis B virus infection. Therefore, the multiple factor model as it applies to animal hepatocarcinogenesis might reasonably include complementary classes of oncogene products. The role of chemicals in the neoplastic process may serve to either create mutant oncoproteins at the DNA level or induce compensatory regeneration due to cytotoxicity, or both.

Our own experimental evidence would suggest that some chemically-induced somatic mutations in biologically-relevant genetic loci my be operat-ing in the emergent tumour cell. These findings are of particular interest in view of recent findings concerning oncogenes in human primary hepatic cancer. Gu *et al.*[13] recently reported that human N-*ras* oncogene sequences were present in the DNA from a high proportion of human liver tumours. Expression of N-*ras* was also markedly enhanced, as was the level of the gene product. Furthermore, c-*myc* was also highly expressed in most tumours, implying that the cooperating activities of the two oncogenes might be responsible for the malignant phenotypic alterations in some cases of human primary liver cancer. Identification of mutations in the N-*ras* oncogene associated with its activation was not reported. It is particularly noteworthy that the technical procedures employed in our experimental studies for the detection and identification of mutations are directly applicable to DNA samples from human tumours, and will greatly facilitate the further character-ization of oncogenes in them. Such analyses will permit direct comparison of oncogene activation and other changes in DNA in human tumours with those induced in well-characterized and defined experimental systems.

The presence of hepatocytes containing mutated oncogene alleles may be phenotypically dormant or may represent only a few cells. The emergence of the neoplatic hepatocyte may occur as a consequence of other cooperative cellular events signalled by viral or chemically-induced cytotoxicity. These latter cellular events may, as in the case of hepatitis infection, or may not, as in the case of compensatory regeneration, involve stable genetic changes at the DNA level. Studies which associate human liver neoplasias with particular genetic changes in known proto-oncogenes will be extremely valuable. When such changes occur, it would be essential to correlate the presence of these mutated genes with exposure to environmental agents of both chemical and viral origin.

References

1. Busby, W. F. and Wogan, G. N. (1984). Aflatoxins. In *Chemical Carcinogens*, Vol. 2, Searle, C. E. (ed.) ACS Monograph 182, Washington, D.C., pp. 945–1136
2. Reynolds, S. H., Stowers, S. J., Maronpot, R. R., Anderson, M. W. and Aaronson, S. A. (1986). Detection and identification of activated oncogenes in spontaneously occurring benign and malignant hepatocellular tumours of the B6C3F1 mouse. *Proc. Natl. Acad. Sci. USA*, **83**, 33–7
3. Reynolds, S. H., Stowers, S. J., Patterson, R. M., Maronpot, R. R., Aaronson, S. A. and Anderson, M. W. (1987). Activated oncogenes in B6C3F1 mouse liver tumours. Implications for risk assessment. *Science*, **237**, 1309–16
4. McMahon, G., Hanson, L., Lee, J.-J. and Wogan, G. N. (1986). Identification of an activated c-Ki-*ras* oncogene in primary liver tumors of rats exposed to aflatoxin B_1. *Proc. Natl. Acad. Sci. USA*, **83**, 9418–22
5. Fasano, O., Birnbaum, D., Edlund, L., Fogh, I. and Wigler, M. (1984). New transforming genes detected by a tumorigenicity assay. *Mol. Cell. Biol.*, **4**, 1695–705
6. Barbacid, M. (1986). Oncogenes and human cancer: cause or consequence? *Carcinogenesis*, **7**, 1037–42
7. Foster, P. L., Eisenstadt, E. and Miller, J. H. (1983). Base substitution mutations induced by metabolically activated aflatoxin B_1. *Proc. Natl. Acad. Sci. USA*, **80**, 2695–8
8. Saiki, R. K., Gelfand, D. H., Stoffel, S., Scharf, S. J., Higuchi, R., Horn, G. T., Mullis, K. B. and Erlich, H. A. (1988). Primer directed enzymatic amplification of DNA with a thermostable DNA polymerase. *Science*, **239**, 487–91
9. McMahon, G., Davis, E. and Wogan, G. N. (1987). Characterization of c-Ki-*ras* oncogene alleles by direct sequencing of enzymatically amplified DNA from carcinogen-induced tumours. *Proc. Natl. Acad. Sci. USA*, **84**, 4974–8
10. Verlaan-de Vries, M., Bogaard, M. E., van den Elst, H., van Boom, J. H., van der Eb, A. J. and Bos, J. L. (1986). A dot-blot screening procedure for mutated *ras* oncogenes using synthetic oligodeoxynucleotides. *Gene*, **50**, 313–20
11. Weinberg, R. A. (1985). The activation of oncogenes in the cytoplasm and nucleus. *Science*, **230**, 770–6
12. Fausto, N. and Shank, P. R. (1983). Oncogene expression in liver regeneration and hepatocarcinogenesis. *Hepatology*, **3**, 1016–23
13. Gu, J.-R., Hu, L.-F., Cheng, Y.-C. and Wan, D.-F. (1986). Oncogenes in human primary hepatic cancer. *J. Cell. Physiol.* Suppl. **4**, 13–20

18
Interactive carcinogenesis in the liver

G. M. WILLIAMS

INTRODUCTION

Carcinogenesis is a complex multi-event and possibly multi-stage process resulting in the emergence of an abnormal population of cells, which is capable of excessive growth and, depending upon the degree of acquired deviation, invasion and metastasis. The process can be divided into two requisite sequences (Fig. 1), neoplastic conversion in which a normal cell is transformed into a neoplastic cell, possibly through stages, and neoplastic development in which clonal expansion of a neoplastic cell gives rise to a neoplasm, which may undergo further change during growth, a phenomenon known as 'progression'[1]. Chemicals act at a number of points in these sequences, both to facilitate and retard the overall process. This chapter describes interactions of chemicals with carcinogens which induce liver neoplasms.

Chemicals that are carcinogenic in aminals by the broad definition of increasing the occurrence of neoplasms are an extremely diverse group of agents, inducing normal body constituents, such as hormones, and exogenous chemicals. In an effort at mechanistic distinction, carcinogens have been categorized into two basic types: DNA-reactive or genotoxic carcinogens that damage DNA through direct chemical interaction and epigenetic carcinogenic agents that do not interact with DNA but produce some other biological effect that underlies their carcinogenicity[1,2]. This distinction is fundamental to the mechanistic understanding of modifying effects on carcinogenesis.

DNA-reactive carcinogens, most of which require enzymatic activation to their reactive species, induce neoplastic conversion of the cell by damaging DNA and producing alterations of gene expression, particularly oncogenes. For some efficient carcinogens, a single exposure will ultimately result in cancer, indicating that neoplastic conversion was readily produced. Others require prolonged administration, which may be necessary for the production of neoplastic conversion through stages, or may be required to facilitate the

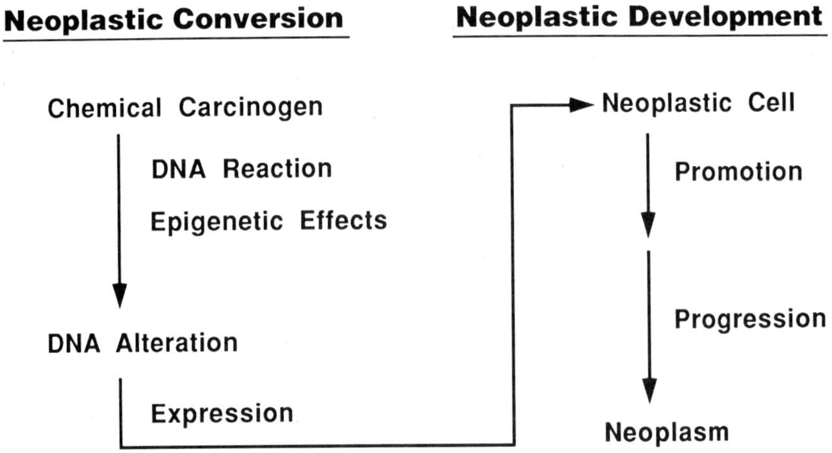

Neoplastic Conversion   **Neoplastic Development**

Chemical Carcinogen   Neoplastic Cell

    DNA Reaction   Promotion

    Epigenetic Effects

                                     Progression

DNA Alteration

    Expression   Neoplasm

Figure 1   Sequences and events in the process of chemical carcinogenesis

sequence of neoplastic development in some way, perhaps through an additional promoting action.

Epigenetic agents yield an increase in neoplasms through a variety of mechanisms. They may enhance the process of neoplastic conversion in an indirect manner by producing epigenetic effects which ultimately lead to genetic alterations. For example, epigenetic agents that are not capable of reacting with DNA may initiate cellular processes leading to generation of reactive species such as activated oxygen[3,4], hydrogen peroxide[5] or S-adenosyl-methionine[6], which could in turn produce genotoxicity. Also, epigenetic agents may operate through effects in the second sequence of events to enhance the development into neoplasms of pre-existing cryptogenic neoplastic cells. As a consequence of enhancement of neoplastic development, certain epigenetic carcinogens can augment the effects of DNA-reactive carcinogens. Thus, an important group of agents that modify the effects of DNA-reactive carcinogens is composed of chemicals that themselves are capable of increasing the occurrence of cancer under specific conditions in the absence of administration of any other carcinogen.

INTERACTIVE EFFECTS

The carcinogenic process can be modified by various intrinsic and extrinsic factors impinging at different steps in the two sequences[7]. Importantly, the same agent can exert several effects and consequently, a given chemical, through one type of action, may be an inhibitor at one step and, through another action, be an enhancer at a different step. Examples in liver carcinogenesis are phenobarbital and butylated hydroxytoluene which inhibit the carcinogenicity of activation-dependent carcinogens when administered together with them, but enhance carcinogenicity when given after liver carcinogens[8-10]. The concentrations or amounts of agents available in specific tissues and the specialized function of a tissue can likewise determine what kind of effect occurs. Additionally, a chemical can be an inhibitor of the carcinogenicity of one agent, but an enhancer of another. Thus, the influences of any agent on the overall process are complex and vary with the specific circumstances of its interaction with a carcinogen. The interactive effects between chemicals in liver carcinogenesis will be discussed for the two sequences of the process. Citations to the general literature may be found in a previous review[7] and mainly references to liver carcinogenesis are given in this chapter. It is well established that dietary factors influence liver carcinogenicity[1] but this review is confined to interactions of chemicals.

INTERACTION IN NEOPLASTIC CONVERSION

Two types of enhancement occur in the sequence of neoplastic conversion: these are syncarcinogenesis, involving two carcinogens, and co-carcino-genesis, involving a carcinogen and a non-carcinogen[7].

Syncarcinogenic effects

The additive or synergistic effect of two or more carcinogens in neoplasm production was defined as syncarcinogenesis[11,12]. Syncarcinogenesis can occur either when two carcinogens are administered concurrently or when they are administered one after the other. Since these two types can have different mechanisms and since the latter type must be clearly identified in order to be distinguished from initiation–promotion, they have been designated as 'combination syncarcinogenesis' and 'sequential syncarcino-genesis', respectively[7].

Generally, syncarcinogenesis occurs only when the two carcinogens have the same target organ[13]. In such situations, syncarcinogenesis can be striking when weakly carcinogenic dosages are used. In the liver, several pairs of genotoxic carcinogens have produced syncarcinogenic effects of the combination[14-16] or sequential[17-20] types. The concomitant or sequential administration of two carcinogens can conversely result in reduction of carcinogenicity[21,22]. This is known to occur when one carcinogen or the first carcinogen, in the case of sequential exposures, is an enzyme inducer.

Enhancement of carcinogenesis by multiple exposures also characterizes co-carcinogenesis and neoplasm promotion. These have been distinguished from syncarcinogenesis on the basis that the co-carcinogen or promoter is ostensibly non-carcinogenic, although 'weak' carcinogenic effects are often overlooked in that assumption. Mechanistically, the critical difference appears to be that co-carcinogens and promoters are not DNA-reactive. Moreover, in sequential syncarcinogenesis the order of administration can be reversed and the combined effect still occurs[23], whereas with co-carcinogenesis and promotion this generally is not the case[23,24]. It is essential that these phenomena be carefully distinguished in protocols of sequential administration in order to properly ascertain the mechanism of an enhancing effect.

Syncarcinogenesis is thought to result from a summation of the irreversible effects of two carcinogens[13], which now appear to be the DNA alterations produced by the agents. In addition, several studies have shown that administration of one carcinogen can inhibit repair of the DNA damage produced by a second[25,26]. Also, in the case of sequential syncarcinogenesis, the enhancement could result from a promoting action of the second carcinogen.

An interesting type of syncarcinogenesis in the liver is that produced by a DNA-reactive and an epigenetic carcinogen. For example, the non-genotoxic liver carcinogen methapyrilene, which induces mitochondrial proliferation[27], enhanced the liver carcinogenicity of 2-acetylaminofluorene when given either after[28] or before[29] the genotoxin. The latter finding provides some evidence for *in vivo* genotoxicity with chronic administration. In some studies, the non-genotoxic peroxisome-proliferating, liver carcinogen clofibrate enhanced the hepatocarcinogenicity of previously-administered diethylnitrosamine[30,31]. This enhancement, however, was not observed in studies in which other genotoxic liver carcinogens were followed by peroxisome proliferators[32-34]. In fact, in some studies, peroxisome proliferators have been reported to inhibit the effects of previously administered DNA-reactive carcinogens[35-37]. The latter observations provide no evidence for summation of the indirect genotoxic effects postulated to be produced by these types of agents[5] with the DNA damage produced by antecedent DNA-reactive carcinogens.

Co-carcinogenesis

Originally, co-carcinogenesis was broadly defined as the augmentation of neoplasm induction brought about by non-carcinogenic factors operating in conjuction with a carcinogen, designated as the 'initiating agent'[38,39]. Co-carcinogenesis thus comprised several kinds of enhancement, including promotion in which the enhancing agent facilitates tumour development after completion of initiation or neoplastic conversion. Subsequently, co-carcinogenesis was distinguished operationally from promotion as the enhancement of carcinogenicity resulting from application of a modifier either just before or together with a carcinogen, while promotion referred to enhancement produced by an agent given after a carcinogen. This distinction is useful to allow a conceptual differentiation between the enhancement of the sequence of neoplastic conversion by co-carcinogenesis and the enhancement of neoplastic development by promotion. From a mechanistic perspective, enhancement of carcinogenesis by an agent given after a genotoxic carcinogen, but while the DNA damage produced by the carcinogen is still persistent, most likely results from increased neoplastic conversion and should be considered a co-carcinogenic action unless proven otherwise. Accordingly, co-carcinogenesis has been proposed to be the enhancement of carcinogenesis resulting from effects produced either immediately before or during carcinogen exposure or at a time after carcinogen exposure when DNA damage is still persistent[7].

Agents with promoting activity can also augment cancer development when given together with a carcinogen. Under these circumstances, it is difficult to ascertain whether the enhancement of carcinogenesis is due to a co-carcinogenic or a promoting action. Accordingly, such agents are probably best regarded as promoters unless it can be demonstrated that the step of neoplastic conversion was facilitated.

Co-carcinogens could operate through a variety of non-genotoxic mechanisms[7]. One of the most extensively studied mechanisms of co-carcinogenesis in the liver is the enhanced conversion of DNA lesions to permanent alterations by stimulation of cell proliferation. Warwick[40] and Craddock[41] and others have shown that partial hepatectomy either immediately before administration of a liver carcinogen or shortly after leads to an increase in tumour occurrence. Enhancement can also be produced by administration of a necrogenic dose of a toxin such as carbon tetra-chloride[42,43] which leads to regenerative proliferation. The basis for this effect is fairly well established to be increased susceptibility of the dividing cells to the genetic effects of carcinogens[44]. If the interval between carcinogen exposure and the onset of proliferation is lengthenend, the effect on carcinogenesis of stimulation of proliferation is diminished[45,46], indicating that repair of DNA damage reduces the potential for neoplastic conversion. Partial hepatectomy, however, does not enhance the carcinogenicity of previously administered liver carcinogens in all cases[47], which, however, may be an artifact stemming from removal by partial hepatectomy of two-thirds of the carcinogen-affected liver.

Modification of biotransformation

Many DNA-reactive carcinogens are pro-carcinogens that require activation by enzyme systems to generate the reactive species that produces their carcino-genic effects[48]. The enzyme systems involved are numerous, but the most important is the cytochrome P-450 monooxygenase system which is abundant in the liver. A wide variety of stimulators and inhibitors of this system has been described[49,50], including hormones and substances that modify the endo-crine system.

Effects on the enzyme systems involved in biotransformation can either decrease or increase the carcinogenicity of activation-dependent genotoxic carcinogens. One of the earliest examples of inhibition of carcinogenesis was the demonstration by Kensler et al.[51] that riboflavin protected against the liver carcinogenicity of aminoazo dyes. Subsequently, it was shown that an hepatic azo reductase that cleaved azo dyes and yielded detoxified products required riboflavin as a cofactor. The preponderance of metabolism of most activation-dependent carcinogens is toward detoxified metabolites[52] and for such carcinogens, enzyme induction usually, but not always, reduces carcinogenicity[7,53]. The enhancement of activities of type-II conjugating systems such as glutathione S-transferase and uridine diphosphate-glucuronyl transferase that serve to detoxify carcinogens seems in particular to be involved in this inhibition[54,55]. Enhancement of detoxification in the liver, although protecting the liver, can result in increased carcinogenicity in the bladder, as seen with modification by butylated hydroxytoluene of 2-acetylaminofluorene carcinogenicity[56]. This is likely due, at least in part, to increased excretion of conjugated metabolites in the urine and release of carcinogen in the bladder.

As mentioned in the discussion of syncarcinogenesis, certain genotoxic carcinogens such as the polycyclic aromatic hydrocarbons, when administered together with other activation-dependent genotoxins can actually reduce their carcinogenicity as a result of effects on biotransformation.

For a number of liver carcinogens, males are more susceptible than females[57], although the converse is the case for some agents[58]. Those sex-dependent differences are due in large part to hormonally-determined differences in biotransformation[59,60]. Thus, orchidectomy prior to 2-acetylaminofluorene administration greatly reduced the susceptibility of male rats[60]. It is possible that chemicals that modify the endocrine system could have interactive effects with liver carcinogens through modification of hepatic biotransformation. This has been documented for neonatal exposures, as will be discussed.

Reduction of the effects of activation-dependent carcinogens can also be produced by inhibitors of enzymes involved in carcinogen activation[7,53]. However, inhibition of metabolism has also been found to increase carcinogenic effects[61]. Moreover, enzyme inhibitors, even when reducing carcinogenicity in primary sites, can produce an increase of neoplasms in secondary sites for the carcinogen[62], probably as a consequence of increased availability of the carcinogen in other organs resulting from reduction of biotransformation in the major organ for metabolism. Several other inhibitors have been described[53], but the exact basis for the effects of certain inhibitors is not always clear because some are also enzyme inducers.

Depletion of cellular substrates involved in activation reactions can also result in inhibition of carcinogenesis. A classic example was delineated in the series of studies by the Weisburgers based on the observation that chloramphenicol inhibited liver carcinogenesis by N-2-fluorenyldiacetamide[63]. In these studies, it was shown that acetanilide, which bears some structural similarity to the nitrophenyl part of chloramphenicol, decreased the liver carcinogenicity of 2-acetylaminofluorene by reducing formation of the proximate N-hydroxy derivative and of the ultimate carcinogenic metabolite, the sulphate ester, largely through reduction of available sulphate by binding to the metabolite p-hydroxyacetanilide[64,65]. Subsequent studies showed that p-hydroxyacetanilide (acetaminophen) inhibited liver carcinogenicity of N-hydroxy-N-2-fluorenylacetamide[66].

Chemical co-carcinogens can enhance neoplastic conversion and, thereby, carcinogenicity through inhibition of detoxification or increasing activation of genotoxic carcinogens[7]. However, only a few agents known to be enzyme inducers have increased the carcinogenicity of activation-dependent carcinogens. Of these, ethanol increased the hepatocarcinogenicity of vinyl chloride[67] and N-nitrosopyrrolidine[68], but had no effect on N'-nitrosonornicotine[68] and decreased the carcinogenicity of dimethylnitrosamine[69] and diethylnitros-amine[70].

Another means by which a chemical may lead to increased activation of a carcinogen is through competition by the agent for detoxification systems. For example, in rats and mice, ethanol inhibits the metabolism of dimethyl-nitrosamine in the liver[71,72]. In this case, first-pass clearance is prevented and more of the carcinogen is distributed to other tissues, similar to the effect with disulfiram[62]. There could, however, be situations in which competition for detoxification systems would lead to enhanced activation.

An important effect of chemicals on carcinogen metabolism is the perman-ent alteration of enzyme systems, known as imprinting, which is produced by chemical exposures during the developmental period[73,74]. Rats exposed to synthetic hormones in the neonatal period have displayed an altered response to N-hydroxy-N-2-fluorenylacetamide later in life[75,76]. This is a potentially important type of modulation that has received relatively little attention as regards carcinogenesis.

Modification of reactive interactions

DNA-reactive carcinogens form electrophiles or radical cations which bind to various cellular nucleophiles, ultimately resulting in neoplastic conversion of the cell (Figure 1). A critical target for such reaction is DNA, hence the designation of carcinogens with this property as DNA-reactive or genotoxic[1]. Epigenetic carcinogens may also indirectly give rise to reactive species[3-6], but by reactions other than biotransformation products of the chemicals themselves.

An agent that competes with target macromolecules for the binding of a reactive carcinogen or an indirectly-generated reactive species could decrease genotoxicity and carcinogenicity. Certain nucleophiles, particularly those containing sulphydryl groups, have been suggested to be capable of inhibiting carcinogenesis on this basis[77]. Also it is possible that antioxidants could act as inhibitors of carcinogenesis in this manner[53]. In vitro studies with butylated hydroxytoluene, which inhibited the liver carcinogenicity of 2-acetylamino-fluorene[9], show inhibition of genotoxicity of the carcinogen to cultured hepatocytes under conditions where modification of biotransformation would be unlikely[78].

Ethoxyquin and, to a lesser extent, butylated hydroxyanisole were found to inhibit liver tumorigenicity of ciprofibrate, a peroxisome proliferator[79]. The interpretation was that the antioxidants scavenged reactive oxygen species, but these agents are also enzyme inducers[53,80] and may have affected the biotransformation of the peroxisome proliferator.

An agent that reduces intracellular levels of nucleophilic substances which compete with DNA for carcinogen binding of reactive species could act as enhancers of the carcinogenicity of DNA-reactive carcinogens of epigenetic agents that generate reactive species. Glutathione, a nucleophile known to bind reactive metabolites of carcinogens, protects the liver against toxicity and carcinogenicity of a variety of chemicals. Diethyl maleate[82,83], which depletes liver glutathione, increased the hepatotoxicity of aflatoxin B_1.

Modification of expression of cellular alteration

The adducts formed in DNA by genotoxic carcinogens can be removed by enzymatic DNA repair systems and this restoration of DNA structure reduces carcinogenic effects. If repair is not complete before the cell replicates its damaged genome, the persisting adducts can result in mispairing of bases and probably other genetic effects such as rearrangements and translocations of segments of DNA, including oncogenes. Thus, an agent that alters repair processes or the rate of cell proliferation can affect the frequency of neoplastic conversion of carcinogen-damaged cells.

The repair of carcinogen-induced alkylation at the O^6 position of guanine is inducible in liver[82,83], but reduction of the effects of a genotoxic carcinogen by induction of repair by another xenochemical has not been demonstrated.

An agent that retards cell proliferation in a tissue can under appropriate conditions reduce the carcinogenicity of a chemical as a consequence of providing a greater interval for the repair of DNA damage. This has not been applied to liver, presumably because the rates of proliferation are normally very low.

Co-carcinogens could produce their effect as a result of inhibition of DNA repair. However, most agents that retard repair also produce a non-specific inhibition of DNA synthesis. As a result, the overall effect is that a longer interval is available for repair prior to replication and, consequently, the inhibition of repair under these conditions has not been shown to result in a greater yield of permanent alterations in DNA. However, 3-aminobenzamide, which inhibits poly(ADP-ribose) polymerase, an enzyme associated with DNA repair, has enhanced the effect of a liver carcinogen[84].

An agent that enhances proliferation in the liver, such as occurs following the production of liver cell necrosis[42,43], can enhance carcinogenesis, probably because the time available for DNA repair is reduced relative to the utilization of the damaged template during replicative DNA synthesis. Hormones and growth factors by stimulating DNA synthesis could possibly act in concert with carcinogens.

INTERACTION IN NEOPLASTIC DEVELOPMENT

Following neoplastic conversion of a cell, further development and proliferation is required for the formation of a tumour (Fig. 1). The facilitation of neoplastic development is a phenomenon known as 'promotion'[38].

Promotion of neoplasia

Promotion was originally defined conceptually as the encouragement of dormant neoplastic cells to develop into growing tumours[38]. Operationally, the phenomenon is usually demonstrated by the enhancing effect on carcinogenesis by a modifier administered after a carcinogen. The first demonstration of this phenomenon in liver was made by Peraino and coworkers[8]. An important concept that requires greater attention is whether any enhancement of carcinogenesis by an agent administered subsequent to a carcinogen can be considered promotion or whether promotion should be restricted to the facilitation of growth and development of dormant neoplastic cells as proposed by Berenblum[38].

In most 'promotion' studies, the second agent is given shortly after a carcinogen. Under these conditions unrepaired DNA adducts are likely to be present and this creates the possibility that stimulation of cell proliferation could enhance neoplastic conversion of cells (Fig. 1) ultimately resulting in increased neoplasm formation. This represents, as discussed, a mechanism of co-carcinogenesis, which is very different in nature from enhanced neoplasm development produced by agents acting on neoplastic cells generated by the carcinogen. Moreover, as also discussed, two carcinogens given in sequence can produce a syncarcinogenic effect. Therefore, when the mechanism of enhancement is uncertain, it would be preferable to use a general term such as 'carcinogenesis enhancement'. In the present discussion promotion will be restricted to the facilitation of development of neoplastic cells into a growing tumour (Fig. 1).

Neoplasm promotion was first established for skin carcinogenesis and the most detailed studies of the phenomenon have been conducted with the phorbol ester series of compounds which are promoters in mouse skin carcinogenesis. A number of chemical promoters for mouse and rat liver have been identified[85-87], although in most cases the demonstration has not been rigorous. In particular, the reverse sequence administrations required to distinguish promotion from syncarcinogenesis have rarely been done[23,24]. Also, interestingly, phenobarbital and DDT, which are quite effective enhancers in mice and rats, did not enhance liver carcinogenesis in hamsters[88-90].

The distinction between co-carcinogenicity and promotion has application in the design of protocols for the study of enhancing effects. Specifically, in many studies of enhancement of liver carcinogenesis, the enhancing agents are administered shortly after a carcinogen, but before abnormal populations have evolved[91-93]. Under these conditions, both co-carcinogenic and promoting effects may contribute to enhancement. In a different type of protocol[94-98], liver altered foci are induced first and then after an interval, the effect of the enhancing agent is delineated on these abnormal cells. Providing that carcinogen-induced DNA damage has been repaired, such protocols should measure specifically promoting effects.

The progeny of initiated or neoplastic cells can remain latent for very long intervals in the skin and other tissues, indicating that host homeostatic factors are able to control such abnormal cells. A variety of mechanisms could be the basis for enhanced development of such latent neoplastic cells into tumours[7,85-87]. An attractive hypothesis for the basis of action of some liver neoplasm promoters is that they may operate by inhibiting intercellular communication. According to this concept, promoters liberate neoplastic cells from tissue constraints, allowing them to proliferate according to their altered genome[85,99]. One form of cell-to-cell communication involves intercellular transfer of molecules, which could be the process by which growth regulating signals are transmitted to neoplastic cells. A variety of promoters have now been shown to produce inhibition or transfer of molecules between cells in culture[100-102], supporting this hypothesis. In particular, several liver-tumour promoters inhibited intercellular molecular exchange between cultured liver cells[103-107]. Also, two liver-tumour promoters were shown to produce structural changes in rat hepatocyte gap junctions[108], the organelle involved in cell–cell communication.

Another possible mechanism of promotion is immunosuppression. A number of studies, however, have shown that immunosuppression does not enhance the carcinogenicity of other chemicals in the liver[109-112].

The cells in pre-neoplastic liver lesions are resistant to the toxic effects of several agents requiring biotransformation[113,114]. Thus cytotoxic exposures have been found to enhance liver carcinogenesis and this has been ascribed to selection of resistant populations[114]. It is possible that in addition to producing neoplastic conversion, DNA-reactive carcinogens may have promoting activity through genotoxic or cytotoxic effects resulting in selective proliferation of altered cells.

Promotion was first identified at a time when promoting agents were not rigorously tested for carcinogenicity and thus promoters were considered to be non-carcinogenic, although even the earliest studies on skin neoplasm promotion with croton oil and phorbol esters revealed weak carcinogenic effects of these agents[115]. It is now established that many agents with promoting activity will increase neoplasia in the absence of deliberate induced initiation when tested for long duration under appropriate conditions. Examples in liver carcinogenesis are phenobarbital, DDT and butylated hydroxytoluene. Such agents have not been found to damage DNA and therefore have been categorized as a type of epigenetic carcinogen[85,103]. It seems likely that their 'carcinogenic' effects are due to a promoting action on cryptogenically-arising neoplastic cells, whose occurrence appears to be the basis for development of spontaneous neoplasm[85,86].

Inhibitors of neoplastic development or anti-promoters have been described for several tissues. A candidate for liver appears to be dihydroepiandrosterone[116].

Neoplastic progression

Neoplastic progression was defined by Foulds[117] as the stepwise development of a neoplasm through qualitatively different stages. So defined, progression includes both neoplastic conversion and neoplastic development as discussed here. However, progression is often used in a more restricted sense to denote the change of a neoplasm from benign to malignant or from low-grade to high-grade malignancy[118]. These latter processes would be part of the sequence of neoplastic development (Fig. 1), as described here. Little is known about the evolution of qualitative changes in a neoplasm, although emergence of new sub-populations seems likely. Proposed mechanisms for the evolution of new cell types within a neoplasm include infidelity of DNA polymerases and hybridization of normal and neoplastic cells. So far, no agent that facilitates progression in liver tumours has been identified, although enhancement of liver carcinogenesis by orotic acid was reported to lead to a greater incidence of metastasizing carcinomas[119].

INTERACTIONS OF AGENTS INVOLVED IN HUMAN LIVER CANCER

The causes of liver cancer in high-incidence regions, such as Asia and Africa, appear to be different from those in low-incidence regions, such as Europe and North America. Nevertheless, the hepatitis B virus (HBV) seems to be implicated in both situations[120–122], although to different degrees. A major focus of research on the role of the virus in liver cancer has been to prove that it is oncogenic[123] and nothing is known about influences on other causative agents. Nevertheless, it is possible that chronic HBV hepatitis could act as a co-carcinogen with environmental carcinogens by provoking replicative DNA synthesis and thereby enhancing the sensitivity of liver cells to the consequences of DNA damage by carcinogens.

Aflatoxins, which are mycotoxins produced by fungi which contaminate foods, have been identified as human carcinogens[124] in high-risk regions. They are genotoxic in many *in vitro* systems, including human liver cells[125]. Conceivably, the DNA damage produced by aflatoxins could in some way facilitate integration of the HBV into host DNA, but this has not been studied. So far, in experimental systems, only discrete changes in DNA (point mutations), have been identified as lesions caused by aflatoxin B_1 and it seems unlikely that these lesions would serve as sites for virus integration[126,127]. Repeated bouts of acute aflatoxicosis could lead to enhanced levels of liver cell proliferation, perhaps facilitating virus integration, but there is no evidence for this concept either.

Heavy consumption of alcohol-containing beverages is a major risk factor for liver cancer in low-incidence areas[128,129]. There are several possible ways in which alcohol could influence cancer development. Ethanol has not been demonstrated to be carcinogenic in animal models[130,131] and thus, it probably influences cancer development in an indirect manner.

As discussed earlier, alcohol has been found to enhance the carcinogenicity of some liver carcinogens while inhibiting others. The enhancement may reflect induction of hepatic biotransformation by ethanol; studies of subcellular preparations from livers of ethanol-treated rats have revealed increased metabolism of carcinogens[132–134]. Thus, ethanol may act as a co-carcinogen, increasing generation of reactive species in the liver.

As another possibility, episodes of alcohol-induced hepatitis and eventually alcoholic cirrhosis could sensitize the liver to the effects of environmental carcinogens by provoking an increased level of liver cell proliferation. This would also represent a co-carcinogenic action.

There has been considerable interest in the possibility that alcohol might act as a promoter of liver cancer. Certainly, ethanol produces several of the effects of promoters, such as changes in cell membranes and induction of specific cytochromes P-450. An enhancing effect of ethanol given after a carcinogen has been observed in some experiments[135,136], but not others[137,138].

Chronic alcohol consumption increases the risk of liver cancer among HBV carriers[139], but the mechanism is not understood. At present, it not possible to ascribe the influence of alcohol on liver cancer to any one of the several possible actions. In fact, the effect may be due to a combination of actions or different actions in different circumstances.

A number of other agents that are liver carcinogens in humans have been identified. These include, prominently, oral contraceptives and vinyl chloride. Interactions of these with the agents discussed has not been established, although ethanol was found to enhance the carcinogenicity of vinyl chloride in an experimental study[67]. The possibility that oral contraceptives act as promoters if supported by observations that liver tumours regress after cessation of use.

In summary, there are several possible ways in which the main elements in liver cancer, HBV, mycotoxins or other chemical carcinogens and ethanol, could interact to lead to the development of the disease.

CONCLUSIONS

Most types of human cancer are clearly multifactorial[140–142], resulting from interactive effects between carcinogens and other elements, often nutritional. Current knowledge suggests that liver cancer in both high- and low-risk regions is very likely a result of interactive carcinogenesis. In regions of high incidence, HBV and aflatoxins seem to be the aetiologic agents. In regions of low incidence, alcohol and possibly HBV appear to be involved. The ways in which these agents could interact are varied[143]. From a public health point of view, attention must be directed to all these agents in preventive efforts.

Control of HBV infection seems possible. Effective vaccines have been developed and are being introduced[144,145].

Prevention of contamination of crops and foods by aflatoxins has been achieved in affluent societies and should be pursued in high-risk areas, but may be difficult to accomplish in these underdeveloped countries. An alternative approach such as inhibition of the effects of aflatoxins on the liver by other agents, especially antioxidants[146,147] deserves consideration. Potential hazards of some of the candidate antioxidants are that they have been found in animal systems to induce or enhance carcinogenesis in several organs, including liver[10]. Given these effects of the antioxidants, it is interesting that none has been associated with human cancer[124], in spite of widespread use as food additives for many years. A number of explanations are possible and have been discussed[148]. In addition, the resistance of hamster liver to enhancement of carcinogenesis by agents effective in rats and mice[88–90] suggests the possibility that human liver might also be resistant. Resistance of human cells to *in vitro* effects of promoters could be studied with existing cell-culture methodologies[85,125].

Excess alcohol consumption is firstly a social problem requiring educational approaches which will have to be begun in childhood. For individuals with a dependency on alcohol, individual intervention efforts are needed and have been proven successful.

Much remains to be done to control the elements involved in liver cancer, but clearly the disease has a high potential for world-wide prevention.

References

1. Williams, G. M. and Weisburger, J. H. (1986). Chemical carcinogens. In Doull, J., Klaassen, C. D. and Amdur, M. O. (eds) *Toxicology: The Basic Science of Poisons*, 3rd edn, pp. 99–173 (New York: Macmillan)
2. Williams, G. M. (1987). Definition of a human cancer hazard. In Banbury Report 25: *Nongenotoxic Mechanisms in Carcinogenesis*, pp. 367–80 (Cold Spring Harbor Laboratory)
3. Kaneko, M. and Leadon, S. A. (1986). Production of thymine glycols in DNA by N-hydroxy-2-naphthylamine as detected by a monoclonal antibody. *Cancer Res.*, **46**, 71–5
4. Kasai, H., Nishimura, S., Kurokawa, Y. and Hayashi, Y. (1987). Oral administration of the renal carcinogen, potassium bromate, specifically produces 8-hydroxydeoxyguanosine in rat target organ DNA. *Carcinogenesis*, **8**, 1959–61
5. Sambasiva, M. and Reddy, J. K. (1987). Peroxisome proliferation and hepatocarcinogenesis. *Carcinogenesis*, **8**, 631–6
6. Barrows, L. R. and Shank, R. C. (1981). Aberrant methylation of liver DNA in rats during hepatotoxicity. *Toxicol. Appl. Pharmacol.*, **60**, 334–45
7. Williams, G. M. (1984). Modulation of chemical carcinogenesis by xenobiotics. *Fund. Appl. Toxicol.*, **4**, 325–44
8. Peraino, C., Fry, R. J. M. and Staffeldt, E. (1971). Reduction and enhancement of phenobarbital of hepatocarcinogenesis induced in the rat by 2-acetylaminofluorene. *Cancer Res.*, **31**, 1506–15
9. Williams, G. M., Maeura, Y. and Weisburger, J. H. (1983). Simultaneous inhibition of liver carcinogenicity and enhancement of bladder carcinogenicity of N-2-fluorenylacetamide by butylated hydroxytoluene. *Cancer Lett.*, **19**, 55–60
10. Maeura, Y. and Williams, G. M. (1984). Enhancing effect of butylated hydroxytoluene on the development of liver altered foci and neoplasms induced by N-2-fluorenylacetamide in rats. *Food Chem. Toxicol.*, **22**, 191–8
11. Nakahara, W. (1970). Mode of origin and characterization of cancer. In Nakahara, W. (ed.) *Chemical Tumor Problems*, pp. 287–330. (Tokyo: Japanese Society for the Promotion of Science)
12. Schmahl, D. (1970). Syncarcinogenesis: Experimental investigations. In Nakahara W. (ed.) *Chemical Tumor Problems*, pp. 1–8. (Japan: Japanese Society for the Promotion of Science)
13. Schmahl, D. (1980). Combination effects in chemical carcinogenesis. *Arch. Toxicol.*, Suppl. **4**, 29–40
14. MacDonald, J. C., Miller, E. C. and Miller, J. A. (1952). The synergistic action of mixtures of certain hepatic carcinogens. *Cancer Res.*, **12**, 50–4
15. Steiner, P. E. (1955). Carcinogenicity of multiple chemicals simultaneously administered. *Cancer Res.*, **15**, 632–5
16. Angsubhakorn, S., Bhamarapravati, N., Romruen, K. and Sahaphong, S. (1981). Enhancing effects of dimethylnitrosamine on aflatoxin B_1 hepatocarcinogenesis in rats. *Int. J. Cancer*, **28**, 621–6
17. Odashima, S. (1959). Development of liver cancers in the rat by 20-methylcholanthrene painting following initial 4-dimethylaminoazobenzene feeding. *Gann*, **50**, 321–45
18. Nakahara, W. and Fukuoka, F. (1960). Summation of carcinogenic effects of chemically unrelated carcinogens, 4-nitroquinoline N-oxide and 20-methylcholanthrene. *Gann*, **51**, 125–37
19. Takayama, S. and Imaizumi, T. (1969). Sequential effects of chemically different carcinogens, dimethylnitrosamine and 4-dimethylaminoazobenzene, on hepatocarcinogenesis in rats. *Int. J. Cancer*, **4**, 373–83
20. Williams, G. M., Katayama, S. and Ohmori, T. (1981). Enhancement of hepatocarcino-

genesis by sequential administration of chemicals: Summation versus promotion effects. *Carcinogenesis*, **2**, 1111–17

21. Richardson, H. L., Stein, A. R. and Borsos-NachtNebel, E. (1952). Tumor inhibition and adrenal histologic responses in rats in which 3'-methyl-4-dimethylaminoazobenzene and 20-methylcholanthrene were simultaneously administered. *Cancer Res.*, **12**, 356–71

22. Hoch-Ligeti, C., Argus, M. F. and Arcos, J. C. (1968). Combined carcinogenic effects of dimethylnitrosamine and 3-methylcholanthrene in the rat. *J. Natl. Cancer Inst.*, **40**, 535–49

23. Williams, G. M. and Furuya, K. (1984). Distinction between liver neoplasm promoting and syncarcinogenic effects demonstrated by reversing the order of administering phenobarbital and diethylnitrosamine either before or after N-2-fluorenylacetamide. *Carcinogenesis*, **5**, 171–4

24. Schwarz, M., Bannasch, P. and Kunz, W. (1983). The effect of pre- and post-treatment with phenobarbital on the extent of gamma-glutamyl transpeptidase positive foci induced in rat liver by N-nitrosomorpholine. *Cancer Lett.*, **21**, 17–21

25. Kleihues, P. and Margison, G. (1976). Exhaustion and recovery of repair excision of O^6-methylguanine from rat liver DNA. *Nature*, **259**, 153–5

26. Pegg, A. E. (1978). Dimethylnitrosamine inhibits enzymatic removal of O^6-methylguanine from DNA. *Nature*, **274**, 182–4

27. Reznik-Schuller, H. M. and Lijinsky, W. (1981). Morphology of early changes in liver carcinogenesis induced by methapyrilene. *Arch. Toxicol.*, **49**, 79–83

28. Furuya, K., Mori, H. and Williams, G. M. (1983). An enhancing effect of the antihistamine drug methapyrilene on rat liver carcinogenesis by previously administered N-2-fluorenylacetamide. *Toxicol. Appl. Pharmacol.*, **70**, 49–56

29. Furuya, K. and Williams, G. M. (1984). Neoplastic conversion in rat liver by the antihistamine methapyrilene demonstrated by a sequential syncarcinogenic effect with N-2-fluorenylacetamide. *Toxicol. Appl. Pharmacol.*, **74**, 63–9

30. Reddy, J. K. and Rao, M. S. (1978). Enhancement by WY-14, 643, a hepatic peroxisome proliferator, of diethylnitrosamine initiated hepatic tumorigenesis in the rat. *Br. J. Cancer.* **38**, 537–43

31. Mochizuki, Y., Furukawa, K. and Sawada, N. (1982). Effects of various concentrations of ethyl-α-p-chlorophenoxyisobutyrate (clofibrate) on diethylnitrosamine-induced hepatic tumorigenesis in the rat. *Carcinogenesis*, **3**, 1027–9

32. Numoto, S., Furukawa, K. and Williams, G. M. (1984). Effects of hepatocarcinogenic peroxisome-proliferating agents clofibrate and nafenopin on the rat liver cell membrane enzymes gamma-glutamyltranspeptidase and alkaline phosphatase and on the early stages of liver carcinogenesis. *Carcinogenesis*, **5**, 1603–11

33 Numoto, S., Mori, H., Furuya, K., Levine, W. G. and Williams, G. M. (1985). Absence of a promoting or sequential syncarcinogenic effect in rat liver by the carcinogenic hypolipidemic drug nafenopin given after N-2-fluorenylacetamide. *Toxicol. Appl. Pharmacol.*, **77**, 76–85

34. Williams, G. M., Maruyama, H. and Tanaka, T. (1987). Lack of rapid initiating, promoting or sequential syncarcinogenic effects of di(2-ethylhexyl)phthalate in rat liver carcinogenesis. *Carcinogenesis*, **8**, 875–80

35. De Angelo, A. B. and Garrett, C. T. (1983). Inhibition of development of preneoplastic lesions in the livers of rats fed a weakly carcinogenic environmental contaminant. *Cancer Lett.*, **20**, 199–205

36. Perera, M. I. R. and Shinozuka, H. (1984). Accelerated regression of carcinogen-induced preneoplastic hepatocyte foci by peroxisome proliferators, BR931, 4-chloro-6-(2,3-xylidino)-2-pyrimidinylthio(N-ß-hydroxyethyl)acetamide, and di-(2-ethylhexyl)phthalate. *Carcinogenesis*, **5**, 1193–8

37. Stäubli, W., Bentley, P., Bieri, F., Fröhlich, E. and Waechter, F. (1984). Inhibitory effect of nafenopin upon the development of diethylnitrosamine-induced enzyme-altered foci within the rat liver. *Carcinogenesis*, **5**, 41–6

38. Berenblum, I. (1974). *Carcinogenesis as a Biological Problem*. Neuberger, A. and Tatum, E. L. (eds) (Elsevier: New York).

39. Sivak, A. (1979). Cocarcinogenesis. *Biochim. Biophys. Acta*, **560**, 67–89

40. Warwick, G. P. (1971). Effect of the cell cycle on carcinogenesis. *Fed. Proc.*, **30**, 1760–5

41. Craddock, V. M. (1971). Liver carcinomas induced in rats by single administration of dimethylnitrosamine after partial hepatectomy. *J. Natl. Cancer Inst.*, **47**, 899–907

42. Pound, A. W., Lawson, T. A. and Horn, L. (1973). Increased carcinogenic action of dimethylnitrosamine after prior administration of carbon tetrachloride. *Br. J. Cancer*, **27**, 451–9

43. Mori, H., Ushimaru, Y., Tanaka, T. and Hirono, I. (1977). Effect of carbon tetrachloride on carcinogenicity of *Petasites japonicus* and transplantability of induced tumors. *Gann*, **68**, 841–5

44. Tong, C., Fazio, M. and Williams, G. M. (1980). Cell cycle-specific mutagenesis at the hypoxanthine-guanine phosphoribosyl transferase locus in adult rat liver epithelial cells. *Proc. Natl. Acad. Sci. USA*, **77**, 7377–9

45. Ishikawa, T., Takayama, S. and Kitagawa, T. (1980). Correlation between time of partial hepatectomy after a single treatment with diethylnitrosamine and induction of adenosine triphosphatase-deficient islands in rat liver. *Cancer Res.*, **40**, 4261–4

46. Hirota, N., Moriyama, S. and Yokoyama, T. (1982). Induction of gamma-glutamyltransferase-positive and nonspecific esterase-positive foci in rat liver by partial hepatectomy following single injection of N-nitrosodiethylamine. *J. Natl. Cancer Inst.*, **69**, 1299–1304

47. Tanaka, T., Mori, H., Hirota, N., Furuya, K. and Williams, G. M. (1986). Effect of DNA synthesis on induction of preneoplastic and neoplastic lesions in rat liver by a single dose of methyl-azoxymethanol acetate. *Chemico-Biol. Interactions*, **58**, 13

48. Miller, E. C. and Miller, J. A. (1981). Mechanisms of chemical carcinogenesis. *Cancer*, **47**, 1055–64

49. Snyder, R. and Remmer, H. (1979). Classes of hepatic microsomal mixed function oxidase inducers. *Pharmacol. Ther.*, **7**, 203–44

50. Conney, A. H. (1982). Induction of microsomal enzymes by foreign chemicals and carcinogenesis by polycyclic aromatic hydrocarbons: G. H. A. Clowes Memorial Lecture. *Cancer Res.*, **42**, 4875–917

51. Kensler, C. J., Sugiura, K., Young, N. F., Halter, C. R. and Rhoads, C. P. (1941). Partial protection of rats by riboflavin with casein against liver cancer caused by dimethylaminoazobenzene. *Science*, **93**, 308–10

52. Weisburger, J. H. and Williams, G. M. (1982). Metabolism of chemical carcinogens. In Becker, F. F. (ed.) *Cancer: A Comprehensive Treatise*, 2nd edn. pp. 241–333 (New York: Plenum)

53. Wattenberg, L. W. (1985). Chemoprevention of cancer. *Cancer Res.*, **45**, 1–8

54. Hesse, S., Jernstrom, G., Martinez, M., Moldeus, P., Christodoulides, L. and Ketterer, B. (1982). Inactivation of DNA-binding metabolites of benzo(a)pyrene and benzo(a)pyrene-7,8-dihydrodiol by glutathione and glutathione S-transferase. *Carcinogenesis*, **3**, 757–60

55. Sparnins, V. L., Venegas, P. L. and Wattenberg, L. W. (1982). Glutathione S-transferase activity by compounds inhibiting chemical carcinogenesis and by dietary constituents. *J. Natl. Cancer Inst.*, **68**, 493–6

56. Maeura, Y., Weisburger, J. H. and Williams, G. M. (1984). Dose-dependent reduction of N-2-fluorenylacetamide-induced liver cancer and enhancement of bladder cancer in rats by butylated hydroxytoluene. *Cancer Res.*, **44**, 1604–10

57. Williams, G. M. (1984). Sex hormones and liver cancer. In Rubin, E. and Damjanov, I. (eds) *Advances in the Biology of Disease*, Vol. 1, pp. 199–201 (Baltimore: Williams & Wilkins)

58. Koepke, S. R., Creassia, D. R., Knutsen, G. L. and Michejda, C. J. (1988). Carcinogenicity of hydroxyalkylnitrosamines in F344 rats: Contrasting behavior of ß- and γ-hydroxylated nitrosamines. *Cancer Res.*, **48**, 1533–6

59. Kato, R. (1979). Characteristics and differences in the hepatic mixed function oxidases of different species. *Pharmacol. Ther.*, **6**, 41–98

60. Katayama, S., Ohmori, T., Maeura, Y., Croci, T. and Williams, G. M. (1984). Early stages of N-2-fluorenylacetamide-induced hepatocarcinogenesis in male and female rats and effect of gonadectomy on liver neoplastic conversion and neoplastic development. *J. Natl. Cancer Inst.*, **73**, 141–9

61. Argus, M. F., Hoch-Ligeti, C., Arcos, J. C. and Conney, A. H. (1978). Differential effects of ß-naphthoflavone and pregnenolone-16 gamma-carbonitrile on dimethylnitrosamine induced hepatocarcinogenesis. *J. Natl. Cancer Inst.*, **61**, 441–9

62. Fiala, E. S., Weisburger, J. H., Katayama, S., Chandrasekaran, V. and Williams, G. M. (1981). The effect of disulfiram on the carcinogenicity of 3,2'-dimethyl-4-aminobiphenyl in Syrian golden hamsters and rats. *Carcinogenesis*, **2**, 965–9

63. Puron, R. and Firminger, H. I. (1965). Protection against induced cirrhosis and hepatocellular carcinoma in rats by chloramphenicol. *J. Natl. Cancer Inst.*, **35**, 29–37

64. Yamamoto, R. S., Glass, R. M., Frankel, H. H., Weisburger, E. K. and Weisburger, J. H. (1968). Inhibition of the toxicity and carcinogenicity of N-2-fluorenylacetamide by acetanilide. *Toxicol. Appl. Pharmacol.*, **13**, 108–17

65. Weisburger, J. H., Yamamoto, R. S., Williams, G. M., Grantham, P. H., Matsushima, T. and Weisburger, E. K. (1972). On the sulfate ester of N-hydroxy-N-2-fluorenylacetamide as a key ultimate hepatocarcinogen in the rat. *Cancer Res.*, **32**, 491–500

66. Yamamoto, R. S., Williams, G. M., Richardson, H. L., Weisburger, E. K. and Weisburger, J. H. (1973). Effect of *p*-hydroxyacetanilide on liver cancer induction by N-hydroxy-N-2-fluorenylacetamide. *Cancer Res.*, **33**, 454–7

67. Radike, M. S., Stemmer, K. L., Brown, P. G., Larson, E. and Bingham, E. (1977). Effect of ethanol and vinyl chloride on the induction of liver tumors: Preliminary report. *Environ. Health Perspect.*, **21**, 153–5

68. McCoy, G. D., Hecht, S. S., Katayama, S. and Wynder, E. L. (1981). Differential effect of chronic ethanol consumption on the carcinogenicity of N-nitrosopyrrolidine and N-nitrosonornicotine in male Syrian golden hamsters. *Cancer Res.*, **41**, 2849–54

69. Gellert, J., Moreno, F., Haydin, M., Oldiges, H., Frenzel, H., Teschke, R. and Strohmeyer, F. (1980). Decreased hepatotoxicity of dimethylnitrosamine following chronic alcohol consumption. *Adv. Exp. Med. Biol.*, **132**, 237–43

70. Habs, M. and Schmahl, D. (1981). Inhibition of the hepatocarcinogenic activity of diethylnitrosamine by ethanol in rats. *Acta Hepatogastroenterol.*, **28**, 242–4

71. Swann, P. F., Coe, A. M. and Mace, R. (1984). Ethanol and dimethylnitrosamine and diethylnitrosamine metabolism and disposition in the rat. Possible relevance to the influence of ethanol on human cancer incidence. *Carcinogenesis*, **5**, 1337–43

72. Anderson, L. M., Harrington, G. W., Jr., Pylypiw, H. M., Hagiwara, A. and Magee, P. N. (1986). Tissue levels and biological effects of N-nitrosodimethylamine in mice during chronic low or high dose exposure with or without ethanol. *Drug Metab. Disposition*, **14**, 733–9

73. Einarson, K., Gustafsson, J. and Stenberg, A. (1973). Neonatal imprinting of liver microsmal hydroxylation and reduction of steroids. *J. Biol. Chem.*, **248**, 4987–97

74. Lucier, G. W. (1976). Perinatal development of conjugative enzyme systems. *Environ. Health Perspect.*, **29**, 7–16

75. Weisburger, J. H., Yamamoto, R. S., Korzis, J. and Weisburger, E. K. (1966). Liver cancer: Neonatal estrogen enhances induction by a carcinogen. *Science*, **154**, 673–4

76. Weisburger, E. K., Yamamoto, R. S., Glass, R. M., Grantham, P. H. and Weisburger, J. H. (1968). Effect of neonatal androgen injection on liver tumor induction by N-hydroxy-N-2-fluorenylacetamide and on the metabolism of the carcinogen in rats. *Endocrinology*, **82**, 685–92

77. Miller, E. C. and Miller, J. A. (1972). Approaches to the mechanism and control of chemical carcinogenesis. In *Environment and Cancer*. pp. 5–39. (The University of Texas Anderson Hospital and Tumor Institute. Williams & Wilkins; Maryland)

78. Chipman, J. K., Davies, J. E. and Paterson, P. (1987). Mechanisms of butylated hydroxytoluene-mediated modulation of 2-acetylaminofluorene mutagenicity in rat and human hepatocyte/*Salmonella* assays. *Mutat. Res.*, **187**, 105–12

79. Rao, M. S., Lalwani, N. D., Watanabe, T. K. and Reddy, J. K. (1984). Inhibitory effect of antioxidants Ethoxyquin and 2 (3)-tert-butyl-4-hydroxyanisole on hepatic tumorigenesis in rats fed ciprofibrate, a peroxisome proliferator. *Cancer Res.*, **44**, 1072–6

80. Furukawa, K., Maeura, Y., Furukawa, N. T. and Williams, G. M. (1984). Induction by butylated hydroxytoluene of rat liver gamma-glutamyl transpeptidase activity in comparison to expression in carcinogen-induced altered lesions. *Chemico.-Biol. Interactions*, **48**, 43–58

81. MgBodile, M. U. K., Holscher, M. and Neal, R. A. (1975). A possible protective role for reduced glutathione in aflatoxin B_1 toxicity: Effect of pretreatment of rats with phenobarbital and 3-methylcholanthrene on aflatoxin toxicity. *Toxicol. Appl. Pharmacol.*, **34**, 128–42

82. Montesano, R., Bresh, H. and Margison, G. P. (1979). Increased excision of O^6-methylguanine from rat liver DNA after chronic administration of dimethylnitrosamine.

Cancer Res., 39, 1798–802

83. Swenberg, J. A., Bedell, M. A., Billings, K. C., Umbenhauer, D. R. and Pegg, A. E. (1982). Cell-specific differences in O⁶-alkylguanine-DNA repair activity during continuous exposure to carcinogen. Proc. Natl. Acad. Sci. USA, 79, 5499–502

84. Takahashi, S., Ohnishi, T., Denda, A. and Konishi, Y. (1982). Enhancing effect of 3-aminobenzamide on induction of gamma-glutamyl transpeptidase positive foci in rat liver. Chemico-Biol. Interactions, 39, 363–8

85. Williams, G. M. (1981). Liver carcinogenesis: The role for some chemicals of an epigenetic mechanism of liver tumor promotion involving modification of the cell membrane. Food Cosmet. Toxicol., 19, 577–83

86. Schulte-Hermann, R. (1985). Tumor promotion in the liver. Arch. Toxicol., 57, 147–58

87. Moore, M. A. and Kitagawa, T. (1986). Hepatocarcinogenesis in the rat: The effect of promoters and carcinogens in vivo and in vitro. Int. Rev. Cytol., 101, 125–73

88. Stenback, F., Mori, H., Furuya, K. and Williams, G. M. (1986). The pathogenesis of dimethylnitrosamine-induced hepatocellular phenobarbital. J. Natl. Cancer Inst., 76, 327–33

89. Diwan, B. A., Ward, J. M., Anderson, L. M., Hagiwara, A. and Rice, J. M. (1986). Lack of effect of phenobarbital on hepatocellular carcinogenesis initiated by N-nitrosodiethylamine or methylazoxymethanol acetate in male Syrian golden hamsters. Toxicol. Appl. Pharmacol., 86, 298–307

90. Tanaka, T., Mori, H. and Williams, G. M. (1987). Enhancement of dimethylnitrosamine induced hepatocarcinogenesis in hamsters by subsequent administration of carbon tetrachloride but not phenobarbital or p,p'-dichlorodiphenyl-trichloroethane. Carcinogenesis, 8, 1171–8

91. Leonard, T. B., Dent, J. G., Graichen, E., Lyght, O. and Popp, J. A. (1982). Comparison of hepatic carcinogen initiation–promotion systems. Carcinogenesis, 3, 851–6

92. Pereira, M. A. (1982). Rat liver foci bioassay. J. Am. Coll. Toxicol., 1, 101–17

93. Tatematsu, M., Hasegawa, R., Imaida, K., Tusda, H. and Ito, N. (1983). Survey of various chemicals for initiating and promoting activities in a short-term in vivo system based on generation of hyperplastic liver nodules in rats. Carcinogenesis, 4, 381–6

94. Watanabe, K. and Williams, G. M. (1978). The enhancement of rat hepatocellular altered foci by the liver tumor promoter phenobarbital: Evidence that foci are precursors of neoplasm and that the promoter acts on carcinogen-induced lesions. J. Natl. Cancer Inst., 61, 1311–14

95. Kitagawa, T. and Sugano, H. (1978). Enhancing effect of phenobarbital on the development of enzyme altered islands and hepatocellular carcinomas initiated by 3'-methyl-4-(dimethylamino) azobenzene or diethylnitrosoamine. Gann, 69, 679–87

96. Mori, H., Tanaka, T., Nishikawa, A., Takahashi, M. and Williams, G. M. (1981). Enhancing effect of barbital on N-2-fluorenylacetamide induced rat liver lesions. Gann, 72, 798–801

97. Remandet, B., Gouy, D., Berthe, J., Mazue, G. and Williams, G. M. (1984). Lack of initiating or promoting activity of six benzodiazepine tranquillizers in rat liver limited bioassays monitored by histopathology and assay of liver and plasma enzymes. Fund. Appl. Toxicol., 4, 152–63

98. Williams, G. M. (1982). Phenotypic properties of preneoplastic rat liver lesions and applications to detection of carcinogens and tumor promoters. Toxicol. Pathol., 10, 3–10

99. Trosko, J. E., Chang, C. and Medcalf, A. (1983). Mechanisms of tumor promotion: potential role of intercellular communication. Cancer Invest., 1, 511–26

100. Trosko, J. E., Yotti, L. P., Warren, S. T., Tsushimoto, G. and Chang, C. (1982). Inhibition of cell–cell communication by tumor promoters. In Hecker, E. et al. (eds.) Carcinogenesis: A Comprehensive Survey, 7, p. 565. (New York: Raven Press)

101. Yamasaki, H., Enomoto, T., Martel, N., Shiba, Y. and Kanno, Y. (1983). Tumour promoter-mediated reversible inhibition of cell–cell communication (electrical coupling). Exp. Cell Res., 146, 297–308

102. Wärngård, L., Flodström, S., Ljungquist, S. and Ahlborg, U. G. (1985). Inhibition of metabolic cooperation in Chinese hamster lung fibroblast cells (V79) in culture by various DDT-analogs. Arch. Environ. Contam. Toxicol., 14, 541–6

103. Williams, G. M. (1980). Classification of genotoxic and epigenetic hepatocarcinogens using

liver culture assays. *Ann. N. Y. Acad. Sci.,* **349**, 273–82

104. Williams, G. M., Telang, S. and Tong, C. (1981). Inhibition of intercellular communication between liver cells by the liver tumor promoter 1,1,1-trichloro-2-2-bis (*p*-chlorophenyl) ethane (DDT). *Cancer Lett.,* **11**, 339–44

105. Telang, S., Tong, C. and Williams, G. M. (1982). Epigenetic membrane effects of a possible tumor promoting type on cultured liver cells by the nongenotoxic organochlorine pesticides chlordane and heptachlor. *Carcinogenesis,* **3**, 1175–8

106. Williams, G. M., Tong, C. and Telang, S. (1984). Polybrominated biphenyls are nongenotoxic and produce an epigenetic membrane effect in cultured liver cells. *Environ. Res.,* **34**, 310–20

107. Ruch, R. J. and Klaunig, J. E. (1986). Antioxidant prevention of tumor promoter induced inhibition of mouse hepatocyte intercellular communication. *Cancer Lett.,* **33**, 137

108. Sugie, S., Mori, H. and Takahashi, M. (1987). Effect of *in vivo* exposure to the liver tumor promoters phenobarbital or DDT on the gap junctions of rat hepatocytes: a quantitative freeze-fracture analysis. *Carcinogenesis,* **8**, 45–51

109. Frankel, H. H., Yamamoto, R. S., Weisburger, E. K. and Weisburger, J. K. (1970). Chronic toxicity of azathioprine and the effect of this immunosuppressant on liver tumor induction by the carcinogen N-hydroxy-N-2-fluorenylacetamide. *Toxicol. Appl. Pharmacol.,* **17**, 462–80

110. Kroes, R., Berkvens, J. M. and Weisburger, J. H. (1975). Immunosuppression in primary liver and colon tumor induction with N-hydroxy-N-2-fluorenylacetamide and azoxymethane. *Cancer Res.,* **35**, 2651–6

111. Weisburger, J. H., Madison, R. M., Ward, J. M., Viguera, C. and Weisburger, E. K. (1975). Modification of diethylnitrosamine liver carcinogenesis with phenobarbital but not with immunosuppression. *J. Natl. Cancer Inst.,* **54**, 1185–8

112. Scherer, E., Van Dijk, W. F. M. and Emmelot, P. (1976). The effect of antilymphocytic and normal horse serum on growth of precancerous foci and development of tumours induced by diethylnitrosamine in rat liver. *Europ. J. Cancer,* **12**, 25–31

113. Williams, G. M., Klaiber, M., Parker, S. E. and Farber, E. (1976). The nature of early-appearing carcinogen-induced liver lesions resistant to iron accumulation. *J. Natl. Cancer Inst.,* **57**, 157–65

114. Farber, E. and Sarma, D. S. R. (1987). Hepatocarcinogenesis: A dynamic cellular perspective. *Lab. Invest.,* **56**, 4–22

115. Van Duuren, B. L. (1969). Tumor-promoting agents in two-stage carcinogenesis. *Prog. Exp. Tumor Res.,* **11**, 31–68

116. Garcea, R., Daino, L., Pascale, R., Frassetto, S., Cozzolino, P., Ruggiu, M. E. and Feo, F. (1987). Inhibition by dehydroepidandrosterone of liver preneoplastic foci formation in rats after initiation–selection in experimental carcinogenesis. *Toxicol. Pathol.,* **15**, 164–9

117. Foulds, L. (1969). *Neoplastic Development.* (New York: Academic Press)

118. Pitot, H. C., Goldsworthy, T., Moran, S., Sirca, A. E. and Weeks, J. (1982). Properties of incomplete carcinogens and promoters in hepatocarcinogenesis. In Slaga, T. J., Sivak, A. and Boutwell, R. K. (eds) *Carcinogenesis, A Comprehensive Survey,* **7**, 85–98 (New York: Raven Press)

119. Laurier, C., Tatematsu, M., Rao, P. M., Rajalakshmi, S. and Sarma, D. S. R. (1984). Promotion by orotic acid of liver carcinogenesis in rats initiated by 1, 2-dimethylhydrazine. *Cancer Res.,* **44**, 2186–90

120. Blumberg, B. S., Larouze, B., London, W. T., Weiner, B., Hesser, J. E., Millman, I., Saimot, G. and Payet, M. (1975). The relation of infection with hepatitis B agent to primary hepatic carcinoma. *Am. J. Pathol.,* **81**, 669–82

121. Omata, M., Ashcavai, M., Liew, C. and Peters, R. L. (1979). Hepatocellular carcinoma in the USA. Etiologic considerations: localization of hepatitis B antigens. *Gastroenterology,* **76**, 279–87

122. Popper, H., Gerber, M. A. and Thung, S. N. (1982). Relation of hepatocellular carcinoma to infection with hepatitis B and related viruses in man and animals. *Hepatology,* **2**, (Suppl.), 15

123. Gerber, M. A. and Thung, S. N. (1985). Molecular and cellular pathology of hepatitis B. *Lab. Invest.,* **52**, 572–90

124. International Agency for Research on Cancer (1987). *IARC Monographs on the*

Evaluation of Carcinogenic Risks to Humans. Overall Evaluations of Carcinogenicity: An Updating of IARC Monographs volumes 1 to 42. Supplement 7, 1–440 (Lyon: IARC)

125. McQueen, C. A., Way, B. M. and Williams, G. M. Genotoxicity of carcinogens in human hepatocytes; application in hazard assessment. *Toxicol. Appl. Pharmacol.,* **96**, 360–6

126. McMahon, G., Davis, E. and Wogan, G. N. (1987). Characterization of c-Ki-ras oncogene alleles by direct sequencing of enzymatically amplified DNA from carcinogen-induced tumors. *Proc. Natl. Acad. Sci. USA,* **84**, 4974–8

127. Armel, P. and Williams, G. M. (1988). The molecular nature of spontaneous and chemically-induced mutations in the hypoxanthine-guanine phosphoribosyl transferase gene in rat liver epithelial cells. *Mutat. Res.,* in press

128. Tuyns, A. J. (1979). Epidemiology of alcohol and cancer. *Cancer Res.,* **39**, 2840–3

129. Lieber, C. S., Seitz, H. K., Garro, A. J. and Wormer, T. M. (1979). Alcohol-related diseases and carcinogenesis. *Cancer Res.,* **39**, 2863–86

130. Ketcham, A. S., Wexler, H. and Mantel, N. (1963). Effects of alcohol in mouse neoplasia. *Cancer Res.,* **23**, 667–70

131. Schmähl, D., Thomas, C., Sattler, W. and Sheld, G. F. (1965). Experimentelle Üntersuchungen zur Syncarcinogenese. 3. Mitteilung. Versuche zur Krebserzeugung bei Ratten bei gleichzeitiger Gabe von Diäthylnitrosamin und Tetrachlorkohlenstoff bzw. Äthylalkohol; zugleich ein experimenteller Beitrag zur Frage der 'Alkoholcirrhose'. *Z. Krebsforch.,* **66**, 526

132. Capel, I. D. and Williams, D. C. (1978). The effect of long term ethanol intake on the hepatic carcinogen metabolising enzyme system of mice. *IRCS Med. Sci.,* **6**, 297.

133. Garro, A. J., Seitz, H. D. and Lieber, C. S. (1981). Enhancement of dimethylnitrosamine metabolism and activation to a mutagen following chronic ethanol consumption. *Cancer Res.,* **41**, 120–4

134. Sohn, O. S., Fiala, E. S., Puz, C., Hamilton, S. R. and Williams, G. M. (1987). Enhancement of rat liver microsomal metabolism of azoxymethane to methylazoxymethanol by chronic ethanol administration: similarity to the microsomal metabolism of N-nitrosodimethylamine. *Cancer Res.,* **47**, 3123–9

135. Takada, A., Nei, J., Takase, S. and Matsuda, Y. (1986). Effects of ethanol on experimental hepatocarcinogenesis. *Hepatology,* **6**, 65–72

136. Driver, H. E. and McLean, A. E. M. (1986). Dose–response relationships for initiation of rat liver tumours by diethylnitrosamine and promotion by phenobarbitone or alcohol. *Food Chem. Toxicol.,* **24**, 241–5

137. Schwarz, M., Buchmann, A., Wiesbech, G. and Kunz, W., (1983). Effect of ethanol on early stages in nitrosamine carcinogenesis in rat liver. *Cancer Lett.,* **20**, 305–12

138. Misslbeck, N. G., Campbell, T. C. and Roe, D. A. (1984). Effect of ethanol consumed in combination with high or low fat diets on the postinitiation phase of hepatocarcinogenesis in the rat. *J. Nutrition,* **114**, 2311–23

139. Ohnishi, K., Ida, S., Iwama, S., Goto, N., Nomura, F., Takashi, M., Mishima, A., Knon, K., Kimura, K., Musha, H., Kotota, K. and Okuda, K. (1982). The effect of chronic habitual alcohol intake on the development of liver cirrhosis and hepatocellular carcinoma; relation to hepatitis B surface antigen carriage. *Cancer,* **49**, 672–7

140. Weisburger, J. H. and Williams, G. M. (1982). Chemical carcinogenesis. In Holland, J. F. and Frei III, E. (eds) *Cancer Medicine,* 2nd edn, pp. 42–95 (Philadelphia: Lea and Febiger)

141. Williams, (1985). Interaction of host and lifestyle factors with occupational chemicals in cancer causation. In Stich, H. F. (ed.) *Carcinogens and Mutagens in the Environment,* Vol. IV, pp. 27–32. (Florida: CRC Press)

142. Williams, G. M. (1985). Types of enhancement of carcinogenesis and influences on human cancer. In Mass, M. J., Kaufmann, D. G., Siegfried, J. M., Steele, V. E. and Nesnow, S. (eds). *Cancer of the Respiratory Tract: Predisposing Factors,* pp. 447–57 (New York: Raven Press)

143. Harris, C. C. and Sun, T. (1984). Multifactoral etiology of human liver cancer. *Carcinogenesis,* **5**, 697–701

144. Blumberg, B. S. and London, W. T. (1985). Hepatitis B virus and the prevention of primary cancer of the liver. *J. Natl. Cancer Inst.,* **74**, 267–73

145. Morio, S., Okamoto, N., Minowa, M., Mori, H. and Nishioka, K. (1987). Preventive effect of HB vaccination against liver cancer: an estimation by simulation. *Gann,* **78**, 899–907

146. Cabral, J. R. R. and Neal, G. E. (1983). The inhibitory effects of ethoxyquin on the carcinogenic action of aflatoxin B_1. *Cancer Lett.*, **19**, 125–32
147. Williams, G. M., Tanaka, T. and Maeura, Y. (1986). Dose-dependent inhibition of aflatoxin B_1 induced hepatocarcinogenesis by butylated hydroxytoluene. *Carcinogenesis*, 7, 1043–50
148. Williams, G. M. (1983). Epigenetic effects of liver tumor promoters and implications for health effects. *Environ. Health Perspect.*, **50**, 177–83

19
Steroid-related liver tumours: experimental induction and modulation

M. METZLER, A. M. TRITSCHER AND G. BLAICH

INTRODUCTION

Epidemiological studies have associated steroidal sex hormones with liver tumours in humans[1]. The long-term use of combined oral contraceptives appears to be related to the development of benign liver adenoma and possibly also hepatocellular carcinomas. Although these lesions are quite rare (about 1–5 per 1 000 000 women), their incidence increases with the dose of the steroid and the age of the user up to 500-fold compared with non-users[2]. Likewise, long-term use of anabolic steroids is linked to an increased incidence of liver lesions including tumours[3].

The mechanisms of the hepatotumorigenic effect of steroidal sex hormones in humans are far from clear. The problems in studying neoplasia and sex hormones include the low incidence of these lesions and the multiple aetiologic factors in the study populations. Therefore, it is preferable to perform mechanistic studies to elucidate the carcinogenic potential of œstrogens and androgens in animals *in vivo* and in isolated cells *in vitro*. The results of such investigations may allow extrapolation to the human situation.

The early stages in the multi-step process of tumorigenesis are operationally separated into the phases of initiation and promotion. Initiation involves a heritable alteration of the genetic material, usually DNA damage, of the future cancer cell, whereas promotion is less well defined and includes any event helping the initiated cell to divide, e.g. by stimulation of cell proliferation.

One of the key issues in the mechanism of hormonal carcinogenesis is the question of whether sex hormones have initiating or promoting potential or both. This chapter will briefly address this issue and provide some recent evidence suggesting that œstrogenic steroids may act as co-carcinogens by modulating the activity of other carcinogenic agents.

STEROIDS AS PROMOTERS OF HEPATOTUMORIGENESIS

There is ample evidence from animal experiments that œstrogens and androgens can act as promoters of hepatocarcinogenesis when administered subsequent to a sub-carcinogenic dose of typical initiators such as diethylnitrosamine. A typical experiment of this kind was reported by Yager et al.[4], who treated female Sprague–Dawley rats with diethylnitrosamine and fed œstradiol (E_2), ethinyloestradiol (EE_2) and mestranol. Afte 9 and 12 months, the liver nodules and carcinomas were scored. EE_2 and mestranol but not E_2 were found to cause a significant increase in hepatocellular nodules and carcinoma.

Similar experiments along these lines have been reviewed[5] recently and have led to the general consensus that œstrogens and androgens are promoters of hepatocarcinogenesis.

STEROIDS AS CARCINOGENS IN *IN VITRO* SYSTEMS

Much effort has been made in several laboratories over the past years to clarify whether steroidal sex hormones can act as initiators of carcinogenesis. According to our present understanding this would require some kind of genetic damage to the cell leading to an irreversible and heritable alteration of the genome. Steroidal œstrogens and androgens have been tested in a number of short-term assays for genotoxicity, and the results have been reviewed[6] recently. It can be concluded that sex hormones, in general, lack the ability to bind to DNA and to induce gene mutations. The inability of steroidal œstrogens and androgens to cause DNA damage in *in vitro* assays is in accordance with *in vivo* studies in rodent liver which failed to show DNA adduct formation[7] or hepatogenotoxicity in the Solt–Farber system[8].

Although there is presently no evidence for DNA-based genotoxic effects of sex hormones in the liver, it should be noted that other forms of genotoxicity cannot yet be ruled out. For example, recent studies in Syrian hamster embryo (SHE) fibroblasts have revealed that these cells are neoplastically transformed *in vitro* by some steroidal and non-steroidal

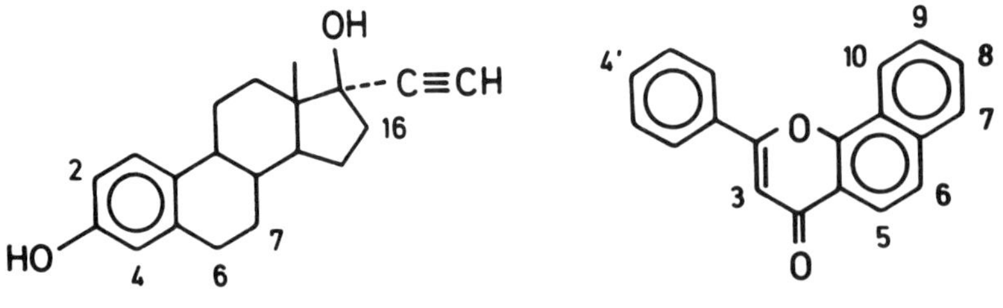

Figure 1 Chemical structures of 17α -ethinylestradiol (EE_2) and 7,8-benzoflavone (BF)

oestrogens in the absence of detectable gene mutations[9,10]. Instead, a numerical chromosomal alteration, i.e. induction of near-diploid aneuploidy, was observed and proposed as a critical event in the process of neoplasia[11]. Aneuploidy induction by various œstrogens was correlated with *in vitro* cell transformation, which in turn appears to be correlated with certain metabolic features rather than with the hormonal potency of the compounds[12]. We have recently demonstrated that reactive metabolites of steroidal and non-steroidal œstrogens bind covalently to tubulin and other proteins of the spindle apparatus *in vitro*, a reaction which might represent the biochemical lesion leading to aneuploidy induction[13]. It should prove interesting to look for aneuploidy induction and binding to microtubular proteins of steroidal sex hormones in hepatocytes and other target cells for hormonal carcinogenesis in order to see whether these compounds can act as chromosomal mutagens.

A NOVEL HAMSTER LIVER TUMOUR MODEL

One of the obstacles in experimental studies of steroid-related liver tumours is the lack of a suitable animal model. Most species are quite resistant towards the hepatotumorigenic effects of sex hormones, yielding at best only low incidences of tumours at high doses of the steroid: for a review see Metzler and Degen[5], and Schuppler and Günzel[14]. Recently however a 100% incidence of multinodular hepatocellular carcinomas was induced in male Syrian golden hamsters by the combined treatment with EE_2 and 7,8-benzoflavone (BF)[15]. The structures of EE_2 and BF are given in Figure 1 and the characteristic features of the new animal tumour model are summarized in Table 1. BF alone did not induce such tumours whereas a very low tumour incidence (about 4%) was observed after prolonged treatment with EE_2 alone. BF could not be replaced by 5,6-benzoflavone but the steroid œstrogen EE_2 could be substituted by the stilbene œstrogens diethylstilbœstrol (DES) or hexestrol (Table 1).

Table 1 Hepatocarcinogenic effects of various sex hormones in the Syrian golden hamster as modulated by 7,8-benzoflavone (BF) according to Li and Li[15]

Treatment	Number of animals with hepatic tumour/total number of animals	Tumour incidence (%)
17α-Ethinyloestradiol + BF	15/15	100
BF alone	0/15	0
Diethylstilbestrol (DES) + BF	12/14	86
DES alone	0/20	0
DES + 5,6-benzoflavone	0/8	0
Hexestrol + BF	7/9	78
5α-Dihydrotestosterone + BF	0/9	0
Progesterone + BF	0/9	0

This novel tumour model has been proposed by Li and Li[15] as an animal model for human liver cancer. It should be helpful for obtaining further insight into the mechanism of steroid-related hepatic neoplasia. As BF is known to interfere with drug-metabolizing enzymes, it may be expected that the combined administration of an oestrogen and BF modulates enzyme activities and thereby alters the metabolism of the oestrogen and/or BF. We have therefore studied the effects of various pre-treatments on the metabolism of EE_2 and BF in hamster liver microsomes.

MODULATION OF ETHINYLOESTRADIOL METABOLISM

Male Syrian golden hamsters were pretreated with EE_2 and BF in the same manner as for tumour induction. Hepatic microsomes were obtained after 12 and 32 weeks of pre-treatment with EE_2 alone, with BF alone and with EE_2 plus BF. The determination of cytochromes P450 and b_5 (Table 2) indicated that EE_2 decreased gross P450 levels whereas BF alone or in combination with EE_2 clearly induced cytochromes P-450 and b_5.

The various microsomes were incubated under identical conditions with [^{3}H]-labelled EE_2 and the extracted metabolites separated by HPLC and identified by gas chromatography (GC)/mass spectrometry (MS). The HPLC tracings of the radioactivity and a quantitative account of the major metabolites are depicted in Figures 2 and 3, respectively. The data indicate that the formation of 2-hydroxy-EE_2, which is the major metabolite in hepatic microsomes from untreated animals, is clearly increased in microsomes from all pre-treated hamsters.

Binding of radioactivity to microsomal protein was determined in all incubations (data not shown) and found to be decreased about two-fold in microsomes from all pre-treated animals as compared with controls.

MODULATION OF 7,8-BENZOFLAVONE METABOLISM

The same microsomes as used for the study of EE_2 metabolism were used to determine the oxidative biotransformation of ^{14}C-labelled BF. With

Table 2 Effect of various pre-treatments on the levels of cytochromes P450 and b_5 in male Syrian golden hamster liver microsomes

| Pre-treatment | Microsomal content (nmol/mg protein) | | Ratio |
	Cytochrome P450	Cytochrome b_5	$P450/b_5$
None	1.03 ± 0.04	0.51 ± 0.03	2.02
EE_2 (12 weeks)	0.63 ± 0.12	0.54 ± 0.06	1.17
BF (32 weeks)	1.42 ± 0.12	0.95 ± 0.04	1.49
EE_2 + BF (12 weeks)	1.68 ± 0.28	1.02 ± 0.20	1.65

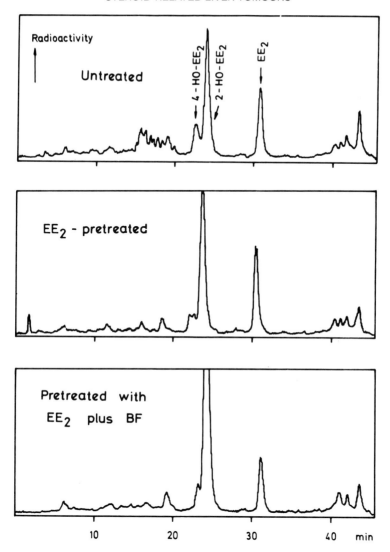

Figure 2 Radio-HPLC of EE_2 metabolites generated by hamster liver microsomes after various pre-treatments. All incubations (1 ml) contained 2 mg microsomal protein and 60 nmol $[^3H]$-E-E_2. Data are the mean values ± standard deviation of three animals.

microsomes from control hamsters, five BF metabolites were clearly separated by HPLC (Figure 4, upper panel). The radioactive peaks were collected and subjected to GC/MS after trimethylsilylation. 6-Hydroxy-BF and 7-hydroxy-BF were unequivocally identified through their mass spectra and co-chromatography with authentic reference compounds in HPLC and GC. The small peak preceding 7-hydroxy-BF in HPLC (metabolite F) was

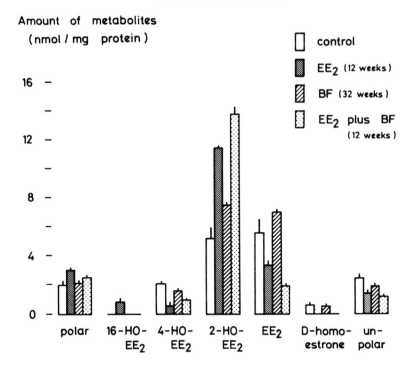

Figure 3 Pattern of oxidative EE_2 metabolites in hamster liver microsomes after various pre-treatments. Details as described in Figure 2

tentatively identified as 4′-hydroxy-BF based on its mass spectrum and the fact that it did not co-chromatograph with any of the reference hydroxy-BFs carrying the hydroxy group in the naphthyl system. Metabolite B was assigned the structure of BF-7,8-dihydrodiol (see Figure 6) on the basis of its mass spectrum and the fact that it was converted to 7-hydroxy-BF upon acid dehydration[16]. According to its mass spectrum, metabolite E was tentatively identified as a dihydroxy-BF, possibly with a catechol structure.

Microsomes from pre-treated hamsters displayed marked differences depending on the kind of pre-treatment. The HPLC chromatograms are given in Figure 4 and the quantitative account in Figure 5. After pre-treatment with EE_2, the amount of 7-hydroxy-BF was increased but the other BF metabolites were not affected. In contrast, pre-treatment with BF led to the formation of three new metabolites (A, C and D in Figure 4). Metabolites A and C are as yet unidentified and metabolite D has the mass spectrum of a dihydroxy-BF, possibly a catechol. It should be noted that microsomes from BF-pre-treated hamster liver had a higher activity than those from controls or EE_2-pre-treated animals, as they oxidized more BF. The same pattern of oxidative metabolites as obtained after BF was observed after pre-treatment

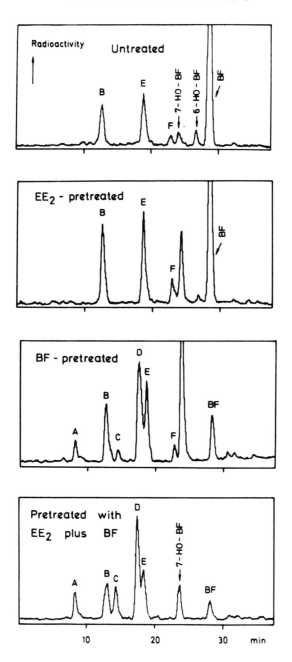

Figure 4 Radio-HPLC of BF metabolites generated by hamster liver microsomes after various pre-treatments. All incubations (1 ml) contained 2 mg microsomal protein and 240 nmol [^{14}C] BF. Data are the mean values ± standard deviation of three animals

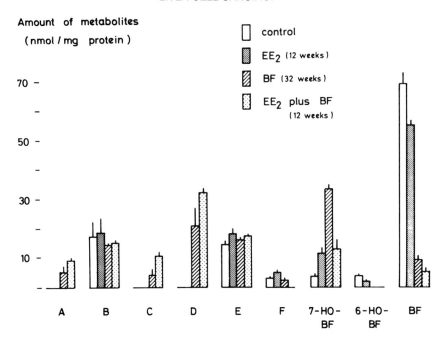

Figure 5 Pattern of oxidative EE$_2$ metabolites in hamster liver microsomes after various pre-treatments. Details as described in Figure 4

with BF plus EE$_2$, with an even higher conversion of BF (Figure 4, lower panel). Studies with increasing concentrations of BF in the microsomal incubations have shown that the combined pre-treatment leads to an at least two-fold higher activity for BF metabolism than pre-treatment with BF alone (data not shown).

Although a complete metabolic scheme of BF cannot be derived before the new metabolites are fully identified, it is clear that pre-treatment with BF and with BF plus EE$_2$ leads to an induction of BF metabolism and to the formation of several new BF metabolites in hepatic microsomes which are not observed in untreated or EE$_2$-treated hamsters. Among these new metabolites are dihydrodiols and catechols (Figure 6) which may serve as precursors of reactive dihydrodiol-epoxides and quinones, respectively. The toxicological significance of these metabolites in the hamster hepatic tumour model remains to be elucidated. If they prove to be genotoxic, then BF would be considered an initiator and EE$_2$ a promoter and also a co-carcinogen, because it enhances the metabolic activation of the initiator.

It is tempting to speculate that the metabolic activation of compounds other than BF, for example aromatic hydrocarbons or of pyrolysis products of proteins ingested with the food, might also be increased by EE$_2$. In this case, the hamster liver tumour model might indeed have some bearing on œstrogen-related hepatotumorigenesis in man.

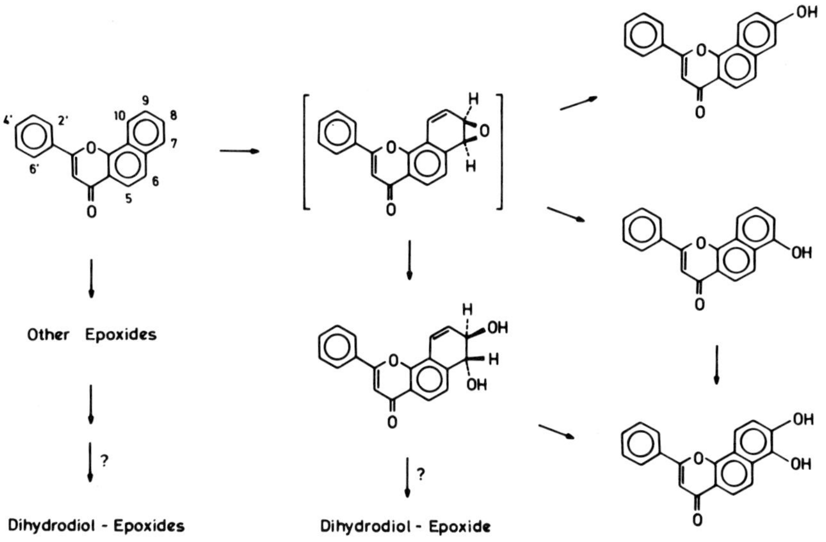

Figure 6 Oxidative pathways in BF metabolism possibly leading to reactive intermediates

CONCLUSION

This chapter has emphasized two aspects of the carcinogenic potential of sex hormones. First, evidence has been reviewed that some sex hormones may, in addition to their promoting capability, act as genotoxic agents in at least certain cell systems. This activity does not involve DNA damage but appears to act on the spindle apparatus resulting in the induction of near-diploid aneuploidy. This activity has not yet been demonstrated in the liver. Secondly, certain œstrogens may have the potential to act as co-carcinogens by enhancing the metabolic activation of environmental or dietary carcinogens. The databases on both aspects need to be broadened before their relevance for the mechanism of œstrogen-associated liver tumour formation in humans can be properly judged.

Acknowledgements

Work from our laboratory cited in this chapter has been supported by the Deutsche Forschungsgemeinschaft (Sonderforschungsbereich 172). The skilful technical assistance of Jutta Colberg, Hella Raabe and Siglinde Stoll is gratefully acknowledged. Synthetic reference compounds for metabolites of ethinyloestradiol and 7,8-benzoflavone were generously provided by Drs. Knuppen (Lübeck, F.R.G.) and Nesnow (EPA, N.C.), respectively. We thank Dr. J. J. Li (Minneapolis) for kindly providing pellets of ethinyloestradiol and the Doktor Robert Pfleger-Stiftung (Bamberg, FRG) for mass spectrometric equipment.

References

1. IARC Monographs on the Evaluation of the Carcinogenic Risk of Chemicals to Humans, Vol. 21 (1979). *Sex Hormones (II)*. (Lyon: International Agency for Research on Cancer)
2. Huggins, G. R. and Zucker, P. K. (1987). Oral contraceptives and neoplasia: 1987 update. *Fertil. Steril.*, **47**, 733–61
3. Evans, D. J. (1978). Liver tumors elicited by specific factors: synthetic androgens and anabolic steroids. In Remmer, H., Bolt, H. M., Bannasch, P. and Popper, H. (eds) *Primary Liver Tumors*, pp. 213–16. (Lancaster: MTP Press)
4. Yager, J. D., Campbell, H. A., Longnecker, D. S., Roebuck, B. D. and Benoit, M. C. (1984). Enhancement of hepatocarcinogenesis in female rats by ethinylestradiol and mestranol but not estradiol. *Cancer Res.*, **44**, 3862–9
5. Metzler, M. and Degen, G. H. (1987). Sex hormones and neoplasia: liver tumors in rodents. *Arch. Toxicol.*, Suppl. **10**, 251–63
6. Degen, G. H. and Metzler, M. (1987). Sex hormones and neoplasia: genotoxic effects in short term assays. *Arch. Toxicol.*, Suppl. **10**, 264–78
7. Caviezel, M., Lutz, W. K., Minini, U. and Schlatter, C. (1984). Interaction of estrone and estradiol with DNA and protein of liver and kidney in rat and hamster *in vivo* and *in vitro*. *Arch. Toxicol.*, **55**, 67–103
8. Schuppler, J., Damme, J. and Schulte-Hermann, R. (1983). Assay of some endogenous and synthetic sex steroids for tumor-initiating activity in rat liver using the Solt–Farber system. *Carcinogenesis*, **4**, 239–41
9. Barrett, J. C., Wong, A. and McLachlan, J. A. (1981) Diethylstilbestrol induces neoplastic transformation without measurable gene mutation at two loci. *Science*, **212**, 1402–4
10. Tsutsui, T., Suzuki, N., Fukuda, S., Sato, M., Maizumi, H., McLachlan, J. A. and Barrett, J. C. (1987). 17ß-estradiol-induced cell transformation and aneuploidy of Syrian hamster embryo cells in culture. *Carcinogenesis*, **8**, 1715–19
11. Tsutsui, T., Maizumi, H., McLachlan, J. A. and Barrett, J. C. (1983). Aneuploidy induction and cell transformation by diethylstilbestrol: a possible chromosomal mechanism in carcinogenesis. *Cancer Res.*, **43**, 3814–21
12. McLachlan, J. A., Wong, A., Degen, G. H. and Barrett, J. C. (1982). Morphological and neoplastic transformation of Syrian hamster embryo fibroblasts by diethylstilbestrol and analogs. *Cancer Res.*, **42**, 3040–5
13. Epe, B., Hegler, J. and Metzler, M. (1987). Site-specific covalent binding of stilbene-type and steroidal estrogens to tubulin following metabolic activation *in vitro*. *Carcinogenesis*, **8**, 1271–5
14. Schuppler, J. and Günzel, P. (1979) Liver tumors and steroid hormones in rats and mice. *Arch. Toxicol.*, Suppl. **2**, 181–95
15. Li, J. J. and Li, S. A. (1984). High incidence of hepatocellular carcinomas after synthetic estrogen administration in Syrian hamsters fed *a*-naphthoflavone: a new tumor model. *J. Natl. Cancer Inst.*, **73**, 543–8
16. Nesnow, S., Bryant, B. J., Rudo, K. and Easterling, R. (1983). Reanalysis and clarification of the structures of *a*-naphthoflavone dihydrodiols formed by uninduced and induced rat liver microsomes from Charles River CD and Sprague–Dawley rats. *Carcinogenesis*, **4**, 425–30

20
Alcohol and liver carcinoma

H. K. SEITZ, U. A. SIMANOWSKI, M. HOERNER AND B. KOMMERELL

Hepatocellular carcinoma (HCC) is common in the alcoholic[1-7]. However, the exact role of ethanol itself, of the ethanol-induced cirrhosis of the liver, of a concomitant hepatitis B virus (HBV) infection, or of a combination of all three has not been determined. Since the importance of hepatic cirrhosis and of HBV infection in the pathogenesis of HCC has been discussed in detail elsewhere in this book, this review will mainly focus on the effect of ethanol itself on hepatocarcinogenesis.

THE EFFECT OF ETHANOL DURING INITIATION AND PROMOTION OF HCC

To study the effect of ethanol on hepatocarcinogenesis, various animal experiments have been performed and it has been shown that ethanol *per se* is not a carcinogen[8]. However, when ethanol is administered chronically to laboratory animals, it can modify carcinogenesis depending on the experimental conditions used[9]. These animal experiments have also clarified that it is ethanol and not contaminants of alcoholic beverages which influence chemically-induced carcinogenesis. Thus, ethanol has to be considered a co-carcinogen or under certain conditions a tumour promoter. In this context it is noteworthy that the administration of ethanol as part of a balanced liquid diet in animal experiments is the only way to guarantee an adequate ethanol intake and account for nutritional factors[10]. If ethanol is given in the drinking water, alcohol intake may be extremely low and nutritional deficiencies may occur which by themselves can influence carcinogenesis[9].

Table 1 summarizes the effect of chronic ethanol ingestion on hepatocarcinogenesis. The majority of these experiments were performed with nitrosamines as tumour inducers; only a few other pro-carcinogens have been studied. Hepatic carcinogenesis with nitrosamines was only enhanced when ethanol was given during promotion[11,12] or when a methyl-deficient diet was administered simultaneously[13]. However, when ethanol was applied prior to, or together with, the pro-carcinogen, carcinogenesis was not affected[14,15] or

Table 1 Effect of ethanol on chemically-induced hepatic carcinogenesis

Authors	Species	Carcinogen[a]	Ethanol administration[b]	Ethanol effect
Griciute et al.[16,17]	Mouse/Rat	DMNA, i.g./NNN, i.g.	40% i.g. with carcinogen	Inhibition[c]
Habs and Schmähl[18]	Rat	DMNA, orally	25% in d.w. with carcinogen	Inhibition
Teschke et al.[14]	Rat	DMNA, i.p.	6% l.d. prior to carcinogen	No effect/inhibition[d]
Gibel[15]	Rat	DENA, i.g.	30% i.g. with carcinogen	No effect[e]
Porta et al.[13]	Rat	DENA, i.p.	25–32% in l.d. and methyl deficiency after carcinogen	Stimulation
Takada et al.[11]	Rat	DENA, i.p., 70% hepatectomy	20% in l.d. after carcinogen	Stimulation
Driver and McLean[12]	Rat	DENA, i.p.	5% in d.w. after carcinogen	Stimulation
Mendenhall and Chedid[21]	Rat	Aflatoxin B₁, i.g.	6% l.d. continuously	No effect[f]
Misslbeck et al.[22]	Rat	Aflatoxin B₁, i.g.	6% l.d. after carcinogen	No effect
Radike et al.[19]	Rat	Vinyl chloride, in air	5% in d.w. prior to and with carcinogen	Stimulation
Weisburger et al.[94]	Rat	N-OH-2AAF, orally	10% in d.w. with carcinogen	No effect

[a]DNMA = dimethylnitrosamine; DENA = diethylnitrosamine; NNN = N-nitronornicotine; N-OH-2AAF = N-hydroxy-2-acetaminofluorene; i.g. = intragastrically; i.p. = intraperitoneally
[b]d.w. = drinking water; l.d. = liquid diet
[c]Occurrence of olfactory neuroepithelioma after alcohol
[d]Similar tumour yield, but prolonged latency period after alcohol
[e]Enhanced oesophageal cancer after alcohol
[f]Stimulation of hepatic peliosis after alcohol

228

even inhibited[14,16-18] by alcohol. The mechanism(s) leading to this observation will be discussed below.

Radike *et al.*[19] found a four-fold increase in vinyl chloride induced hepatic cancer as well as a change in histology of the tumours after chronic ethanol consumption in the rat. This was associated with severe mitochondrial damage due to the combined effect of vinyl chloride and ethanol[20]. These data seem of particular interest because of two unusual human accidents in the vinyl chloride industry. One chemical worker consumed large quantities of ethanol in addition to his exposure to vinyl chloride and developed both angiosarcoma and HCC, while his colleague, a non-drinker, developed 'only' angiosarcoma of the liver[5].

When aflatoxin B_1 was used for tumour induction, no effect of ethanol on hepatocarcinogenesis was noted[21,22], although a significant increase in the occurrence of hepatic peliosis was observed in the rat[21]. One epidemiological study[23] on aflatoxin exposure demonstrated that the daily consumption of 24 g of ethanol or more increases the risk of developing HCC induced by 4 µg of dietary aflatoxin B_1 by a factor of 35.

In general, ethanol may increase the susceptibility of various tissues to chemical carcinogens by a variety of mechanisms. Among these are activating chemical carcinogens, altering the metabolism and/or distribution of carcinogens, interfering with the repair of carcinogen-mediated DNA alkylation and the immune response, stimulating cellular regeneration, and exacerbating dietary deficiencies[9,24] (Figure 1).

Alcohol and microsomal metabolism of pro-carcinogens

Many environmental carcinogens exist in their pro-carcinogenic form and require metabolic activation by microsomal cytochrome P-450-dependent

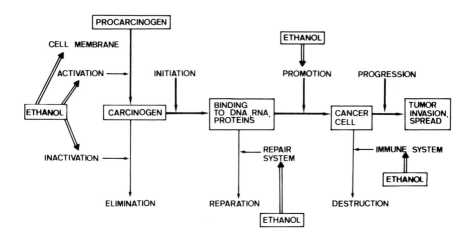

Figure 1   Simplified scheme of two-step carcinogenesis and possible sites of action of ethanol

enzymes. Induction of microsomal enzyme activities increases the mutagenic effect of many compounds in the Ames Salmonella mutagenesis assay[25]. Ethanol is a well-known microsomal enzyme inducer in the liver and in other tissues[10,24,26,27] and chronic consumption results in the appearance of a distinct form of cytochrome P-450 in the liver[24,28]. This specific cytochrome P-450 has a preferential affinity towards aniline and 7-ethoxycoumarin[29] and is the major P-450 responsible for the low K_m-dimethylnitrosamine (DMN) demethylase activity[30,31]. Thus, in the alcoholic subject, the metabolism of a great number of drugs and xenobiotics is accelerated. In addition, the capacity of hepatic and intestinal microsomes to activate a variety of chemical pro-carcinogens to mutagens, including polycyclic hydrocarbons[32-36] (Figure 2), 2-aminofluorene[33,35,36], amino acid pyrolysates[33,35,37] and nitrosamines[38-41] (Figure 3) is increased following chronic ethanol ingestion. The enhanced intestinal activation of pro-carcinogens after ethanol consumption (Figure 4) can increase the bioavailability of these compounds and may ultimately lead to increased concentrations of carcinogens in the portal vein and in the liver.

Although the microsomal cytochrome P-450-dependent biotransformation system is essential for the activation of most chemical pro-carcinogens, induction of this enzyme system does not necessarily entail an increased

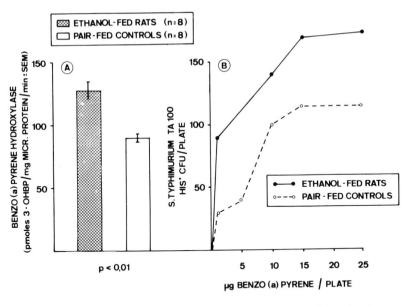

Figure 2 (A) Effect of chronic ethanol consumption on the activity of hepatic microsomal benzo(a)pyrene hydroxylase in female rats. (B) Effect of chronic ethanol consumption on the hepatic microsomal activation of benzo(a)pyrene to a mutagen in female rats using the Ames Salmonella mutagenesis test. Each point is an average of the number of his$^+$ colonies of *Salmonella typhimurium* strain TA 100 present on duplicate plates. The levels of spontaneous his$^+$ revertants have been subtracted. Microsomes were from pools of 3 animals pair-fed either an ethanol containing or a control diet. The microsomal protein content per plate was 0.4 mg. For all amounts of benzo(a)pyrene[34] used, $p < 0.01$

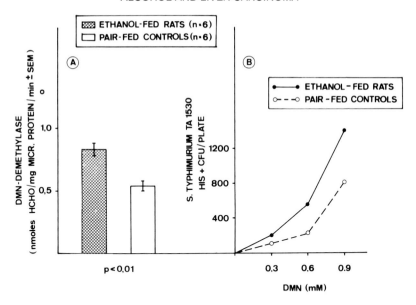

Figure 3 (A) Effect of chronic ethanol consumption on the activity of hepatic microsomal DMN demethylase measured at 1 mM DMN in the rat. (B) Effect of chronic ethanol consumption on the hepatic microsomal activation of DMN to a mutagen in the rat using the Ames Salmonella mutagenesis test: 2 mg of microsomal protein was incubated with 5 mM NADPH and an average of 2×10^9 CFU of nitrosomethylurea-pretreated *Salmonella typhimurium* TA 1530 at 37°C for 15 min. The numbers of his$^+$ CFU were assayed by overlaying, in duplicate, 0.2 ml aliquots of the reaction mixture on histidine deficient medium. The data are averages of two sets of experiments, i.e. 4 plates/point[38]

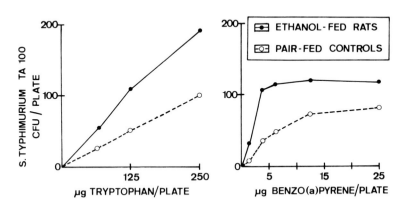

Figure 4 Effect of chronic ethanol consumption on the intestinal microsomal activation of tryptophan pyrolysate and benzo(a)pyrene to mutagens in the rat using the Ames Salmonella mutagenesis test. Each point is an average of the number of his$^+$ colonies of *Salmonella typhimurium* TA 100 present on duplicate plates. The levels of spontaneous revertants have been subtracted. In each case the microsomes were from pools of 3 animals pair-fed either an ethanol-containing or a control diet. The microsomal protein concentration was 0.4 mg for the tryptophan, and 0.5 mg for the benzo(a)pyrene experiment[32,33]

cancer risk. This is probably related to the fact that detoxification may also be induced. Microsomal metabolism of some compounds, such as benzo(a)-pyrene, gives rise to multiple products and the components of the microsomal enzyme system and associated enzymes, such as epoxide hydratase and glutathione transferase are also involved in the detoxification of many of the same chemicals that require activation and may also be inducible by ethanol (Figure 1). Ultimately, what is probably most critical in the relationship between enzyme activities and carcinogenesis is the relative effect of the inducer such as ethanol on the steady-state level of activated carcinogens. In aflatoxin B_1-induced hepatocarcinogenesis, for example, chronic ethanol ingestion led to an enhanced activation of the pro-carcinogen[42,43], but did not increase the level of DNA-bound aflatoxin B_1 in the liver of male F344 rats[44]. This lack of DNA-binding is in good agreement with the fact that ethanol does not influence aflatoxin B_1-induced cancer occurrence in animals[21,22].

Alcohol and nitrosamine metabolism

Nitrosamines have been detected in alcoholic beverages[9,24,45]. Since ethanol and nitrosamines are both metabolized via cytochrome P-450 dependent enzymes it is not surprising that the two compounds interact.

Ethanol and DMN are metabolized by a similar cytochrome P-450 species in hepatic microsomes. Therefore, ethanol is capable of inhibiting competitively the activity of hepatic low K_m DMN demethylase[46-48]. On the other hand, chronic ethanol consumption increases microsomal DMN-demethylase activity[38] as a result of induction of a specific ethanol-metabolizing cytochrome P-450 species with strong affinity for DMN. Thus, alcoholism results in an enhanced microsomal capacity to activate DMN to a mutagen in the Ames test[38]. Such an enhanced activation had already been observed with DMN concentrations < 0.3mM, which may be of pathophysiological relevance[38]. However, no increase in the methylation of hepatic DNA was noted when [^{14}C]DMN was administered to ethanol-fed and control rats[49] or when the mutagenicity of DMN was tested in vivo using the host-mediated assay[50]. In addition, as already pointed out, ethanol feeding did not stimulate nitrosamine-induced hepatocarcinogenesis[14-18]. The lack of an ethanol-mediated co-carcinogenicity may possibly be related either to the fact that inactivating enzymes are also enhanced by chronic ethanol consumption or that the presence of ethanol in the liver during pro-carcinogen application prevents the hepatic activation of the nitrosamine.

When DMN is administered orally the liver can exert a first-pass clearance up to a DMN dose of $30 \mu g/kg$ body weight[46]. At higher doses, the hepatic enzymes are saturated, and methylation in other organs such as kidney and œsophagus occurs. Ethanol, when given to rats in low amounts, equivalent to an adult male drinking half a litre of beer, prevents the first-pass clearance by competing for the hepatic microsomal enzyme. As a result, more nitrosamine bypasses the liver, and nitrosamine-sensitive extrahepatic organs are exposed to greater levels of the pro-carcinogen (Figure 5). Measurements of DMN metabolism in liver slices and in œsophageal epithelium suggest that the

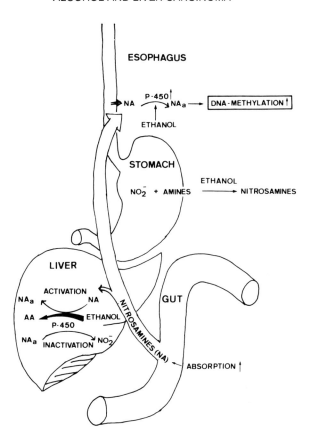

Figure 5 Ethanol and nitrosamine metabolism. Ethanol catalyses nitrosamine production in the stomach and favours its absorption in the intestine. In the presence of ethanol hepatic nitrosamine activation and its hepatic uptake is inhibited since ethanol competes for the cytochrome P-450 binding site. Therefore more nitrosamine reaches the systemic circulation, and extrahepatic tissues such as the œsophagus are exposed to higher nitrosamine concentrations. Since ethanol increases cytochrome P-450 also in the œsophagus and since this nitrosamine-activating enzyme system has a lower K_m (and therefore an increased affinity to nitrosamines), nitrosamine activation to a carcinogen is enhanced even in the presence of ethanol

changes in alkylation of œsophageal DNA can be the result of selective inhibition of DMN metabolism in the liver and kidney[46]. The interaction between nitrosamine and vitamin A metabolism will be discussed below.

These biochemical data on the interaction between ethanol and nitrosamine metabolism in hepatic and extrahepatic tissue may explain, at least in part, why ethanol when given prior to, or during, initiation does not stimulate nitrosamine-induced hepatocarcinogenesis but enhances the development of extrahepatic tumours such as carcinoma of the œsophagus[15,51], the nasal cavity[52,53], and the trachea[52].

Alcohol and DNA metabolism

There are two effects of ethanol on DNA metabolism that might be associated with co-carcinogenic activity, namely its effect on sister chromatid exchanges (SCEs) and on DNA repair. In some way, ethanol may also affect DNA integration of genetic material from HBV.

Obe and Ristow[54] have reported that acetaldehyde, the first metabolite of ethanol, induces SCEs in tissue cultures. In addition, they found an elevation of chromosomal aberrations in the lymphocytes of alcoholics[55]. The potential significance of these observations with respect to tumour promotion is related to the hypothesis that compounds with SCEs activity may act as promoters[56]. By increasing the frequency of SCEs, such compounds could theoretically enhance recessive mutations being converted from a heterozygous to a homozygous state and thereby lead to tumour development.

A second mechanism by which alcohol abuse may increase the risk of developing cancer is by inhibiting the capacity of cells to repair carcinogen-induced DNA damage. It was reported that DMN-induced hepatic DNA alkylation persisted for longer periods in ethanol-fed animals than in controls[57]. This effect appeared to be specific for O^6-methylguanine (O^6-MeG) repair. The enzyme responsible for the repair of O^6-MeG adducts is O^6-MeG transferase, which transfers methyl or ethyl groups from the O^6 position of guanine to a cysteine residue located in the enzyme, which in turn inactivates the transferase[58-60]. Chronic ethanol consumption was found to reduce this enzyme activity significantly[57]. Since alkylation at the O^6 position of guanine is associated with both mutagenesis and carcinogenesis[61-63], the apparent decreased O^6-MeG transferase activity in alcohol-fed rats could be an important mechanism in alcohol-associated cancer risk. It should be noted that two other studies failed to detect an effect of dietary ethanol on the repair of DMN-induced O^6-MeG adducts[64,65]. However, these studies have been criticized and it was suspected that because of the low caloric intake, under-nourishment may have occurred.

Alcohol as a tumour promoter in the liver

It has been shown in experimental animals that ethanol can also act as tumour promoter in the liver. At 8 weeks after a single injection of diethyl-nitrosamine (DENA), Takada et al. gave an ethanol-containing diet to 70% hepatectomized rats[11]. After 32 weeks the numbers of visible nodules per liver as well as the numbers of enzyme-altered foci positive for γ-glutamyltrans-peptidase were significantly increased in the ethanol group and were similar to a pentobarbital control group. These results indicate that ethanol, similar to pentobarbital, acts as a promoter in chemically-induced hepatic carcinogenesis and this may be of some practical importance with respect to HBV carriers who additionally consume large amounts of alcohol.

In another experiment, Driver and McLean[12] gave ethanol (unfortunately as 5% solution in the drinking water) to rats after initiation of hepatocarcino-genesis with DENA. Again, an enhancement of cancer development with ethanol as promoter was noted.

Alcohol and dietary deficiencies

In chronic alcoholics, 50% of the daily caloric intake may be in the form of ethanol. Alcoholic beverages, however, lack essential nutrients and nutritional deficiencies therefore are common in this population. With respect to hepatocarcinogenesis, recent studies in rats have suggested that ethanol may be co-carcinogenic because of methyl deficiency[13]. In addition, deficiency of vitamin A and pyridoxine may also play a role.

It is well known that chronic alcoholism, at least in rodents, increases the requirement for methyl groups[66-68] and that dietary methyl deficiency enhances the activity of several hepatocarcinogens[69,70]. It must be pointed out, however, that primates are less affected by ethanol-associated lipotrope deficiencies than rodents[71].

Methionine, obtained in the diet and synthesized by several reactions in the body, is the sole precursor of S-adenosylmethionine, the primary methyl donor in the body. Disruption in methionine metabolism and methylation reactions may be involved in the cancer process[72]. S-adenosylmethionine is involved in the methylation of a small percentage of cytosine bases of DNA[72]. Recent findings suggest that enzymatic DNA methylation is an important component of gene control and may serve as a silencing mechanism for gene function. Some carcinogens interfere with enzymatic DNA methylation, and thus may allow oncogene activation[73-75]. Demethylation may be a necessary,

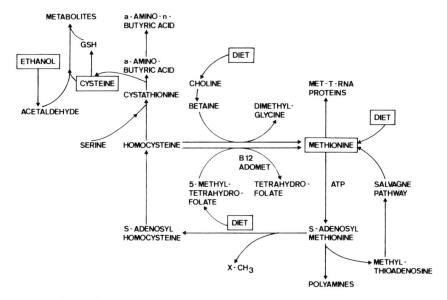

Figure 6 Effect of ethanol on the metabolism of methionine. Acetaldehyde traps cysteine which leads to a decrease of homocysteine, a precursor of methionine. As a result, methionine concentrations may also decrease, especially when the diet lacks methyl groups (methionine, choline), cysteine and folate/B_{12} (necessary to convert homocysteine to methionine). In addition, as a side product α-amino-n-butyric acid accumulates. This amino acid is increased in the alcoholic but also in the state of malnutrition

but not always sufficient condition for enhanced transcription. DNA hypomethylation has been observed in many cancer cells and tumours[72]. Figure 6 illustrates the effect of ethanol on methionine metabolism and the importance of methionine in the intermediary metabolism.

Vitamin A deficiency is also very common in the alcoholic. Chronic ethanol consumption decreases vitamin A concentrations in the liver of experimental animals[76] and in humans[77]. As a possible mechanism an increased microsomal cytochrome P-450 dependent degradation of retinol as well as an increased mobilization of retinol as retinol esters from the liver into the circulation has been discussed[24]. It was found that retinol can compete with DMN for its activation in liver microsomes[24]. It is therefore conceivable that a lowering of hepatic vitamin A, by diminishing this inhibition, may indirectly favour activation of chemical carcinogens, particularly in view of the fact, as discussed before, that chronic ethanol intake results in the induction of a type of cytochrome P-450 that selectively activates DMN and presumably other pro-carcinogens of this type.

Wynder has related pyridoxine (vitamin B₆) deficiency to enhanced liver tumour formation[78]. Pyridoxine deficiency also occurs in alcoholic subjects, and acetaldehyde has been incriminated in the accelerated destruction of this vitamin[79]. In addition to its key function in haematopoiesis, vitamin B₆ has been shown to play an important role in the induction of an antibody response against various antigens[80]; this may influence tumour development indirectly by modifying the immune response to HBV infection.

Deficiencies of other vitamins and trace elements such as riboflavin, vitamin E, vitamin C and zinc have also been observed in alcoholic subjects and seem to be associated with enhanced extrahepatic carcinogenesis (for a review see refs 7, 10 and 24).

THE ROLE OF ETHANOL-ASSOCIATED CIRRHOSIS IN HCC

HCC in alcoholics is commonly thought to be associated with cirrhosis of the liver. Indeed, the incidence of cirrhosis in patients with HCC has been reported to vary between 16 and 80%[81], with most reports indicating a 55–80% association. Cirrhosis may contribute to the development of HCC independently of alcohol. HCC in alcoholics without cirrhosis is a rare event. In a retrospective study by Lieber et al.[7], only 1 out of 15 patients with HCC in a non-cirrhotic liver did not consume alcohol. However, serological markers for HBV infection were not completely determined and therefore the significance of this study is limited. The importance of cirrhosis of the liver as a precursor of HCC has been discussed in detail elsewhere in this book.

HBV INFECTION IN THE ALCOHOLIC

It has been suggested that hepatitis B virus (HBV) infection is more common in alcoholic than in non-alcoholic populations, and therefore could contribute to the increased incidence of HCC. Indeed, an increased prevalence of serologic markers of HBV infection was reported in alcoholics[82]. These results have been confirmed in alcoholics from the same and different geographical areas[83-86]. An increased prevalence of anti-HBV antibodies was also observed in an unselected outpatient alcoholic population, which was comparable to results obtained from an inpatient population with alcoholic liver disease[87]. Brechot et al.[88] reported that among 51 subjects with various stages of alcoholic liver disease, 19 had one or more serological markers of HBV in their serum, 8 had HBV DNA in their livers, and in 5 the DNA was integrated in their genome. Integrated HBV DNA sequences in the liver have been reported in a number of subjects[88,89], particularly in chronic HBV carriers. Brechot et al.[88] evaluated 20 subjects with alcoholic cirrhosis and HCC, all of whom had HBV DNA integrated into the genome of the neoplastic liver cells. However, only 9 exhibited serological markers for HBV infection. These results are consistent with the data from Shafritz et al.[89] in a group of South Africans with HCC and from Ohnishi et al.[90] who noted that hepatocarcinogenesis was hastened significantly in HbsAg carriers if they continue to drink. On the other hand autopsy studies and prospective epidemiological studies have contradicted an association between alcoholism and HBV infection[91-93]. Both of these studies have been criticized on methodological grounds.

Whether the increased incidence of HBV infection in the alcoholic merely reflects the socio-economic status of the alcoholic, whether it is a consequence of increased exposure to HBV infection from blood transfusions, or whether it results from an enhanced susceptibility to HBV, remains to be determined.

CONCLUSION

In summary, the alcoholic subject seems to be at jeopardy for HCC for several reasons. These include direct effects of ethanol during tumour initiation and promotion due to enzyme induction, alteration of the DNA repair and the immune system and dietary deficiencies as well as the production of hepatic cirrhosis and the possible facilitation of infection with HBV.

Acknowledgements

This paper is dedicated to Hans Popper in grateful remembrance. Original studies have been supported by the Deutsche Forschungsgemeinschaft (Se 333/1,2,4-1,6-1,2).

References

1. Austin, H., Delzell, E., Grufferman, S., Levine, R. and Morrison, A. S. (1986). A case control study of hepatocellular carcinoma and the hepatitis B virus, cigarette smoking, and alcohol consumption. *Cancer Res.*, **46**, 962-6

2. Hakulinnen, T., Lehtimäki, L., Lehtonen, M. and Teppo, M. (1974). Cancer morbidity among male cohorts with increased alcohol consumption in Finland. *J. Natl. Cancer Inst.*, **52**, 1711–14

3. Hardell, L., Bengtsson, N. O. and Jonsson, U. (1984). Aetiological aspects on primary liver cancer with special regard to alcohol organic solvents and acute intermittent porphyria. An epidemiologic investigation. *Br. J. Cancer*, **50**, 389–97

4. Keller, A. Z. (1967). Cirrhosis of the liver, alcoholism and heavy smoking associated with cancer of the mouth and the pharynx. *Cancer*, **20**, 1015–22

5. Tamburro, C. H. and Lee, H. M. (1981). Primary hepatic cancer in alcoholics. *Clin. Gastroenterol.*, **10**, 457–77

6. Yu, M. C., Mack, T., Hanisch, R., Peters, R. L. and Henderson, B. E. (1983). Hepatitis, alcohol consumption, cigarette smoking, and hepatocellular carcinoma in Los Angeles. *Cancer Res.*, **43**, 6077–9

7. Lieber, C. S., Seitz, H. K., Garro, A. J. and Worner, T. M. (1979). Alcohol-related diseases and carcinogenesis. *Cancer Res.*, **39**, 2863–86

8. Ketcham, A. S., Wexler, H. and Mantel, N. (1963). Effects of alcohol in mouse neoplasia. *Cancer Res.*, **23**, 667–70

9. Seitz, H. K. and Simanowski, U. A. (1988). Alcohol and carcinogenesis. *Ann. Rev. Nutr.*, **8**, 99–119

10. Seitz, H. K. and Simanowski, U. A. (1987). Metabolic and nutritional effects of ethanol. In Hathcock, J. N. (ed.) *Nutritional Toxicology*, Volume II. pp. 63–103. (London: Academic Press)

11. Takada, A., Nei, J., Takase, S. and Matsuda, Y. (1986). Effects of ethanol on experimental hepatocarcinogenesis. *Hepatology*, **6**, 65–72

12. Driver, H. E. and McLean A. E. M. (1986). Dose–response relationship for initiation of rat liver tumors by diethylnitrosamine and promotion by phenobarbitone and alcohol. *Food Chem. Toxicol.*, **24**, 241–5

13. Porta, E. A., Markell, N. and Dorado, R. D. (1985). Chronic alcoholism enhances hepatocarcinogenesis of diethylnitrosamine in rats fed a marginally methyl-deficient diet. *Hepatology*, **5**, 1120–5

14. Teschke, R., Minzlaff, M., Oldiges, H. and Frenzel, H. (1983). Effect of chronic alcohol consumption on tumor incidence due to dimethylnitrosamine administration. *J. Cancer Res. Clin. Oncol.*, **106**, 58–64

15. Gibel, W. (1967). Experimentelle Untersuchungen zur Synkarzinogenese beim Ösophaguskarzinom. *Arch. Geschwulstforsch.*, **30**, 181–9

16. Griciute, L., Castegnaro, M. and Bereziat, J. C. (1981). Influence of ethyl alcohol on carcinogenesis with N-nitrosodiethylamine. *Cancer Lett.*, **13**, 345–52

17. Griciute, L., Castegnaro, M., Bereziat, J. C. and Cabral, J. R. P. (1986). Influence of ethyl alcohol on the carcinogenic activity of N-nitrosonornicotine. *Cancer Lett.*, **31**, 267–75

18. Habs, M. and Schmähl, D. (1981). Inhibition of the hepatocarcinogenic activity of diethylnitrosamine (DENA) by alcohol in rats. *Acta Gastroenterol.*, **28**, 242–4

19. Radike, M. J., Stemmer, K. L., Brown, P. B., Larson, E. and Bingham, E. (1977). Effect of ethanol and vinyl chloride on the induction of liver tumors. *Environ. Health Perspect.*, **21**, 153–5

20. Miller, M. L., Radike, M. J., Andringa, A. and Bingham, E. (1982). Mitochondrial changes in hepatocytes of rats chronically exposed to vinyl chloride and ethanol. *Environ. Res.*, **29**, 272–9

21. Mendenhall, C. L. and Chedid, L. A. (1980). Peliosis hepatis: its relationship to chronic alcoholism, aflatoxin B_1 and carcinogenesis in male Holtzman rats. *Dig. Dis. Sci.*, **25**, 587–92

22. Misslbeck, N. G., Campbell, T. C. and Roe, D. A. (1984). Effect of ethanol consumed in combination with high or low fat diets on the postinitiation phase of hepatocarcinogenesis in the rat. *J. Nutr.*, **114**, 2311–23

23. Bulatao-Jayme, J., Almero, E. M., Castro, C. A., Jardeleza, T. H. and Salamat, L. A. (1982) A case controlled dietary study of primary liver cancer risk from aflatoxin exposure. *Int. J. Epidemiol.*, **11**, 112–19

24. Lieber, C. S., Garro, A. J., Leo, M. A., Mak, K. M. and Worner, T. M. (1986). Alcohol and cancer. *Hepatology*, **6**, 1005–19

25. Ames, B. N., McCann, J. and Yamasaki, E. (1975). Methods for detecting carcinogens and

mutagens with the *Salmonella*/mammalian microsomes mutagenicity test. *Mut. Res.,* **31,** 347–64

26. Lieber, C. S. (1985). Ethanol metabolism and pathophysiology of alcoholic liver disease. In Seitz, H. K. and Kommerell, B. (eds) *Alcohol Related Diseases in Gastroenterology.* pp. 19–47. (Springer-Verlag: Berlin, Heidelberg, New York, Tokyo)

27. Seitz, H. K. (1985). Alcohol effects on drug–nutrient interactions. *Drug Nutr. Interactions,* **4,** 143–63

28. Koop, D. R., Morgan, E. T., Tarr, G. and Coon, M. (1982). Purification and characterization of a unique isoenzyme of cytochrome P-450 from liver microsomes of ethanol treated rabbits. *J. Biol. Chem.,* **57,** 8472–80

29. Elves, R. G., Ueng, T. H. and Alvares, A. P. (1984). Comparative effects of ethanol administration on hepatic monooxygenases in rats and mice. *Arch. Toxicol.,* **55,** 258–64

30. Yang, C. S., Koop, D. R., Wang, T. and Coon, M. J. (1985). Immunochemical studies on the metabolism of nitrosamines by ethanol-inducible cytochrome P-450. *Biochem. Biophys. Res. Commun.,* **128,** 1007–13

31. Ko, I. Y., Park, S. S., Song, B. J., Patten, C., Tan, Y., Hah, Y. C., Yang, C. S. and Gelboin, H. V. (1987). Monoclonal antibodies to ethanol-induced rat liver cytochrome P-450 that metabolizes aniline and nitrosamines. *Cancer Res.,* **47,** 3101–9

32. Seitz, H. K., Garro, A. J. and Lieber, C. S. (1978). Effect of chronic ethanol ingestion on intestinal metabolism and mutagenicity of benzo(a)pyrene. *Biochem. Biophys. Res. Commun.,* **85,** 1061–6

33. Seitz, H. K., Garro, A. J. and Lieber, C. S. (1981). Enhanced pulmonary and intestinal activation of procarcinogens and mutagens after chronic ethanol consumption in the rat. *Europ. J. Clin. Invest.,* **11,** 33–8

34. Seitz, H. K., Garro, A. J. and Lieber, C. S. (1981). Sex dependent effect of chronic ethanol consumption in rats on hepatic microsome mediated mutagenicity of benzo(a)pyrene. *Cancer Lett.,* **13,** 97–102

35. Seitz, H. K., Garro, A. J. and Lieber, C. S. (1983). Increased activation of procarcinogens by microsomes of various tissues induced by chronic ethanol ingestion. In Lieber, C. S. (ed.) *Biological Approach to Alcoholism: update 1980,* pp. 131–41 (Research Monograph No. 11, DHHS, Publ. No. (ADM) 83–1261)

36. Steele, C. M. and Ioannides, C. (1986). Differential effects of chronic alcohol administration to rats on the activation of aromatic amines to mutagens in the Ames test. *Carcinogenesis,* **7,** 825–9

37. Loury, D. J., Kado, N. Y. and Byard, J. L. (1985). Enhancement of hepatocellular genotoxicity of several mutagens from amino acid pyrolysates and broiled foods following ethanol pretreatment. *Food Chem. Toxicol.,* **23,** 661–7

38. Garro, A. J., Seitz, H. K. and Lieber, C. S. (1981). Enhancement of dimethylnitrosamine metabolism and activation to a mutagen following chronic ethanol consumption. *Cancer Res.,* **41,** 120–4

39. McCoy, G. D., Chen, C. H. B., Hecht, S. S. and McCoy, E. C. (1979). Enhanced metabolism of nitrosopyrrolidine in liver fractions isolated from chronic ethanol-consuming hamsters. *Cancer Res.,* **39,** 793–6

40. Neis, J. M., TeBrömmelstroet, B. W. J., VanGemert, P. J. L., Roelofs, H. M. J. and Henderson, P. T. (1985). Influence of ethanol induction on the metabolic activation of genotoxic agents by isolated rat hepatocytes. *Arch. Toxicol.,* **57,** 217–21

41. Smith, B. A. and Guttman, M. R. (1984). Differential effect of chronic consumption by the rat on microsomal oxidation of hepatocarcinogens and their activation to mutagens. *Biochem. Pharmacol.,* **33,** 2901–10

42. Toskulkao, C. and Glinsukon, T. (1986). Effect of ethanol on the *in vivo* covalent binding and *in vitro* metabolism of aflatoxin B_1 in rats. *Toxicol. Lett.,* **30,** 151–7

43. Toskulkao, C., Yoshida, T., Glinsukon, T. and Kuroiwa, Y. (1986). Potentiation of aflatoxin B_1-induced hepatotoxicity in male Wistar rats with ethanol pretreatment. *J. Toxicol. Sci.,* **11,** 41–51

44. Marinovich, M. and Lutz, W. K. (1985). Covalent binding of aflatoxin B_1 to liver DNA in rats pretreated with ethanol. *Experientia,* **41,** 1338–40

45. Spiegelhalder, B., Eisenbrand, G. and Preussmann, R. (1979). Contamination of beer with trace quantities of N-nitrosodimethylamine. *Food Cosmet. Toxicol.,* **17,** 29–31

46. Swann, P. F., Coe, A. M. and Mace, R. (1984). Ethanol and dimethylnitrosamine and diethylnitrosamine metabolism and disposition in the rat. *Carcinogenesis*, **5**, 1337–43
47. Peng, R., Yong Tu, Y. and Yang, C. S. (1982). The induction and competitive inhibition of a high affinity microsomal nitrosodimethylamine demethylase by ethanol. *Carcinogenesis*, **3**, 1457–61
48. Tomera, J. F., Skipper, P. L., Wishnok, J. S., Tannenbaum, S. R. and Brunengraber, H. (1984). Inhibition of N-nitrosodimethylamine metabolism by ethanol and other inhibitors in the isolated perfused rat liver. *Carcinogenesis*, **5**, 113–16
49. Kouros, M., Mönch, W. and Reiffer, F. J. (1983). The influence of various factors on the methylation of DNA by the esophageal carcinogen N-nitrosomethylbenzylamine. I. The importance of alcohol. *Carcinogenesis*, **4**, 1081–4
50. Glatt, H., DeBalle, L. and Oesch, F. (1981). Ethanol or acetone pretreatment of mice strongly enhanced the bacterial mutagenicity of dimethylnitrosamine in assays mediated by liver subcellular fractions, but not in host mediated assays. *Carcinogenesis*, **2**, 1057–61
51. Gabrial, G. N., Schrager, T. F. and Newberne, P. M. (1982). Zinc deficiency, alcohol, and retinoid: association with esophageal cancer in rats. *J. Natl. Cancer Inst.*, **68**, 785–9
52. McCoy, G. D., Hecht, S. S., Katayama, S. and Wynder, E. L. (1981). Differential effect of chronic ethanol consumption on the carcinogenicity of N-nitrosopyrrolidine and N-nitrosonornicotine in male Syrian golden hamsters. *Cancer Res.*, **41**, 2849–54
53. Castonguay, A., Rivenson, A., Trushin, N., Reinhardt, J. and Spathopoulos, S. (1984). Effect of chronic ethanol consumption on the metabolism and carcinogenicity of N-nitrosonornicotine in F344 rats. *Cancer Res.*, **44**, 2285–90
54. Obe, G. and Ristow, H. (1977). Acetaldehyde but not alcohol induces sister chromatid exchanges in Chinese hamster cells *in vitro*. *Mut. Res.*, **56**, 211–13
55. Obe, G. and Ristow, H. (1979). Mutagenic, cancerogenic and teratogenic effects of alcohol. *Mut. Res.*, **65**, 229–59
56. Kinsella, A. and Radman, M. (1978). Tumor promoter induces sister chromatid exchanges: relevance to mechanisms of carcinogenesis. *Proc. Natl. Acad. Sci. USA*, **75**, 6149–53
57. Garro, A. J., Espina, N., Farinati, F. and Salvagnini, M. (1986). The effect of chronic ethanol consumption on carcinogen metabolism and on O^6-methylguanine transferase-mediated repair of alkylated DNA. *Alcohol. Clin. Exp. Res.*, **10**, 73S–77S
58. Pegg, A. E. and Perry, W. (1981). Alkylation of nucleic acids and metabolism of small doses of dimethylnitrosamine in the rat. *Cancer Res.*, **41**, 3128–32
59. Pegg, A. E., Wiest, L. and Foote, R. S. (1983). Purification and properties of O^6-methylguanine-DNA transmethylase from rat liver. *J. Biol. Chem.*, **258**, 2327–33
60. Harris, A. L., Karran, P. and Lindahl, T. (1983) O^6-methylguanine-DNA methyltransferase of human lymphoid cells: structural and kinetic properties and absence in repair deficient cells. *Cancer Res.*, **43**, 3247–52
61. Kleihues, P., Doejer, G. and Keefer, L. K. (1979). Correlation of DNA methylation by methyl(acetoxymethyl)nitrosamine with organspecific carcinogenicity in rats. *Cancer Res.*, **39**, 5136–40
62. Lewis, J. G. and Swenberg, J. A. (1980). Differential repair of O^6-methylguanine in DNA of rat hepatocytes and nonparenchymal cells. *Nature*, **288**, 185–7
63. Newbold, R. F., Warren, W. and Medcalf, A. S. C. (1980). Mutagenicity of carcinogenic methylating agents is associated with a specific DNA modification. *Nature*, **283**, 596–9
64. Schwarz, M., Wiesbeck, G., Hummel, J. and Kunz, W. (1982). Effect of ethanol on dimethylnitrosamine activation and DNA synthesis in rat liver. *Carcinogenesis*, **3**, 1071–5
65. Belinsky, S. A., Bedell, M. A. and Swenberg, J. A. (1982). Effect of chronic ethanol diet on the replication, alkylation and repair of DNA from hepatocytes and nonparenchymal cells following dimethylnitrosamine administration. *Carcinogenesis*, **3**, 1293–7
66. Finkelstein, J. D., Cello, J. P. and Kyle, W. E. (1974). Ethanol-induced changes in methionine metabolism in rat livers. *Biochem. Biophys. Res. Commun.*, **61**, 525–31
67. Tuma, D. J., Barak, A. J. and Schafer, D. F. (1973). Possible interrelationship of ethanol metabolism and choline oxidation in the liver. *Can. J. Biochem.*, **51**, 117–20
68. Uthus, E. O., Skurdal, D. N. and Cornatzer, W. E. (1976). Effect of ethanol ingestion on choline phosphotransferase and phosphatidylethanolamine methyltransferase activities in liver microsomes. *Lipids*, **11**, 641–4
69. Rogers, A. E. and Newberne, P. M. (1980). Lipotrope deficiency in experimental

carcinogenesis. *Nutr. Cancer,* **2**, 104–12

70. Mikol, Y. B., Hoover, K. L. and Creasia, D. (1983). Hepatocarcinogenesis in rats fed methyl-deficient, amino acid defined diets. *Carcinogenesis,* **4**, 1619–29

71. Lieber, C.S., Leo, M. A. and Mak, K. M. (1985). Choline fails to prevent liver fibrosis in ethanol-fed baboons but causes toxicity. *Hepatology,* **5**, 561–72

72. Van der Westhuyzen, J. (1985). Methionine metabolism and cancer. *Nutr. Cancer,* **7**, 179–83

73. Riggs, A. D. and Jones, P. A. (1983). 5-methylcytosine, gene regulation and cancer. *Adv. Cancer Res.,* **40**, 1–30

74. Hoffman, R. M. (1984). Altered methionine metabolism, DNA methylation and oncogene expression in carcinogenesis. A review and synthesis. *Biochem. Biophys. Acta,* **738**, 49–87

75. Felsenfeld, G. and McGhee, J. (1982). Methylation and gene control. *Nature,* **296**, 602–3

76. Sato, M. and Lieber, C. S. (1981). Hepatic vitamin A depletion after chronic ethanol consumption in baboons and rats. *J. Nutr.,* **111**, 2015–23

77. Leo, M. A. and Lieber, C. S. (1982). Vitamin A depletion in alcoholic liver injury in man. *N. Engl. J. Med.,* **307**, 597–601

78. Wynder, E. L. (1976). Nutrition and cancer. *Fed. Proc.,* **35**, 1309–16

79. Lumeng, L. and Li, T. K. (1974). Vitamin B$_6$ metabolism in chronic alcohol abuse. *J. Clin. Invest.,* **53**, 693–704

80. Axelrod, A. E. and Trakatellis, A. C. (1964). Relationship of pyridoxine to immunologic phenomenon. *Vitamin Horm.,* **22**, 591–607

81. Chan, C. H. (1975). Primary carcinoma of the liver. *Med. Clin. North Am.,* **59**, 989–94

82. Mills, P. R., Rennington, T. H., Kay, P., MacSween, R. N. M. and Watkinson, G. (1979). Hepatitis B antibody in alcoholic cirrhosis. *J. Clin. Pathol.,* **32**, 778–82

83. Hislop, W. S., Follett, E. A. C., Bouchier, I. A. D. and MacSween, R. N. M. (1981). Serological markers of hepatitis B in patients with alcoholic liver disease: a multicentre survey. *J. Clin. Pathol.,* **34**, 1017–19

84. Orholm, M., Aldersvile, J., TageJensen, U., Schglichting, I., Nielsen, J., Hardt, F. and Christoffersen, P. (1981). Prevalence of hepatitis B virus infection among alcoholic patients with liver disease. *J. Clin. Pathol.,* **34**, 1378–80

85. Gluud, C., Aldersvile, J., Henriksen, J., Kryger, P. and Mathiesen, L. (1982). Hepatitis A and B virus antibodies in alcoholic steatosis and cirrhosis. *Clin. Pathol.,* **35**, 695–7

86. Chevilotte, G., Durbec, J. P., Gerolami, A., Berthezene, P., Bidart, J. M. and Camatte, R. (1983). Interaction between hepatitis B virus and alcohol consumption in liver cirrhosis. *Gastroenterology,* **85**, 141–5

87. Gluud, C., Gluud, B. and Aldersvile, J. (1984). Prevalence of hepatitis B virus infection in out-patient alcoholics. *Infection,* **12**, 72–4

88. Brechot, C., Nalpas, B., Courouce, A. M., Duhamel, G., Callard, P., Cornot, F., Tiollais, P. and Berthelot, P. (1982). Evidence that hepatitis B virus has a role in liver cell carcinoma in alcoholic liver disease. *N. Engl. J. Med.,* **306**, 1384–7

89. Shafritz, D. A., Shouval, D. and Sherman, H. I. (1981). Integration of hepatitis B virus DNA into the genome of liver cells in chronic liver disease and hepatocellular carcinoma. *N. Engl. J. Med.,* **305**, 1067–73

90. Ohnishi, K., Iida, S. and Iwama, S. (1982). The effect of chronic habitual alcohol intake on the development of liver cirrhosis and hepatocellular carcinoma: relation to hepatitis B surface antigen carriers. *Cancer,* **49**, 672–7

91. Omata, M., Ashcavai, M., Liew, C. and Peters, R. L. (1979). Hepatocellular carcinoma in the USA: etiologic considerations. *Gastroenterology,* **76**, 280–7

92. Goudeau, A., Maupas, P., Dubois, F., Coursaget, P. and Bougnoux, P. (1981). Hepatitis B infection in alcoholic liver disease and primary hepatocellular carcinoma in France. *Prog. Med. Virol.,* **27**, 26–34

93. Yarrish, R. L., Werner, B. G. and Blumberg, B. S. (1980). Association of hepatitis B virus infection with hepatocellular carcinoma in American patients. *Int. J. Cancer,* **26**, 711–15

94. Weisburger, J. H., Yamamoto, R. S. and Pai, S. R. (1964). Ethanol and the carcinogenicity of N-hydroxy-N-2-fluorenyl-acetamide in male and female rats. *Toxicol. Appl. Pharmacol.,* **6**, 363 (abstract)

21
Metabolism of chemical carcinogens

F. OESCH, L. SCHLADT, H. R. GLATT AND H. THOMAS

INTRODUCTION

Many natural as well as man-made foreign compounds, including pharmaceuticals, possess aromatic and olefinic structural elements. Although several of these compounds are chemically little reactive *per se*, they may exert carcinogenic effects after metabolic activation by microsomal monooxygenases present in many mammalian tissues. These enzymes catalyze the formation of electrophilic epoxides from the parent compound, which may spontaneously react with cellular nucleophiles, e.g. deoxyribonucleic acid, ribonucleic acid and protein. If these damages are not efficiently repaired the cellular homeostasis may be disturbed leading to cytotoxic, mutagenic and/or carcinogenic effects. The effects of a given compound depend on several properties, e.g. its chemical reactivity, geometry and lipophilicity. Furthermore, several enzymes are able to metabolize epoxides: for example, enzymatic conversion of epoxides by epoxide hydrolases leads to chemically unreactive *trans*-dihydrodiols[1-5]. At least three different forms of epoxide hydrolases with different substrate specificities are involved in epoxide metabolism: microsomal epoxide hydrolase, cholesterol epoxide hydrolase and cytosolic epoxide hydrolase[6]. Glutathione S-transferases open the epoxide ring by adding the elements of glutathione[2,3,5,7,8]. Epoxide reductases convert the derivative back to the mother compound[9,10]. Furthermore, non-enzymatic isomerizations of the epoxides can occur[2,3,5].

The role of epoxide hydrolases, dihydrodiol dehydrogenase and glutathione S-transferases in the control of reactive metabolites will now be discussed.

ROLE OF MICROSOMAL EPOXIDE HYDROLASE

As mentioned above, reactive epoxides can be derived from aromatic and olefinic precursor compounds by the action of microsomal monooxygenases. Different members of this enzyme superfamily differ substantially from each other with respect to preferential site of oxidative attack in substrate molecules thus generating various sets of reactive metabolites. Some of them may be detoxified by second-step enzymes, whilst other metabolites might be converted to even more reactive compounds by the same second or third step enzyme(s). The polycyclic hydrocarbon benzo(a)pyrene is metabolized by monooxygenases to the 7,8-oxide, which is hydrolyzed by microsomal epoxide hydrolase. The resulting benzo(a)-pyrene-7,8-diol can serve as a substrate for a second attack by monooxygenases producing benzo(a)pyrene-7,8-diol-9,10-oxide[1,2]. This metabolite is not detoxified by epoxide hydrolase and was shown to be an ultimate carcinogen[11-14]. Thus, a single enzyme can play multiple roles in activating some metabolites, but also producing precursors for reactive species from other metabolites[15]. The situation is complicated by the fact that inducers may shift the preferential site of attack of monooxygenases on a given compound. Microsomes from untreated or phenobarbitone-treated animals preferentially oxidize benzo(a)pyrene at the 4,5-position. The product is readily converted by microsomal epoxide hydrolase to mutagenically-inactive diol. However, microsomes of 3-methylcholanthrene-induced animals produce the 7,8-oxide at a much higher rate, which is the precursor for the above-mentioned ultimate carcinogen. Thus, treatment with inducers may also affect mutagenicity of a given compound[1,2,8].

Mutagenesis of chemicals is also species dependent. This was shown with benzo(a)pyrene as a mutagenic compound, with rat and mouse liver microsomes as sources of enzymes and using *Salmonella typhimurium* mutants. With mouse liver microsomes the observed mutagenic potency of benzo(a)pyrene was several-fold higher than with rat microsomes[16]. This may be due to differences in enzymatic activities in the two species: mouse liver monooxygenases exert about two-fold higher activity with benzo(a)-pyrene as substrate. This results in a higher amount of reactive epoxide metabolites. On the other hand activity of mouse liver epoxide hydrolase, measured with styrene oxide as substrate, is only one-seventh of rat liver microsomal epoxide hydrolase[16]. This explanation is supported by the fact that either induction of rat liver monooxygenases by 3-methylcholanthrene or inhibition of rat liver microsomal epoxide hydrolase by trichloropropene oxide increased mutagenicity of benzo(a)pyrene mediated by rat liver microsomes[16].

The role of microsomal epoxide hydrolase in benzo(a)pyrene mutagenesis was further investigated using *S. typhimurium* TA 98 and post-mitrochondrial supernatant of two different rat strains. When the same metabolic activation was performed with post-mitochondrial supernatant from Fischer rats, the mutation rate was considerably higher compared to Sprague–Dawley rats. The monooxygenase activity as well as the contributions of the various monooxygenase forms were similar for the two strains. Only microsomal epoxide hydrolase activity was markedly lower in Fischer rats, which should result in a higher accumulation of monofunctional epoxides, for the mutagenicity of which (especially the 4,5-oxide) this strain is very susceptible. This interpretation is supported by the fact that after treatment of animals with phenobarbitone the differences in mutagenicity disappeared. Phenobarbitone led to a similar induction of 'overall' monooxygenase activity in both strains, whereas microsomal epoxide hydrolase activity was increased more in the Fischer rats than in Sprague–Dawley rats, thus leading to the observed decrease in mutagenicity[17].

ROLE OF DIHYDRODIOL DEHYDROGENASE IN COMPARISON TO THAT OF CYTOSOLIC AND MICROSOMAL EPOXIDE HYDROLASES

In contrast to microsomal epoxide hydrolase only limited data exist about the role of its cytosolic counterpart in mutagenicity. Cytosolic epoxide hydrolase differs from microsomal epoxide hydrolase in molecular weight, several biochemical properties investigated, subcellular distribution and inducibility[6,18]. It was reported that the mutagenicity of allylbenzene oxide, styrene oxide and 4-chlorophenylglycidylether in *S. typhimurium* strain TA 100 was decreased by addition of cytosolic protein. Reduction of mutagenicity by the addition of cytosol from three species correlated with the cytosolic epoxide hydrolase activity observed in those species (mouse $>$ guinea pig $>$ rat)[19].

We have investigated the effect of purified cytosolic epoxide hydrolase on mutagenicity of benz(*a*)anthracene 5,6-oxide using *S. typhimurium* TA 100. Mutagenicity of this compound could be inactivated, but in comparison with purified microsomal epoxide hydrolase relatively large amounts of the cytosolic enzyme were required[20]. The metabolites of polycyclic hydrocarbons that seem to be responsible for most of the carcinogenic and mutagenic effects induced by these compounds are vicinal dihydrodiol epoxides[11,13,21–27]. Mutagenicity and DNA-binding experiments with *trans*-7,8-dihydro-7,8-dihydroxy-benzo(*a*)pyrene indicate that some inactivation is caused by the presence of glutathione[28–30] but not by microsomal epoxide hydrolase[15,30–32]. The latter may be a result of the short half-life of the investigated diol-epoxide in an aqueous environment. Therefore, we have studied the diol-epoxide of the above mentioned benz(*a*)anthracene. The non-bay-region diol-epoxide benz(*a*)anthracene-8,9-diol 10,11-oxide has a half-life of many hours, is mutagenic[33,34] and it is often the major DNA-binding metabolite derived from the parent compound *in vivo* and *in vitro*[26,27,35,36]. In contrast to the 5,6-oxide of benz(*a*)anthracene (see above) neither microsomal nor cytosolic epoxide hydrolase could inactivate the 8,9-diol 10,11-oxide of this compound[20].

However, mutagenicity of the diol-epoxide was decreased by dihydrodiol dehydrogenase whereas this enzyme had no effect on mutagenicity of benz(*a*)anthracene 5,6-oxide. Relatively high amounts of the enzyme, purified from rat liver cytosol, were needed for this inactivation[20]. Differences in isoenzyme pattern, dihydrodiol dehydrogenase activity among species, organs and physiological states may cause corresponding differences in susceptibility for mutagenic compounds.

ROLE OF GLUTATHIONE S-TRANSFERASES

Other enzymes, which play an important role in detoxification of mutagenic compounds are the glutathione S-transferases. Several glutathione S-transferases occur in rat liver cytosol. They differ in molecular weight, composition of subunits, isoelectric point and substrate specificity. With r-7, t-8-

dihydroxy-t-9, 10-oxy-7,8,9,10-tetrahydrobenzo(*a*)pyrene and benz(*a*)anthracene-8,9-diol 10,11-oxide enzyme catalyzed formation of glutathione conjugates were observed[35,36]. Furthermore, mutagenicity and DNA-binding experiments using *trans*-7,8-dihydro-7,8-dihydroxybenzo(*a*)pyrene and an activating system have shown that some inactivation occurs when glutathione was added[28,30,37].

We have tested the influence of purified glutathione S-transferases A, B, C, and X on the mutagenicity of the above-mentioned benz(*a*)anthracene 5,6-oxide and benz(*a*)anthracene-8,9-diol 10,11-oxide. In contrast to the epoxide hydrolases and the dihydrodiol dehydrogenase, the four tested glutathione S-transferases decreased mutagenicity of both benz(*a*)anthracene metabolites. The ability to inactivate mutagenicity of benz(*a*)anthracene 5,6-oxide decreased in the order glutathione S-transferase X > C > A > B. However, about 1000-fold higher concentrations of enzymes were required for inactivation of the diol-epoxide.

COMPARISON OF THE EFFECTIVENESS OF THE DISCUSSED ENZYMES IN THE CONTROL OF TWO PROTOTYPE EPOXIDES

In order to quantify the contribution of the various enzymes to the inactivation of the two benz(*a*)anthracene epoxides the amount of enzyme required for 50% reduction in mutagenicity was estimated (Table 1). When intrinsic enzyme activities and the relative amounts of enzymes present in the liver are considered and subcellular compartmentalization is disregarded, the glutathione S-transferase can play a more important role in the inactivation of the two epoxides than dihydrodiol dehydrogenase or the epoxide hydrolases. Amongst the glutathione S-transferases, large differences in efficiency of detoxification occur. In rat liver the forms C, because of its quantitative abundance, and X, because of its high efficiency in inactivating, appear to be able to contribute most to the inactivation of the two epoxides. It should be kept in mind that such an estimate is rather crude, when different types of enzymes are compared, because of differences in cofactor concentration, in pH optima and in other environmental factors which may lead to substantial differences between enzyme activities *in vivo* and *in vitro*.

Microsomal epoxide hydrolase was tested in the mutagenicity experiments as the free purified enzyme, whereas *in vivo* it is situated in the endoplasmic reticulum and in other membranes[38]. This may be of great advantage in comparison with cytosolic enzymes, since it increases the opportunities for reaction with epoxides, which are generated in these membranes and tend to stay there because of their relative lipophilicity[28]. Dihydrodiol dehydrogenase may inactivate diol-epoxides, but may also sequester precursor dihydrodiols, an effect that has not been taken into account in the experimental model used. In spite of these limitations, the data presented here on the more efficient *in vitro* inactivation of epoxides by glutathione S-transferases than by the other enzymes indicate that it is quite likely that glutathione S-transferases also play an important role in the *in vivo* inactivation of epoxides and that glutathione S-transferase X is especially important.

Table 1   Relative contribution of various purified enzymes to the inactivation of two prototype epoxides, compared with the relative amounts of these enzymes in the liver[a]

Enzyme	Enzyme concentration in liver[b] (μg/mg tissue)	Amounts of enzyme required for a 50% reduction in mutagenicity			
		Benzo(a)anthracene 5,6-oxide		Benz(a)anthracene-8,9-diol 10,11-oxide	
		(μg/incubation)	(mg liver equivalents)	(μg/incubation)	(mg liver equivalents)
Microsomal epoxide hydrolase	0.5	0.7	1.3	inactive (≥ 170)	≥300[c]
Cytosolic epoxide hydrolase	0.16	4	30	inactive (≥ 30)	≥200[c]
Glutathione transferase A	0.5	0.11	0.2	110	200
Glutathione transferase B	2.2	0.5	0.2	130	60
Glutathione transferase C	1.1	0.02	0.017	30	20
Glutathione transferase X	0.25	0.003	0.011	6	20
Dihydrodiol dehydrogenase	0.45	inactive (≥3)	≥1000[c]	70	170

[a]Data taken from refs 20 and 39
[b]Values refer to untreated adult males of the species from which the enzyme was purified
[c]Determinable only as an upper limit from the experiment

247

CONCLUSION

Most chemical carcinogens show *per se* a low chemical reactivity and need a further metabolic activation to the ultimate carcinogenic species. The enzyme pattern responsible for the generation and disposition of reactive metabolites constitutes an important contribution to the metabolic control of chemical carcinogenesis. Especially well studied is the group of enzymes reponsible for the control of reactive epoxides.

Epoxides can be derived from many natural and man-made compounds, which possess olefinic or aromatic double bonds by the action of microsomal monooxygenases. Enzymes controlling the concentration of such epoxides are an important factor contributing to the control of chemical carcinogens. Enzymes involved in biosynthesis and further metabolism of epoxides differ in quantity as well as in substrate specificity between organs, developmental stages, sexes and animal species. Differences in susceptibilities between species and individuals are often causally linked to these metabolic differences.

Acknowledgements

We thank Mrs. I. Böhm for typing the manuscript and the Deutsche Forschungsgemeinschaft (SFB 302) for financial support.

References

1. Guenthner, T. M. and Oesch, F. (1981). Microsomal epoxide hydrolase and its role in polycyclic aromatic hydrocarbons biotransformation. In Gelboin, H. and Ts'o, P. O. P. (eds) *Polycyclic Hydrocarbons and Cancer*, pp. 183–212 (New York: Academic Press)
2. Jerina, D. M. and Daly, J. W. (1974). Arene oxides: A new aspect of drug metabolism. *Science*, **185**, 573–82
3. Oesch, F. (1973). Mammalian epoxide hydrases. Inducible enzymes catalysing the inactivation of carcinogenic and cytotoxic metabolites derived from aromatic and olefinic compounds. *Xenobiotica*, **3**, 305–40
4. Oesch, F. (1979). Enzymes as regulator of toxic reactions by electrophilic metabolites. In Chambers, P. L. and Gunzel, P. (eds) *Mechanism of Toxic Action on Some Target Organs*, pp. 215–27 (Heidelberg: Springer-Verlag)
5. Sims, P. and Grover, P. L. (1974). Epoxides in polycyclic aromatic hydrocarbon metabolism and carcinogenesis. *Adv. Cancer Res.*, **20**, 165–274
6. Timms, C., Oesch, F., Schladt, L. and Wörner, W. (1984). Multiple forms of epoxide hydrolase. In Mitchell, J. F., Paton, W. and Turner, P. (eds) *Proceedings of the 9th International Congress of Pharmacology*, pp. 231–7 (London: Macmillan Press)
7. Arias, I. M. and Jakoby, W. B. (1976). *Proc. Foundation Series*, **6** (New York: Raven Press)
8. Oesch, F. (1980). Species differences in activating and inactivating enzymes related to *in vitro* mutagenicity mediated by tissue preparations. In Clemmesen, J., Conning, D. M., Henschler, D. and Oesch, F. (eds) *Quantitative Aspect of Risk Assessment in Chemical Carcinogenesis*. (Heidelberg: Springer-Verlag)
9. Booth, J., Hewer, A., Keysell, G. R. and Sims, P. (1975). Enzymic reduction of aromatic hydrocarbon epoxides by the microsomal fraction of rat liver. *Xenobiotica*, **5**, 197–203
10. Sugimura, M., Yamazoe, Y., Kamutaki, T. and Kato, R. (1980). Reduction of epoxy derivatives of benzo(*a*)pyrene by microsomal cytochrome P-450. *Cancer Res.*, **40**, 2910–14

11. Slaga, T. J., Viaja, A., Berry, D. L., Bracken, W. M., Buty, S. F. and Scribner, J. D. (1976). Skin-tumor initiating ability of benzo(a)pyrene 4,5-, 7,8- and 9,10-oxide, 7,8-diol-9,10-epoxides and 7,8-diol. *Cancer Lett.,* **2**, 115-22

12. Kapitulnik, J., Wislocki, P. G., Levin, W., Yagi, H., Thakker, D. R., Akagi, H., Koreeda, M., Jerina, D. M. and Conney, A. H. (1978). Marked differences in the carcinogenic activity of optically pure (+)- and (-)-*trans*-7,8-dihydrobenzo(a)pyrene in newborn mice. *Cancer Res.,* **38**, 2661-5

13. Levin, W., Wood, A. W., Wislocki, P. G., Chang, R. L., Kapitulnik, J., Mah, H. D., Yagi, H., Jerina, D. M. and Conney, A. H. (1978). Mutagenicity and carcinogenicity of benzo(a)-pyrene and benzo(a)pyrene derivatives. In Gelboin, H. V. and Ts'o, P. O. P. (eds) *Polycyclic Hydrocarbons and Cancer,* Vol. I, pp. 183-94 (New York: Academic Press)

14. Slaga, T. J., Bracken, W. J., Gleason, G., Levin, W., Yagi, H., Jerina, D. M. and Conney, A. H. (1979). Marked differences in the skin tumor-initiating activities of the optical enantiomers of the diastereomeric benzo(a)pyrene 7,8-diol-9,10-oxides. *Cancer Res.,* **39**, 67-71

15. Bentley, P., Oesch, F. and Glatt, H. R. (1977). Dual role of epoxide hydratase in both activation and inactivation. *Arch. Toxicol.,* **39**, 65-75

16. Oesch, F. and Glatt, H. R. (1976). Evaluation of the importance of enzymes involved in the control of mutagenic metabolites. In Montesano, R., Bartsch, H. and Tomatis, L. (eds) *Chemical Carcinogenesis,* pp. 255-95 (Lyon: IARC Scientific Publications)

17. Oesch, F., Raphael, D., Schwind, H. and Glatt, H. R. (1977). Species differences in activating and inactivating enzymes related to the control of mutagenic metabolites. *Arch. Toxicol.,* **39**, 97-108

18. Schladt, L., Hartmann, R., Timms, C., Strolin-Benedetti, Dostert, P. and Oesch, F. (1987). Concomitant induction of cytosolic but not microsomal epoxide hydrolase with peroxisomal ß-oxidation by various hypolipidemic compounds. *Biochem. Pharmacol.,* **36**, 345-51

19. El-Tantaway, M. A. and Hammock, B. D. (1980). The effect of hepatic microsomal and cytosolic subcellular fractions on the mutagenic activity of epoxide-containing compounds in the Salmonella assay. *Mutation Res.,* **79**, 59-71

20. Glatt, H. R., Cooper, C. S., Grover, P. L., Sims, P., Bentley, P., Merdes, M., Waechter, F., Vogel, K., Guenthner, T. M. and Oesch, F. (1982). Inactivation of a diol epoxide by dihydrodiol dehydrogenase but not by two epoxide hydrolases. *Science,* **215**, 1507-9

21. Sims, P., Grover, P. L., Swaisland, A., Pal, K. and Hewer, A. (1974). Metabolic activation of benzo(a)pyrene proceeds by a diol-epoxide. *Nature,* **252**, 226-8

22. Huberman, E., Sachs, L., Yang, S. K. and Gelboin, H. V. (1976). Identification of mutagenic metabolites of benzo(a)pyrene in mammalian cells. *Proc. Natl. Acad. Sci. USA,* **73**, 607-11

23. Newbold, R. F. and Brookes, P. (1976). Exceptional mutagenicity of benzo(a)pyrene diol epoxide in cultured mammalian cells. *Nature,* **261**, 52-4

24. Wislocki, P. G., Wood, A. W., Chang, R. L., Levin, W., Yagi, H., Hernandez, O., Jerina, D. M. and Conney, A. H. (1976). High mutagenicity and toxicity of a diol epoxide derived from benzo(a)pyrene. *Biochem. Biophys. Res. Commun.,* **68**, 1006-12

25. Hecht, S. S., LaVoie, E., Mazzorese, R., Amin, S., Bedenko, V. and Hoffman, D. (1978). 1,2-Dihydro-1,2-dihydroxy-5-methylchrysene a major activated metabolite of the environmental carcinogen 5-methylchrysene. *Cancer Res.,* **38**, 2191-8

26. Vigny, P., Kindts, M., Duguesne, M., Cooper, C. S., Grover, P. L. and Sims, P. (1980). Metabolic activation of benz(a)anthracene: fluorescence spectral evidence indicates the involvement of a non-'bay-region' diol epoxide. *Carcinogenesis,* **1**, 33-41

27. MacNicoll, A. D., Cooper, C. S., Ribeiro, O., Pal, K., Hewer, A., Grover, P. L. and Sims, P. (1981). The metabolic activation of benz(a)anthracene in three biological systems. *Cancer Lett.,* **11**, 243-9

28. Glatt, H. R. and Oesch, F. (1977). Inactivation of electrophilic metabolites by glutathione transferases and limitation of the system due to subcellular localization. *Arch. Toxicol.,* **39**, 87-96

29. Guenthner, T. M., Jernström, B. and Orrenius, S. (1980). On the effect of cellular nucleophiles on the binding of metabolites of 7,8-dihydroxy-7,8-dihydrobenzo(a)pyrene and 9-hydroxy-benzo(a)pyrene to nuclear DNA. *Carcinogenesis,* **1**, 407-18

30. Glatt, H. R., Billings, R., Platt, K. L. and Oesch, F. (1981). Improvement of the correlation of bacterial mutagenicity with carcinogenicity of benzo(a)pyrene and four of its major

metabolites by activation with intact liver cells instead of cell homogenate. *Cancer Res.,* **41**, 270–7

31. Glatt, H. R. (1976). Die Bedeutung verschiedener aktivierender und inaktivierender Stoffwechselschritte für die Mutagenität des Karzinogens Benzo(*a*)pyren. (Thesis: University of Basel)

32. Wood, A. W., Levin, W., Lu, A. Y. H., Yagi, H., Hernandez, O., Jerina, D. M. and Conney, A. H. (1976). Metabolism of benzo(*a*)pyrene derivatives to mutagenic products by highly purified hepatic microsomal enzymes. *J. Biol. Chem.,* **251**, 4882–90

33. Malaveille, C., Kuroki, T., Sims, P., Grover, P. L. and Bartsch, H. (1977). Mutagenicity of isomeric diol-epoxides of benzo(*a*)pyrene and benz(*a*)anthracene in *S. typhimurium* TA 98 and TA 100 and in V79 Chinese hamster cells. *Mutat. Res.,* **44**, 313–26

34. Wood, A. W., Chang, R. L., Levin, W., Lehr, R. E., Schaefer-Ridder, M., Karle, J. M., Jerina, D. M. and Conney, A. H. (1977). Mutagenicity and cytotoxicity of the bay region 1,2-epoxides. *Proc. Natl. Acad. Sci. USA,* **74**, 2746–50

35. Cooper, C. S., MacNicoll, A. D., Ribeiro, O., Gervasi, O. P., Hewer, A., Walsh, C., Pal, K., Grover, P. L. and Sims, P. (1980). The involvement of a non-'bay-region' diol epoxide in the metabolic activation of benz(*a*)anthracene in hamster embryo cells. *Cancer Lett.,* **9**, 49–53.

36. Cooper, C. S., Hewer, A., Ribeiro, O., Grover, P. L. and Sims, P. (1980). The enzyme-catalysed conversion of *anti*-benzo(*a*)pyrene-7,8-diol 9,10-oxide into a glutathione conjugate. *Carcinogenesis,* **1**, 1975–80

37. Hesse, S., Jernström, B., Marinez, M., Guenthner, T., Orrenius, S., Christodoulides, L. and Ketterer, B. (1980). Inhibition of binding of benzo(*a*)pyrene metabolites to nuclear DNA by glutathione and glutathione S-transferase B. *Biochem. Biophys. Res. Commun.,* **94**, 612–17

38. Stasiecki, P., Oesch, F., Bruder, G., Jorasch, E. D. and Franke, W. W. (1980). Distribution of enzymes involved in metabolism of polycyclic aromatic hydrocarbons among rat liver endomembranes and plasma membranes. *Eur. J. Cell Biol.,* **21**, 79–92

39. Glatt, H. R., Friedberg, T., Grover, P. L., Sims, P. and Oesch, F. (1983). Inactivation of a diol-epoxide and a K-region epoxide by glutathione S-transferases high efficiency of the new form X. *Cancer Res.,* **43**, 5713–17

22
Conjugation reactions in carcinogen metabolism and their permanent alterations after initiation of hepatocarcinogenesis

K. W. BOCK

Most carcinogens enter the body as biologically inactive compounds which are then metabolized to electrophilic, ultimate carcinogens[1]. The balance between phase-I (functionalization) and phase-II (conjugation) reactions determines the accumulation of these electrophiles in cells. The present review focuses on three selected topics: (a) Examples are given for the roles of conjugation in both detoxication and toxication of carcinogens. (b) Using the glucuronyltransferase enzyme family as an example the connection between conjugation of endo- and xenobiotics and co-regulation with other drug metabolizing enzymes is stressed. For more detailed information on other conjugation reactions the reader is referred to recent comprehensive reviews on glutathione conjugation[2,3], on sulphation[3–5] and on N-acetylation[6]. (c) After initiation of hepatocarcinogenesis, permanent alterations in the pattern of drug metabolizing enzymes, including conjugating enzymes, are found which are part of the toxin-resistance phenotype of initiated hepatocytes[7]. These alterations emphasize the multiple roles of activating and inactivating reactions in determining both genotoxicity and (non-genotoxic) cytotoxicity of carcinogens at cancer pre-stages.

ROLES OF CONJUGATING REACTIONS IN METABOLISM AND DISPOSITION OF CARCINOGENS

The roles of conjugation reactions (phase II) in carcinogen metabolism can be appreciated best in the context of overall metabolism and disposition of carcinogens in which a number of nucleophilic and electrophilic metabolites are generated in phase I (Figure 1). Reactive electrophilic metabolites of

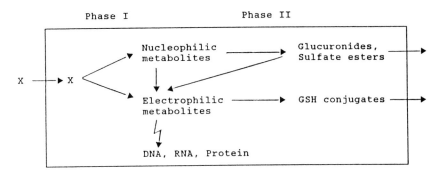

Figure 1 Scheme of cellular xenobiotic metabolism

carcinogens may interact with DNA and can therefore be considered as ultimate carcinogens[1]. They are controlled by glutathione transferases and, in the case of epoxides, by epoxide hydrolases. The more stable and more abundant nucleophilic metabolites are controlled by, for example, glucuronyl transferases, sulfotransferases and N-acetyltransferases. It is noteworthy that some nucleophiles such as phenols and quinols can be readily converted to electrophilic phenol radicals and semiquinones[8]. Therefore, the control of both nucleophiles and of electrophiles is important in detoxication. It is the balance between phase I and II reactions which largely determines the accumulation of toxic electrophiles in cells. Although this scheme generally holds true, there are some notable exceptions: (a) Carcinogens such as aromatic amines which contain functional groups are often conjugated without prior phase-I metabolism. (b) Many sulphate and glutathione conjugates are unstable and can be readily converted to reactive electrophiles. Examples are: N-hydroxy-2-acetylaminofluorene-O-sulphate[1], the sulphate ester of 7-hydroxymethylbenz(a)anthracene[9] and of N-nitroso-2-hydroxymorpholine, formed in the metabolism of N-nitroso-diethanolamine[10], S-2-bromoethyl-glutathione, formed in the metabolism of dibromoethane[11]. These unstable conjugates can be considered as proximal carcinogens. (c) In some instances conjugates are stable transport forms of carcinogens which are subsequently activated at the target site and thus determine the target of carcinogenicity; for example in 2-naphthylamine-induced bladder cancer[1] and in colon cancer induced by 3,2'-dimethyl-4-aminobiphenyl[12]. Moreover, glutathione conjugation is involved in the conversion of many halogenated alkanes and alkenes to nephrotoxic metabolites, for example in the metabolism of 1,2-dichloroethane[13,14]. Detailed studies on the metabolism and biliary excretion of the rat liver carcinogen, benzidine, indicate that a labile N-glucuronide of acetylbenzidine is a major metabolite in the first 3 h. Later, the glucuronide of N-hydroxybenzidine is formed which is highly mutagenic after ß-glucuronidase treatment. Moreover, the stable glucuronide of 3-hydroxy-N,N'-diacetylbenzidine is the major conjugate excreted in urine[15]. The benzidine study illustrates the complexity of the process converting lipid-soluble compounds into water-soluble and excretable metabolites.

252

ROLES OF MULTIPLE ISOZYMES AND THEIR DIFFERENTIAL INDUCTION USING RAT LIVER UDP-GLUCURONYLTRANSFERASE ISOZYMES AS EXAMPLES

Glucuronide formation represents a major and often the final excretory pathway of a variety of lipid-soluble xenobiotics and of endogenous compounds such as bilirubin and various steroids[16]. The firmly membrane-bound glucuronyltransferases (GTs) are found in the endoplasmic reticulum and the nuclear envelope. The enzyme transfers the glucuronic acid moiety from UDP-glucuronic acid to a large number of functional groups, such as aliphatic and phenolic hydroxyl groups, carboxylic acids, amines etc. The water-soluble glucuronides are actively secreted from cells, for example at the biliary canalicular membrane. They can be hydrolysed by ß-glucuronidases in the intestine and then undergo enterohepatic circulation.

GTs represent a family of isozymes (Table 1). In rat liver the inducible GT isozymes appear to be preferentially induced by four prototype inducers (3-methylcholanthrene (MC), phenobarbital, pregnenolone 16α-carbonitrile (PCN) and clofibrate) which also control gene expression of different P-450 isozyme families (P-450I, P-450II etc.[29]). Some GT isozymes such as GT-1 are widely distributed in tissues whereas others are more restricted in their distributions[16,31]. GT isozymes exhibit different but overlapping substrate specificity for endo- and xeno-biotics (Table 2). For example, the bladder carcinogen 4-aminobiphenyl is conjugated by 3α-hydroxysteroid GT or androsterone GT[32]. Similarly, 17ß-hydroxysteroid GT or testosterone GT

Table 1 Glucuronosyltransferase (GT) isozymes of rat liver

Isozyme	Substrate for identification	Inducer	M_r (ref.) (kDa)	cDNA (ref.)
Inducible enzymes[a]				
GT-1	PAH phenols and polyphenols	3-Methylcholanthrene	55[17–19]	+[20]
GT-2A	Morphine	Phenobarbital	56[17,21]	
GT-2B	4-Hydroxybiphenyl	Phenobarbital	?	+[22]
GT-3	Digitoxigenin monodigitoxoside	Pregnenolone 16α-carbonitrile	?[23]	
GT-4	Bilirubin	Clofibrate, phenobarbital	54[24,25]	
Steroids[b]				
17ß-OH-steroid GT	Testosterone	–	50[18]	+[26]
3α-OH-steroid GT	Androsterone	–	52[18]	+[27,28]
Aromatic steroid GT	Œstrone	–	?[18]	

[a]Inducible isozymes were numbered similar to the numbering system adopted for inducible P-450 isozyme families[29]. [b]In the case of constitutive steroid GTs, nomenclature is based on generally agreed substrates[30]

Table 2 Substrate specificity of glucuronyltransferase (GT) isozymes[a]

Isozyme	Substrate
GT-1	PAH phenols and polyphenols
	N-OH-2-naphthylamine
	4-Methylumbelliferone
	1-Naphthol
	4-Nitrophenol
	Serotonin
3α-OH-steroid GT	Androsterone
	Etiocholanolone
	Lithocholic acid
	4-Aminobiphenyl
17ß-OH-steroid GT	Testosterone
	Œstradiol (at C_{17})
	1-Naphthol
	4-Nitrophenol

[a]Taken from refs 17–19

efficiently conjugates many planar phenols such as 4-nitrophenol and 1-naphthol[18]. This isozyme is mainly responsible for conjugation of these phenols in untreated rat liver. However, in MC-treated rats phenol glucuronidation is mainly carried out by GT-1, an isozyme which is scarce in untreated liver. The latter isozyme efficiently conjugates planar phenolic and polyphenolic metabolites of PAHs such as 3-hydroxybenzo(a)pyrene and benzo(a)pyrene-3,6-quinol[19,33]. It is noteworthy that GT-1 appears to recognize the size and shape of PAHs[34]. For example, the planar PAH phenol 8-hydroxybenzo(a)pyrene is not a preferred substrate of GT-1. Benzo(a)pyrene-3,6-quinol glucuronidation proceeds in two sequential steps whereby the mono- and di-glucuronide is formed[33]. Monoglucuronide, and in particular diglucuronide, formation are markedly MC-inducible (10- and 40-fold, respectively). However, more work is needed to elucidate whether several MC-inducible GT forms are responsible for the widely different induction factors. Interestingly benzo(a)pyrene-3,6-quinol and other quinols are involved in toxic quinone/quinol redox cycles[8]. Quinols are formed from the corresponding quinones by several reductases, for example by P-450 reducase[35] and by NAD(P)H quinone reductase or DT diaphorase[36]. They are rapidly autoxidized with the generation of reactive oxygen species and semiquinones. The semiquinone step is bypassed by the quinone reductase which is MC-inducible. Hence the latter reaction and conjugation with glucuronic acid or glutathione may be considered as detoxication reactions. This is supported by mutagenicity studies of benzo(a)pyrene-3,6-quinone using the Ames test and tester strain TA 104. Addition of UDP-glucuronic acid or of glutathione to the Ames test markedly decreased mutagenicity of the quinone (B. S. Bock-Hennig and K. W. Bock, unpublished). It is noteworthy that glucuronidation of benzo(a)pyrene-7,8-dihydrodiol (an intermediate in the pathway leading to the bay-region diol epoxide) is only marginally induced by MC[31].

Genetic evidence using MC-inducible and non-inducible inbred strains of mice suggest that GT-1 and P-450I are controlled by a common receptor, the Ah receptor[37]. The pleiotropic response controlled by this Ah receptor may represent an adaptive programme which has evolved to efficiently detoxify PAHs.

Studies utilizing cDNA clones encoding GT-1 demonstrated that MC-treatment enhances the transcriptional rate of GT-1[20] *Cis*-acting drug regulatory elements of 10 base pairs have been identified upstream the 5' flanking region of the P-450I gene[38]. Therefore it would be interesting to investigate whether similar regulatory elements are responsible for transcriptional activation of GT-1.

PERMANENT ALTERATIONS OF CONJUGATING ENZYMES AFTER INITIATION OF HEPATOCARCINOGENESIS

The pattern of drug metabolizing enzymes, including conjugating enzymes, is permanently altered after initiation of hepatocarcinogenesis[7,39-41]. Permanently increased GT-1 activities and immunoreactive GT-1 protein have been demonstrated in liver foci after treatment with a variety of carcinogens[42-44]. Selective increases of GT-1 activities, including benzpyrene-3,6-quinol mono- and di-glucuronide formation, have also been detected in liver nodules and some differentiated hepatocellular carcinomas produced by feeding 2-acetyl-aminofluorene[45]. The molecular basis for increased GT-1 was studied in more detail by immunoblot analysis using two kinds of antibodies: (a) broad-spectrum antibodies to the GT-1 holoenzyme which recognize testosterone GT and androsterone GT in addition to GT-1; (b), more selective antibodies (provided by Thomas R. Tephly, Iowa), who used the electroeluted GT-1 polypeptide from polycrylamide gels as antigen to produce the antibody[19]. It was found that in normal liver both antibodies recognize similar MC-inducible polypeptides at M_r = 55000. However, a minor MC-inducible polypeptide at M_r = 53000 has also been recognized[45]. When GT-1 was analysed in several nodules and differentiated hepatocellular carcinomas produced by feeding a diet containing 2-acetylaminofluorene this minor GT-1 polypeptide at M_r = 53000 was preferentially increased in liver nodules[45]. In differentiated hepatocellular carcinomas either the M_r = 55000 or the M_r = 53000 polypeptide was preferentially stained. The M_r = 53000 polypeptide was also increased after short-term treatment with 2-acetylaminofluorene (0.02% in the diet for 1 week). It remains to be solved whether the M_r = 53000 polypeptide represents a second MC-inducible GT-isozyme or a post-transcriptional modification of a common GT-1 isozyme. Since GT-1 is a glycoprotein[20] post-transcriptional modifications are conceivable. Preliminary evidence suggests that in liver nodules produced by feeding N-nitrosomorpholine, the M_r = 55000 is increased, i.e. that formation of the M_r = 53000 polypeptide may be related to treatment with 2-acetylaminofluorene.

Permanently increased GT-1 activities in liver nodules have to be distinguished from adaptive increases of this isozyme after treatment with inducers. GT activity in liver foci can be further enhanced by treatment with inducers[46].

This additional increase of enzyme activity is reversible. It is important to investigate the mechanisms responsible for the permanent alterations of enzymes in liver foci and nodules. In the case of the MC-inducible quinone reductase its gene has been found to be hypomethylated in liver nodules[47]. It may be interesting to study whether a similar mechanism is underlying the permanent increase of GT-1.

The permanent alterations in the pattern of drug metabolizing enzymes may have functional implications. As shown in Table 3, enzymes which often lead to toxication of chemicals have been found to be permanently decreased in nodules whereas those enzymes and transport proteins are increased which often lead to detoxification. This altered pattern is consistent with the toxin-resistance phenotype of initiated hepatocytes[7]. When the liver is exposed to complete carcinogens their cytotoxicity preferentially damages normal hepatocytes. The mito-inhibitory and necrogenic action of carcinogens on normal liver cells may therefore stimulate regenerative growth of initiated hepatocytes, as observed in the Solt–Farber model[50]. Selective growth of rare, initiated hepatocytes favours the probability that these hepatocytes may be hit a second or third time[7,51]. This phenomenon may provide a hint as to how, by successive selection mechanisms, the cell may eventually acquire the properties of autonomous, invasive and metastasizing growth.

The balance between phase I and II enzymes critically determines the accumulation of genotoxic and of cytotoxic (non-genotoxic), electrophilic metabolites and may thus influence initiation and promotion of hepatocarcinogenesis in many ways. At the stage of initiation the cytotoxic and necrogenic action of carcinogens stimulates regenerative growth of hepatocytes and renders them more susceptible to the genotoxic action of carcinogens. At the

Table 3 Permanent alterations of proteins involved in drug metabolism and disposition in rat liver nodules[a]

Altered enzyme (protein)	Relative nodular activity
Phase I	
Cytochrome P-450	*0.02*
Aryl hydrocarbon hydroxylase	*0.5–0.3*[b]
NAD(P)H quinone reductase (cytosol)	13
Aldehyde dehydrogenase (cytosol)	40
Epoxide hydrolase (microsomal)	5
Phase II	
Sulphotransferase	*0.06*
Glucuronyltransferase (GT-1)	5–10[b]
GSH transferase	5
GSH transferase P	34
Others	
γ-Glutamyltranspeptidase	100–170[b]
Glycoprotein P (mdr gene product)	Increases[c]

[a–c]Data taken from refs 48, 39 and 49, respectively. Decreased relative activity is indicated by italicized numbers.

stage of promotion cytotoxicity may stimulate selective growth of toxin-resistant hepatocytes.

CONCLUSIONS

1. Conjugation reactions represent key steps in the conversion of lipid-soluble compounds into water-soluble and excretable metabolites. However, besides its role in detoxication, conjugation may also lead to activation of carcinogens. Moreover, conjugation often determines the target of toxicity.
2. Conjugating enzymes exist as enzyme families, exemplified by the glucuronyltransferase family. They consist of isozymes with different but overlapping substrate specificity for endo- and xeno-biotics and with differential inducibility by xeno-biotics. Some conjugating enzymes appear to be co-regulated with phase-I drug metabolizing enzymes as part of adaptive programmes.
3. After initiation of hepatocarcinogenesis drug metabolizing enzymes, including conjugating enzymes, are permanently altered. These alterations contribute to the toxin-resistance phenotype of initiated hepatocytes.

Acknowledgements

The author wishes to thank the Deutsche Forschungsgemeinschaft for financial support.

References

1. Miller, E. C. and Miller, J. A. (1981). Searches for ultimate carcinogens and their reactions with cellular macromolecules. *Cancer*, **47**, 2327–45
2. Mannervik, B. (1985). The isoenzymes of glutathione transferase. *Adv. Enzymol.*, **57**, 357–417
3. Armstrong, R. N. (1987). Enzyme-catalyzed detoxication reactions: Mechanism and stereochemistry. *CRC Crit. Rev. Biochem.*, **22**, 39–88
4. Jacoby, W. B., Sekura, R. D., Lyon, E. S., Marcus, C. J. and Wang, J. L. (1980). In Jacoby, W. B. (ed.) *Enzymatic Basis of Detoxication*, **2**, pp. 199–228. (New York: Academic Press)
5. Mulder, G. J. (1981). In Mulder, G. J. (ed.) *Sulfation of Drugs and Related Compounds* (Boca Raton, Florida: CRC Press)
6. Weber, W. W. and Hein, D. W. (1985). N-acetylation pharmacokinetics. *Pharmacol Rev.*, **37**, 25–79
7. Farber, E., (1984). Cellular biochemistry of the stepwise development of cancer with chemicals. *Cancer Res.*, **44**, 5463–74
8. Lorentzen, R. J. and Ts'o, P. O. P. (1977). Benzo(a)pyrenedione/benzo(a)pyrenediol oxidation–reduction couples and the generation of reactive reduced molecular oxygen. *Biochemistry*, **16**, 1467–73
9. Watabe, T., Hakamata, Y., Hiratsuka, A. and Ogura, K. (1986). A 7-hydroxymethyl sulphate ester as an active metabolite of the carcinogen, 7-hydroxymethylbenz(a)anthracene. *Carcinogenesis*, **7**, 207–14
10. Denkel, E., Sterzel, W. and Eisenbrand, G. (1986). *In vivo* activation of N-nitrosodiethanolamine and other N-nitroso-2-hydroxyalkylamines by alcohol dehydrogenase and sulfotransferase. In Bartsch, H., O'Neil, I. and Schulte-Hermann, R. (eds) *Relevance of*

N-nitroso Compounds to Human Cancer: Exposure and Mechanisms. IARC Scientific Publications No. 84, pp. 83–86 (New York: Oxford University Press)

11. Van Bladeren, P. J., Breimer, D. D., Rotteveel-Smijs, G. M. T., De Jong, R. A. W., Buijs, W., Van Der Gen, A. and Mohn, G. R. (1980). The role of glutathione conjugation in the mutagenicity of 1,2-dibromoethane. *Biochem. Pharmacol.,* **29**, 2975–82

12. Weisburger, J. H. (1971). Colon carcinogens: Their metabolism and mode of action. *Cancer,* **28**, 60–70

13. Anders, M. W., Lash, L. H. and Elfarra, A. A. (1986). Nephrotoxic amino acid and glutathione S-conjugates: Formation and renal activation. In Koscis, J. J., Jollow, D. J., Witmer, C. M., Nelson, J. O. and Snyder, R. (eds) *Biological Reactive Intermediates III.* pp. 443–55. (New York: Plenum Press)

14. Dekant, W., Metzler, M. and Henschler, D. (1986). Identification of S-1,2-dichlorovinyl-N-acetyl-cysteine as a urinary metabolite of trichloroethylene: A possible explanation for its nephrocarcinogenicity in male rats. *Biochem. Pharmacol.,* **35**, 2455–8

15. Lynn, R. K., Garvie-Gould, C. T., Milam, D. F., Scott, K. F., Eastman, C. L., Ilias, A. M. and Rodgers, R. M. (1984). Disposition of the aromatic amine, benzidine, in the rat: Characterization of mutagenic urinary and biliary metabolites. *Toxicol. Appl. Pharmacol.,* **72**, 1–14

16. Dutton, G. J. (1980). *Glucuronidation of Drugs and Other Compounds.* (Boca Raton, Florida: CRC Press)

17. Bock, K. W., Josting, D., Lilienblum, W. and Pfeil, H. (1979). Purification of rat liver glucuronyltransferase. Separation of two enzyme forms inducible by 3-methylcholanthrene or phenobarbital. *Eur. J. Biochem.,* **98**, 19–26

18. Falany, C. N. and Tephly, T. R. (1983). Separation, purification and characterization of three isozymes of UDP-glucuronyltransferase from rat liver microsomes. *Arch. Biochem. Biophys.,* **227**, 248–58

19. Bock, K. W., Schirmer, G., Green, M. D. and Tephly, T. R. (1988). Properties of a 3-methylcholanthrene-inducible phenol UDP-glucuronosyltransferase from rat liver. *Biochem. Pharmacol.,* **37**, 1439–43

20. Iyanagi, T., Haniu, M., Sogawa, K., Fujii-Kuriyama, Y., Watanabe, S., Shively, J. E. and Anan, K. F. (1986). Cloning and characterization of cDNA encoding 3-methylcholanthrene inducible rat mRNA for UDP-glucuronyltransferase. *J. Biol. Chem.,* **261**, 15607–14

21. Buik, J. F. and Tephly, T. R. (1986). Isolation and purification of rat liver morphine UDP-glucuronosyltransferase. *Mol. Pharmacol.,* **30**, 558–65

22. Mackenzie, P. I. (1987). Rat liver UDP-glucuronyltransferase. Identification of cDNAs encoding two enzymes which glucuronidate testosterone, dihydrotestosterone, and ß-estradiol. *J. Biol. Chem.,* **262**, 9744–9

23. Meyerinck von, L., Coffmann, B. L., Green, M. D., Kirkpatrick, R. B., Schmoldt, A. and Tephly, T. R. (1985). Separation, purification, and characterization of digitoxigenin-monodigitoxoside UDP-glucuronosyltransferase activity. *Drug Metab. Dispos.,* **13**, 700–4

24. Roy Chowdhury, J., Roy Chowdhury, N., Falany, C. N., Tephly, T. R. and Arias, T. M. (1986). Isolation and characterization of multiple forms of rat liver UDP-glucuronate glucuronosyltransferase. *Biochem. J.,* **233**, 827–37

25. Scragg, I., Celier, C. and Burchell, B. (1985). Congenital jaundice in rats due to the absence of hepatic bilirubin UDP-glucuronyltransferase enzyme protein. *FEBS Lett.* **183**, 37–42

26. Harding, D., Wilson, S. M., Jackson, M. R., Burchell, B., Green, M. D. and Tephly, T. R. (1987). Nucleotide and deduced amino acid sequence of rat liver 17ß-hydroxysteroid UDP-glucuronyltransferase. *Nucl. Acids Res.,* **15**, 3936

27. Jackson, M. R. and Burchell, B. (1986). The full length coding sequence of rat liver androsterone UDP-glucuronyltransferase cDNA and comparison with other members of this gene family. *Nucl. Acids Res.,* **14**, 779–95

28. Mackenzie, P. I. (1986). Rat liver UDP-glucuronosyltransferase. Sequence and expression of a cDNA encoding a phenobarbital-inducible form. *J. Biol. Chem.,* **261**, 14112–17

29. Nebert, D. W. and Gonzalez, F. Y. (1987). P450 Genes: structure, evolution and regulation. *Annu. Rev. Biochem.,* **56**, 945–93

30. Bock, K. W., Burchell, B., Dutton, G., Hänninen, O., Mulder, G. J., Owens, I. S., Siest, G. and Tephly, T. R. (1983). UDP-glucuronosyltransferase: Guidelines for consistent interim terminology and assay conditions. *Biochem. Pharmacol.,* **32**, 953–5

31. Bock, K. W., von Clausbruch, U. C., Kaufmann, R., Lilienblum, W., Oesch, F., Pfeil, H. and Platt, K. L. (1980). Functional heterogeneity of UDP-glucuronyltransferase in rat tissues. *Biochem. Pharmacol.,* **29**, 495–500
32. Green, M. D. and Tephly, T. R. (1987). N-glucuronidation of carcinogenic aromatic amines catalyzed by rat hepatic microsomal preparations and purified rat liver uridine 5′-diphosphate-glucuronosyltransferases. *Cancer Res.,* **47**, 2028–31
33. Lilienblum, W., Bock-Hennig, B. S. and Bock, K. W. (1985). Protection against toxic redox-cycles between benzo(a)pyrene-3,6-quinone and its quinol by 3-methylcholanthrene-inducible formation of the quinol mono- and diglucuronide. *Mol. Pharmacol.,* **27**, 451–8
34. Lilienblum, W., Platt, K. L., Schirmer, G., Oesch, F. and Bock, K. W. (1987). Regioselectivity of rat liver microsomal UDP-glucuronosyltransferase activities toward phenols of benzo(a)pyrene and dibenz(a,h)anthracene. *Mol. Pharmacol.,* **32**, 173–7
35. Bock, K. W., Lilienblum, W. and Pfeil, H. (1980). Conversion of benzo(a)pyrene-3,6-quinone to quinol glucuronides with rat liver microsomes or purified NADPH-cytochrome *c* reductase and UDP-glucuronosyltransferase. *FEBS Lett.,* **121**, 269–72
36. Lind, C., Hochstein, P. and Ernster, L. (1982). DT-diaphorase as a quinone reductase: A cellular control device against semiquinone and superoxide radical formation. *Arch. Biochem. Biophys.,* **216**, 178–85
37. Owens, I. S. (1977). Genetic regulation of UDP-glucuronosyltransferase induction by polycyclic aromatic compounds in mice. *J. Biol. Chem.,* **252**, 2827–33
38. Sogawa, K., Fujiisawa-Sehara, A., Yamane, M. and Fujii-Kuriyama, Y. (1986). Location of regulatory elements responsible for drug induction in the rat cytochrome P-450*c* gene. *Proc. Natl. Acad. Sci. USA,* **83**, 8044–8
39. Bock, K. W., Lilienblum, W., Pfeil, H. and Eriksson, L. C. (1982). Increased UDP-glucuronyltransferase activity in preneoplastic liver nodules and Morris hepatomas. *Cancer Res.,* **42**, 3747–52
40. Aström, A., DePierre, J. W. and Eriksson, L. C. (1983). Characterization of drug-metabolizing systems in hyperplastic nodules from the livers of rats receiving 2-acetylaminofluorene in their diet. *Carcinogenesis,* **4**, 577–81
41. Yin, Z., Sato, K., Tsuda, H. and Ito, N. (1982). Changes in activities of uridine diphosphate-glucuronyl-transferase during chemical hepatocarcinogenesis. *Gann,* **73**, 239–48
42. Fischer, G., Ullrich, D., Katz, N., Bock, K. W. and Schauer, A. (1983). Immunohistochemical and biochemical detection of uridine-diphosphate-glucuronyltransferase (UDP-GT) activity in putative preneoplastic liver foci. *Virchows Arch.,* **42**, 193–200
43. Fischer, G., Schauer, A., Bock, K. W., Ullrich, D. and Katz, N. R. (1983). Immunohistochemical demonstration of increased UDP-glucuronyltransferase in putative preneoplastic foci. *Naturwissenschaften,* **70**, 153–4
44. Fischer, G., Ullrich, D. and Bock, K. W. (1985). Effects of N-nitrosomorpholine and phenobarbital on UDP-glucuronyltransferase in putative preneoplastic foci of rat liver. *Carcinogenesis,* **6**, 605–9
45. Bock, K. W., Schirmer, G. and Eriksson, L. C. (1988). UDP-glucuronosyltransferase: Adaptive responses and permanent alterations in preneoplastic liver. In Miners, J. O. *et al.* (eds) *Microsomes and Drug Oxidations: 7th International Symposium in Adelaide 1987.* (London: Taylor and Francis), pp. 287–94
46. Bock, K. W., Lilienblum, W., Ullrich, D. and Fischer, G. (1984). Differential induction of UDP-glucuronosyltransferases and their 'permanent induction' in preneoplastic rat liver. *Biochem. Soc. Transact.,* **12**, 55–9
47. Williams, J. B., Lu, A. Y. H., Cameron, R. G. and Pickett, C. B. (1986). Rat liver NAD(P)H: quinone reductase. *J. Biol. Chem.,* **261**, 5524–8
48. Eriksson, L. C., Blanck, A., Bock, K. W. and Mannervik, A. (1987). Metabolism of xenobiotics in hepatocyte nodules. *Toxicol. Pathol.,* **15**, 27–42
49. Thorgeirsson, S. S., Huber, B. E., Sorrell, S., Fojo, A., Pastan, I. and Gottesman, M. M. (1987). Expression of the multidrug-resistant gene in hepatocarcinogenesis and regenerating rat liver. *Science,* **236**, 1120–2
50. Solt, D. and Farber, E. (1976). New principle for the analysis of chemical carcinogenesis. *Nature,* **263**, 701–3
51. Scherer, E. (1984). Neoplastic progression in experimental hepatocarcinogenesis. *Biochim. Biophys. Acta,* **738**, 219–36

23
The role of DNA damage, repair and replication in hepatocarcinogenesis

J. A. SWENBERG

The relationships between hepatocarcinogenesis and the chemical induction of DNA adducts, their potential to cause base-mispairing during DNA synthesis and their persistence in genomic DNA has been the focus of many investigations. Of particular interest to researchers conducting high-dose carcinogenicity bioassays is the quantitative relationship between the doses employed in bioassays and environmental exposures that are several orders of magnitude lower. It is well known that enzymatic processes involved in metabolic activation, detoxification, and DNA repair can exhibit saturable kinetics, so that non-linearities in dose-response can occur[1]. Such non-linearities can either increase or decrease the effect per unit dose of the carcinogen. It will only be possible to make accurate predictions of effects of low exposure when the dose-response relationships of the critical events involved in carcinogenesis are understood. Conversely, one can only determine which events play a critical role in hepatocarcinogenesis by examining the relationship between these events and the dose–response for tumour induction. By employing similar exposure regimens in mechanistic and carcinogenesis studies over wide dose ranges, it should be possible to determine which factors are quantitatively related to the induction of liver cancer.

While it is not practical to conduct carcinogenesis bioassays at low doses because of their lack of sensitivity, by understanding the relationship between these critical factors and carcinogenesis, it should be possible to incorporate such data obtained at low doses into the process of high- to low-dose extrapolation and thereby improve accuracy. This chapter will review the relationship between carcinogen exposure and DNA adduct formation and repair. Data on the molecular dose of a DNA adduct that is associated with a given exposure regimen should provide a method for integrating non-linearities in absorption, distribution, metabolic activation, detoxication, and DNA repair (Figure 1). Target-site molecular dosimetry should provide a more predictive index for extrapolation of carcinogenic risk than measures of external exposure.

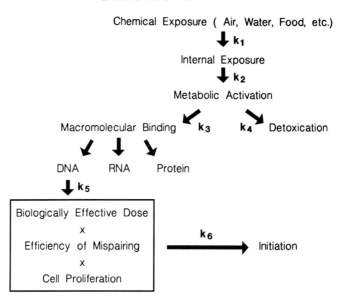

Figure 1 Schematic of events involved in determining the dose–response relationship for DNA adducts and initiations in hepatocarcinogenesis. The amount absorbed (k_1), distributed to the liver (k_2), metabolized to an electrophile (k_3) and detoxified (k_4) determine the formation of DNA adducts. The number of DNA adducts may be reduced prior to scheduled DNA synthesis by DNA repair and cell death (k_5). Those adducts that persist to the time of DNA synthesis constitute the biologically effective dose and each has its own efficiency for causing a base-pair mismatch that results in a mutation. When such mutations occur at critical sites in the genome (k_6), initiation occurs

A large body of evidence suggests that mutations caused by DNA replication over promutagenic DNA adducts represent a critical factor involved in the chemical induction of cancer. The efficiency of a given DNA adduct to cause base-mispairing during DNA replication differs greatly. *In vitro* studies, using purified DNA polymerases, demonstrate mispairing efficiencies for specific DNA adducts ranging from inserting a wrong nucleotide as often as 50% of the time, to doing so less than once in a million replications. It is therefore obvious that the efficiency for causing base-pair mismatch must be factored into the weighting of DNA adduct molecular dosimetry data. Many carcinogens produce multiple types of DNA adducts. Both the quantity and the potential for causing mutations should be considered when evaluating the role of DNA adducts in carcinogenesis.

DOSE – RESPONSE RELATIONSHIPS FOR DNA ADDUCTS

The shape of a dose–response curve for DNA adducts can be linear or non-linear, with the latter being either supra-linear or sub-linear. A supra-linear dose–response curve is characterized by having a greater effect per unit dose

THE ROLE OF DNA DAMAGE

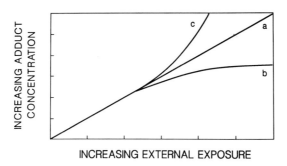

Figure 2 Relationship for DNA adduct concentration for simple linear (a), supra-linear (b) and sub-linear (c) dose–responses

at low versus high exposure (Figure 2, curve b). Supra-linear curves are frequently associated with saturation of metabolic activation. One of the best known examples of supra-linear dose–responses for liver tumour incidence is the induction of vinyl chloride angiosarcomas[2]. Proportionately smaller increases in tumour incidence occur at exposures above 200 ppm. No data on the dose–response relationship for vinyl chloride DNA adducts have been reported. Appleton *et al.*[3] demonstrated that covalent binding of single doses of aflatoxin B_1 to DNA was also supra-linear, whereas binding to protein and RNA was linear. The authors suggested that this might be due to saturation of the nuclear mixed-function oxidase system. Such saturation is however confined to relatively high doses of aflatoxin B_1. It should be emphasized that

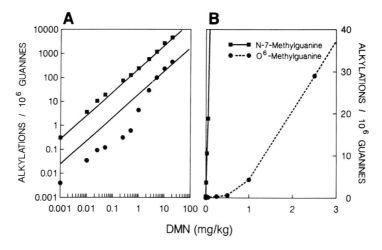

Figure 3 Effect of DNA repair on the dose response curve (A, log–log; B, linear) for a single dose of DMN. O^6-Methylguanine (●) increases at a greater rate per unit dose at doses above 0.5 mg/kg, while N-[7]methylguanine (■) is proportional to dose over more than four orders of magnitude. The solid line for O^6-methylguanine represents the theoretical amount forward. Data from Pegg and Hui[7]

in the case of simple saturation of activation, exposures below saturation will have linear, first-order kinetics.

Carcinogens that do not saturate any of the biotransformation or DNA repair pathways should also exhibit a linear relationship for DNA adducts versus external exposure (Figure 2, curve a). Neumann[4] has demonstrated a linear dose–response for *trans*-diaminostilbene DNA adducts in liver from rats exposed to single doses ranging from 5×10^{-10} to 1.8×10^{-4} moles/kg. Similar data have been reported by Dunn[5] for acid hydrolysable DNA adducts of benzo(a)pyrene from 10^{-7} to 10^{-3} g/mouse. This differed from the data of Adriaenssens *et al.*[6], who demonstrated a sub-linear dose–response for benzo(a)pyrene. The major non-linearity occurred at doses of benzo(a)pyrene that were higher than those employed by Dunn[5]. Non-linearities, such as reported by Adriaenssens *et al.*[6], result from saturation of detoxification or DNA repair, so that at high exposures a greater amount of DNA adducts is formed per unit dose (Figure 2, curve c). Pegg and Hui[7] demonstrated such an effect in rats treated with 0.001 to 20 mg/kg DMN (Figure 3). This non-linearity was due to saturation of the specific DNA repair protein for O^6-methylguanine, O^6-methylguanine DNA-methyltransferase (O^6-MT). N^7-Methylguanine was linear with respect to the administered dose of DMN, while O^6-methylguanine had a sharp increase in slope at doses of 0.5 mg/kg or higher. This is shown in log–log (Figure 3A) and linear (Figure 3B) plots.

More complex dose–response curves can also be envisioned, but clear examples have not been reported. Saturation of activation, detoxification, and DNA repair could all occur at different doses, leading to dose–response curves with several non-linearities.

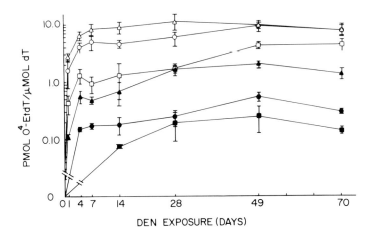

Figure 4 Accumulation of O^4-EtdT during continuous exposure of rats to 0.4 (■), 1 (●) (▲), 10 (□) 40 (○) or 100 (△) ppm DEN. Adduct concentrations are expressed versus time of exposure 1, 4, 7, 14, 28, 49 or 70 days. Note the log-scale of the y-axis. Bars, mean ± S.E. for three to four animals. The O^4-EtdT concentrations were below the limit of detection of the radio-immunoassay (<0.2 pmole O^4-EtdT μmole dT) for exposure of 0.4 ppm DEN, for 1, 4, and 7 days and 1 ppm DEN for 1 day. From Boucheron[9]

All of the above examples have been for single-dose studies. The same principles hold true for multiple-dose studies; however, these are also complicated by potential induction of biotransformation and DNA repair pathways, by dilution from cell proliferation and by loss from cell death. The latter two are frequent complications of high exposure[8]. Only two molecular dosimetry studies of liver DNA adducts have been reported following multiple exposure. Boucheron et al.[9] exposed rats via their drinking water to six concentrations of diethylnitrosamine (DEN) ranging from 0.4 to 100 ppm for 1–70 days. A linear dose–response was present for the major DNA adduct, O^4-ethyldeoxythymidine (O^4-EtdT) for 0.4–40 ppm at 49 and 70 days of DEN exposure (Figure 4). A less than linear concentration of O^4-EtdT was present in rats exposed to 100 ppm DEN that was due to increased cell loss and dilution associated with cytotoxicity[10]. At earlier exposure times (2–7 days), the response was sub-linear, suggesting possible saturation of DNA repair at higher exposures[9]. O^4-EtdT concentrations in the two higher exposure groups reached 54–74% of their steady-state concentration by 7 days, whereas the adducts only attained ca. 25% of their steady-rate concentration from 1 to 10 ppm DEN. Proportionately less O^4-EtdT was present in livers of rats exposed to the lowest concentration of DEN (0.4 ppm). More sensitive methods will be needed to conduct molecular dosimetry studies on O^4-EtdT at even lower concentrations to fully characterize the shape of the chronic dose–response for this DNA adduct of DEN. Such studies have a high priority because the data will be comparable with carcinogenesis bioassay data that also show non-linearity at low exposures[11,12].

The second molecular dosimetry study was conducted by Beland et al.[13] using 2-acetylaminofluorene (2-AAF) exposed mice. This study utilized 30-

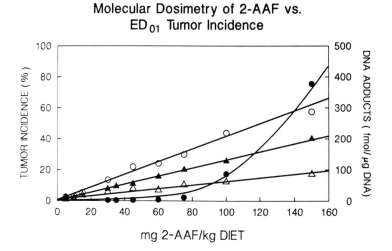

Figure 5 Dose–response relationship for DNA adducts in the liver (Δ) and bladder (O) and neoplasms of the liver (▲) and bladder (●) for mice exposed to 2-acetylaminofluorene. From Beland et al.[13]

day dietary exposures to 2-AAF at the concentrations used in the ED_{01} assay (30 to 150 ppm), a study that evaluated the dose–response for bladder and liver tumours in 24 192 mice[14]. In addition, the Beland et al.[13] study employed lower exposures of 5, 10, and 15 ppm 2-AAF. Both liver and bladder DNA adducts were linearly related to external exposure over the concentrations evaluated (Figure 5). This corresponded to the linear dose–response for liver tumours, but was markedly different from the sub-linear response for bladder tumours. Using a similar protocol, Cohen (personal communication) has shown that hepatic cell proliferation was not affected by 2-AAF exposure, whereas increased proliferation was present in bladder epithelium at high exposures.

HETEROGENEITY OF RESPONSE

The extent of DNA adduct formation varies between liver lobes, within liver lobules, between hepatocytes, endothelial cells, and Kupffer cells, as well as in different parts of the genome. Only a few investigations have examined many of these parameters; however, the data suggest that they may be chemical- or class-specific.

Lobe specificity is thought to be related to streamlining of blood flow. In the case of rats exposed to DEN, the left lobe develops more neoplasia, γ-glutamyl transpeptidase positive (GGT+) foci, and O^4-EtdT, followed by the right median and the right anterior lobes[15,16]. In contrast, the anterior lobe of 2-AAF-exposed rats exhibits the greatest number of DNA adducts[17] and iron-deficient foci[18].

Differences have also been demonstrated within the liver lobule. This appears to be the result of differences in localization of enzymes involved in biotransformation. Nitrosamines, such as DMN and DEN, are preferentially metabolized by the centrilobular hepatocytes. Evidence for this includes centriboluar necrosis and greater DNA alkylation, as demonstrated by immunohistochemistry[19]. No preferential localization was demonstrated for the direct-acting nitrosamide, ethylnitrosourea (ENU). The periportal region exhibits the greatest response to 2-AAF. DNA adducts are localized in hepatocytes of this region[20] and, on prolonged exposure, oval cell proliferation occurs there.

Pre-neoplastic foci and neoplasms of hepatocytes have decreased capacity for activating many carcinogens including DEN[20] and 2-AAF[19]. In contrast, ENU, an ethylating agent that does not require metabolic activation, alkylates DNA in nodular and non-nodular liver[21].

Several carcinogens have been evaluated for cell specificity of response. Dimethylhydrazine (SDMH) and DMN exposure regimens that primarily induce angiosarcomas cause increased concentrations of promutagenic DNA adducts[22–24] and replication[24,25] in non-parenchymal cells. Carcinogens that primarily induce hepatocellular carcinoma produce greater numbers of DNA adducts in hepatocytes. In the case of simple alkylating agents such as DMN, DEN and NNK, the cell-specific differences in individual adduct concentrations are dependent on the amount of O^6-MT. This DNA repair protein has

5-fold greater activity in rat hepatocytes than in non-parenchymal cells[26]. In addition, O^6-MT is induced by exposure to the alkylating agents, so that during chronic exposure, the activity is 12-fold greater. This results in vastly different rates for repair between cell types, with hepatocytes retaining only small amounts of O^6-alkylguanine relative to non-parenchymal cells. In contrast, no cell type differences in repair of O^4-alkylthymidine have been demonstrated. The net result is that O^4-EtdT represents the predominant promutagenic DNA adduct in hepatocytes of rats chronically exposed to DEN, while O^6-methylguanine is the most prevalent promutagenic DNA adduct in non-parenchymal cells. O^4-methyldeoxythymidine is formed in small amounts, but is repaired less rapidly in hepatocytes than O^6-methylguanine. It, therefore, accumulates to concentrations similar to O^6-methylguanaine on continuous exposure to SDMH[27].

Cell-specific differences in DNA adduct concentration are less prominent in 2-AAF-exposed rat livers. Hepatocytes have approximately twice the number of DNA adducts compared to non-parenchymal cells[28]. Both hepatocytes and non-parenchymal cells exhibit biphasic repair of the 2-AAF adduct. DNA adduct concentrations were similar in bile duct cells and non-parenchymal cells; however, the bile duct cells did not exhibit the rapid initial loss of the adducts.

CONCLUSIONS

Hepatocarcinogenesis is a highly complex, multi-stage process that involves different responses depending on the species, dose of carcinogen, exposure regimen and cell type. Investigations on DNA alkylation, repair and replication suggest that these factors play a critical role in determining the site, tumour type and dose–response following exposure to hepatocarcinogens. Data can be collected and compared between high and low exposure and across different species. This would permit greater utilization of biological data and knowledge of mechanism that should improve our ability to accurately predict human risk for chemical exposures.

References

1. Swenberg, J. A., Richardson, F. C., Boucheron, J. A., Deal, F. H., Belinsky, S. A., Charbonneau, M. and Short, B. G. (1987). High to low dose extrapolation: Critical determinants involved in the dose–response of carcinogenic substances. *J. Environ. Hlth. Perspect.*, **76**, 57–63

2. Purchase, I. F. H., Stafford, J. and Paddle, G. M. (1987). Vinyl chloride: An assessment of the risk of occupational exposure. *Food Chem. Toxicol.*, **25**, 187–202

3. Appleton, B. S., Goetchius, M. P. and Campbell, T. C. (1982). Linear dose–response curve for the hepatic macromolecular binding of aflatoxin B_1 in rats at very low exposures. *Cancer Res.*, **42**, 3659–62

4. Neumann, H.-G. (1980). Dose-response relationship in the primary lesion of strong electrophilic carcinogens. *Arch. Toxicol.*, Suppl. **3**, 69–77

5. Dunn, B. P. (1983). Wide-range linear dose–response curve for DNA binding of orally administered benzo(a)pyrene in mice. *Cancer Res.*, **43**, 2654–8

6. Adriaenssens, P. I., White, C. M. and Anderson, M. W. (1983). Dose–response relationships for the binding of benzo(a)pyrene metabolites to DNA and protein in lung, liver, and forestomach of control and butylated hydroxyanisole-treated mice. *Cancer Res.*, **43**, 3712–19

7. Pegg, A. E. and Hui, G. (1978). Formation and subsequent removal of O^6-methylguanine from deoxyribonucleic acid in rat liver and kidney after small doses of dimethylnitrosamine. *Biochem. J.*, **173**, 739–48

8. Swenberg, J. A. and Short, B. G. (1987). The influence of cytotoxicity on the induction of tumors. *Banbury Report: Nongenotoxic Mechanisms in Carcinogenesis*, **25**, 151–8. (Cold Spring Harbor Laboratory)

9. Boucheron, J. A., Richardson, F. C., Morgan, P. H. and Swenberg, J. A. (1987). Molecular dosimetry of O^4-ethyldeoxythymidine in rats continuously exposed to diethylnitrosamine (DEN). *Cancer Res.*, **47**, 1577–81

10. Deal, F. H., Richardson, F. C. and Swenberg, J. A. (1988). Dose–response of hepatocyte replication following continuous exposure to diethylnitrosamine. *Cancer Res.*, in press

11. Peto, R., Gray, R., Brantom, P. and Grasso, P. (1984). Nitrosamine carcinogenesis in 5120 rodents: Chronic administration of sixteen different concentrations of NDEA, NDMA, NPYR and NPIP in the water of 4400 inbred rats with parallel studies on NDEA alone of the effect of age of starting (3, 6, or 20 weeks) and of species (rats, mice, hamsters). In O'Neill, I. K., Borstell, R. C., Miller, C. T., Long, J. and Bartsch, H. (eds) *N-Nitroso Compounds: Occurrence, Biological Effects and Relevance to Human Cancer*, IARC Scientific Publications No. 57. (Lyon: IARC)

12. Zeise, L., Wilson, R. and Crouch, E. A. C. (1987). Dose–response relationships for carcinogens: A review. *Environ. Hlth. Perspect.*, **73**, 259–308

13. Beland, F. A., Fullerton, N. F., Kinourchi, T. and Poirier, M. C. (1987). DNA adduct formation during continuous feeding of 2-acetylaminofluorene at multiple concentrations. In *Proceedings of the Meeting on Methods to Detect DNA Damaging Agents in Man*, Helsinki, Finland, September 1987

14. Staff, J. A. and Mehlman, M. A. (1979). *Innovation in Cancer Risk Assessment (ED_{01} Study)*. 246 pp. (Park Forest South: Pathtox Publishers)

15. Dyroff, M. C., Richardson, F. C., Popp, J. A., Bedell, M. A. and Swenberg, J. A. (1986). Correlation of O^4-ethyldeoxythymidine accumulation, hepatic initiation and hepatocellular carcinoma induction in rats continuously administered diethylnitrosamine. *Carcinogenesis*, **7**, 241–6

16. Richardson, F. C., Boucheron, J. A., Dyroff, M. C., Popp, J. A. and Swenberg, J. A. (1986). Biochemical and morphologic studies of heterogeneous lobe responses in hepatocarcinogenesis. *Carcinogenesis*, **7**, 247–51

17. Poirier, M. C., Hunt, J. M., True, B. and Laishes, B. A. (1983). Kinetics of DNA adduct formation and removal in liver and kidney of rats fed 2-acetylaminofluorene. In Rydshöm, J., Montelius, J. and Bongtsson, M. (eds) *Extrahepatic Drug Metabolism and Chemical Carcinogenesis*, pp. 479–88 (Amsterdam: Elsevier)

18. Williams, G. M. and Watanabe, K. (1978). Quantitative kinetics of development of N-2-fluorenylacetamide-induced, altered (hyperplastic) hepatocellular foci resistant to iron accumulation and of their reversion or persistence following removal of carcinogen. *J. Natl. Cancer Inst.*, **61**, 113–18

19. Menkveld, G. J., Van Der Laken, C. J., Hermsen, T., Kriek, E., Scherer, E., and Engelse, L. D. (1985). Immunohistochemical localization of O^6-ethyldeoxyguanosine and deoxyguanosin-8-yl-(acetyl)aminofluorene in liver sections of rats treated with diethylnitrosamine, ethylnitrosourea or N-acetylaminofluorene. *Carcinogenesis*, **6**, 263–70

20. Huitfeldt, H. S., Spangler, E. F., Hunt, J. M. and Poirier, M. C. (1986). Immunohistochemical localization of DNA adducts in rat liver tissue and phenotypically altered foci during oral administration of 2-acetylaminofluorene. *Carcinogenesis*, **7**, 123–9

21. Scherer, E., Jenner, A. A. J. and Engelse, L. D. (1987). Immunocytochemical studies on the formation and repair of O^6-alkylguanine in rat tissues. In Bartsch, H., O'Neill, I. and Schulte-Hermann, R. (eds) *Proceedings of the 9th International Meeting on N-Nitroso Compounds: The Relevance of N-Nitroso Compounds to Human Cancer*. IARC Scientific Publications No. 84, pp. 55–8. (Lyon: IARC)

22. Lewis, J. G. and Swenberg, J. A. (1980). Differential repair of O^6-methylguanine in DNA of rat hepatocytes and non-parenchymal cells. *Nature*, **288**, 185–7

23. Bedell, M. A., Lewis, J. G., Billings, K. C. and Swenberg, J. A. (1982). Cell specificity in hepatocarcinogenesis: Preferential accumulation of O^6-methylgunaine in target cell DNA during continuous exposure of rats to 1,2-dimethylhydrazine. *Cancer Res.,* **42**, 3079–83

24. Lindamood, C., Bedell, M. A., Billings, K. C. and Swenberg, J. A. (1982). Alkylation and *de novo* synthesis of liver cell DNA from C3Hf mice during chronic DMN exposure. *Cancer Res.,* **42**, 4153–7

25. Lewis, J. G. and Swenberg, J. A. (1982). The effect of 1,2-dimethylhydrazine and diethylnitrosamine on cell replication and unscheduled DNA synthesis in target and nontarget cell populations in rat liver following chronic administration. *Cancer Res.,* **42**, 89–92

26. Swenberg, J. A., Bedell, M. A., Billings, K. C., Umbenhauer, D. R. and Pegg, A. E. (1982). Cell specific differences in O^6-alkykguanine DNA repair activity during continuous carcinogen exposure. *Proc. Natl. Acad. Sci. USA,* **79**, 5499–502

27. Richardson, F. C., Dyroff, M. C., Boucheron, J. A. and Swenberg, J. A. (1985). Differential repair of O^4-alkylthymidine following exposure to methylating and ethylating hepatocarcinogens. *Carcinogenesis*, **6**, 625–9

28. Poirier, M. C., Beland, F. A., Deal, F. H. and Swenberg, J. A. (1988). DNA adduct formation and removal in specific cell populations within the liver during chronic dietary administration of 2-acetylaminofluorene. *Carcinogenesis*, submitted for publication

Section 4
Biology of chemical hepatocarcinogenesis

24
The biochemical–molecular pathology of the stepwise development of liver cancer: new insights and problems

E. FARBER*, Z -Y. CHEN, L. HARRIS, G. LEE, J. S. RINAUDO, W. M. ROOMI, J. ROTSTEIN AND E. SEMPLE

INTRODUCTION

As is readily apparent from other chapters in this volume, primary liver cancer, despite its relatively uncommon occurrence in Western countries, constitutes a major medical problem world-wide, since it is first or second in incidence of cancer in many African and Asian countries. As with any chronic disease in humans affecting an internal organ, the sequence of tissue, cellular and molecular changes, including the stepwise pathophysiological modulations, during the long development of liver cancer, are poorly understood. This paucity of solid data on pathogenesis is true, regardless of the aetiology. Whether the liver cancer shows a very strong association with hepatitis B virus, as in some countries, or more complex associations with other possible aetiological agents, in addition to hepatitis B virus, as in other countries, has made little difference in our understanding of pathogenesis to date. Our understanding of how cancer develops over the many years remains primitive and largely speculative. This is in no small part due to our misconception that studies of the beginning and the end will lead by themselves to a reconstruction of the complex series of changes that constitute the 'middle'. The viewing of the last frame and the first of a movie will rarely if ever allow one to reconstruct accurately the essence of the movie.

This difficulty naturally favours increasing attention and concentration on possible relevant surrogate models of liver carcinogenesis in experimental animals. The purposes of studies of hepatocarcinogenesis in experimental models are several (Table 1). In this communication, we shall concentrate on

*Dedicated to the memory of Hans Popper, Honorary President of this Symposium. Hans was a source of inspiration and critical discussion for me since my first association with him in 1949–1950. The fruits of his dedication, devotion and energy in hepatology will be evident to all of us for many years to come.

273

Table 1 Purposes of experimental models of the pathogenesis of hepatocellular carcinoma

1.	To study the cellular and molecular pathogenesis of hepatocellular carcinoma, as a guide for, and surrogate of, the human disease
2.	To study the basic response patterns of a mammalian liver and their mechanisms to selective environmental perturbations such as chemicals and viruses
3.	To obtain new leads as to possible ætiological agents for human liver cancer
4.	To develop reliable and relevant test systems for possible environmental contaminants for humans
5.	To study the organization and control of the normal liver and its structural and functional constituents by selective perturbations

the first, the experimental system as a model for the human disease. Models of disease should suggest possible steps and mechanisms leading to hypotheses that can be explored in humans. The majority of studies on models to date have been with rats and mice, although increasing attention is being given to ducks, the woodchuck and squirrels infected with DNA hepatitis viruses. No detailed pathogenetic insights have been generated so far with the latter animals and therefore they will not be discussed. With respect to the other species, the pattern of liver cell cancer development in the rat appears to mimic quite closely that in the human, including the biology and histopathology of the end-stage cancers[1]. The major exception, so far, is the appearance of ductular-oval cell proliferation in some rat models (Table 2), a tissue response that does not seem to be commonly seen in liver carcinogenesis in humans. The pattern in the mouse has some resemblances to that in humans but also differences[2].

However, regardless of the specific details of any model in any species, one general overall pattern dominates. In every model, liver cell cancers are the

Table 2 Models of liver cancer development in the rat

Model	Description
A.	Single agent
(i)	Long-term continuous exposure to a carcinogen[a]
(ii)	Intermittent chronic exposure[a]
(iii)	The stop model
(iv)	Chronic exposure to peroxisome proliferators (hypolipidaemic agents, phthalates, halogenated hydrocarbons)
B.	Initiation–promotion–progression
(v)	Chronic enzyme induction model[b]
(vi)	Resistant hepatocyte model[a]
(vii)	Choline–methionine-deficient model[a]
(viii)	Orotic acid model[b]
C.	Dietary deficiency
(ix)	Choline-devoid low methionine diet without added carcinogens[a]

[a]Models in which ductular-oval cell proliferation occurs
[b]Models in which ductular-oval cell proliferation is not seen

end stages of very prolonged multistep processes in which new focal populations of hepatocytes are regularly seen. This prolonged multi-step pattern is also seen in the majority of instances of human liver cell cancer where it has been studied. As we shall note below, even the appearance of cancer in an apparently normal-looking liver does not rule out the likely possibility that the liver contained many focal non-malignant nodules that underwent remodelling before the time of appearance of cancer. Thus, a major challenge in the study of liver cell cancer is the identification and analysis of the essential nature of benign precursor lesions and their role, if any, in the cellular evolution to cancer[3,4].

STRATEGY OF CANCER DEVELOPMENT

Based upon the evidence from nine different models of liver carcinogenesis in the rat with the use of many different chemical carcinogens and promoters or a dietary deficiency (Table 2), an overall seemingly basic pattern of liver cancer development is emerging[1,5-8]. This pattern consists of two fundamental sequences: (a) the genesis of benign focal proliferations of hepatocytes (hyperplastic nodules, 'neoplastic' nodules, *hepatocyte nodules*) probably due to clonal expansion, a small subset of which persists and shows 'spontaneous' hepatocyte proliferation but no other evidence of neoplasia and certainly no evidence of cancer; and (b) the very slow evolution of the subset of persistent focal hepatocyte proliferations (*persistent hepatocyte nodules*, 'adenomas') through a stepwise process to an ultimate malignant hepatocellular carcinoma with cytological and histological earmarks of malignancy, with invasion and with metastasis[9-14]. Each of these two sequences is made up of several steps. In many models (i, ii, iv, v, vii in Table 2), these two sequences show so much overlap that it is impossible to determine which step precedes or follows any other step during carcinogenesis. As with any multi-step process, be it physical, chemical or biological, synchrony of step development is crucial to a sequential analyses[5-7]. The following outline is made possible by the presence of good-to-fair synchrony in a few models, especially the resistant hepatocyte, the orotic acid and probably the stop models.[15].

It should be emphasized that there may be more than one sequence in the pathogenesis of liver cell cancer. This sequence to be discussed, from original hepatocytes, is an established one. Possible suggested additional sequences[16], such as from ductular-oval cell proliferation[17], must be kept in mind.

Sequence A: Agent-dependent genesis of clonal hepatocyte nodules

In every model of liver carcinogenesis in the rat that has been studied in detail, a critical lesion at the crossroads is a focal proliferation of hepatocytes[18] (as many as a thousand or more per liver), a few of which persist and show 'spontaneous' proliferation of hepatocytes. We consider this step to be critical, since a key biological option, *proliferation* versus *remodelling*, is made at this time. The majority of nodules elect the option of remodelling and only a small minority, perhaps 1–2%, persist as such, continue to show hepatocyte proliferation, now 'spontaneous', and slowly evolve toward liver cell cancer. However, this second option, persistence, is not absolute, but rather relative, since most of the persistent nodules, now 5 to 15 per liver, show slow remodelling and only 1 or 2 persist for several months to evolve towards cancer.

Genesis of sequence A

The essential steps in this sequence are the initial induction of a new phenotype (and probably also a new genotype) in a rare hepatocyte (*initiation*) and the subsequent clonal expansion of these rare altered hepatocytes to generate benign focal proliferations, hepatocyte nodules (*promotion*). Thus, with the majority of chemical carcinogens and probably with other ætiological agents as well (choline-deficient diet, radiations?), the formation of the persistent benign focal proliferations, the clonal nodules, is a reflection of the classical pattern of chemical carcinogenesis, initiation and promotion.

'Initiation' is a two-step process in which some change is induced in a rare hepatocyte by an activated form of a carcinogen, presumably via an interaction with DNA. This change generates a new constitutive phenotype if a round of cell proliferation occurs. The initial interaction is readily repaired if cell proliferation does not occur or if it is inhibited or delayed for several days[1]. Cell proliferation for initiation may be triggered by the induction of cell death by the carcinogen or by other hepato-necrogenic agents or by partial hepatectomy. The obligatory dependence on cell proliferation for initiation is striking[19]. It has obvious implications concerning the role of cytotoxicity and concomitant liver inquiry in the development of liver cell cancer. Since a round of cell proliferation is necessary for initiation in other cells and tissues and with viruses or radiations as well as with chemicals[20,21], its role in the non-proliferating adult liver could be of major importance as a determinant in establishing the frequency of liver cancer in some geographical areas in the world.

In the rat, initiation with many different chemical carcinogens is associated with the constitutive appearance in a rare hepatocyte, usually 1 per 10^5 or 10^6 hepatocytes, of a new phenotype, a *resistance phenotype*[22], with a highly characteristic biochemical pattern (Table 3). This pattern includes large decreases in the enzymes that activate carcinogens and other xenobiotics (phase I) and appreciable increases in enzymes and other components, such as glutathione, active in detoxification (phase II). The phenotype of the initiated hepatocytes in the rat does *not* include any measurable degree of spontaneous or autonomous cell proliferation. Thus, no expansion of the individual initiated cells occurs until a suitable environment is created by a promoting regimen. The only known way so far that this is accomplished in the liver of the rat is by providing a stimulus for cell proliferation while, at the same time, proliferation by all hepatocytes other than the few initiated ones is inhibited, i.e. by *differential inhibition*.

It should be pointed out that the resistance phenotype is associated with a

Table 3 Biochemical pattern associated with the resistance phenotype in hepatocyte nodules in rats

A.	*Decrease* in xenobiotic metabolizing and activating components
	Cytochromes P-450
	Mixed function oxygenases
	Sulphotransferases
	Aldehyde dehydrogenase
	Lipid peroxidation
B.	*Increase* in detoxification components
	Glutathione
	Glutathione-S-transferases including glutathione-S-transferase 7-7 (P)
	UDP-glucuronyl transferase-I
	γ-glutamyltransferase
	Epoxide hydrase (epoxide hydrolase)
	DT-diaphorase (quinone reductase)
	P-glycoprotein (multi-drug resistance, *mdr*)

'ground glass' appearance of the hepatocytes in the nodules. This change is not unlike that seen in the 'ground glass hepatocytes' in hepatitis B carriers and in livers surrounding hepatocellular carcinomas in humans. A major change in the ground glass cells is a large increase in smooth endoplasmic reticulum that shows 'hypertrophic hypoactive' properties[23,24], i.e. decreases in phase I components.

The resistance phenotype in the initiated hepatocytes has several similarities to the phenotype in some human cancer cells when they become resistant to chemotherapeutic agents ('multi-drug resistance, *mdr*')[25-28].

'Promotion'[29] is the process whereby an initiated tissue or organ develops focal proliferations (nodules, papillomas, polyps, etc.), one or more of which act as precursors for subsequent steps in the carcinogenic process[30].

During the clonal expansion of the initiated hepatocytes to form hepatocyte nodules, one sees the appearance of small microscopic islands or foci. With some models (e.g. vi, Table 2), the foci rapidly expand by proliferation to generate macroscopic nodules within a few days. With other models (e.g. v, viii, ix, Table 2) the expansion is slow, lasting many weeks.

The foci or islands are frequently called 'preneoplastic', even though very few (less than 1%) develop into hepatocyte nodules in several models and even fewer can be related to an ultimate cancer. Thus, they contain, *as a population*, the few preneoplastic cells.

The hepatocyte nodules demonstrate two basic sets of properties that appear to be fundamental to our understanding of the development of liver cancer. These are: (a) *a characteristic biochemical phenotype*, and (b) *the availability of at least two physiological–biological options – remodelling versus persistence*.

In (a), as indicated above, the hepatocytes in the nodules have a special resistance phenotype (Table 3) that enables them to grow and expand in an environment that is inhibitory to cell proliferation of the large body of hepatocytes surrounding the nodules. When the liver is stimulated to proliferate by partial hepatectomy or by a necrogenic agent such as CCl₄, and when exposed at the same time to a carcinogen such as 2-acetylaminofluorene[11] or other carcinogens[31], only the resistance hepatocytes proliferate to generate nodules. This 'differential inhibition' is a major mechanism for promotion in liver cancer development in the rat[30]. Phenobarbital[32] and orotic acid[33] also may promote liver cancer development by this mechanism.

Thus, the acquisition of a resistance phenotype during initiation and its use in the selection process during promotion to generate nodules is fundamental to the development of nodules as early steps in hepatocarcinogenesis in several instances.

It is perhaps noteworthy that a similar differential has been suggested to be operative in the pathogenesis of hepatocelluar carcinoma in humans in association with hepatitis B virus[34]. London and Blumberg[34] proposed that hepatitis B virus infection may generate a few resistant hepatocytes (R cells) and such R cells would be capable of differential selection for growth by virtue of the inhibitory effects of the virus on the majority of hepatocytes (S cells) that are susceptible or sensitive to the cytopathic–cytotoxic effects of the virus. This suggestion, so close in principle to that previously suggested for chemical hepatocarcinogenesis in the rat[35], has been discussed by others in relation to the pathogenesis of human liver cancer[36-38]. It is interesting that Chisari et al.[39] have recently reported that liver neoplasms in transgenic mice containing the DNA for a large surface antigen of human hepatitis B virus are somehow resistant to the accumulation in the endoplasmic reticulum of the antigen. Conceivably, this resistance phenomenon might be related to the proposed R and S hepatocytes in the human liver of patients with hepatitis B infection.

In (b), a characteristic and critical property of the hepatocyte nodules is the availability of two major options — remodelling by differentiation and persistence[1]. The remodelling is associated with changes in the biochemistry, architecture, organization and ultrastructure of the nodules such that they become very similar if not identical to normal mature liver and the nodules as such 'disappear'[40]. The information for this spontaneous remodelling, a complex genetic expression, must be built into the genome. It indicates the fundamental physiological nature of the hepatocyte nodule[7]. Whether the remodelled hepatocytes can be selected again for expansion is not known.

The persistence of a few nodules appears to indicate a block or delay in remodelling by differentiation. This minor option sets the stage for the truly carcinogenic sequence, the nodule to cancer sequence.

The occurrence of remodelling to normal-looking liver could well be the basis for the appearance of liver cell cancer in a normal-appearing liver. The seeming normality could be only apparent, and could be the result of remodelling in an earlier grossly-distorted or altered liver.

The time period for sequence A lasts from several weeks to a few months depending on the model. With the resistance hepatocyte (vi) model, initiation is apparently complete within 48 to 72 hours and promotion is complete at 6 weeks. With the orotic acid (viii) or phenobarbital (v) models, initiation is also within 1 to 3 days but promotion requires from 10 to 20 weeks.

Sequence B: Agent-independent nodule to cancer process

The 'nodule to cancer' sequence contains the steps that are most directly relevant to cancer. Despite this, this *progression stage* has received little attention, is poorly studied and, of the sequences in carcinogenesis, is least understood either phenomenologically or mechanistically. Its existence is only now beginning to be appreciated as an important target phase for cancer prevention[41].

'Progression' is the process whereby one or more focal proliferations, such as papillomas and polyps and hepatocyte nodules in the case of the liver, undergo a slow cellular evolution to malignant neoplasia[30]. Included are the series of changes which malignant neoplasms may undergo as they become more malignant and more prone to show invasion and then metastases.

Beginning with the earliest persistent hepatocyte nodule as the first step in this *precancerous* sequence (Table 4), one observes a characteristic phenotype including reproducible biological behaviour and a slow series of changes leading ultimately to cancer. During this sequence, there occurs a further decrease in the number of hepatocyte nodules, as several of the persistent nodules show slow remodelling to normal-looking liver. This slow remodelling diminishes further the persistent nodule population, such that often only 1 to 3 nodules are clearly evident in the whole liver by the time unequivocal cancer can be identified.

A study in our laboratory just being completed shows that the synchrony that is seen so characteristically in the resistant hepatocyte (vi) model during sequence A persists. Sequence B has now been found to show an unusual degree of synchrony of the series of progressive changes as a function of time preceding the appearance of cancer.

The time period for sequence B is usually about 10–15 months. Although the first step, persistent hepatocyte nodules, is seen at 6 weeks post-initiation, cancer can be recognized at about 10–11 months with metastases at 11–12 months. This time frame is seen in the resistance hepatocyte model with diethylnitrosamine as initiating carcinogen.

The changes so far documented in sequence B include (Table 4) (a) persistence of the characteristic resistance phenotype in the nodule[42], (b) 'spontaneous' hepatocyte proliferation in the nodules, increasing with time over several months[9], (c) normal diurnal rhythm of nodule hepatocyte proliferation[9], (d) a balance between cell proliferation and cell loss in nodules[9,43], (e)

Table 4 Properties of persistent hepatocyte nodules as a function of time during sequence B

1.	Persistence of resistance phenotype
2.	'Spontaneous' hepatocyte proliferation
3.	Normal response to phenobarbital and normal diurnal rhythm
4.	Balance between cell proliferation and cell loss
5.	Progressive loss of binding of some ligands
6.	New pattern of growth on transplantation to spleen
7.	Appearance of 'nodules in nodules'
8.	Appearance of hepatocellular carcinoma with invasion and later metastasis
9.	Imbalance between cell proliferation and cell loss

a 'normal' proliferative response of nodule hepatocyte to a strong mitogenic stimulus, partial hepatectomy (PH)[9], (f) a progressive loss in the binding and response to some ligands[44], (g) a new characteristic pattern of growth on transplantation to the spleen[10], (h) the appearance of new focal cell populations in nodules, so-called 'nodules in nodules'[45], and (i) finally appearance of hepatocellular carcinoma inside nodules[11]. Some of these may show invasion and/or metastasis. These changes seem to be associated with a large increase in cell proliferation relative to cell loss.

Persistence of resistance phenotype in the precancerous persistent nodules

The biochemical pattern of the small subset of persistent nodules is similar to that of the earlier nodules in respect to phase 1 and phase 2 drug metabolizing components[42]. This is also true with respect to the nodular growth in the spleen derived from the persistent hepatocyte nodules[42].

Spontaneous hepatocyte proliferation in persistent nodules. The most important new property of the persistent hepatocyte nodules, beginning at the earliest time point, is seemingly 'spontaneous' hepatocyte proliferation[9]. At 2 months post-initiation, the nodules show a labelling index of 4% and this increases to about 8% by 6 months. This is in contrast to the hepatocytes in the liver surrounding the nodules which show a growth fraction of about 0.4%.

When labelling continues for a week or so with radioactive thymidine in a mini-pump, from 60 to 80% of the hepatocytes in the persistent nodules become labelled, even at 2 months. Thus the majority of hepatocytes are cycling but asynchronously, with only 4% in S phase at any random hourly period[9].

Normal response to partial hepatectomy and normal diurnal rhythm. The hepatocytes in the persistent nodules show at least some normal control patterns. The cell cycle of nodule hepatocytes shows a diurnal rhythm similar to normal liver hepatocytes[9]. Also, the nodule hepatocytes respond to the mitogenic stimulus of partial hepatectomy both quantitatively and qualitatively as do normal control or surrounding liver hepatocytes.

Balance between cell proliferation and cell loss in the precancerous persistent nodules. Not only is there about a 10-fold increase in cell proliferation over the surrounding liver in the nodules, but there is another new phenomenon — cell loss or cell death[9]. Cell loss or cell death during the promotion phase of nodule formation was virtually absent with growth fraction of over 80%[46]. In the early persistent nodules, there now appears cell loss or cell death as a quantitatively important property of nodules. The 4% growth fraction is almost balanced by a 3% cell loss, thus accounting for a slow rate of enlargement of the nodules[9]. This appears to be the first clear-cut appearance of cell death in hepatocyte foci and nodules in the sequence in the resistant hepatocyte model (vi model) and is present throughout the whole nodule-to-cancer sequence as well as in the cancers themselves. This balance between cell proliferation and cell loss appears to persist throughout much of sequence B until the appearance of cancer. Once cancer appears, the balance is seriously disturbed and one observes a much faster growth of the cancer as compared to the preceding nodules.

Progressive loss of binding of some ligands. The hepatocytes in the persistent nodules as well as earlier nodules show a decrease in the capacity to bind epidermal growth factor, asialo-orosomucoid and lipoprotein apoprotein[44] as well as desialylated glycoproteins[47] and asialofetuin[48]. In contrast to these findings are those of Eriksson and co-workers who reported a large increase in the binding capacity of hepatocyte nodules to transferrin[49].

New pattern of growth on transplantation to spleen. The persistent nodules also show another new property — generation of nodules and hepatocellular carcinoma on transplantation to the spleen[10]. This is in contrast to the behaviour of the early nodules. The early nodules, most of which will remodel by differentiation, grow slowly in the spleen with a pattern resembling normal liver hepatocytes, with gradual replacement of the splenic pulp by liver but without nodules or cancer.

Appearance of nodules-in-nodules. As emphasized some years ago by Popper, new hepatocyte populations arise frequently as nodules inside nodules[45]. These new cells have obvious and histological differences from cytological the hepatocytes in the larger nodule. Although direct proof that such nodules within nodules are the precursors of liver cancer is missing, their common occurrence late in the nodule-to-cancer sequence, their histological appearance and the presence of metastasizing hepatocellular carcinoma inside nodules[11,14] makes them highly suspect as precursors for cancer.

There is increasing evidence that unequivocal hepatocellular carcinoma showing metastasis to the lung can be seen entirely within the confines of a late persistent nodule[11,14]. It is known that hepatocyte nodules are precursors for hepatocellular carcinoma in at least five studies with different models[14]. This observation provides clear convincing evidence that cancer can arise inside hepatocyte nodules. Whether this is an obligatory requirement for liver cell cancer is, of course, not known. These observations however indicate the utility of studying the nodule-to-cancer sequence as one established sequence. This is particularly so in view of our recent evidence that many of the steps in the cancer-to-nodule sequence appear to be quite well synchronized as a function of time as one carefully examines the nodules between 2 months and 12 months.

Appearance of hepatocellular carcinoma with invasion and later metastasis. As already noted, as one studies the nodules carefully as a function of time, one can see increasing numbers of new populations inside the nodules and in some instances some of these are obviously hepatocellular carcinoma, even showing metastasis to the lung. This is a difficult area to be examined with great certainty unless one can find that the primary cancer is confined entirely within an hepatocyte nodule. In the case of the resistant hepatocyte model, we have now increasing evidence that many late nodules have carcinoma within them.

Imbalance between liver cell proliferation and cell loss. A new perspective is evident during the nodule-to-cancer sequence. In the precancerous nodules, the overall growth of the nodules is severely restricted by the existence of a

Table 5 Biochemical phenotype of hepatocyte nodules induced by genotoxic agents in the rat

1. Resistance phenotype including P-170 glycoprotein
2. Altered iron metabolism
3. Altered glycolytic enzymes
4. Alterations in pentose shunt including increase in glucose-6-phosphate dehydrogenase

level of cell loss by cell death almost as large as the level of cell proliferation. This balance is reminiscent of the response of normal liver to a primary mitogenic stimulus[50]. The increase in hepatocytes in the liver of normal animals after administration of a primary mitogen is succeeded shortly by the return of the liver to its 'resting level' with loss of the extra cells. These studies, as well as those with lead nitrate by Columbano et al.[43], indicate the existence of a homeostatic mechanism that operates in the liver to maintain a steady-state level of cell number. Conceivably, the same control could be operating in the precancerous nodules to limit and restrict their rate of growth[51].

This homeostatic balance appears to be lost with malignancy. Although hepatocellular carcinomas, like so many other carcinomas, show regional necrosis associated with ischaemia, it appears that the physiological balance between cell proliferation and cell loss is lost or disturbed. Thus, the key factor in the precancer-to-cancer sequence might be the imbalance between cell loss and cell proliferation rather than the stimulation of cell proliferation.

SPECIES DIFFERENCES — RAT, MOUSE AND HUMAN

The most intensely studied carcinogenic process has been in the rat. However, a few studies in the mouse and even fewer in the human indicate some basic similarities as well as some differences.

Biologically, it has been documented that at least some benign focal hepatocyte proliferations in humans (adenomas), undergo regression with disappearance[52,53]. These adenomas, most often induced by contraceptive or anabolic steroids, resemble the hepatocyte nodules in the rat in respect to architecture, histologic and cytologic appearance[1,54]. Whether the regression of the adenomas is by remodelling to normal-looking liver is not known but is possible.

Table 6 Biochemical patterns in precancerous liver nodules

Pattern I
Decrease in phase I
Altered iron metabolism (see Table 7)
Increase in phase II

Pattern II
Decrease in phase I
Altered iron metabolism (see Table 7)
No increase in phase II

Table 7 Altered iron metabolism in hepatocyte nodules

Decrease in:
Iron uptake and/or concentration
Total iron
Total heme
Heme enzymes
   cytochromes P-450
   cytochrome b_5
   catalase
   tryptophan 2,3-dioxygenase
Heme binding protein (cytosolic)

Increase In:
Heme oxygenase
Transferrin receptors (by 60 times)

Biochemically, the benign focal hepatocyte proliferations, the early (remodelling) and the persistent hepatocyte nodules, appear to show characteristic similarities and differences among the three species.

In the rat (Table 5), the nodules induced by the majority of chemical carcinogens, the 'genotoxic' carcinogens and by exposure to a choline devoid diet, show a highly characteristic and common pattern, regardless of the nature of the initiating and promoting exposure. The phase I components show a large decrease while the phase II show an increase (Pattern I, Table 6)[42,55]. In addition, there are characteristic changes in some enzymes in glycolysis and in the pentose shunt[56-58]. Also, a common pattern of iron metabolism is seen (Table 7).

With nodules and cancers induced in rat by some hypolipidaemic agents, the phase I enzymes were considerably decreased but the phase II components were not[59,60] (Table 8).

In the mouse, nodules and cancers as a group show the decrease in phase I enzymes (Group A in Table 3) but *not* the increase in phase II components (Group B in Table 3)[60-63]. This pattern is designated pattern II (Table 6).

Table 8 Phenotypic patterns in precancerous nodules in three species

Species	Pattern*
Rat	
Genotoxic chemicals	I
Non-genotoxic chemicals	II
Mouse	
All (few)	II
Human	
Few examples	I and II

*See Table 6

In the human[64,65], from two studies, it appears that the phase I enzymes are again very much decreased in hepatocellular carcinoma[64] but the phase II components seem to be variable[64,65].

Thus, from the few studies in mice and even fewer in humans, in comparison to the several in rats, it appears that a common pattern might be emerging. The new focal proliferations, either precancerous or cancerous, consistently show large decrease in phase I enzymes with variable levels of phase II.

The basis for the decrease in phase I, at least in rats and mice, is possibly related to an underlying disturbance in iron metabolism (Table 7). This hypothesis[55,60,63,66–74] is consistent with the total body of knowledge we have at this time. Eriksson et al.[74] have suggested that at the root of the disturbed iron metabolism could be a defect in the proton pump in the nodules.

ONCOGENES AND LIVER CANCER

A popular current hypothesis is that 'turning on' of a proto-oncogene or a mutation in a proto-oncogene is somehow involved in cancer development and/or in the expression of malignant properties in some cancers[75–77]. Since this area of cancer research is in its formative stage, our speculation base far exceeds our knowledge base by orders of magnitude. Whether any or all oncogenes play roles in the carcinogenic process, i.e. in the *development of cancer*, remains to be established. Since some proto-oncogenes are normally related to the proliferative cell cycle (c-*fos*, c-*myc*, c-*myb*, c-H-*ras*, c-k-*ras*, P-53 etc.), others to growth factors including growth factor receptors (e.g. see ref. 78) and still others to signal transduction from the cell membrane, it is predictable that altered gene expression of these important genes in one or more steps in the complex process of cancer development would occur. Whether they are mechanistically involved in the genesis of any of the steps in cancer development remains unclear. Since the carcinogenic process involves both common and diverse phenotypic expressions at different steps, it is not evident yet whether increased or altered expression of one or more proto-oncogenes is involved in the major common features or perhaps in epiphenomena that could be involved as modulators such as enhanced growth.

In the liver, the cell-cycle related oncogenes and other genes show characteristic 'ebbs and flows' as they do in many other cells[79,80]. This has been studied quite well in the liver of the rat[81] but almost not at all in the mouse. Yet, hepatocyte neoplasms quite commonly contain mutated H-*ras* proto-oncogenes in the mouse but quite uncommonly or rarely in the rat.

In B6C3F mice, 33/48 spontaneously occurring liver neoplasms contained activated oncogenes with at least 28/33 having activated H-*ras* genes[82–85]. With single doses of N-hydroxy-2-acetylaminofluorene, vinyl chloride or 1-hydroxy-2',3'-dehydroestragole given at day 12 of development[86] and with seven other carcinogens[87], activated *ras* genes were detected in each liver tumour. Also, with single doses of diethylnitrosamine at 12 or 15 days of age, DNA from 14/33 liver tumours in the same strain of mouse revealed activated H-*ras* proto-oncogenes[88].

In the rat (F-344), in contrast, only 1/28 diethylnitrosamine-induced liver tumours showed positive evidence of activated proto-oncogenes by transfection with NIH 3T3 cells[88]. Similar negative or low-incidence results were found with other liver cancers in rats[14,87,89]. Several Morris hepatomas and some primary hepatocellular carcinomas induced with a chemical carcinogen were found to contain elevated levels of mRNA for c-*myc*, c-H-*ras* and c-Ki-*ras* proto-oncogenes[90]. These results were found in a study that was not controlled for cell proliferation. Increased expression of c-*fos* was found in carcinogen-induced liver cancer and in regenerating liver[91]. A variety of mouse hepatocellular neoplasms were found to express elevated levels of several proto-oncogenes[92]. The expressions were variable with no consistent pattern and again were not controlled for cell proliferation.

An activated H-*ras* proto-oncogene was found in 1/5 rat liver carcinomas induced by a quinoline derivative[93]. Artifactual activation of a proto-oncogene, c-*raf*, was found in a chemically-induced hepatocellular carcinoma from a rat during the transfection process[94].

A high frequency of transforming genes in aflatoxin B_1-induced rat-liver tumours induced morphologic transformation of NIH 3T3 cells[89]. Two tumours were shown to contain an activated K-*ras* gene.

Early focal collections of altered putative initiated hepatocytes (foci of altered hepatocytes positive for γ-glutamyltransferase) in the rat did not differ from other hepatocyte populations in the expressions of c-*myc* and c-H-*ras* proto-oncogenes[95]. Persistent hepatocyte nodules, precancerous lesions in the rat, displayed a pattern of expression of mRNAs of 10 cell-cycle related genes, including c-*fos*, c-*myc*, c-Ha-*ras*, c-Ki-*ras*, that was completely expected on the basis of the degree of cell proliferation[96]. The time sequence pattern was virtually identical in the precancerous lesions and in normal rat liver when cell proliferation was stimulated by partial hepatectomy.

The results of appropriate critical control experiments, including the induction of non-neoplastic cell proliferation after exposure to chemical carcinogens, will be awaited with considerable interest by the scientific community. These should help to decide whether these various changes in genes and gene expressions are intimately involved at discrete reproducible steps during the development of liver cancer. Included must be a rational testable hypothesis if this interesting field is not to remain largely in the realm of speculation.

The published studies on oncogenes and carcinogenesis in animals seem to suggest that if point mutations of *ras* genes are important mechanistically in the carcinogenic process, they may be involved during initiation and/or promotion but not in the progression from nodules to cancer[88]. In the lung[87], skin[98] and liver[83,85,86] the initiated *ras* genes occur equally in early focal proliferations, so-called 'benign neoplasms', and in carcinomas. This suggestion of involvement early in the process[88] would seem to be in apparent conflict with some clinical studies in which activated proto-oncogenes, including members of the *ras* family, are found in advanced stages of cancer but not in earlier ones[99].

Parenthetically, it should be pointed out that the term 'oncogene' or 'cancer gene' is an unfortunate one, since it is difficult to accept the concept that biological evolution would select for a property or set of properties that would kill the host and the species. The 'proto-oncogenes' are conserved to a major degree for long time spans in evolution. It is more attractive to consider them as important in cancer only because they are involved in key rate-limiting steps in many biological processes both 'normal' (so-called) and 'pathological' (so-called). This concept is receiving more support by the increasing number of reports of the involvement of each specific proto-onco-genes in various aspects of normal development, differentiation, cell proliferation and response patterns to injury and to other important processes in many different diseases, not only in cancer.

PERSPECTIVES: THE PREVENTION OF LIVER CANCER

It is evident from the studies in animals that focal hepatocyte proliferations, variously designated as adenomas or more accurately hepatocyte nodules, are a critical relatively early common lesion in the development of liver cancer. The slow evolution from nodule to cancer is an agent-independent process and occurs 'spontaneously'. Thus, it should be possible to modulate this process without knowing anything about the preceding exposure, whether chemical or viral. In fact, this is experimentally quite feasible. Feo and associates[100] have found that the administration of S-adenosyl-methionine has a striking inhibitory effect on the development of liver cancer from hepatocyte nodules initiated by diethylnitrosamine and promoted by 2-acetylamino-fluorene plus partial hepatectomy with and without phenobarbital. We have also found that extra dietary choline may have a similar effect on liver cancer development. Thus, it appears to be feasible to inhibit the nodule to cancer sequence, sequence B. It is not unlikely that this may be so, regardless of whether the early events are induced by chemicals or viruses.

In addition, a recent study[101] indicates the feasibility of diagnosing early proliferative changes in the liver long before any cancer develops.

Thus, a reasonable approach to cancer prevention becomes (a) the early diagnosis of preneoplasia or precancer, and (b) the inhibition or delay of the precursor to product evolution. The further development of this approach and its possible use in the human may offer an opportunity to prevent cancer until the truly widespread use of appropriate vaccines against hepatitis B virus becomes practical.

References

1. Farber, E. and Sarma, D. S. R. (1987). Biology of disease: hepatocarcinogenesis: a dynamic cellular perspective. *Lab. Invest.*, **56**, 4–22
2. Farber, E. (1987). Pathogenesis of experimental liver cancer: comparison with humans. *Arch. Toxicol.*, Suppl, **10**, 281–8
3. Farber, E. (1973). Carcinogenesis — cellular evolution as a unifying trend. (Presidential address.) *Cancer Res.*, **33**, 2537–50
4. Farber, E. (1973). Hyperplastic liver nodules. *Methods Cancer Res.*, **7**, 345–75
5. Foulds, L. (1969). *Neoplastic Development*, Vol. 1 (London: Academic Press)

6. Foulds, L. (1975). *Neoplastic Development*, Vol. 2 (London: Academic Press)
7. Farber, E. and Cameron, R. (1980). The sequential analysis of cancer development. *Adv. Cancer Res.*, **35**, 125–226
8. Farber, E. (1987). Some emerging general principles in the pathogenesis of hepatocellular carcinoma. *Cancer Surveys*, **5**, 695–718
9. Rotstein, J. B., Sarma, D. S. R. and Farber, E. (1986). Sequential alterations in growth control and cell dynamics of hepatocytes in early precancerous steps in hepatocarcinogenesis. *Cancer Res.*, **46**, 2377–85
10. Tatematsu, M., Lee, G., Hayes, M. A. and Farber, E. (1987). Progression of hepatocarcinogenesis: differences in growth and behaviour of transplants of early and late hepatocyte nodules in the spleen. *Cancer Res.*, **47**, 4699–705
11. Solt, D. B., Medline, A. and Farber, E. (1977). Rapid emergence of carcinogen-induced hyperplastic lesions in a new model for the sequential analysis of liver carcinogenesis. *Am. J. Pathol.*, **88**, 595–618
12. Ogawa, K., Medline, A. and Farber, E. (1979). Sequential analysis of hepatic carcinogenesis. A comparative study of the ultrastructure of preneoplastic, malignant, prenatal, postnatal and regenerating liver. *Lab. Invest.*, **41**, 22–35
13. Ogawa, K., Medline, A. and Farber, E. (1979). Sequential analysis of hepatic carcinogenesis. The comparative architecture of preneoplastic, malignant, prenatal, postnatal and regenerating liver. *Br. J. Cancer*, **40**, 782–90
14. Farber, E. (1984). Cellular biochemistry of the stepwise development of cancer with chemicals: G. H. Clowes Memorial Lecture. *Cancer Res.*, **44**, 5463–74
15. Bannasch, P. (1986). Preneoplastic lesions as endpoints in carcinogenicity testing. I. Hepatic preneoplasia. *Carcinogenesis*, **7**, 689–95
16. Farber, E. (1963). Ethionine carcinogenesis. *Adv. Cancer Res.*, **7**, 383–474
17. Sell, S., Hunt, J. M., Knoll, B. J. and Dunsford, H. A. (1987). Cellular events during hepatocarcinogenesis in rats and the question of premalignancy. *Adv. Cancer Res.*, **48**, 37–111
18. Farber, E., Eriksson, L. C., Roomi, M. W., Cameron, R. G. and Hayes, M. A. (1984). Chemical carcinogenesis: hepatocyte nodules with a special phenotype as a common step at the crossroads. *Toxicol. Pathol.*, **12**, 288–90
19. Columbano, A., Rajalakshmi, S. and Sarma, D. S. R. (1982). Requirement of cell proliferation for the initiation of liver carcinogenesis as assayed by three different procedures. *Cancer Res.*, **42**, 2079–83
20. Craddock, V. M. (1976). Cell proliferation and experimental liver cancer. In Cameron, H. M., Linsell, D. A. and Warrick, G. P. (eds.) *Liver Cell Cancer*, pp. 152–201. (Amsterdam: Elsevier)
21. Grisham, J. W., Kaufman, W. K. and Kaufman, D. G. (1983). The cell cycle and chemical carcinogenesis. *Surv. Synth. Pathol. Res.*, **1**, 46–66
22. Farber, E. (1987). Resistance phenotype in the initiation and promotion of chemical hepatocarcinogenesis. *Chemica Scripta*, **27A**, 131–3
23. Hutterer, F., Schaffner, F., Klion, F. M. and Popper, H. (1968). Hypertrophic hypoactive smooth endoplasmic reticulum: a sensitive indicator of hepatotoxicity by dieldrin. *Science*, **161**, 1017–19
24. Hutterer, F., Klein, F. M., Wengraf, A., Schaffner, R. and Popper, H. (1969). Hepatocellular adaptation and injury: structural and biochemical changes following dieldrin and methyl butter yellow. *Lab. Invest.*, **20**, 455–64
25. Batist, G., de Muys, J. M., Cowan, K.-H. and Myers, C. E. (1986). Purification and characterization of a novel glutathione-S transferase (GST) in multi-drug resistant (*mdr*) human breast cancer cells. *Proc. Am. Assoc. Cancer Res.*, **27**, 270
26. Tulpule, A., Batist, G., Sinha, B., Katki, A., Myers, C. E. and Cowan, K. H. (1986). Similar biochemical changes associated with pleomorphic drug resistance (PDR) in human MCF-7 breast cancer cells and xenobiotic resistance induced by carcinogens. *Proc. Am. Assoc. Cancer Res.*, **27**, 271
27. Thorgeirsson, S. S., Huber, B. E., Sorrell, S., Fajo, A., Pastan, I. and Gottesman, M. M. (1987). Expression of the multidrug resistant gene in hepatocarcinogenesis and regenerating rat liver. *Science*, **236**, 1120–2
28. Fairchild, C. R., Ivy, S. P., Rushmore, T., Lee, G., Koo, P., Goldsmith, M. E., Myers, C.

E., Farber, E. and Cowan, K. H. (1987). Carcinogen-induced *mdr* overexpression is associated with xenobiotic resistance in rat preneoplastic liver nodules and hepatocellular carcinomas. *Proc. Natl. Acad. Sci. USA,* **84**, 7701–5

29. Sarma, D. S. R., Rao, P. M. and Rajalakshmi, S. (1986). Liver tumor promotion by chemicals: models and mechanisms. *Cancer Surveys,* 5, 781–98

30. Farber, E. (1982). Sequential events in chemical carcinogenesis. In Becker, F. F. (ed.) *Cancer: A Comprehensive Treatise*, pp. 485–506. (New York: Plenum Press)

31. Tatematsu, M., Murasaki, G., Nakanishi, K., Miyoto, Y., Shinohara, Y., and Ito, N. (1979). Sequential quantitative studies in hyperplastic nodules in the liver of rats treated with carcinogenic chemicals. *Gann,* **70**, 125–30

32. Eckl, P. M., Meyer, S. F., Rive, W., Whitcomb, W. R. and Jirtle, R. L. (1988). Phenobarbital reduces EGF receptors and the ability of physiological concentrations of calcium to suppress hepatocyte proliferation. *Carcinogenesis,* **9**, 479–83

33. Laconi, E., Li, F., Semple, E., Rao, P. M., Rajalakshmi, S. and Sarma, D. S. R. (1988). Inhibition of DNA synthesis in primary cultures of hepatocytes by orotic acid. *Carcinogenesis,* **9**, 675–7

34. London, W. T. and Blumberg, B. S. (1981). Hepatitis B virus and primary hepatocellular carcinoma. In Birchinal, J. H. and Oettgen, H. F. (eds.) *Cancer Achievements, Challenges and Prospects for the 1980s*, pp. 161–83. (New York: Grune and Stratton)

35. Solt, D. B. and Farber, E. (1976). New principle for the analysis of chemical carcinogenesis. *Nature,* **263**, 702–3

36. Popper, H., Gerber, M. A. and Thung, S. N. (1982). The relation of hepatocellular carcinoma to infection with hepatitis B and related viruses in man and animals. *Hepatology,* **2**, 1s–9s

37. Harris, C. C. and Sun, T-t. (1984). Multifactorial etiology of human liver cancer. *Carcinogenesis,* **5**, 697–701

38. Harris, C. C. and Sun, T-t. (1986). Interactive effects of chemical carcinogenesis and hepatitis B virus in the pathogenesis of hepatocellular carcinoma. *Cancer Surveys,* **5**, 765–80

39. Chisari, F. V., Filippi, P., Buras, J., McLachlan, A., Popper, H., Pinkert, C. A., Palmitter, R. D. and Brinster, R. L. (1987). Structural and pathological effects of synthesis of hepatitis B virus large envelope polypeptide in transgenic mice. *Proc. Natl. Acad. Sci. USA,* **84**, 6909–13

40. Tatematsu, M., Nagamine, Y. and Farber, E. (1983). Redifferentiation as a basis for remodelling of carcinogen-induced hepatocyte nodules to normal appearing liver. *Cancer Res.,* **43**, 5049–58

41. Farber, E. (1988). Approaches to cancer prevention: introduction and perspectives. *Proc. Am. Assoc. Cancer Res.,* **29**, 527

42. Roomi, M. W., Ho, R. K., Sarma, D. S. R. and Farber, E. (1985). A common biochemical pattern in hepatocyte nodules generated in four different models in the rat. *Cancer Res.,* **45**, 564–71

43. Columbano, A., Ledda-Columbano, G. M., Coni, P. P., Feo, G., Liguori, C., Santa-Cruz, G. and Pani, P. (1985). Occurrence of cell death (apoptosis) during the invalution of liver hyperplasia. *Lab. Invest.,* **52**, 670–5

44. Harris, L., Preat, V. and Farber, E. (1987). Patterns of ligand binding to normal regenerating preneoplastic and neoplastic rat hepatocytes. *Cancer Res.,* **47**, 3954–8

45. Popper, H., Sternberg, S. S., Oser, B. C. and Oser, M. (1960). The carcinogenic effect of aramite in rats. A study of hepatic nodules. *Cancer,* **13**, 1035–46

46. Rotstein, J., Macdonald, P. D. M., Rabes, H. M. and Farber, E. (1984). Cell cycle kinetics of rat hepatocytes in early putative preneoplastic lesions in hepatogenesis. *Cancer Res.,* **44**, 2913–17

47. Stockert, R. J. and Becker, F. F. (1980). Diminished hepatic binding of protein for desialylated glycoproteins during chemical hepatocarcinogenesis. *Cancer Res.,* **40**, 3632–4

48. Evarts, R. P., Marsden, E., Hanna, P., Wirth, P. J. and Thorgeirsson, S. S. (1984). Isolation of preneoplastic rat liver cells by centrifugal elutriation and binding to asialoglycoprotein. *Cancer Res.,* **44**, 5718–24

49. Eriksson, L. C., Torndal, U-B. and Andersson, G. N. (1986). The transferrin receptor nodules: binding properties, subcellular distribution and endocytosis. *Carcinogenesis,* **7**, 1467–74

50. Schulte-Hermann, R. (1979). Reactions of the liver to injury. In Farber, E. and Fisher, M. M. (eds.) *Toxic Injury of the Liver*, p. 385. (New York: Marcel Dekker)

51. Farber, E., Rotstein, J., Harris, L., Lee, G. and Chen, Z -Y. (1988). Cell proliferation and cell loss in liver carcinogenesis: a new hypothesis. In Feo, F. (ed.) *Chemical Carcinogenesis: Models and Mechanisms*. (New York: Plenum), in press

52. Edmondson, H. A., Reynolds, T. B. and Henderson, B. (1977). Regression of liver cell adenomas associated with oral contraceptives. *Ann. Intern. Med.*, **86**, 180–2

53. Ishak, K. G. (1981). Hepatic lesions induced by anabolic and contraceptive steroids. *Semin., Liver Disease*, **1**, 116–28

54. Ishak, K. G. (1987). New developments in diagnostic liver pathology. In Farber, E. Phillips, M. J. and Kaufman, N. (eds.) *Pathogenesis of Liver Diseases*, pp. 223–373 (Baltimore: Williams and Wilkins)

55. Stout, D. L. and Becker, F. F. (1987). Heme enzyme patterns in rat liver nodules and tumors. *Cancer Res.*, **47**, 963–6

56. Bannasch, P., Hacker, H. J., Klimek, F. and Mayer, D. (1984). Hepatocellular glycogenosis and related pattern of enzymatic changes during hepatocarcinogenesis. *Adv. Enzyme Regul.*, **22**, 97–121

57. Bannasch, P., Moore, M. A., Klimek, F. and Zerban, H. (1982). Biological markers of preneoplastic foci and neoplastic nodules in rodent liver. *Toxicol. Pathol.*, **10**, 19–34

58. Schulte-Hermann, R., Timmermann-Trosiener, I. and Schuppler, J. (1984). Aberrant expression of adaptation to phenobarbital may cause selective growth of foci of altered cells in rat liver. In Börzsönyi, M., Day, N. E., Lapis, K. and Yamasaski, H. (eds.) *Models, Mechanisms and Etiology of Tumour Promotion*, IARC Scientific Publication No. 56, pp. 67–75 (Lyon: IARC)

59. Rao, M. S., Kokkinakis, D. M., Subbaro, V. and Reddy, J. K. (1987). Peroxisome proliferator-induced hepatocarcinogenesis: levels of activating and detoxifying enzymes in hepatocellular carcinomas induced by ciprofibrate. *Carcinogenesis*, **8**, 19–23

60. Roomi, M. W. (1987). Molecular Pathology of Rat Hepatic Nodules. PhD. Thesis, University of Surrey, Guildford, England.

61. Becker, F. F. and Stout, D. L. (1984). A constitutive deficiency in the monooxygenase system of spontaneous mouse liver tumors. *Carcinogenesis*, **5**, 785–8

62. Roomi, M. W., Lee, G. and Farber, E. (1986). The biochemical pattern exhibited by mouse hepatocyte nodules (HN) appears to be different than that seen in rat HN. *Fed. Proc.*, **45**, 687

63. Stout, D. L. and Becker, F. F. (1986). Heme enzyme patterns in genetically and chemically induced mouse liver tumors. *Cancer Res.*, **46**, 2756–9

64. El Mouelhi, M., Didolkar, M. S., Elias, E. G., Gungerich, F. P. and Kaufmann, F. I. (1987). Hepatic drug-metabolizing enzymes in primary and secondary tumors of human liver. *Cancer Res.*, **47**, 460–6

65. Gerber, M. A. and Thung, S. N. (1980). Enzyme patterns in human hepatocellular carcinoma. *Am. J. Pathol.*, **98**, 395–9

66. Williams, G. M. and Yamamoto, R. S. (1972). Absence of stainable iron from preneoplastic and neoplastic lesions in rat liver with 8-hydroxyquinoline-induced siderosis. *J. Natl. Cancer Inst.*, **49**, 685–92

67. Roomi, M. W., Cameron, R. G. and Farber, E. (1984). Is the reduced cytochrome P-450 content in hepatic nodules a reflection of decreased heme synthesis? *Proc. Canad. Fed. Biol. Soc.*, **27**, 161

68. Eriksson, L. C., Torndal, U-B. and Andersson, G. N. (1986). The transferrin receptor in hepatocyte nodules: binding properties, subcellular distribution and endocytosis. *Carcinogenesis*, **7**, 1467–74

69. Stout, D. L. and Becker, F. F. (1986). Xenobiotic metabolizing enzymes in genetically and chemically initiated mouse liver tumors. *Cancer Res.*, **46**, 2693–6

70. Roomi, M. W., Cameron, R. G. and Farber, E. (1987). Association between decreased cytochrome P-450 content and heme synthesis in rat hepatocyte nodules. *Fed. Proc.*, **46**, 973

71. Stout, D. L. and Becker, F. F. (1988). Normal heme synthesis in hepatic cancers despite reduced 5-aminolevulinic acid synthetase activity and iron uptake. *Proc. Am. Assoc. Cancer Res.*, **29**, 19

72. Roomi, M. W., Bacher, M. A., Gibson, G. G., Parke, D. V. and Farber, E. (1988). Decreased expression of cytochrome P-452 in the resistance phenotype characteristic of putative preneoplastic hepatocyte nodules during hepatocarcinogenesis. *Biochem, Biophys. Res. Commun.,* **152**, 921–5

73. Roomi, M. W., Vincent, S. H., Farber, E. and Muller-Eberhard, U. (1988). Decreased cytosolic levels of the heme binding Z protein in rat hepatocyte nodules and hepatocellular carcinomas. *Cancer Lett.,* in press.

74. Eriksson, L. C., Rissler, P., Andersson, N., Möller, C., Norstedt, G. and Andersson, G. (1988). The expression of cell surface receptors in regenerating and neoplastic liver tissue. *Proc. Europ. Meet. Experimental Carcinogenesis,* in press.

75. Barbacid, M. (1986). Oncogenes and human cancer: cause or consequence? *Carcinogenesis,* **7**, 1037–42

76. Barbacid, M. (1986). Mutagens, oncogenes and cancer. *Trends Genet.,* **2**, 188–92

77. Barbacid, M. (1987). *ras* genes. *Annu. Rev. Biochem.,* **56**, 779–828

78. Heldin, C. E. and Westermark, B. (1984). Growth factors: mechanism of action and relation to oncogenes. *Cell,* **37**, 9–20

79. Denhardt, D. T., Edwards, D. R. and Parfett, C. L. J. (1986). Gene expression during the mammalian cell cycle. *Biochem. Biophys. Acta,* **865**, 83–125

80. Kaczmarek, L. (1986). Biology of disease: protooncogene expression during the cell cycle. *Lab. Invest.,* **54**, 365–76

81. Thompson, N. L., Mead, J. E., Braun, L., Goyette, M., Shank, P. R. and Fausto, N. (1986). Sequential protooncogene expression during rat liver regeneration. *Cancer Res.,* **46**, 3111–17

82. Fox, T. R. and Watanabe, P. G. (1985). Detection of a cellular oncogene in spontaneous liver tumors in B6CF mice. *Science,* **288**, 596–7

83. Reynolds, S. H., Stowers, S. J., Maronpot, R. R., Aaronson, S. A. and Anderson, M. W. (1986). Detection and identification of activated oncogenes in spontaneously occurring benign and malignant hepatocellular tumors of B6C3F1 mouse. *Proc. Natl. Acad. Sci. USA,* **83**, 33–7

84. Fox, T. R., Schumann, A. M. and Watanabe, P. G. (1987). Activation of a cellular proto-oncogene in spontaneous liver tumor tissue of the B6C3F$_1$ mouse. *Arch. Toxicol.,* Suppl., **10**, 217–27

85. Reynolds, S. H., Stowers, S. J., Patterson, R., Maronpot, R. R., Aaronson, S. A. and Anderson, M. W. (1987). Activated oncogenes in B6C3F$_1$ mouse liver tumors: implications for risk assessment. *Science,* **237**, 1309–16

86. Wiseman, R. W., Stowers, S. J., Miller, E. C., Anderson, M. W. and Miller, J. A. (1986). Activating mutations of the Ha-*ras* proto-oncogene in chemically induced hepatomas of the male B6C3F$_1$ mouse. *Proc. Natl. Acad. Sci. USA,* **83**, 5825–9

87. Wiseman, R. W., Stewart, B. C., Grenier, D., Miller, E. C. and Miller, J. A. (1987). Characterization of c-Ha-*ras* proto-oncogene in chemically induced hepatomas of the B6C3F$_1$ mouse. *Proc. Am. Assoc. Cancer Res.,* **28**, 147

88. Stowers, S. J., Wiseman, R. W., Ward, J. M., Miller, E. C., Miller, J. A., Anderson, M. W. and Eva, A. (1988). Detection of activated proto-oncogenes in N-nitrosodiethylamine-induced liver tumors: a comparison between B6C3F$_1$ mice and Fischer 344 rats. *Carcinogenesis,* **9**, 271–6

89. McMahon, G., Hanson, L., Lee, J. and Wogan, G. N. (1986). Identification of an activated c-Ki-*ras* oncogene in rat liver tumors induced by aflatoxin B$_1$. *Proc. Natl. Acad. Sci. USA,* **83**, 9418–22

90. Cote, G. J., Lastra, B. A., Cook, J. R., Huang, D-P. and Chiu, J-F. (1985). Oncogene expression in rat hepatomas and during hepatocarcinogenesis. *Cancer Lett.,* **26**, 121–7

91. Corral, M., Tichonicky, L., Gugen-Guillouzo, C., Corcos, D., Raymondjean, M., Paris, B., Kruh, J. and Defer, N. (1985). Expression of c-*fos* oncogene during hepatocarcinogenesis, liver regeneration and in synchronized HTC cells. *Exp. Cell Res.,* **160**, 427–34

92. Dragani, T. A., Manenti, G., Della-Porta, G., Gattoni-Celli, S. and Weinstein, I. B. (1986). Expression of retroviral sequences and oncogenes in murine hepatocellular tumors. *Cancer Res.,* **46**, 1915–19

93. Ishikawa, F., Takaku, F., Nagao, M., Hayashi, K., Takayama, S. and Sigimura, T. (1985). Activated oncogenes on a rat hepatocellular carcinoma induced by 2-amino-3-

methylimidazo[4,5-f]quinoline. *Gann,* **76,** 425–8

94. Ishikawa, F., Takaku, F., Hayashi, K., Nagao, M. and Sugimura, T. (1986). Activation of rat c-*raf* during transfection of hepatocellular carcinoma DNA. *Proc. Natl. Acad. Sci. USA,* **83,** 3209–12

95. Beer, D. G., Schwarz, M., Sawada, N. and Pitot, H. C. (1986). Expression of H-*ras* and c-*myc* proto-oncogenes in isolated γ-glutamyltranspeptidase-positive rat hepatocytes and in hepatocellular carcinomas induced by diethylnitrosamine. *Cancer Res.,* **46,** 2435–41

96. Lee, G. and Farber, E. (1988). Expression of cell cycle dependent (CCD) gene in hepatocyte nodules during hepatocarcinogenesis. *Proc. Am. Assoc. Cancer Res.,* **29,** 143

97. Maronpot, R. R., Reynolds, S. H. and Anderson, M. W. (1987). Activation of the k-*ras* proto-oncogene in rat and mouse lung tumors induced by chronic exposure to tetranitromethane. *Cancer Res.,* **47,** 3212–19

98. Balmain, A., Ramsden, M., Bowden, G. T. and Smith, J. (1984). Activation of the mouse cellular Harvey-*ras* gene in chemically induced benign skin papillomas. *Nature,* **307,** 658–60

99. Brodeur, G. M. (1987). The involvement of oncogenes and suppressor genes in human neoplasia. *Adv. Pediatr.,* **34,** 1–44

100. Feo, F., Garcea, R., Daino, L., Pascale, R., Frassetto, S., Cozzolino, R., Vannini, M. G., Ruggiu, M. E., Simile, M. and Puddu, M. (1988). S-adenosylmethionine antipromotion and antiprogression effort in hepatocarcinogenesis; its association with inhibition of gene expression. In Feo, F., Pani, P., Columbano, A. and Garcea, R. (eds.) *Chemical Carcinogenesis: Models and Mechanisms,* (New York: Plenum Press) in press

101. Semple, E., Hayes, M. A., Rushmore, T. H., Harris, L. and Farber, E. (1987). Mitogenic activity in platelet-poor plasma from rats with persistent liver nodules or liver cancer. *Biochem. Biophys. Res. Commun.,* **148,** 449–55

25
Regulation of liver growth: A comparison between liver regeneration and carcinogenesis

N. FAUSTO AND J. E. MEAD

INTRODUCTION

The analysis of the mechanisms that regulate the proliferation of liver cells is a biological problem with direct applications in clinical medicine. From a basic science perspective, understanding these mechanisms is of special interest because hepatocytes, although quiescent in livers of adult humans and animals, do not lose their proliferative capacity. Using hepatocytes one can study, both *in vivo* and in primary culture, the steps that enable a non-replicating cell to enter the cell cycle and progress to DNA synthesis within its physiological state. This is in contrast with the usual systems employed for cell cycle studies which make use of continuously proliferating cell lines that lack corresponding *in vivo* models.

Liver cell replication plays an important role in determining the outcome and patient survival in many hepatic diseases. Yet, the management of these conditions is limited to supportive therapy. The long range expectation of experimental studies of liver regeneration is that the work will lead to the identification of factors which can be used clinically to modulate cell proliferation (positively or negatively) in patients with liver disease. Moreover, as hepatocyte proliferation is essential for the development of hepatocellular carcinomas regardless of cause, it is expected that successful interference with cell proliferation should ultimately stop the neoplastic process.

In experimental animals, hepatocyte proliferation can be easily triggered by resection of part of the organ (partial hepatectomy) or in response to hepatic cell death, although non-necrotizing agents can also induce a replicative response. We have used liver regeneration after partial hepatectomy in rats to study the control of liver cell replication. The operation (resection of 70% of the liver) consists in the removal of entire lobes by ligating their vascular pedicles[1]. The liver lobes that remain in place are intact: there is no cut surface or wound and consequently no healing or inflammatory phenomena. Some important properties of liver regeneration after partial hepatectomy in rats should be emphasized:

1. The growth response is rapid and perfectly regulated.
2. Initially, only hepatocytes replicate, but non-parenchymal cells also divide after a lag of 2–3 days[2].
3. Hepatocyte replication does not start until 12–14 hours after the operation; it is a reasonably synchronous process which reaches a maximum 24 hours after partial hepatectomy[3].
4. The growth process ceases in about 10 days, when the original liver mass is restored (± 10%).
5. The lobes removed at the operation do not grow back; the growth response takes place in the lobes not removed at surgery (compensatory growth).

Liver regeneration after partial hepatectomy is the 'purest' system for the study of liver cell replication *in vivo*. It corresponds to situations in clinical medicine where a portion of the liver containing a tumour nodule is resected or to cases in which the organ is split for transplantation into two donors[4]. More often, however, hepatocyte replication occurs in livers in which necrosis and inflammation are present. It is our belief that the knowledge gained by studying liver regeneration after partial hepatectomy can be applied to these more complex situations, both in humans and in experimental animals.

GROWTH REGULATORY SIGNALS DURING LIVER REGENERATION

The most fascinating problem in liver regeneration is identifying the signals that control the response. Given its precise regulation and predictable end point, it is most likely that the growth process involves both positive and negative signals, that is, those which trigger hepatocyte DNA replication and others which terminate the replicative wave[5,6]. To identify such signals, one can search for the signals themselves or look for their potential effects on the target cells. We adopted the second strategy and assumed that the pattern of expression of proto-oncogenes could provide clues regarding the signals sensed by hepatocytes as they enter the cell cycle and eventually replicate. This indeed proved to be the case.

The expression of proto-oncogenes after partial hepatectomy has 3 major characteristics: it is specific (*fos, myc, p53* and *ras* genes are involved but not *src, mos* or *abl*), it is sequential (following the sequence *fos, myc, p53, ras*) and it is regulated (for each gene there is a limited defined period of time when expression is increased)[7]. Based on these results we proposed that the pre-replicative phase of liver regeneration involves a priming phase corresponding to the entrance of hepatocytes into the cell cycle (associated with elevated expression of c-*fos* and c-*myc* and perhaps other proto-oncogenes) and a second phase in which primed hepatocytes progress to the S phase[5,8]. Given the precise nature of the regenerative response, we postulated that in the progression phase, both positive and negative signals involving autocrine or paracrine circuits may be activated. Thus, a basic tenet of this hypothesis is that the actual control of liver regeneration resides in the liver through mediators produced by hepatocytes and/or non-parenchymal cells. We searched for such mediators and determined whether several growth factors which have been recently purified and fully characterized could play a role in liver regeneration. We found that the transforming growth factors α and ß (TGF-α and TGF-ß)[9,10] may regulate liver regeneration by acting respectively as a stimulator and inhibitor of hepatocyte DNA replication.

TRANSFORMING GROWTH FACTORS α AND ß (TGF-α AND TGF-ß) AS GROWTH MODULATORS IN THE REGENERATING LIVER

TGF-α

Little TGF-α mRNA is detected in normal livers, livers of sham-operated rats or regenerating livers at 1–12 hours after partial hepatectomy. After approx-

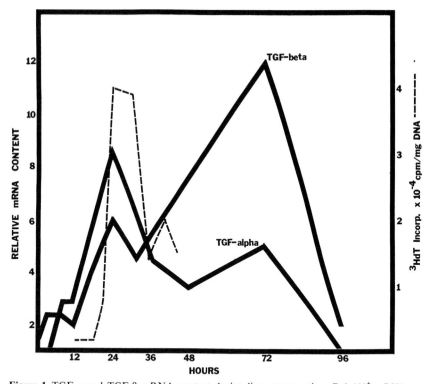

Figure 1 TGF-α and TGF-ß mRNA content during liver regeneration. Poly(A)$^+$ mRNA was isolated from livers of partially hepatectomized rats at the times indicated on the abscissa and hybridized with [^{32}P]TGF-α and [^{32}P]TGF-ß probes using the Northern blot technique. The ordinate (left hand) shows TGF-α and TGF-ß mRNA content in regenerating livers determined by densitometric scanning of the gels expressed as relative amounts in relationship to those of normal (or sham-operated) rats. The dashed line shows the time of DNA synthesis during liver regeneration (right-hand ordinate)

Table 1 Differential effects of transforming growth factors α and ß in the liver

Parameter	TGF-α	TGF-ß
Maximal mRNA expression during liver regeneration	24 hours	72 hours
Localization of mRNA	hepatocytes	non-parenchymal cells (endothelial)
Type of receptor	same as EGF	specific
Modulation of receptor during liver regeneration	down-regulation	induction of high affinity sites (?)
Effect on hepatocytes in culture	stimulates DNA synthesis	inhibits DNA synthesis

imately 12 hours of regeneration, TGF-α mRNA begins to increase (Figure 1) with a time course which parallels almost exactly the curve for the incorporation of [^{3}H]TdR into DNA in regenerating livers. (Mead and Fausto[43]). The mRNA reaches a maximum (9–10 fold above normal) at 24 hours, the time of the peak of DNA synthesis, with a second elevation of lesser magnitude at 72 hours. Northern blot analysis of RNA obtained from hepatocytes and non-parenchymal cells purified from regenerating livers showed that TGF-α mRNA is made by hepatocytes. We then turned to the analysis of the effects of TGF-α on hepatocytes in culture and demonstrated that:

1. TGF-α stimulates DNA synthesis in isolated hepatocytes in primary culture.
2. The stimulation is greater than that caused by EGF which is considered as a probable 'physiological' mediator of DNA synthesis.
3. TGF-α induces its own mRNA in cultured hepatocytes.

These effects point to the possibility that TGF-α functions as an autocrine stimulator of hepatocyte proliferation[6]. This notion is strengthened by the finding that hepatocytes contain receptors for TGF-α (same receptors as for EGF), and that the number of TGF-α/EGF receptors decreases during liver regeneration[11] at the same time that the abundance of the TGF-α/EGF receptor mRNA increases[12]. This suggests that down-regulation of the receptor induced by a ligand may occur in the regenerating liver. Since liver and serum EGF concentrations do not change in the first 24 hours after partial hepatectomy while TGF-α mRNA and peptide show a significant increase, we propose that the 'physiological' ligand for the receptor during liver regeneration might be TGF-α and not EGF.

TGF-ß

In contrast to TGF-α, TGF-ß is a potent inhibitor of hepatocyte proliferation[13-15]. Approximately 40 pM/ml is sufficient to block 50% of the DNA response elicited by EGF or TGF-α in cultured hepatocytes[16]. Surprisingly however, TGF-ß mRNA also increases during liver regeneration (Figure 1) suggesting that the synthesis of an inhibitor is activated in a tissue stimulated to undergo non-neoplastic growth. In contrast to TGF-α, TGF-ß mRNA reaches a maximum 72 hours after partial hepatectomy, that is, 2 days later than the peak of hepatocyte DNA synthesis (Figure 1). A further distinction between the regulation of the two growth factors in the liver (Table 1) is that their site of synthesis differs: while TGF-α mRNA is present in hepatocytes, TGF-ß mRNA is synthesized in non-parenchymal cells and is most abundant in sinusoidal cells[16]. Although hepatocytes do not make TGF-ß mRNA (and presumably do not synthesize the corresponding peptide) they contain receptors for the factor and respond to it. Preliminary results indicate that the affinity of receptors for TGF-ß in rat liver may increase after partial hepatectomy, starting at 12–24 hours after the operation (Gruppuso, Mead and Fausto, submitted). Thus, TGF-ß appears to function as a paracrine inhibitor of hepatocyte DNA synthesis which is activated during liver regeneration, perhaps to prevent uncontrolled proliferation[16]. A similar function for TGF-ß has been postulated in the case of growth stimulated lymphocytes[17]. Opposing effects of TGF-α and TGF-ß in modulating growth have also been described in mouse keratinocytes in culture[18].

LOCAL REGULATION AND HUMORAL FACTORS IN HEPATIC GROWTH

If TGFs made locally in the liver do indeed control some key steps of the regenerative response after partial hepatectomy, it is necessary to reconcile these findings with well-known views regarding humoral control of liver regeneration[19]. In the first place, the time course of their actions indicates that TGFs do not trigger the process but rather act later, probably on hepatocytes which have already advanced from G_0 to G_1. Thus, humoral factors might initiate regeneration perhaps by inducing a 'primed' state in hepatocytes which then become competent to enter the cell cycle. At some point in this sequence, hepatocytes begin to synthesize and/or respond to TGFs. However, the existence of factors in the serum of partially hepatectomized animals capable of inducing hepatic DNA synthesis, is not in itself proof that such serum factors are responsible for the initiation of liver regeneration. For instance, it is conceivable that factors which appear in the serum are actually synthesized and released by the regenerating liver. Additionally, factors which are normally metabolized in the liver may accumulate in the serum of partially hepatectomized animals as a result of the decreased hepatic mass.

As mentioned earlier, hepatocyte proliferation in humans most commonly occurs in livers where necrotic and inflammatory processes are also present. None of the existing experimental models approximates the complexity of these clinical situations. Nevertheless, it is of interest to speculate whether the regulatory mechanisms which we have described for liver regeneration after partial hepatectomy would be similar to liver growth which occurs after administration of necrogenic agents to rats. More likely than not, the triggering event for the regenerative response in injured livers is a local rather than a humoral stimulus. It has been shown that after carbon tetrachloride administration to rats, proto-oncogene expression in the liver follows the same sequence as that observed after partial hepatectomy although with a different time course[20]. It seems reasonable to expect that, despite the differences which may exist in the mechanisms which trigger liver growth after partial hepatectomy and necrogenic injury, TGFs would be active participants in both types of growth. Moreover, in cases where hepatic fibrosis is a major component of the response to injury, TGF-ß is likely to function as an important mediator since this growth factor induces the synthesis of collagens and fibronectin[21].

THE EXISTENCE OF 'STEM CELLS' IN ADULT LIVER AND THEIR IMPLICATION FOR STUDIES OF LIVER INJURY AND CARCINOGENESIS

In the compensatory growth which follows partial hepatectomy, DNA replication occurs at least once in almost 95% of hepatocytes (in the young rat)[22]. Thus, in this growth response hepatocyte proliferation is not confined to a special cellular compartment that might contain 'stem cells'. However, during growth of the liver induced by necrogenic agents, such as carbon tetrachloride and galactosamine, a rather unique kind of cell can be detected[23-25]. These cells resemble bile ductular cells morphologically but, in contrast to typical biliary cells, they are capable of synthesizing alpha-fetoprotein (AFP) and albumin. In fact, the increase in AFP which takes place in the liver after galactosamine administration[25] (and probably also after carbon tetrachloride injury) is primarily due to the synthesis of AFP by these epithelial cells. Such cells have phenotypic traits of both immature and fully differentiated hepatocytes yet differ from hepatocytes in their size, overall morphology and ultrastructure.

Two major questions arise regarding these cells: (a) their site of origin and (b) their biological potential. Matters dealing with the origin of the cells and their identification during development of the liver will not be explored here. Suffice to say however, that in the liver of early mouse embryos, AFP-containing precursor cells generate both hepatocytes and intra-hepatic bile ducts[26]. The question of the biological potential of liver epithelial cells is better discussed in the context of hepatocarcinogenesis and the issue of cell lineages in liver neoplasia. It is a common observation that such cells (generally referred to as 'oval cells') become abundant in the liver of animals given a diverse range of chemical carcinogens[27,28]. At the same time, it is also known that the proliferation of oval cells, although a frequent phenomenon, is not required for liver carcinogenesis. However, in azo dye carcinogenesis transition between these cells and hepatocytes can be observed even by light microscopy[29,30].

Liver epithelial cells obtained from normal and carcinogen-treated animals have been the subject of extensive studies during the last few years. They have been purified, characterized, maintained in culture, probed with monoclonal antibodies, and transformed by chemicals and oncogenes[31-41]. The general

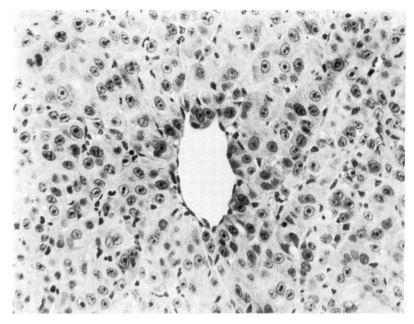

Figure 2 Well-differentiated hepatocellular carcinoma produced by the subcutaneous injection into nude mice of oval cells transfected with the EJ oncogene

conclusions from these studies are that liver epithelial cells: (a) have pheno-typic traits and biological potential which place them in the category of stem cells for the hepatocytic lineage; and (b) proliferate mostly under conditions where hepatocyte replication is inhibited (hence the term 'facultative stem cells').

We have examined the biological potential of epithelial cells which proliferate in the liver of rats fed a carcinogenic diet containing 0.5% ethionine and is deficient in choline. These cells were purified by centrifugal elutriation from livers of rats fed the carcinogenic diet for 2–6 weeks. The methods for cell isolation (which have been published in detail) involved digestion of the liver with collagenase and treatment of the undigested remnant with pronase, DNase and collagenase[31,32]. After separation of the cell suspension by centrifugal elutriation, the final fraction was completely free of hepatocytes but contaminated with about 10% Kupffer cells. These cells were placed in culture and became immortalized and clonogenic, a further assurance that no hepatocytes were present in the cultures. Although immortalized, the cells are not tumorigenic and do not grow in soft agar. After the 50th passage the cells can grow in soft agar if EGF is present but even then, they are not tumorigenic in nude mice[40].

We transfected cells from the liver epithelial cell line LE/6 at its 25th passage with plasmids containing the normal c-Ha-*ras* gene or the activated oncogene EJ-*ras*[40,41]. Markers for drug selection ('neo' gene) were introduced either by co-transfection with another plasmid or by the transfection with

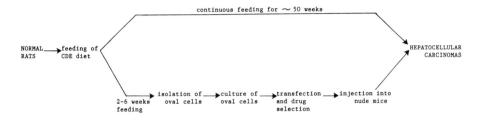

Figure 3 Outline of studies comparing the induction of hepatocellular carcinomas *in vivo* in rats fed a carcinogenic diet and the production of similar tumours by oncogene-transfected oval cells

single vectors containing both *ras* and *neo* genes. The epithelial cells transfected with neo genes or the normal c-*ras* gene did not produce tumours when inoculated into nude mice. In contrast, cells from the same line transfected with the EJ-*ras* gene (the activated oncogene from c-Ha-*ras*, isolated from a bladder carcinoma cell line) produced tumours upon injection in nude mice. Most importantly, all of the tumours were hepatocytic and at least 4/8 tumours proved to be well-differentiated hepatocellular carcinomas (Figure 2)[40]. The hepatocellular carcinomas and the cell lines derived from them have now been extensively characterized as to their histochemical properties, presence of mRNAs for AFP and albumin, and reactivity to various monoclonal antibodies which recognize different cell types in rat liver[41]. The results of these experiments leave little doubt that liver epithelial cells transfected with an oncogene have the capacity to generate hepatocellular carcinomas which are practically identical to those which develop *in vivo* in the liver of rats treated with chemical carcinogens (Figure 3).

SUMMARY

During liver regeneration after partial hepatectomy fully differentiated hepatocytes undergo DNA synthesis. Together with the replication of non-parenchymal cells and the synthesis of cell matrix, hepatocyte proliferation restores the organ to its original mass. We postulate that after partial hepatectomy, the progression of 'primed' hepatocytes into DNA synthesis is regulated by TGF-α acting as a positive autocrine mediator and that the eventual cessation of hepatocyte DNA synthesis is modulated by TGF-ß, acting as a negative paracrine mediator. These growth factors are also likely to regulate some phases of liver growth occurring after necrogenic injury. However, in certain types of injury and models of carcinogenesis (perhaps in cases when hepatocyte replication is inhibited) a special type of liver epithelial cell proliferates. Such cells appear to function as facultative stem cells and when transformed by oncogenes give rise to hepatocellular carcinomas. Although such cells have been studied mainly in relationship to liver carcinogenesis, they may be a component of the response of the liver to common types of injury. Similar cells have been recently identified in liver specimens from patients with various non-neoplastic hepatic diseases[42].

300

References

1. Higgins, G. M. and Anderson, R. M. (1931). Experimental pathology of the liver. 1. Restoration of the liver of the white rat following surgical removal. *Arch. Pathol.,* **12,** 1986–2002
2. Grisham, J. W. (1962). Morphologic study of deoxyribonucleic acid synthesis and cell proliferation in regenerating rat liver: autoradiography with thymidine-H^3. *Cancer Res.,* **22,** 842–9
3. Bucher, N. L. R. and Malt, R. (1971). *Regeneration of Liver and Kidney.* (Boston: Little, Brown & Co.)
4. Kam, I., Lynch, S., Svanas, G., Todo, S., Polimeno, L., Francavilla, A., Penkrot, R. J., Takaya, S., Ericzon, B. G., Starzl., T. E. and Van Thiel, D. H. (1987). Evidence that host size determines liver size: studies in dogs receiving orthotopic liver transplants. *Hepatology,* **7,** 362–6
5. Fausto, N., Mead, J. E., Braun, L., Thompson, N. L., Panzica, M., Goyette, M., Bell, G. I. and Shank, P. R. (1987). Protooncogene expression and growth factors during liver regeneration. *Symp. Fundam. Cancer Res.,* **39,** 69–86
6. Fausto, N. and Mead, J. E. (1989). Regulation of liver growth: protooncogenes and transforming growth factors. *Lab. Invest.,* **60,** 4–13
7. Thompson, N. L., Mead, J. E., Braun, L., Goyette, M., Shank, P. R. and Fausto, N. (1986). Sequential protooncogene expression during rat liver regeneration. *Cancer Res.,* **46,** 3111–17
8. Fausto, N. and Shank, P. R. (1987). Analysis of protooncogene expression during liver regeneration and hepatocarcinogenesis. In Okuda, K. and Ishak, K. G. (eds.) *Neoplasms of the Liver,* pp. 57–69. (Tokyo: Springer-Verlag)
9. Roberts, A. B. and Sporn, M. B. (1985). Transforming growth factors. *Cancer Surveys,* **4,** 683–705
10. Goustin, A. S., Leof, E. B., Shipley, G. D. and Moses, H. L. (1986). Growth factors and cancer. *Cancer Res.,* **46,** 1015–29
11. Earp, H. S. and O'Keefe, E. J. O. (1981). Epidermal growth factor receptor number decreases during rat liver regeneration. *J. Clin. Invest.,* **67,** 1580–3
12. Johnson, A. C., Garfield, S. H., Merlino, G. T. and Pastan, I. (1988). Expression of epidermal growth factor receptor proto-oncogene mRNA in regenerating rat liver. *Biochem. Biophys. Res. Commun.,* **150,** 412–18
13. Nakamura, T., Tomita, Y., Hirai, R., Yamaoka, K., Kaji, K. and Ichihara, A. (1985). Inhibitory effect of transforming growth factor-ß on DNA synthesis of adult rat hepatocytes in primary culture. *Biochem. Biophys. Res. Commun.,* **133,** 1042–50
14. Carr, B. I., Hayashi, I., Branum, E. L. and Moses, H. L. (1986). Inhibition of DNA synthesis in rat hepatocytes by platelet-derived type ß transforming growth factor. *Cancer Res.,* **46,** 2330–4
15. McMahon, J. B., Richards, W. L., del Campo, A. A., Song, M-K. H. and Thorgeirsson, S. S. (1987). Differential effects of transforming growth factor ß on proliferation of normal and malignant rat liver epithelial cells in culture. *Cancer Res.,* **46,** 4665–71
16. Braun, L., Mead, J. E., Panzica, M., Mikumo, R., Bell, G. I. and Fausto, N. (1988). Transforming growth factor ß mRNA increases during liver regeneration: A possible paracrine mechanism of growth regulation. *Proc. Natl. Acad. Sci. USA,* **85,** 1539–43
17. Kehrl, J. H., Wakefield, L. M., Roberts, A. B., Jakowlew, S., Alvarez-Mon, M., Derynck, R., Sporn, M. B. and Fauci, A. S. (1986). Production of transforming growth factor-beta by human T lymphocytes and its potential role in the regulation of T cell growth. *J. Exp. Med.,* **163,** 1037–50
18. Coffey, R. J. Jr., Sipes, N. J., Bascom, C. C., Graves-Deal, R., Pennington, C. Y., Weissman, B. E. and Moses, H. L. (1988). Growth modulation of mouse keratinocytes by transforming growth factors. *Cancer Res.,* **48,** 1596–1602
19. Moolten, F. L. and Bucher, N. L. R. (1967). Regeneration of rat liver: transfer of a humoral agent by cross circulation. *Science,* **158,** 272–3
20. Goyette, M., Petropoulos, C. J., Shank, P. R. and Fausto, N. (1984). Regulated transcription of c-Ki-*ras* and c-*myc* during compensatory growth of rat liver. *Mol. Cell. Biol.,* **4,** 1493–8
21. Sporn, M. B., Roberts, A. B., Wakefield, L. M. and de Crombrugghe, B. (1987). Some

recent advances in the chemistry and biology of transforming growth factor-beta. *J. Cell Biol.,* **105**, 1039–45

22. Fabrikant, J. I. (1969). Size of proliferating pools in regenerating liver. *Exp. Cell Res.,* **55**, 277–9

23. Petropoulos, C. J., Yaswen, P., Panzica, M. and Fausto, N. (1985). Cell lineages in liver carcinogenesis: possible clues from studies of the distribution of α-fetoprotein RNA sequences in cell populations isolated from normal, regenerating and preneoplastic livers. *Cancer Res.,* **45**, 5762–8

24. Engelhardt, N. V., Baranov, V. N., Lazareva, M. N. and Goussev, A. I. (1984). Ultrastructural localization of alpha-fetoprotein (AFP) in regenerating mouse liver poisoned with CCl₄. *Histochemistry,* **80**, 401–7

25. Kuhlmann, W. D. and Wurster, K. (1980). Correlation of histology and alpha₁-fetoprotein resurgence in rat liver regeneration after experimental injury by galactosamine. *Virchows Arch. (A) Path. Anat. Histol.,* **387**, 47–57

26. Shiojiri, N. (1981). Enzymo- and immunocytochemical analyses of the differentiation of liver cells in the prenatal mouse. *J. Embryol. Exp. Morph.,* **62**, 139–52

27. Fausto, N., Thompson, N. L. and Braun, L. (1987). Purification and culture of oval cells from rat liver. In Pretlow, T. G. II and Pretlow, T. P. (eds.) *Cell Separation. Methods and Selected Applications,* Vol. 4, pp. 45–77. (Orlando: Academic Press)

28. Kuhlman, W. D. (1978). Localization of alpha-fetoprotein and DNA-synthesis in liver cell populations during experimental hepatocarcinogenesis in rats. *Int. J. Cancer,* **21**, 368–80

29. Inaoka, Y. (1967). Significance of the so-called oval cell proliferation during azo-dye hepatocarcinogenesis. *Gann,* **58**, 355–66

30. Farber, E. (1956). Similarities in the sequence of early histological changes induced in the liver of the rat by ethionine, 2-acetylaminofluorene and 3′-methyl-4-dimethylaminoazobenzene. *Cancer Res.,* **16**, 142–9

31. Yaswen, P., Hayner, N. T. and Fausto, N. (1984). Isolation of oval cells by centrifugal elutriation and comparison with other cell types purified from normal and preneoplastic livers. *Cancer Res.,* **44**, 324–31

32. Hayner, N. T., Braun, L., Yaswen, P., Brooks, M. and Fausto, N. (1984). Isozyme profiles of oval cells, parenchymal cells and biliary cells isolated by centrifugal elutriation from normal and preneoplastic livers. *Cancer Res.,* **44**, 332–8

33. Sirica, A. E. and Cihla, H. P. (1984). Isolation and partial characterization of oval and hyperplastic bile ductular cell-enriched populations from the livers of carcinogen and non-carcinogen-treated rats. *Cancer Res.,* **44**, 3454–66

34. Germain, L., Goyette, R. F. and Marceau, N. (1985). Differential cytokeratin and α-fetoprotein expression in morphologically distinct epithelial cells emerging at the early stage of rat hepatocarcinogenesis. *Cancer Res.,* **45**, 673–81

35. Sells, M. A., Katyal, S. L., Shinozuka, H., Estes, L. W., Sell, S. and Lombardi, B. (1981). Isolation of oval cells and transitional cells from the livers of rats fed the carcinogen D,L-ethionine. *J Natl. Cancer Inst.,* **66**, 355–62

36. Tsao, M-S., Grisham, J. W., Nelson, K. G. and Smith, J. D. (1985). Phenotypic and karyotypic changes induced in cultured rat hepatic epithelial cells that express the 'oval' cell phenotype by exposure to N-methyl-N′-nitro-N-nitrosoguanidine. *Am. J. Pathol.,* **118**, 306–15

37. Sell, S., Karnasuta, C. and Dunsford, H. A. (1987). Monoclonal antibodies identify two possible lineages of hepatocellular carcinomas in rats induced by diethylnitrosamine. *Fed. Proc.,* **3**, 2503

38. Hixson, D. C. and Allison, J. P. (1985). Monoclonal antibodies recognizing oval cells induced in the livers of rats by N-2-fluorenylacetamide or ethionine in a choline-deficient diet. *Cancer Res.,* **45**, 3750–60

39. Tsao, M-S. and Grisham, J. W. (1987). Hepatocarcinomas, cholangiocarcinomas and hepatoblastomas produced by chemically transformed cultured rat liver epithelial cells. A light and electron-microscopic analysis. *Am. J. Pathol.,* **127**, 168–81

40. Braun, L., Goyette, M., Yaswen, P., Thompson, N. L. and Fausto, N. (1987). Growth in culture and tumorigenicity after transfection with the *ras* oncogene of liver epithelial cells from carcinogen-treated rats. *Cancer Res.,* **47**, 4116–24

41. Goyette, M., Faris, R., Braun, L., Hixson, D. and Fausto, N. (1988). Liver epithelial cells

transfected with the *ras* oncogene produce differentiated hepatocellular carcinomas. Submitted for publication

42. Manivel, J. C., Swanson, P. E., Hagen, K., Wick, M. R. and Snover, D. C. (1988). Role of isolated cytokeratin positive liver cells in hepatocellular and ductal regeneration. Annual Meeting, International Academy of Pathology, Abstr. No. 355

43. Mead, J. E. and Fausto, N. (1989). *Proc. Natl. Acad. Sci.,* **86**, 1558–62

26
Cell proliferation and clonal development in hepatocarcinogenesis

H. M. RABES

Exposure of an organism to a hepatocarcinogen leads to initiation of selected hepatocytes. At first these cells are morphologically undetectable, and in most organs initiated cells escape detection even at later stages. In the rodent liver, however, foci of altered hepatocytes become apparent at a short time interval after initiation. There are two possibilities of how they could develop: either by a simultaneous expression in a few neighbouring hepatocytes of an aberrant enzymatic phenotype, for instance ATPase deficiency, or γ-glutamyl transferase positivity, or by clonal amplification with a single initiated hepatocyte as the cell of origin. The second possibility would imply that an initiated hepatocyte is endowed with an increased growth potential as compared with normal adult hepatocytes. Many observations suggest that foci of altered hepatocytes are putative pre-neoplastic[1] with an increased risk of liver cancer formation. However, the possibility has to be kept in mind that carcinomas may also arise from other precursor cells than localized in these foci. In a few foci, subpopulations may develop which could again originate by clonal selection from the amplified pre-neoplastic cell group and might form a nodule as a neoplastic, but pre-malignant population. The next step, in only a single or a few selected nodules, might be the start of hepatoma growth, a process which is putatively again clonal. At further stages, clonal selection might play a role also in the development of metastases. A schematic presentation of putative clonal steps during carcinogenesis in the liver is shown in Figure 1. This review is aimed at summarizing some recent data on cell proliferation and clonal selection steps during chemical liver carcinogenesis.

Initiation is a cell cycle-dependent event. Craddock and Frei[2] showed that a single injection of N-methyl-N-nitrosourea (MNU), a self-decomposing alkylating agent, induced liver tumours most effectively when given 24 hours after partial hepatectomy when the maximum number of cells is in DNA synthesis. On the basis of similar experimental data models for initiation of liver carcinogenesis have been developed, all of which combine an exposure

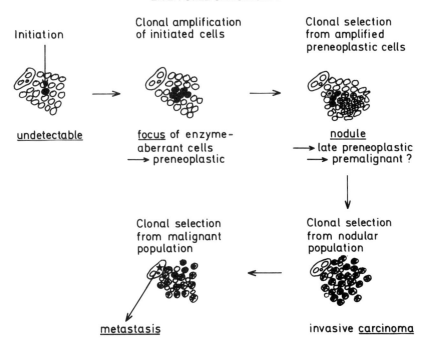

Figure 1 Scheme of putative clonal selection steps during hepatocarcinogenesis

of a single dose of a carcinogen with partial hepatectomy or toxic liver cell loss[3]. The regenerative response is obviously required for the initiating action of the carcinogen in the liver[4,5]. However, a critical evaluation of the cell kinetics after partial hepatectomy in rat liver revealed that regeneration is only a partially synchronized process. DNA synthesis starts at 15–18 hours, with a maximum at 20–27 hours in the periportal areas. Later, the wave of DNA synthesis proceeds to intermediary and perivenous parts of the lobule[6]. It remains difficult to relate in such system the initiation probability to a defined cell cycle period. With the use of hydroxyurea as a synchronizing agent, when applied continuously from 14 to 24 hours after partial hepatectomy, it was possible to delineate exactly the period of highest transformation sensitivity in the liver *in vivo*. Foci of altered hepatocytes developed at the maximum rate after N-methyl-N-nitrosourea given during late G_1/early S-phase of the cell cycle[7]. This is in agreement with data from Kaufman *et al.*[8], who obtained the same result after cell-cycle modification by hydrocortisone treatment and subsequent MNU exposure.

Alkylating carcinogens lead to adduct formation at critical sites of DNA bases, some of which are pro-mutagenic, e.g. O^6-alkylguanine or O^4-alkylthymine[9]. It has been shown that these pro-mutagenic lesions might induce base mispairing during DNA synthesis and thus might lead to permanent mutations[10]. The quantitatively most prominent pro-mutagenic lesion O^6-alkylguanine is repaired by an error-free O^6-alkylguanine DNA transferase[11].

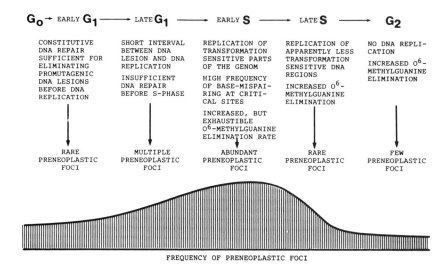

Figure 2 Summary of possible relations between DNA adduct formation, DNA repair and the cell cycle during initiation of hepatocarcinogenesis

Though the activity of this enzyme increases in rat liver after partial hepatectomy[12], the repair is not sufficient as the time interval between adduct formation and DNA synthesis is apparently too short to remove the pro-mutagenic lesion and thus prevent base-mispairing and mutation. A summary of this hypothesis is given in Figure 2.

However, not all hepatocytes in early S-phase are potential target cells for initiation. An analysis of early S-phase cells after partial hepatectomy in different parts of the liver lobule revealed that hepatocytes localized in the periportal and intermediary part of the liver lobule are more inclined to being initiated by MNU in early S-phase than cells localized at the efferent hepatic vein. Although the G_1–S transit rate of periportal and perivenous cells is similar at 16–18 hours and at 22–24 hours, respectively, a single injection of MNU at these time points after partial hepatectomy induces significantly more pre-neoplastic foci when given at 16 hours, at which time periportal hepatocytes are at G_1–S boundary[13].

We assume that besides proliferation, an additional requirement for effective initiation is clonogenic potential, and that periportal hepatocytes exceed in adult animals perivenous cells in clonogenicity.

Foci of altered hepatocytes after carcinogen exposure might represent the clonal progeny of initiated cells. With the analytical methods provided by use of chimeric or mosaic animals, this hypothesis can be tested. A few years ago a strain of mice with a mutant expression of the enzyme phosphoglycerate kinase (PGK) became available. Mutant PGK has faster electrophoretic mobility and can thus be separated from the wild-type enzyme, and the relative proportions of both enzymes can be determined[14]. The gene for PGK is X-chromosomal. Mating of male mice bearing the mutant gene for PGK, PGK-1A, with normal female mice with the wild-type PGK-1B, results in a female offspring, the cells of which contain both the parental mutant PGK-1A and the maternal wild-type PGK-1B. Due to early embryonic random inactivation of one of the two cellular X-chromosomes[15], the female F_1-generation consists of a mosaic of cells either expressing the maternal or the paternal X-chromosome, and thus the different PGKs. From such heterozygous female mice, small samples punched with cannulas of a diameter of 300 μm from cryostat liver sections 40-μm thick, reveal a PGK pattern of 11–61% PGK-1B, and between 10 and 47 coherent patches of cells expressing a single PGK type. This results in a calculated average patch size of 8 hepatocytes per patch[16]. In these female mosaic mice foci of altered hepatocytes were induced by feeding 2-acetylaminofluorene. ATPase-deficient foci were localized in cryostat sections. In congruent unstained frozen serial sections of 40-μm thickness, samples were obtained from normal and focus areas and the proportion of mutant and wild type PKG was determined. In contrast to samples obtained from normal liver, which always showed the expression of both PGK-1A and 1B, liver samples from altered hepatic foci and pre-neoplastic nodules contained either exclusively PGK-1A or PGK-1B with contamination of the opposite PGK enzyme at an average of 1.1%[16]. This result suggests that the majority of altered hepatic foci and pre-neoplastic nodules originate by clonal growth from a single cell.

As even the smallest foci which could be studied accurately with this method showed a selective expression of only one of the two enzyme allo-types, it has to be concluded that even these early pre-neoplastic foci are of single-cell origin.

It has been argued that these clonal growths might not be the result of exposure to chemical carcinogens, but merely be related to the high incidence of spontaneously occurring hepatomas in mice of C3H background. In order to meet this argument, experiments with mouse aggregation chimeras, composed of Swiss Albino and NMRI origin, were used for similar experiments. Swiss Albino mice expressed the glucose phosphate-isomerase Gpi-1A, and NMRI the allozyme Gpi-1B, which can be separated in electrophero-grams. In these mice, ATPase-deficient foci and nodules were induced by 2-acetylaminofluorene feeding. The Gpi pattern was determined in ATPase-deficient lesions and surrounding liver tissue. In normal liver, both Gpi-1A and 1B were present in the samples of a diameter of 300 μm and a thickness of 40 μm punched from unstained cryostat sections. In ATPase-deficient foci, however, either Gpi-1A or Gpi-1B was selectively expressed (Figure 3; Fundele, Krietsch and Rabes, unpublished observations). It is evident from these results that ATPase-deficient foci and nodules are indeed monoclonal in origin, irrespective of the mouse strain used.

In the meantime, morphological studies have confirmed the hypothesis of monoclonal origin of pre-neoplastic foci. Howell et al.[17] used female mice heterozygous for the sparse-fur strain. In this strain, histochemical techniques can be applied in heterozygotes to differentiate in the liver section between liver cells expressing the normal and abnormal form of the X-linked ornithine

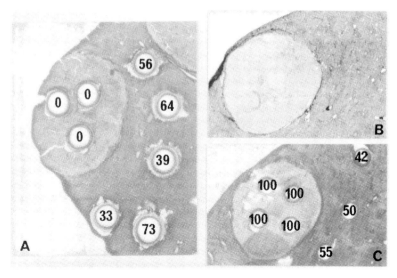

Figure 3 Glucose phosphate isomerase (Gpi) pattern (percent Gpi-1A) in normal liver and ATPase-deficient pre-neoplastic liver nodules of chimeric mice composed of Swiss Albino (Gpi-1A) and NMRI (Gpi-1B) cells after 2-acetylaminofluorene exposure. Pre-neoplastic populations show a selective expression of either Gpi-1A (A) or Gpi-1B (C) in contrast to the phenotypically normal surrounding liver tissue. (A and C), 40-μm cryostat sections, counterstained for ATPase after taking punches of 300-μm diameter for Gpi-determination. (B), 8-μm ATPase-stained serial section adjacent to the section of (C), for comparison (Fundele, Krietsch and Rabes, unpublished observations)

carbamoyl transferase. Liver tumours and pre-stages were induced by N-nitrosodiethylamine. In contrast to the mixed ornithine carbamoyl transferase pattern in normal liver of heterozygous female mice, small foci and larger pre-neoplastic nodules revealed either a selective expression of the normal, or the mutant ornithine carbamoyl transferase. Iannaccone and his co-workers[18,19] came to the same conclusions using chimeric rats containing two cell populations genetically distinguished by alleles of the major histocompatibility complex. With monoclonal antibodies directed to distinctive class I MHC alloantigens they showed that γ-glutamyltransferase positive foci in the liver induced by N-nitrosodiethylamine and subsequent phenobarbital promotion expressed only one of the two alleles.

The fact that even the smallest foci which might have escaped the biochemical determinations reported for PGK- or Gpi-heterozygotes showed a consistent homogeneous enzyme expression, is a strong argument in favour of the hypothesis that liver tumours are clonal growths from their earliest stage, starting at initiation.

These findings imply that an initiated hepatocyte will be or become endowed with a proliferative advantage over normal adult hepatocytes, or, expressed in the terms of Cerutti in a recent review[20], initiated cells might become promotable, might become capable of responding to promoters of carcinogenesis, and thus proliferate. This endogenous growth advantage or promotability by exogenous factors leads to clonal growth of initiated hepatocytes in a stable proliferation-controlled organ. In a strict sense, even the earliest enzyme aberrant lesions should then be classified as aberrantly growing populations. This does not imply, however, that each focus is on a one-way street to hepatoma formation. Clonal growth is not synonymous with neoplasia; a stop of promotion or a loss of promotability may even result in regression of early lesions[21].

A crucial point in the development of foci is the fact that clonal homogeneity of an incipient focus is rapidly lost. DNA cytophotometry in single ATPase-deficient foci, induced in rat liver by a single dose of N-methyl-N-nitrosourea, showed a homogeneity of DNA content at early stages. Foci contain exclusively either diploid or tetraploid cells, with a preference of purely diploid ones[22]. However, at advanced stages, homogeneity is lost. Larger ATPase-deficient foci contain a mixture of di- and tetraploid cells and an increased number of cells in DNA synthesis[22,23]. This increasing heterogeneity indicates that enzyme aberrant pre-neoplastic populations may already possess the attributes of genetic instability. Nowell[24] proposed this term to explain the increasing diversification of tumour phenotypes and the development of tumour sub-populations with different growth and differentiation characteristics. The results discussed here indicate that similar processes may operate already early in pre-neoplastic foci and nodules. It is not possible to apply the methods of aggregation chimeras or mosaic animals for solving the question of sub-clonal progression in pre-neoplastic foci. As early stages

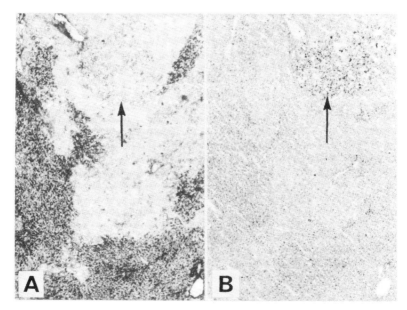

Figure 4 Development of a highly proliferating putative clonal sub-population (arrows) in an ATPase-deficient pre-neoplastic focus in rat liver. (A), ATPase-stained section after continuous feeding of diethylnitrosamine. (B), serial section, [^{3}H]thymidine autoradiogram after seven injections of [^{3}H]thymidine at 6-hour intervals to label the growth fraction (Rabes et al.[25], reprinted by permission of *Cancer Research*)

are clonal, subsequent clonal deviations cannot be evaluated with this method. However, in autoradiograms published already more than 15 years ago, sub-populations of excessive proliferative activity were demonstrated in ATPase-deficient foci[25], focus in focus or nodule in nodule as Farber and Cameron[26] have called them. This could be an equivalent of subclonal progression during pre-neoplasia (Figure 4).

A method to test a possible genetic instability of pre-neoplastic cells and development of sub-clones is the cytogenetic approach. It is impossible to study cytogenetics in pre-neoplastic foci *in vivo*. However, because of the proliferative advantage of pre-neoplastic hepatocytes, they can be propagated *in vitro* under conditions which eliminate contaminating normal adult hepatocytes. After a few weeks in primary culture, foci or proliferating cells are formed which are mechanically isolated and sub-cultured. Some of them give rise to established cell lines, which can be studied with respect to growth characteristics, tumorigenicity and chromosomal aberrations[27]. The instability of the karyotype can be demonstrated with the loss of chromosomes during subsequent passages. Besides numerical chromosomal instability cell lines obtained from pre-neoplastic liver cells show during their progression *in vitro* remarkable structural aberrations from the normal karyotype[28] (Holecek, Kerler and Rabes, in press[29]).

The fact that numerical and some structural chromosomal aberrations were found already in early passages of pre-neoplastic cells *in vitro*, suggests their preexistence *in vivo* and selection by the passages *in vitro*. It is tempting to assume that clonal selection processes as observed *in vitro* reflect similar clonal selection steps *in vivo* on the way from pre-neoplasia into hepatocarcinoma. Though still speculative, this concept is supported by the fact that initiated liver cells show a proliferative advantage, form a clonal progeny and are, during progression, unstable with respect to cytology, metabolism, intercellular contacts, karyotype, gene expression and genomic structure. In a few pre-neoplastic cell populations, such instability in connection with the enhanced proliferative activity might be responsible for the generation of a malignant clone.

Acknowledgements

Original work reported in this review was supported by grants from Deutsche Forschungsgemeinschaft and Dr. Mildred Scheel-Stiftung für Krebsforschung.

References

1. Bannasch, P. (1986). Preneoplastic lesions as end points in carcinogenicity testing. I. Hepatic preneoplasia, *Carcinogenesis*, **7**, 689–95
2. Craddock, V. M. and Frei, F. V. (1974). Induction of liver cell adenomata in the rat by a single treatment with N-methyl-N-nitrosourea given at various times after partial hepatectomy. *Br. J. Cancer*, **30**, 503–11
3. Warwick, E. (1971). Effect of the cell cycle on carcinogenesis. *Fed. Proc.*, **30**, 1760

4. Cayama, E., Tsuda, H., Sarma, D. S. R. and Farber, E. (1978). Initiation of chemical carcinogenesis requires cell proliferation. *Nature (London)*, **275**, 60–2
5. Rabes, H. M. (1979). Proliferative Vorgänge während der Frühstadien der malignen Transformation. *Verh. Dtsch. Ges. Path.*, **63**, 18–39
6. Rabes, H. M. (1978). Kinetics of hepatocellular proliferation as a function of the microvascular structure and functional state of the liver. In *Ciba Foundation Symposium 55 (new series). Hepatotrophic Factors*, pp. 31–59. Elsevier–Excerpta Medica–North Holland (New York–Amsterdam–Oxford)
7. Rabes, H. M., Müller, L., Hartmann, A., Kerler, R. and Schuster, Ch. (1986). Cell cycle-dependent initiation of ATPase-deficient populations in adult rat liver by a single dose of N-methyl-N-nitrosourea. *Cancer Res.*, **46**, 465–650
8. Kaufman, W. K., Kaufman, D. G., Rice, J. M. and Wenk, M. L. (1981). Reversible inhibition of rat hepatocyte proliferation by hydrocortisone and its effect on cell cycle-dependent hepatocarcinogenesis by N-methyl-N-nitrosourea. *Cancer Res.*, **41**, 4653–60
9. Saffhill, R., Margison, G. P. and O'Connor, P. J. (1985). Mechanisms of carcinogenesis by alkylating agents. *Biochem. Biophys. Acta*, **823**, 111–45
10. Abbott, P. J. and Saffhill, R. (1979). DNA synthesis with methylated poly(dC–dG) templates: evidence for a competitive nature to miscoding by O^6-methylguanine. *Biochem. Biophys. Acta*, **562**, 51–61
11. Pegg, A. E., Wiest, L., Foote, R. S., Mitra, S. and Perry, W. (1983). Purification and properties of O^6-methylguanine-DNA transmethylase from rat liver. *J. Biol. Chem.*, **258**, 2327–33
12. Schuster, Ch., Rode, G. and Rabes, H. M. (1985). O^6-methylguanine repair of methylated DNA *in vitro*: Cell cycle-dependent action of rat liver methyltransferase. *J. Cancer Res. Clin. Oncol.*, **110**, 98–102
13. Maguire, S. and Rabes, H. M. (1987). Transformation sensitivity in early S phase and clonogenic potential are target cell characteristics in liver carcinogenesis by N-methyl-N-nitrosourea. *Int. J. Cancer*, **39**, 385–9
14. Bücher, Th., Bender, W., Fundele, R., Hofner, H. and Linke, I. (1980). Quantitative evaluations of electrophoretic allo- and isozyme patterns. *FEBS Lett.*, **115**, 319–24
15. Lyon, M. F. (1974). Mechanisms and evolutionary origins of variable X chromosome activity in mammals. *Proc. R. Soc. Lond. (B)*, **187**, 243–68
16. Rabes, H. M., Bücher, Th., Hartmann, A., Linke, I. and Dünnwald, H. (1982). Clonal growth of carcinogen-induced enzyme-deficient preneoplastic cell populations in mouse liver. *Cancer Res.*, **42**, 3220–7
17. Howell, S., Wareham, K. A. and Williams, F. D. (1985). Clonal origin of mouse liver cell tumours. *Am. J. Pathol.*, **121**, 426–32
18. Iannaccone, P. M., Weinberg, W. C. and Deamant, F. D. (1987). On the clonal origin of tumours: a review of experimental models. *Int. J. Cancer*, **39**, 778–84
19. Weinberg, W. C., Berkwits, L. and Iannaccone, P. M. (1987). The clonal nature of carcinogen-induced altered foci of γ-glutamyl transpeptidase expression in rat liver. *Carcinogenesis*, **8**, 565–70
20. Cerutti, P. A. (1988). Response modification creates promotability in multistage carcinogenesis. *Carcinogenesis*, **9**, 519–26
21. Tatematsu, M., Nagamine, Y. and Farber, E. (1983). Redifferentiation as a basis for remodelling of carcinogen-induced hepatocyte nodules to normal-appearing liver. *Cancer Res.*, **43**, 5049–58
22. Sarafoff, M., Rabes, H. M. and Dörmer, P. (1986). Correlations between ploidy and initiation probability determined by DNA cytophotometry in individual altered hepatic foci. *Carcinogenesis*, **7**, 1191–6
23. Mori, H., Tanaka, T., Sugie, S., Takahashi, M. and Williams, G. M. (1982). DNA content of liver cell nuclei of N-2-fluorenylacetamide-induced altered foci and neoplasms in rats and human hyperplastic foci. *J. Natl. Cancer Inst.*, **69**, 1277–81
24. Nowell, P. C. (1976). The clonal evolution of tumour cell populations. *Science*, **194**, 23–8
25. Rabes, H. M., Scholze, P. and Jantsch, B. (1972). Growth kinetics of diethylnitrosamine-induced, enzyme-deficient 'preneoplastic' liver cell populations *in vivo* and *in vitro*. *Cancer Res.*, **32**, 2577–86
26. Farber, E. and Cameron, R. (1980). The sequential analysis of cancer development. *Adv. Cancer Res.*, **32**, 125

27. Kerler, R. and Rabes, H. M. (1988). Preneoplastic rat liver cells *in vitro*: Slow progression without promoters, hormones, or growth factors. *J. Cancer Res. Clin. Oncol.,* **114**, 113–23

28. Holecek, B. and Rabes, H. M. (1986). Cytogenetic analysis of normal and diethylnitrosamine-initiated preneoplastic hepatocytes. *J. Cancer Res. Clin. Oncol.,* **111** (Suppl.), S95

29. Holecek, B. U., Kerler, R. and Rabes, H. M. (1989). Chromosome analysis of a diethylnitrosamine-induced tumorigenic and a non-tumorigenic liver cell line. *Cancer Res.,* **49** (In press)

27
The regulation of cell-surface receptors in chemical hepatocarcinogenesis

L. C. ERIKSSON, U.-B. TORNDAL AND G. N. ANDERSSON

INTRODUCTION

Work with animal models and tissue cultures for the study of mechanisms involved in chemical carcinogenesis has pointed out that the processes taking place in the target cells are very much dependent on, and regulated by, the cellular environment, humoral as well as cellular matrix and cell-to-cell contact. The expression of cell receptors is assumed to determine the ability of the cell to respond to some of these environmental signals regulating cellular behaviour. Major alterations in receptor activity have been noted during functional states of the cell, such as regeneration, foetal and neonatal proliferation, ligand exposure as well as in states of tumour development[1-11]. The mechanisms involved in regulation of receptor expression, translocation or receptor modulation and the functional consequences of the alterations are very complex and not known in great detail. Processes involved are receptor synthesis and transport, availability of ligand, receptor–ligand binding, complex formation, endocytosis, dissociation of receptor–ligand complexes, degradation of receptor, receptor recycling and receptor modulation.

The transferrin receptor and the asialoglycoprotein receptor both are altered in proliferating hepatocytes and in preneoplastic liver cells, where an increase in transferrin receptor and a decrease in asialoglycoprotein receptor binding have been described[4,11,12,34]. The transferrin receptor is involved in uptake of iron by binding to, and internalizing, diferric transferrin by mechanisms of endocytosis[6,13]. The internalized complex reaches the endosomes and iron is released in the acidic compartment for uncoupling of receptor–ligand complexes. The apotransferrin–transferrin receptor complexes recirculate to the cell surface where the ligand is released in the neutral pH outside the cell, making the receptor ready to bind two new molecules of diferric transferrin. Liver nodules exhibit a storage deficiency upon exposure to excess of iron[14] and are low in iron-containing enzymes[15] and in total cellular heme[16] and heme binding protein[17].

The function of the asialoglycoprotein receptor is controversial and not known. It has been proposed that it sequesters galactose and galactosamine terminated glycoproteins from the blood for degradation in the lysosomes. The receptor–ligand complex is internalized by endocytosis, the acid-sensitive complex is dissociated in the endosomal compartment, whereafter the ligand goes to the lysosomes for degradation, while the receptor recirculates to the cell surface[18]. Both receptors are transmembrane glycoproteins with the carboxyterminal on the outside of the cell[19-21] and they are both internalizing glycoproteins by endocytosis. Still, their regulation in proliferating cells is very different. Is there a common denominator explaining this contradiction?

In this presentation alterations in transferrin receptor and asialoglycoprotein receptor expression during rat liver regeneration and hepatocarcinogenesis are discussed. Attempts are made to explain the mechanisms of receptor alterations as well as their functional relevance.

MATERIALS AND METHODS

Liver nodules and carcinomas were produced in male Wistar rats by intermittent feeding with 2-acetylaminofluorene[22]. Partial hepatectomy was performed as described by Higgins and Andersson[23]. Receptor binding was quantitated in a total membrane fraction (TPF) to estimate the total cell content of accessible binding sites. We also prepared a microsomal fraction

Table 1   Relative expression of binding sites for diferric transferrin (Fe_2Tf) and asialoorosomucoid (ASOR) in total particulate fraction and in a low-density membrane fraction enriched in endosomes in normal liver, regenerating liver and in liver nodules. The specific receptor content in normal liver is normalized to 1

Ligand or fraction	Relative receptor expression		
	Normal liver	Regenerating liver	Liver nodules
Fe_2Tf			
TPF	1	20	60
RM	1	3	31
LDMF	1	2.2	8
ASOR			
TPF	1	0.60	0.54
RM	1	0.93	0.52
LDMF	1	0.67	0.24

TPF = Total particulate fraction; RM = residual microsomes; LDMF = low-density membrane fraction.
The specific binding (pmoles Fe_2Tf or ASOR bound/mg of protein) in normal liver tissue sub-fractions was: For diferric transferrin, TPF, 5.2; RM, 14.8; LDMF, 608. For ASOR, TPF, 1.1; RM, 1.4; LDMF, 18.

and a fraction enriched in Golgi-derived membranes as well as endocytic vesicles, low-density membrane fraction. The fractionation procedures have been described in detail[11]. Radioiodinated ligands were used for the binding studies. Binding of diferric transferrin was measured according to Eriksson *et al.*[11]. Asialoglycoprotein receptors were measured by binding of asialooorosomucoid as described by Hudgin *et al.*[24]. ATP-driven proton pump activity was measured by the acridine orange method according to Stone *et al.*[35].

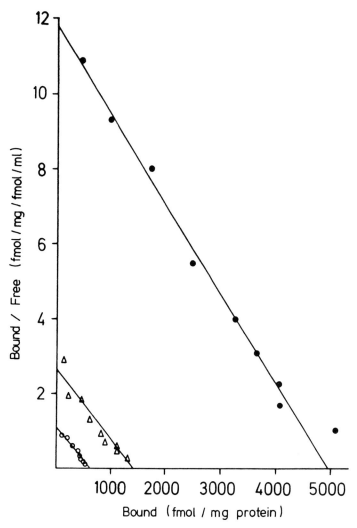

Figure 1 Scatchard analysis of the binding of diferric transferrin to low-density membrane fraction in normal liver (O—O), regenerating liver (Δ – Δ) and liver nodules (●—●). Lines were fitted using least squares fit

RESULTS AND DISCUSSION

The binding of diferric transferrin to different subfractions in normal, regenerating and nodular livers is shown in Table 1. The distribution of binding sites was heterogeneous within the cell, with a significant enrichment in an endosome-enriched low-density membrane fraction (LDMF). The pattern of intracellular distribution of diferric transferrin binding sites was almost the same in regenerating liver and in liver nodules, but the total number of receptors was increased. In nodules, the total receptor content exceeded the normal binding by 60-fold. It can be noted that the relative induction of binding sites was less pronounced in the endosome-enriched fraction in regenerating liver as well as in nodules, indicating receptor re-localization. It is interesting to see that in membranes from nodular tissue the binding to the residual microsome fraction, containing mostly endoplasmic reticulum membranes without contaminating Golgi vesicles, was higher than expected, suggesting an increase in *de novo* synthesis of transferrin binding protein.

Scatchard analysis (Figure 1) showed homogeneous receptor populations in all tissues, with straight and parallel lines. Only the number of binding sites varied in the different tissues. No significant differences could be detected in binding affinity or specificity[11]. Cross-linking experiments using disuccin-imidyl suberate showed that the radioactive ligand was associated to the same peptide bands in preparations from all three liver tissues[11]. We conclude that the properties of the binding protein in normal liver, regenerating liver and

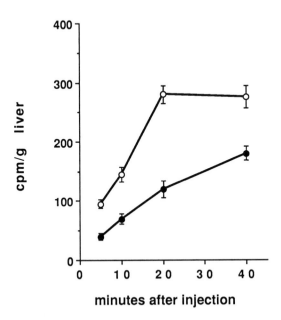

Figure 2 Uptake of [^{59}Fe]diferric transferrin in homogenates from normal liver (O—O) and liver nodules (●—●) after intra-mesenteric injection of the radioactive tracer

liver nodules are very similar, but that the number of available sites for binding is increased in regenerating liver and in liver nodules.

Uptake of iron in livers after intra-mesenteric injection of [^{59}Fe]diferric transferrin into normal and nodule-bearing rats (Figure 2) showed that the rate of accumulation of radioactivity in homogenates from liver nodules was significantly slower than that in normal liver, in spite of the increased number of available binding sites in the nodular liver tissue. It is obvious that initial rate of iron uptake was not proportional to the amount of binding sites. There are several possible explanations for the reduced uptake of iron such as receptor re-localization, deficient mechanisms of endocytosis, subnormal rate of receptor–ligand dissociation etc.

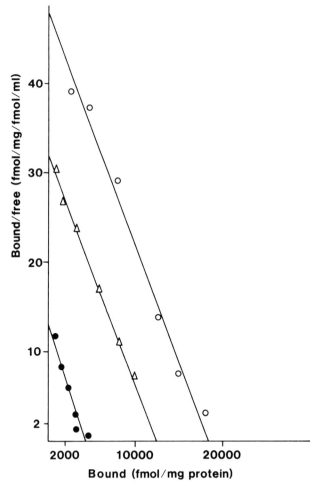

Figure 3 Scatchard analysis of asialoorosomucoid binding in low-density membrane fraction from normal liver (O—O), regenerating liver (Δ—Δ) and liver nodules (●—●). Lines were fitted using least squares fit

Regarding the asialoglycoprotein receptor measured as asialoorosomucoid binding, the highest specific binding was seen in the endosome enriched low-density membrane fraction as was true for the transferrin binder. In regenerating and nodular liver tissue the total binding to cellular membranes was reduced to around half that of normal cells. The binding in the endosome-enriched fraction of liver nodules showed a reduction of specific ligand binding down to 25% of that of normal low-density membranes. Scatchard analysis again showed homogeneous receptor populations in all three tissues, with no differences in binding affinity (Figure 3). Only the number of binding sites was altered. In contrast to what was found for diferric transferrin receptor, where no structural receptor changes were evident, disuccinimidyl suberate cross-linking experiments revealed major alterations in cross-linkable asialoorosomucoid-containing complexes (Figure 4). In normal and regenerating liver preparations, a 250000, a 110000 and an

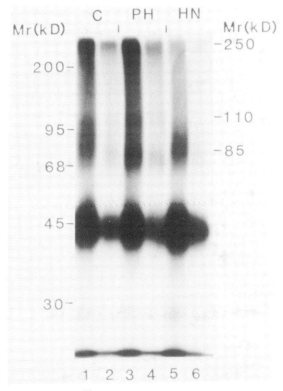

Figure 4 Affinity cross-linking of [^{125}I]ASOR to a low-density membrane fraction prepared from normal rat liver (lanes 1 and 2), regenerating liver (lanes 3 and 4) and from liver nodules (lanes 5 and 6). The incubations in lane 2, 4 and 6 contained in addition to the radioactive ligand also a 100-fold excess of unlabelled ligand. The samples were cross-linked using disuccinimidyl suberate and electrophoresed on 7.5% polyacrylamide gels containing SDS. On the left side of the autoradiogram are indicated the sizes of molecular weight standards. The positions of specifically-labelled and cross-linked receptor–ligand complexes are indicated on the right side

85000 M_r complex were found, while in the nodules the larger, presumably oligomeric complexes were not seen. It has been reported[25,26] that ligand binding to the asialoglycoprotein receptor is dependent on the formation of a hexameric receptor complex. Insufficient oligomerization therefore can be assumed to reduce the number of available binding sites even in the presence of a normal amount of receptor monomer. In fact it was recently shown by Steer *et al.*[5] that antibodies raised against the asialoglycoprotein receptor detected normal amounts of the receptor on the surface of Hep G2 cells in spite of an almost complete lack of ligand binding. The authors also found reduced cell surface sialylation and suggested defect receptor sialylation as a reason for reduced receptor affinity.

Asialoorosomucoid uptake studies *in vivo*, using intra-mesenteric injection of [^{125}I]asialoorosomucoid (Figure 5) showed a low uptake of ligand in nodular cells compared to normal cells. The differences noted reflect the difference in receptor binding activity between the two tissues. It is noteworthy that the decay of radioactivity in the nodular homogenates was also slower than normal, indicating a reduced internalization, dissociation and/or degradation of ligand. The variation with time in the blood levels of radioactivity is consistent with an almost complete single passage elimination of the ligand in the normal rat, while the capacity to bind the injected ligand in the nodule-bearing rats was significantly lower, allowing a substantial amount of the ligand to pass the liver without binding. The appearance of radioactivity in the blood at later time points represented degradation products of the injected ligand.

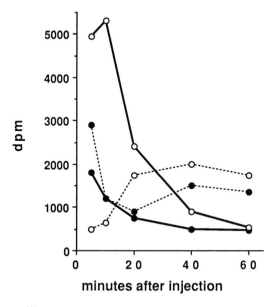

Figure 5 Uptake of [^{125}I]ASOR in homogenates from normal liver (O—O) and liver nodules (●—●) after intra-mesenteric injection of the radioactive tracer (cpm/mg of protein). Dashed lines represent the blood-levels (cpm/25 μl) of radioactivity at indicated time points

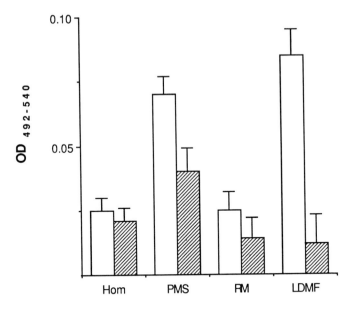

Figure 6 The proton pump activity measured as acridine orange spectral change ($OD_{462-540}$/min/mg of protein) in homogenate (Hom), post-mitochondrial supernatant (PMS), residual microsomes free from Golgi membrane and endosomes by flotation (RM) and low-density membrane fraction containing endosomes (LDMF) prepared from normal liver (open bars) and from liver nodules (filled bars)

It is suggested that intracellular dissociation of iron from the transferrin receptor and of the asialoglycoprotein receptor from the asialoglycoprotein receptor requires an acidic pH in the endosomes[13]. Elevation of endosomal pH by weak bases reduces intracellular accumulation of iron as well as increases the number of diferric transferrin binding sites and decreases the number of binding sites for asialoglycoprotein on the cell surface[27]. Is the acidification of the endosome compartment the common denominator, explaining the receptor alterations seen in liver nodules?

Figure 6 shows the activity of the proton pumps in normal and nodular liver tissue measured as spectral changes in acridine orange upon binding of protons. The difference between nodular and normal specific activity in the total particulate fraction was not very substantial, but in the low-density, endosome-enriched, membrane fraction the nodular activity was one-fifth of that found in normal liver, i.e. protonization of nodular endosomes was significantly decreased. The acidification of the endosomal and lysosomal compartments in the cell is maintained by several proton pumping membrane enzyme complexes. One of them is the ATP-driven proton-translocation pump that is abundant in lysosomal membranes. In this context it is also important to mention the transmembrane NADH diferric transferrin reductase, described in plasma-membrane fractions isolated from liver cells by Sun *et al.*[28]. This enzyme is a transmembrane, presumably 50-kDa, protein that uses intracellular NADH to reduce electron acceptors on the outside of

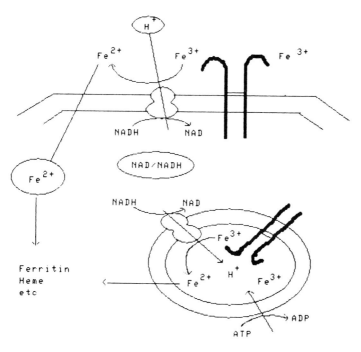

Figure 7 Schematic presentation of NADH diferric transferrin reductase and diferric transferrin receptor on the cell membrane and in endosomes. The uptake of iron via endocytosis and the acidification of the endosome compartment as well as the reduction of ferric iron is shown. See text for more details

the cell and while doing so also pumps out protons from the cytoplasm to the extracellular room[29]. It is reasonable to assume that this enzyme, a constitutive component of the plasma membrane, also could be present in the membranes of endosomes, which are derived from the cell membrane by invagination and endocytosis.

One of the most potent electron acceptors for the redox system is diferric transferrin, although other electron acceptors could be used as well[29]. Diferric transferrin reductase activity is dependent on the transferrin receptor and the activity follows the transferrin receptor expression in the cell systems investigated so far, with the exception of most tumours and tumour cell lines[30]. The trivalent iron bound to transferrin is very firmly associated with its carrier protein. The dissociation constant has been determined to between 10^{-22} and 10^{-20} at neutral pH[31]. In the acidic pH of the endosomes, pH 5.5, the trivalent iron dissociates but cannot pass the membrane in its trivalent form to reach the intracellular end points for heme synthesis in the mitochondria or for storage in ferritin. After reduction to divalent iron, membranes can be readily passed. In Figure 7 a schematic simplification is drawn to illustrate the possible role of the NADH diferric transferrin reductase activity for uptake of iron to the cell both via the transferrin receptor-mediated pathway and via direct uptake through the cell membrane of reduced iron.

Hypothetically the diverse alterations in expression of diferric transferrin and asialoglycoprotein binding sites in liver nodules could be explained by a common mechanism including reduced acidification of the endosome compartment for uncoupling of receptor ligand. The increase in pH will result in a slow and insufficient dissociation of iron in the endosomes. The holotransferrin–receptor complex will therefore recirculate to the cell surface without having delivered iron to the cell. The reduced uptake of iron will consequently create intracellular iron deficiency with a compensatory increase in transferrin receptor *de novo* synthesis and a reduction of intracellular ferritin. If diferric transferrin NADH reductase activity, as in several other neoplastic or transformed cells, should be low, this could partially explain the reduced proton pump activity, but also the reduced formation of ferrous iron able to pass cellular membranes. For asialoglycoprotein receptor recycling a reduction of endosomal pH results in a reduced dissociation of receptor–ligand in the endosome compartment, with a reduction in recycling as the complex will proceed to the lysosomes for degradation or remain in the endosomal vacuom. To this relocalization of binding sites will add the impaired oligomerization of the receptor monomer suggested by our cross-linking data and work using receptor antibodies[5].

The transferrin receptor as well as the diferric transferrin reductase has been strongly correlated to cell proliferation in several cell systems[6,29]. This is true also for diferric transferrin[32], which has been described as a growth factor for cells cultured in serum-free media[29,33]. It has been speculated that the function of the diferric transferrin–receptor complex is not only to supply the cell with iron for internal metabolism but also to provide an electron acceptor for the transplasma membrane redox system, the activity of which by far exceeds that of iron uptake[29]. The conversion of ferric iron to ferrous iron by the redox system will not only maintain the intracellular pH on a reasonable level by pumping protons out of the cytoplasm, but also increase the NAD/NADH ratio. High pH and high levels of NAD in the cytoplasm both promote growth. In order to characterize the proton pump insufficiency in nodular liver tissue, the proton pumps and the transplasma NADH diferric transferrin reductase activity is now being characterized.

SUMMARY

The expression of cell-surface receptors is assumed to determine the ability of the cell to respond to environmental signals regulating cellular behaviour. Major alterations in receptor activity have been noted during different functional states of the cell, i.e. regeneration, foetal and neonatal growth, ligand exposure as well as in states of tumour development. Alterations in transferrin receptor and asialoglycoprotein receptor expression during liver regeneration and hepatocarcinogenesis have been presented. Attempts have

324

been made to explain the mechanisms of the receptor alterations as well as their functional relevance.

Transferrin is a well-known growth factor in several cell systems. It has been proposed that the growth-promoting effect depends on the supply of iron to the cell and/or on the role of transferrin in the transmembrane NADH diferric transferrin redox system of the cell membrane. Iron uptake as well as the reductase activity is dependent on the expression of the transferrin receptor on the surface of the cell. We have shown in membrane preparations from regenerating liver and liver nodules an increase in the number of diferric transferrin binding sites. In spite of this increase in receptor density, the rate of uptake of iron was reduced in liver nodules. This contradiction has been discussed in the light of our recent finding that the proton pump, acidifying the endosome compartment, is very significantly reduced in liver nodular endosome preparations.

The expression of asialoglycoprotein receptor on the surface of rapidly proliferating cells has been reported to be most significantly reduced. This is true also for regenerating liver and liver nodules. In the latter tissue the binding of ligand to the cell surface binders almost disappears. In this presentation we have illustrated the receptor expression and intracellular relocalization in liver nodules and suggested a possible mechanism for the noted alterations. Our data are consistent with altered ligand dissociation due to reduced protonization of endosome compartment of the cell and consequent reduction of receptor recycling. Furthermore cross-linking experiments indicate incomplete oligomerization of the receptor, which may well contribute to the modulation of asialoglycoprotein receptor binding activity in liver nodules.

Acknowledgements

The work was financially supported by grants from the Swedish Medical Research Council and the Swedish Cancer Society. Göran Andersson is a fellow of the Swedish Cancer Society.

References

1. Collins, J. C., Stockert, R. J. and Morell, A. G. (1984). Asialoglycoprotein receptor expression in murine pregnancy and development. *Hepatology,* **4**, 80–3
2. Theilmann, L., Teicher, L., Schildkraut, C. S. and Stockert, R. (1983). Growth-dependent expression of a cell surface glycoprotein. *Biochem. Biophys. Acta,* **762**, 475–7
3. Howard, D. J., Stockert, R. J. and Morell, A. G. (1982). Asialoglycoprotein receptors in hepatic regeneration. *J. Biol. Chem.,* **257**, 2856–8
4. Evarts, R. P., Marsden, E., Hanna, P., Wirth, P. J. and Thorgeirsson, S. S. (1984). Isolation of preneoplastic rat liver cells by centrifugal elutriation and binding to asialofetuin. *Cancer Res.,* **44**, 5718–24
5. Steer, C. J., Weiss, P., Huber, B. E., Wirth, P. J., Thorgeirsson, S. S. and Ashwell, G. (1987). Ligand-induced modulation of the hepatic receptor for asialoglycoproteins in the human hepatoblastoma cell line, Hep G2. *J. Biol. Chem.,* **262**, 17524–9
6. Huebers, H. A. and Finch, C. A. (1987). The physiology of transferrin and transferrin receptors. *Physiol. Rev.,* **67**, 520–82

7. Aisen, P., Leibman, A. and Pinkowitz, R. A. (1974). The anion-binding functions of transferrin. *Adv. Exp. Med. Biol.*, **48**, 125–40

8. Sutherland, R. D., Delia, D., Schneider, C., Newman, R., Kemshead, J. and Greaves, M. (1980). Ubiquitous cell-surface glycoprotein on tumor cells is proliferation-associated receptor for transferrin. *Proc. Natl. Acad. Sci. USA*, **78**, 4515–19

9. Trowbridge, I. S. and Omary, M. B. (1981). Human cell surface glycoprotein related to cell proliferation is the receptor for transferrin. *Proc. Natl. Acad. Sci. USA*, **78**, 3039–43

10. Harris, L., Preat, V. and Farber, E. (1987). Patterns of ligand binding to normal, regenerating, preneoplastic and neoplastic rat hepatocytes. *Cancer Res.*, **47**, 3954–8

11. Eriksson, L. C., Torndal, U-B. and Andersson, G. N. (1986). The transferrin receptor in hepatocyte nodules: binding properties, subcellular distribution and endocytosis. *Carcinogenesis*, **7**, 1467–74

12. Huber, B. E., Glowinski, I. B. and Thorgeirsson, S. S. (1986). Transcriptional and posttranscriptional regulation of the asialoglycoprotein receptor in normal and neoplastic rat liver. *J. Biol. Chem.*, **261**, 12400–7

13. Morgan, E. H., Smith, G. D. and Peters, T. J. (1986). Uptake and subcellular processing of $^{59}Fe-^{125}I$-labelled transferrin by rat liver. *Biochem. J.*, **237**, 163–73

14. Williams, G. M. and Yamamoto, R. S. (1972). Absence of stainable iron from preneoplastic and neoplastic rat liver with 8-hydroxyquinoline-induced siderosis. *J. Natl. Cancer Inst.*, **49**, 685–92

15. Stout, D. L. and Becker, F. F. (1987). Heme enzyme pattern in rat liver nodules and tumors. *Cancer Res.*, **47**, 963–6

16. Roomi, M. W., Cameron, R. G. and Farber, E. (1984). Is the reduced cytochrome P-450 content in hepatocyte nodules a reflection of decreased heme synthesis? *Can. Fed. Biol. Soc.*, **27**, 161

17. Roomi, M. W., Vincent, S. H., Farber, E. and Müller-Eberhardt, U. (1989) Decreased cytosolic levels of the heme binding Z protein in rat hepatocyte nodules and hepatocellular carcinomas. *Cancer Letters*, in press

18. Breitfeld, P. P., Simmons Jr, C. F., Strous, G. J. A. M., Geuze, H. J. and Schwartz, A. L. (1985). Cell biology of the asialoglycoprotein receptor system: A model of receptor-mediated endocytosis. *Int. Rev. Cytol.*, **99**, 47–95

19. McClelland, A., Kuhn, L. C. and Ruddle, R. H. (1984). The human transferrin receptor gene: genomic organization, and the complete primary structure of the receptor deduced from a cDNA sequence. *Cell*, **39**, 267–74

20. Schneider, C., Owen, M. J., Banville, D. and Williams, J. G. (1984). Primary structure of human transferrin receptor deduced from the mRNA sequence. *Nature (London)*, **311**, 675–8

21. Drickamer, K., Mamon, J. F., Binns, G. and Leung, J. O. (1984). Primary structure of the rat liver asialoglycoprotein receptor. Structural evidence for multiple polypeptide species. *J. Biol. Chem.*, **259**, 770–8

22. Eriksson, L. C., Torndal, U-B. and Andersson, G. N. (1983). Isolation and characterization of endoplasmic reticulum and Golgi apparatus from hepatocyte nodules in male Wistar rats. *Cancer Res.*, **43**, 3335–47

23. Higgins, G. M. and Anderson, R. M. (1931). Experimental pathology of the liver. I. Restoration of the liver of the white rat following partial surgical removal. *Arch. Pathol.*, **12**, 186–202

24. Hudgin, R. L., Pricer, W. E., Ashwell Jr, G., Stockert, R. J. and Morell, A. G. (1974). The isolation and properties of a rabbit liver binding protein specific for asialoglycoproteins. *J. Biol. Chem.*, **249**, 5536–43

25. Halberg, D. F., Wager, R. E., Farell, D. C., Hildreth, IV, J., Quensenberry, M. S., Loeb, J. A., Holland, E. C. and Drickamer, K. (1987). Major and minor forms of rat liver asialoglycoprotein receptor are independent galactose-binding proteins. Primary structure and glycosylation heterogeneity of minor receptor forms. *J. Biol. Chem.*, **262**, 9828–38

26. Loeb, J. A. and Drickamer, K. (1987). The chicken receptor for endocytosis of glycoproteins contains a cluster of N-acetyl-glucosamine-binding sites. *J. Biol. Chem.*, **262**, 3022–9

27. Zijderhand-Bleekemolen, J. E., Schwarz, A. L., Slot, J. W., Strous, G. J. and Geuze, H. J. (1987). Ligand- and weak base-induced redistribution of asialoglycoprotein receptors in hepatoma cells. *J. Cell. Biol.*, **104**, 1647–54

28. Sun, I. L., Navas, P., Crane, F. L., Morré, D. J. and Löw, H. (1987). NADH diferric transferrin reductase in liver plasma membrane. *J. Biol. Chem.,* **262,** 15915–21
29. Crane, F. L., Sun, I. L., Clark, M. G., Grebing, C. and Löw, H. (1985). Transplamamembrane redox systems in growth and development. *Biochim. Biophys. Acta,* **811,** 233–364
30. Sun, I. L., Crane, F. L., Chou, J. Y., Löw, H. and Grebing, C. (1983). Transformed liver cells have modified transplasma membrane redox activity which is sensitive to adriamycin. *Biochem. Biophys. Res. Commun.,* **116,** 210–16
31. Aisen, P. and Leibman, A. (1978). Thermodynamic and accessibility factors in the specific binding of iron to human transferrin. In Blauer, G. and Sundi, H. (eds.) *Transport by Proteins,* pp. 277–90. (Berlin: Walter de Grayter)
32. Barnes, D. and Sato, G. (1980). Serum-free cell culture: a unifying approach. *Cell,* **22,** 649–54
33. Crane, F. L., Löw, H., Navas, P. and Morré, D. J. (1987). Redox control of cell growth. In Ramirez, J. (ed.) *Plasma Membrane Electron Transport,* pp. 3–17. (Madrid: Consejo Superior de Investigaciones Cientificas)
34. Andersson, G. N., Rissler, P. and Eriksson, L. C. (1988). Asialoglycoprotein receptors in rat liver nodules. *Carcinogenesis,* **9,** 1623–8
35. Stone, D. K., Xie, X-S. and Racker, E. (1983). An ATP-driven proton pump in clathrin-coated vesicles. *J. Biol. Chem.,* **258,** 4059–62

28
Carbohydrate metabolism in hepatic pre-neoplasia

D. MAYER, F. KLIMEK, H. J. HACKER, G. SEELMANN-EGGEBERT
AND P. BANNASCH

INTRODUCTION

Since the fundamental work of Warburg[1,2] it has been known that cancer cells are characterized by an aberrant carbohydrate metabolism which is manifested in a high aerobic glycolysis as a common feature of tumour cells[3]. Further investigations on a broad spectrum of transplantable hepatomas with different growth rates and different stages of differentiation[4] revealed a positive correlation between glycolysis and tumour growth rate[5-7], a decrease in glycogen metabolism, an increase in pentose phosphate pathway[8-11] and a decrease in gluconeogenesis in most of the tumours studied. Furthermore, it became evident that isoenzymes, which were normally present in hepatocytes of adult animals, were decreased or even lost whereas isoenzymes, normally present in foetal hepatocytes, were increased[12-16] in most of the tumours studied.

While these investigations provided important knowledge on the altered metabolism of fully-developed tumours they did not give information on processes preceding the manifestation of tumours. Another methodological approach using cytochemical techniques was adapted to elucidate *in situ* some aspects of pre-neoplasia and of the processes leading to the appearance of a tumour. Thus, the development of hepatocellular tumours was found to be preceded by a series of characteristic prestages. Focal lesions characterized by an excessive storage of glycogen (glycogen storage foci) are so far considered to represent the earliest alterations detectable in the livers of carcinogen-treated rats[17-19]. In later stages of carcinogenesis, these foci gradually lose their glycogen and progress through a sequence of lesions to hepatocellular adenomas (neoplastic nodules) and hepatocellular carcinomas[20,21]. Using enzyme histochemical and immunocytochemical methods a large number of alterations in enzyme activities[22-23] and enzyme protein content[34-38] could be observed in carcinogen-induced early liver lesions. Some of the alterations could be determined quantitatively by biochemical microanalysis of the micro-dissected lesions[38-41]. The present communication gives a summary on alterations in carbohydrate metabolism in pre-neoplastic liver cells.

MODELS USED

Rat liver

Most of the results described were obtained from male Sprague-Dawley rats treated for a limited time period ('stop experiment') with N-nitroso-morpholine (NNM) in their drinking water as described earlier[31,32,36,39,40]. Groups of NNM-treated animals and respective untreated controls were sacrificed sequentially at the end of carcinogen treatment and up to two years after withdrawal of the carcinogen. The advantage of such stop experiments has been discussed earlier[40]. All animals were invariably sacrificed without prior starvation between 9 and 11 a.m. in order to avoid diurnal variations of glycogen content and activities of related enzymes[42,43]. The livers were rapidly removed and shock-frozen in liquid isopentane at –140°C to –150°C.

Liver cell lines

It was found earlier that homogenates from carcinogen-treated livers are only of limited usefulness for biochemical studies of pre-neoplasia[44,45]. On the other hand, micro-dissection and biochemical microanalysis of pre-neoplastic lesions is very time-consuming. Since the amount of tissue gained from dissection is very small (<1 μg per lesion)[39] biochemical studies on the regulation of carbohydrate metabolism in such lesions are extremely difficult. We therefore established epithelial liver cell lines which revealed properties similar to pre-neoplastic liver cells induced in vivo[46-48]. These cell lines could be used successfully as an in vitro model to study the phenomenon of glycogen storage.

ENZYME HISTOCHEMICAL PATTERN OF PRE-NEOPLASTIC AND NEOPLASTIC LESIONS IN RAT LIVER

The appearance of hepatocellular carcinomas (HC) in carcinogen-treated rats is preceded by a number of focal lesions such as glycogen storage foci (GSF), mixed-cell foci (MCF), amphophilic foci (APF), tigroid cell foci (TCF), basophilic cell foci (BF) and hepatocellular adenomas (HA). The morphology of these lesions and their position in the sequence of cellular alterations have been described in detail[17,18,25,40,49,50]. So far, the earliest pre-neoplastic lesion occurring during hepatocarcinogenesis is the glycogen storage focus which is composed of large clear or acidophilic cells accumulating excessive amounts of glycogen. During neoplastic transformation these populations gradually lose their glycogen and develop through MCF to BF or directly to HA which

Table 1 Enzyme histochemical pattern of pre-neoplastic and neoplastic lesions induced in rat liver in stop experiments with N-nitrosomorpholine*

Parameter	GSF	MCF	TCF	APF	BF	HA	HC
Basophilia	n.c.	n.c. or ↑	↑	n.c.	↑↑	↑	↑↑
Glycogen	↑↑	↑ or ↓	↓	↓	↓↓	↑↓	↓↓
Synthase	n.c.	n.c. or (↓)	↓	↓	↓	↓ or n.c	↓↓
Phosphorylase	↓	↓	↓	↓	↓	↓	↓
Adenylate cyclase	↓	↓	n.c. or ↑	n.d.	↓	↓	↓(↑)
Glucose-6-phosphatase	↓	↓	n.c.	↑↓	↓	↓	↓
Glucose-6-phosphate dehydrogenase	↑↑	↑↑	↑	↑	↑↑	↑↑	↑
Glyceraldehyde-3-phosphate dehydrogenase	(↑)	↑	↑	↑	↑	↑↑	↑↑
Pyruvate kinase	↑	↑↓	n.d.	n.d.	↓	↑↓	↑↓
Hexokinase	n.c.	n.c.	n.d.	n.d.	↑	↑	↑↑

Key:
GSF, glycogen storage focus; MCF, mixed-cell focus; TCF, tigroid cell focus; APF, amphophilic focus; BF, basophilic focus; HA, hepatocellular adenoma; HC, hepatocellular carcinoma. Lesions were induced in adult male Sprague-Dawley rats by NNM[25,31,32,36]; TCF were induced by aflatoxin B₁ (ref. 49). n.c., no change; (↑), very slight increase; ↑, slight increase; ↑↑, strong increase; (↓), very slight decrease; ↓, slight decrease; ↓↓, strong decrease; ↑↓, heterogeneity of enzyme activity, some cells increased, some decreased; n.d., not determined

sometimes may still contain considerable amounts of glycogen. The end stage, the HC, is usually basophilic and free of glycogen. TCF and AF preferentially occur when low carcinogen doses are given. They must be considered members of a sequence of lesions which finally also lead to HA[49,50]. However, it has not been clarified so far whether they also develop from GSF.

In order to get insight into the mechanisms leading to a focal glycogenosis in early stages and to a loss of glycogen in late stages of hepatocarcinogenesis, we investigated a number of key enzymes of carbohydrate metabolism by enzyme histochemical methods[31,33,51–54] in the lesions mentioned above (see Table 1). The enzymes chosen were: glycogen synthase (EC 2.4.1.11) and glycogen phosphorylase (EC 2.4.1.1), which are the two glycogen metaboliz-ing enzymes; glucose-6-phosphate dehydrogenase (EC 1.1.1.49), the key enzyme of pentose phosphate pathway; low K_m hexokinase (EC 2.7.1.30) and pyruvate kinase (EC 2.7.1.40), which are the first and the last key enzymes in glycolysis; glyceraldehyde-3-phosphate dehydrogenase (EC 1.2.1.12), another glycolytic enzyme; glucose-6-phosphatase (EC 3.1.3.9), which sometimes is considered the final enzyme in gluconeogenesis; and adenylate cyclase (EC 4.6.1.1), a superordinate enzyme system which is involved in the regulation of glycogen degradation via several protein kinases and of glycolysis via phosphorylation of pyruvate kinase. The results are summarized in Table 1.

All lesions observed showed typical alterations of enzyme activities compared to the normal surrounding tissue. Thus, the typical enzyme histochemical pattern of early lesions like GSF was characterized by a decrease in phosphorylase, adenylate cyclase and glucose-6-phosphatase, and by an increase in glucose-6-phosphate dehydrogenase, glyceraldehyde-3-phosphate dehydrogenase and pyruvate kinase. Synthase was unchanged or only slightly increased and hexokinase was low in these lesions. With progression of the lesions to a more basophilic stage when the glycogen content was gradually reduced, the enzyme alterations persisted or became even more prominent. In contrast, synthase activity was reduced. Hexokinase, which is present only in very low activities in normal hepatocytes, and early foci like GSF and MCF, showed a considerable increase in activity in late lesions like BF, HA and HC. The activity of pyruvate kinase strikingly correlated with the glycogen content of the cells. Single cells of MCF, HA and HC which still contained glycogen, revealed high pyruvate kinase activity whereas glycogen-free basophilic cells exhibited only low pyruvate kinase activity[38]. Adenylate cyclase was consistently decreased in all types of lesions except TCF. Sometimes HC cells showed an adenylate cyclase activity localized in vesicles[32]. The significance of this finding is not clear.

MICRO-DISSECTION AND BIOCHEMICAL MICROANALYSIS OF RAT LIVER LESIONS

A precise biochemical analysis and quantification of part of the alterations of carbohydrate metabolism was possible with the help of a laser dissection technique that permitted a distinct localization and cutting out of even very small foci[33,39,40]. By means of this methodological approach the changes in glycogen content and in glucose-6-phosphate dehydrogenase and pyruvate kinase activities were measured in pre neoplastic and neoplastic lesions (Table 2). On average, the glycogenotic foci contained about 100% more glycogen than normal liver tissue or tissue of NNM-treated animals surrounding the foci. Individual foci contained up to the 3-fold amount of glycogen compared to normal hepatocytes. In the MCF the overall glycogen content was not distinguishable from that of the normal liver parenchyma because in these lesions the cells excessively storing glycogen were cancelled out by glycogen-poor, basophilic cells.

Concerning glucose-6-phosphate dehydrogenase it is evident from Table 2 that the enzyme activity was about the same in normal liver and in tissue of normal appearance from carcinogen-treated livers. The enzyme activity was increased about 3-fold in GSF and about 6-fold in MCF. Although large variations were obvious, particularly between small and large GSF, the increase in activity compared to normal tissue was significant.

The pronounced zonation of pyruvate kinase within the liver lobule which was also observed with enzyme histochemical[38] and immunohistochemical[34] techniques is reflected in the data obtained by micro-dissection (Table 2; see also ref. 55). The activity in zone 3 as defined by Rappaport[56] was about 1.8-fold higher in normal rat liver and 1.5-fold in tissue of normal appearance

Table 2 Biochemical microanalysis of glycogen content and glucose-6-phosphate dehydrogenase and pyruvate kinase activity in pre-neoplastic and neoplastic lesions induced in rat liver by N-nitrosomorpholine*

Tissue	Glycogen (% of dry weight)	Glucose-6-phosphate dehydrogenase (U/g dry weight)	Pyruvate kinase (U/g dry weight)
Control liver	9.93 ± 1.43	2.62 ± 1.28	87 ± 20 [a] 157 ± 29 [b]
NNM liver of normal appearance	9.04 ± 1.50	2.89 ± 1.48	99 ± 29 [a] 142 ± 29 [b]
GSF	20.43 ± 4.11	8.71 ± 4.47	169 ± 42
MCF	9.15 ± 3.79	17.00 ± 4.74	106 ± 34
BF	n.d.	n.d.	52 ± 24

*Abbreviations as in Table 1. Data represent means ± S.D. of up to 90 samples. [a]Zone 1 according to Rappaport[56]; [b]Zone 3 according to Rappaport. n.d. = not determined

of NNM-treated liver than in zone 1. The activity in GSF was only slightly increased compared to zone 3, and about 1.8-fold compared to zone 1. The surprising decrease of pyruvate kinase activity in basophilic cells as observed enzyme histochemically and immunohistochemically was confirmed by the biochemical assay. The activities found in MCF were dependent on their glycogen content and represented about 63% of that observed in GSF. In BF pyruvate kinase activity was one-third of that in GSF. In glycogen-rich HA, pyruvate kinase was 304 ± 46 U/g dry weight; in glycogen-poor HC, it was 37 ± 28 U/g dry weight.

Using a somewhat different technical approach and a different animal model, Fischer and co-workers[41] quantified the activities of glucose-6-phosphatase, hexokinase and glucokinase. In the livers of rats which were treated with 2-acetylamino-fluorene (AAF) for 165 days and then kept on normal diet, pre-cancerous lesions occurred which from their morphology may be comparable to larger focal lesions and the HA described above. Fischer *et al.* described a gradual decrease of glucose-6-phosphatase activity in these lesions to about 50% of normal tissue and a concomitant reduction of the liver specific glucokinase to less than 10% of the activity observed in the surrounding tissue (Table 3). Hexokinase activity slowly increased during the process of carcinogenesis reaching about twice the activity observed in normal surrounding tissue. Since in our model (Table 1) hexokinase appeared only in BF and HA, its expression may be considered a late event during the process of hepatocarcinogenesis.

IMMUNOCYTOCHEMICAL PATTERN OF ENZYMES IN PRE-NEOPLASTIC AND NEOPLASTIC LESIONS IN RAT LIVER

The alterations in enzyme activities described above may be due either to alterations in the amount of enzyme protein or to a modulation of the activity

Table 3 Microbiochemical analysis of glucose-6-phosphatase, hexokinase and glucokinase in micro-dissected pre-neoplastic liver lesions and surrounding liver tissue after administration of 2-AAF for 165 days*

Days after start of 2-AAF administration	Glucose-6-phosphatase (U/g dry weight)		Hexokinase (U/g dry weight)		Glucokinase (U/g dry weight)	
	pre-cancerous tissue	surrounding tissue	pre-cancerous tissue	surrounding tissue	pre-cancerous tissue	surrounding tissue
165	6.10 ± 3.57	9.10 ± 2.96[a] / 5.02 ± 2.82[b]	5.33 ± 1.36	4.70 ± 0.53	5.06 ± 0.80	9.21 ± 2.38
180	5.56 ± 3.46	8.98 ± 2.92[a] / 5.50 ± 2.81[b]	7.08 ± 3.23	4.37 ± 0.88	4.73 ± 0.78	8.95 ± 2.19
350	5.52 ± 2.26	9.87 ± 2.50	11.53 ± 0.98	5.62 ± 0.62	1.08 ± 0.02	10.99 ± 2.30
420	4.94 ± 3.55	10.70 ± 3.54	10.88 ± 3.27	4.43 ± 0.98	0.76 ± 1.05	10.57 ± 1.59

*Data taken from Fischer et al.[41].
[a]Periportal area; [b]Pericentral area

334

Table 4 Immunocytochemical pattern of enzymes in pre-neoplastic and neoplastic lesions induced in rat liver in stop experiments with N-nitrosomorpholine*

Parameter	GSF	MCF	BF	HA	HC
Phosphorylase	↑	↑↓	↓	↑↓	↓
Glucose-6-phosphate dehydrogenase†	↑↑	↑↑	↑	↑↑	↑
Pyruvate kinase (L-form)	↑↑	↑↓	↓	↑↓	↓

*Abbreviations as in Table 1. ↑, slight increase; ↑↑, strong increase; ↓, slight decrease; ↑↓, heterogeneity of enzyme protein content.
†According to ref. 35

by, for example, phosphorylation/dephosphorylation processes or inhibiting/activating protein factors. For some enzymes described above, the mechanism could be clarified.

Antibodies raised against glucose-6-phosphate dehydrogenase[35] and liver-type pyruvate kinase[34,38] revealed a direct correlation between enzyme activity as detected by enzyme histochemistry and amount of enzyme protein stained by the antibodies (Table 4). This points to an enzyme induction in the case of glucose-6-phosphate dehydrogenase in all lesions studied. Using electrophoretic techniques we earlier found that the increase in glucose-6-phosphate dehydrogenase activity was not accompanied by an isoenzyme expression[44]. In the case of L-pyruvate kinase there was an increase in enzyme protein in early lesions and a loss of enzyme protein in late lesions. No M_2-type pyruvate kinase could be detected in the tumours by the respective antibody. This is in contrast to transplantable hepatomas which usually contain high levels of M_2-pyruvate kinase.

A completely different correlation between enzyme activity and enzyme protein was observed in the case of phosphorylase[36]. Although the enzyme activity was markedly reduced in all lesions, a strong reaction with an antibody raised against phosphorylase was observed in all cells containing glycogen. In lesions where the glycogen was lost, like in BF and HC, no enzyme protein was detectable by the antibody. It can be concluded that the decrease in phosphorylase in GSF was due to a defect in the cascade of phosphorylation processes resulting in active phosphorylase. Alteration in gene expression leading to a loss of phosphorylase protein was a late event in the process of hepatocarcinogenesis.

POTENTIAL SIGNIFICANCE OF ENZYME ALTERATIONS FOR GLUCOSE AND GLYCOGEN METABOLISM IN PRE-NEOPLASTIC HEPATOCYTES

Glycogen accumulation phase

The data presented show that glycogen accumulation is more probably due to a disturbance in glycogen degradation than to increased synthesis. The reduction in phosphorylase activity in this phase is not caused by a loss in enzyme protein but by a disturbance in the activation cascade leading over several phosphorylation steps which are activated by cyclic AMP to active phosphorylase. The decrease in adenylate cyclase activity fits into this pattern since a reduction in cAMP-production would lead to a decrease in cAMP-dependent activation of phosphorylase.

On the other hand cAMP inactivates pyruvate kinase via a cAMP-dependent protein kinase. Loss in cAMP-synthesis would result in activation of pyruvate kinase. However, not only activation of pyruvate kinase but also increase in pyruvate kinase protein due to enzyme induction, was observed. This points, together with the increase in glyceraldehyde-3-phosphate dehydrogenase activity, to an overall increase in the glycolytic capacity of glycogen storage cells. The rise in glucose-6-phosphate dehydrogenase activity which also proved to be due to increased enzyme expression suggests that the cells switch over simultaneously to pentose phosphate pathway, too.

Glycogen reduction phase

The drastic reduction in glycogen content and in synthase activity in mixed cell and basophilic foci suggests a phasing out of glycogen metabolism in such cells. Since only little phosphorylase activity is detectable in glycogen-rich as well as glycogen-poor cells, it is not understood how glycogen is degraded. The lysosomal enzyme α-glucosidase is not increased in these cells (Klimek, unpublished data). The enzymatic capacities for glycolysis and pentose phosphate pathway are even increased in glycogen-poor cells thus confirming their intermediary stage between glycogen storage foci and hepatocellular tumours[18,25]. Although we do not know anything about the intracellular metabolic fluxes along the various pathways in the foci, the results presented suggest that glucose is preferably consumed by enzymes of glycolysis and pentose phosphate pathway. The reduction of pyruvate kinase activity in basophilic cells (Table 2) is not easily understood in this context. However, the residual pyruvate kinase activity in basophilic cells represents 30–50% of that observed in normal liver and might therefore be sufficient for an increased glycolytic metabolism.

LIVER CELL LINES AS *IN VITRO* MODELS FOR HEPATOCARCINOGENESIS

Epithelial liver cell lines transformed *in vitro* have been used by a number of authors to study some aspects of liver cell transformation. Three different ways have been followed to obtain transformed liver cells. Either hepatocytes have been initiated *in vivo* by a hepatocarcinogen and thereafter transformed cells have been selected by prolonged culturing *in vitro*[57,58] or cell lines have been established from primary cultures of hepatocytes and treated *in vitro* with carcinogens[60-66]. In some cases, spontaneous malignant transformation of liver cells in culture has been observed[67-69]. Such cell lines have usually

Table 5 Growth characteristics and phenotypic properties of two epithelial liver cell lines and Morris hepatoma 3924A

Characteristic	C_1I	C_2I	MH3924A
Doubling time (hours)	28	28	16
Final cell density (25 cm² growth area)	1.3×10^6	1.2×10^6	4.5×10^6
Colony forming efficiency (% of plated cells)	86	65	81
Growth on dishes	confluent	confluent	criss-cross
Growth in soft agar	(+)	–	+++
Growth in nude mice	–	–	+
γ-glutamyltranspeptidase	++	+	n.d.
Albumin synthesis	–	–	–
α-Fetoprotein synthesis	–	–	n.d.

n.d. = not determined; + = weak; +++ = strong; – = negative

been used for phenotypic and karyotypic characterization, for evaluation of transformation markers[65,70], for studying proliferation kinetics and for morphological characterization of the resulting tumours.

We have recently cloned several epithelial liver cell lines[46] from a primary culture of normal adult hepatocytes. The cell lines themselves were not tumorigenic after transplantation, but they could be transformed malignantly with hepatocarcinogens. The cell lines were characterized concerning their morphology, their cellular origin and their transformation state[46–48]. Table 5 summarizes some aspects of transformation of the two cell lines (C_1I and C_2I); for comparison we used Morris hepatoma 3924A, a de-differentiated, rapidly-growing hepatoma.

The cell lines exhibited some parameters which are usually considered as transformation markers, such as γ-glutamyltranspeptidase expression or growth in low serum concentration. On the other hand, they showed contact inhibition growth, no or only low anchorage-independent growth, and they did not produce tumours after transplantation into athymic nude mice.

A characterization of the two cell lines according to their pattern of key enzymes of carbohydrate metabolism is given in Table 6. The pattern showed a striking similarity with that observed in pre-neoplastic cells occurring *in vivo*. Besides a reduction in phosphorylase, glucokinase, fructose-1,6-bisphosphatase and glucose-6-phosphatase, a strong increase in hexokinase, glucose-6-phosphate dehydrogenase and pyruvate kinase was observed. It has not been clarified so far which pyruvate kinase isoenzyme is expressed in C_1I and C_2I cells. Pyruvate kinase was also strongly increased in MH3924A cells due to the expression of the M_2-type of the enzyme in this tumour. Regarding these enzyme alterations it is obvious that transformation *in vitro* is accompanied by similar alterations in enzyme expression as *in vivo*. The two cell lines were therefore considered pre-neoplastic cells.

Table 6 Activity of enzymes of carbohydrate metabolism in C_1I, C_2I, MH3924A and normal rat liver. Data are presented as percent of normal liver

Enzyme	Normal liver	C_1I	C_2I	MH3924A
Glycogen phosphorylase a	100	8.3	5.6	9.3
Glycogen phosphorylase a + b	100	13.7	12.0	10.6
Glycogen synthase I	100	100	24	32
Glycogen synthase I + D	100	186	57	68
Hexokinase	100	5720	3674	8302
Glucokinase	100	155	59	200
Glucose-6-phosphatase	100	27	19	13
Fructose-1, 6-bisphosphatase	100	0	0	0
Glucose-6-phosphate dehydrogenase	100	1449	1530	1303

REGULATION OF GLYCOGEN SYNTHESIS AND DEGRADATION IN PRE-NEOPLASTIC LIVER CELL LINES

One of the most prominent differences between C_1I and C_2I cells was their glycogen content. C_1I accumulated large amounts of glycogen whereas C_2I revealed only low concentrations of glycogen (Table 7). The two cell lines were, therefore, considered to be a suitable model for studying some aspects of biochemical regulation of glycogen metabolism and for obtaining some insight into the processes leading to glycogen storage. Glycogen synthase and phosphorylase are the two enzymes directly involved in the synthesis and degradation of glycogen. Both enzymes exist in two or more interconvertible forms. Glycogen metabolism is known to be mediated through the covalent modification of glycogen synthase and phosphorylase by phosphorylation and dephosphorylation processes[71-74]. The activation of glycogen synthesis involves the conversion of the phosphorylated inactive synthase D into dephosphorylated active synthase I. Recently, Tan[75] has described an intermediate form R which may be active *in vivo* in the presence of physiological levels of glucose-6-phosphate. The glucose-6-phosphate-dependent D-form is supposed to be inactive *in vivo*. Interconversion of the enzyme forms is

Table 7 Glycogen and glucose-6-phosphate content of cells. Cells are grown for 5 days. For determination of glycogen and glucose-6-phosphatase the cell layers and normal rat liver slices were frozen in liquid nitrogen. Data represent means ± S.D. of at least 5 different samples

Cells	Glycogen (mg/mg protein)	Glucose-6-phosphate (μmol/g wet weight)
C_1I (glycogen-storing)	0.25 ± 0.04	0.73
C_2I (glycogen-poor)	0.05 ± 0.03	0.042
MH 3924A	not detectable	0.045
Normal rat liver	0.17 ± 0.04	0.20

Table 8 Kinetic data of glycogen phosphorylase*

Cells	Phosphorylase a			Phosphorylase a + b	
	Specific activity (mU/min) (% of normal liver)	K_m (glucose-1-phosphate) (mM)	$K_{i(app)}$ (mM glucose-6-phosphate)	Specific activity (mU/min) (% of normal liver)	K_m (glucose-1-phosphate) (mM)
C₁† (glycogen-storing)	17.3 ± 0.7 (8.3)	2.4 ± 0.4	0.45	29.3 ± 0.9 (13.7)	2.4 ± 0.3
C₂† (glycogen-poor)	11.7 ± 0.1 (5.6)	3.4 ± 0.1	0.19	25.7 ± 0.7 (12.0)	2.8 ± 0.1
MH 3924A	19.5 ± 0.7 (9.3)	1.9 ± 0.3	0.55	22.7 ± 0.7 (10.6)	2.3 ± 0.3
Normal rat liver	208.3 ± 3.8 (100)	2.8 ± 0.2	>25	213.5 ± 2.5 (100)	3.1 ± 0.2

*Samples were obtained as described in text. Data represent means ± S.D. of ≥3 different samples.
†Confluent cells

Table 9 Kinetic data of glycogen synthase

Cells	Synthase I specific activity (mU/min) (% of normal liver)	Synthase R specific activity (mU/min) (% of normal liver)	Synthase I + D specific activity (mU/min) (% of normal liver)	$K_{m(app)}$ (mM uridine diphosphoglucose)	Synthase I + D $A_{0.5}$ (mM glucose-6-phosphate)
C_1* (glycogen storing)	0.25 ± 0.11 (100)	0.92 ± 0.04 (65)	5.2 ± 0.1 (189)	0.18 ± 0.01	0.79 ± 0.08
C_2* (glycogen-poor)	0.06 ± 0.03 (24)	0.07 ± 0.05 (54)	1.6 ± 0.1 (56)	0.15 ± 0.01	1.05 ± 0.25
MH 3924A	0.08 ± 0.05 (32)	n.d.	1.9 ± 0.1 (67)	0.14 ± 0.01	0.79 ± 0.11
Normal rat liver	0.25 ± 0.10 (100)	1.42 ± 0.16 (100)	2.8 ± 0.1 (100)	0.37 ± 0.04	0.17 ± 0.06

*Confluent cells

n.d. = not determined

performed by various synthase kinases and synthase phosphatase. Glycogen phosphorylase activation and inactivation are mediated by phosphorylase kinase and phosphorylase phosphatase. It has generally been agreed that only the phosphorylated *a*-form of phosphorylase is able to catalyze phosphorolysis of glycogen *in vivo* whereas dephosphorylated phosphorylase *b* is completely inactive[73,76].

Kinetic analysis of phosphorylase from C_1I, C_2I, MH3924A and normal liver revealed that, in contrast to the enzyme from normal liver, phosphorylase *a* from the cell lines can be competitively inhibited by physiological concentrations of glucose-6-phosphate (Table 8). K_m values for glucose-1-phosphate were not changed. It is suggested that in the cell lines the liver type phosphorylase is replaced by an isoenzyme which might be characteristic for transformed cells. This assumption was supported by the finding that, in the Western blot, phosphorylase from the cell lines did not (or only weakly) cross-react with the antibody raised against phosphorylase from normal liver and by isoelectric focusing which revealed different isoelectric points for the enzymes from liver, C_1I and MH3924A.

Table 9 shows that the increase in synthase activity in C_1I cells is due to the glucose-6-phosphate-dependent form rather than to the active form I. Enzyme kinetics of synthase revealed that the K_m values for uridine diphosphoglucose of the enzymes from the cell lines were somewhat lower than those for the enzyme from normal liver. On the other hand, the glucose-6-phosphate concentration necessary for activation of synthase at saturation concentrations of uridine diphosphoglucose was considerably higher (Table 9). This means that the enzymes from the cell lines are less sensitive to glucose-6-phosphate than synthase from normal liver.

Determination of the intracellular glucose-6-phosphate level showed that glycogen-rich C_1I cells contained much more glucose-6-phosphate than glycogen-poor C_2I and glycogen-free MH3924A cells and than normal liver from well-fed rats (Table 7). On a theoretical basis, glucose-6-phosphate was high enough to inhibit phosphorylase *a* and to activate synthase R in C_1I, but not in C_2I and MH3924A cells (Tables 8 and 9). We therefore suggest that glycogen storage in pre-neoplastic C_1I cells is due to a high intracellular glucose-6-phosphate concentration which activates synthase R and inhibits phosphorylase *a*. The high intracellular glucose-6-phosphate level may be due to high hexokinase and low glucose-6-phosphatase activity.

CONCLUSIONS

The data presented show that transformation of hepatocytes *in vivo* and *in vitro* is accompanied by a similar pattern of alterations of enzyme activities of carbohydrate metabolism. These alterations indicate a shift from the gluconeogenic metabolism in normal liver to glycolysis and pentose phosphate pathway in pre-neoplastic and neoplastic hepatocytes. Glycogen accumulation may be explained, on one hand, by a disturbance in glycogen degradation manifested in a strong reduction of glycogen phosphorylase activity, while on the other hand, the results from the *in vitro* model indicate not only that alterations in specific enzyme activities are involved but also that changes in the concentration of metabolites like glucose-6-phosphate, acting as allosteric activator of synthase, are causally related to glycogen storage.

Acknowledgements

The authors wish to express their appreciation to Erika Fislinger, Ditmar Greulich, Iris Letsch, Elsbeth Schneider and Erwin Zang for excellent technical assistance and to Brigitte Pétillon for typing the manuscript. The work was supported by the Deutsche Forschungsgemeinschaft.

References

1. Warburg, O. (1926). *Über den Stoffwechsel der Tumoren*. (Berlin: Julius Springer)
2. Warburg, O. (1967). Über die Ursache des Krebses. In *Molekulare Biologie des malignen Wachstums*, 17. Colloquium der Gesellschaft für Physiologische Chemie. pp 1–16. (Berlin: Springer)
3. Aisenberg, A. C. (1961). *The Glycolysis and Respiration of Tumors*. (London and New York: Academic Press)
4. Morris, H. P. (1965). Studies on the development, biochemistry and biology of experimental hepatomas. *Adv. Cancer Res.*, **9**, 228–96
5. Weber, G., Morris, H. P., Love, W. C. and Ashmore, J. (1961). Comparative biochemistry of carbohydrate metabolism in Morris hepatoma 5123. *Cancer Res.*, **21**, 1406–11
6. Sweeney, M. J., Ashmore, J., Morris, H. P. and Weber, G. (1963). Comparative biochemistry of hepatomas. IV. Isotope studies of glucose and fructose metabolism in liver tumors of different growth rates. *Cancer Res.*, **23**, 995–1002
7. Burk, D., Wood, M. and Hunter, J. (1967). On the significance of glycolysis for cancer growth. *J. Natl. Cancer Inst.*, **38**, 839–63
8. Ashmore, J., Weber, G and Landau, B. R. (1958). Isotope studies on the pathways of glucose-6-phosphate metabolism in Novikoff hepatoma. *Cancer Res.*, **18**, 974–9
9. Weber, G. (1968). Carbohydrate metabolism in cancer cells and the molecular correlation concept. *Naturwissenschaften*, **55**, 418–29
10. Weber, G. (1982). Differential carbohydrate metabolism in tumor and host. In Arnott, M. S., van Eys, J. and Wang, Y.-M. (eds.) *Molecular Interrelations of Nutrition and Cancer*. pp 191–208. (New York: Raven Press)
11. Weber, G. and Morris, H. P. (1963). Comparative biochemistry of hepatomas. III. Carbohydrate enzymes in liver tumors of different growth rates. *Cancer Res.*, **23**, 987–94
12. Criss, W. E. (1971). A review of isoenzymes in cancer. *Cancer Res.*, **31**, 1523–42
13. Weinhouse, S. (1972). Glycolysis, respiration and anomalous gene expression in experimental hepatomas. *Cancer Res.*, **32**, 2007–16
14. Schapira, F. (1973). Isoenzymes and cancer. *Adv. Cancer Res.*, **18**, 77–153
15. Sato, K., Morris, H. P. and Weinhouse, S. (1973). Characterization of glycogen synthetases and phosphorylases in transplantable rat hepatomas. *Cancer Res.*, **33**, 724–33
16. Sato, K., Satoh, K., Sato, T., Imai, F. and Morris, H. P. (1976) Isoenzyme patterns of glycogen phosphorylase in rat tissues and transplantable hepatomas. *Cancer Res.*, **36**, 487–95
17. Bannasch, P. and Müller, H. A. (1964). Lichtmikroskopische Untersuchungen über die Wirkung von N-Nitrosomorpholin auf die Leber von Ratte und Maus. *Arzneim. Forsch. (Drug Res.)*, **14**, 805–14
18. Bannasch, P. (1968). The cytoplasm of hepatocytes during carcinogenesis. Electron and light microscopical investigations of the nitrosomorpholine-intoxicated rat liver. *Rec. Res.*

Cancer Res., **19**, 1–100. (Berlin–Heidelberg–New York: Springer)

19. Bannasch, P. (1986). Preneoplastic lesions as end points in carcinogenicity testing. I. Hepatic preneoplasia. *Carcinogenesis*, **7**, 689–95

20. Bannasch, P. (1980). Dose-dependence of early cellular changes during liver carcinogenesis. *Arch. Toxicol.*, Suppl. **3**, 111–28

21. Bannasch, P., Moore, M., Klimek, F. and Zerban, H. (1982). Biological markers of preneoplastic foci and neoplastic nodules in rodent liver. *Toxicol. Pathol.*, **10**, 19–34

22. Gössner, W. and Friedrich-Freksa, H. (1964). Histochemische Untersuchungen über die Glucose-6-Phosphatase in der Rattenleber während der Cancerisierung durch Nitrosamine. *Z. Naturforsch.*, **19b**, 862–4

23. Friedrich-Freksa, H., Papadopulu, G. and Gössner, W. (1969). Histochemische Untersuchungen der Cancerogenese in der Rattenleber nach zeitlich begrenzter Verabfolgung von Diäthylnitrosamin. *Z. Krebsforsch.*, **72**, 240–53

24. Epstein, S., Ito, N., Merkow, L. and Farber, E. (1967). Cellular analysis of liver carcinogenesis: the induction of large hyperplastic nodules in the liver with 2-fluorenylacetamide or ethionine and some aspects of their morphology and glycogen metabolism. *Cancer Res.*, **27**, 1702–11

25. Bannasch, P., Mayer, D. and Hacker, H. J. (1980). Hepatocellular glycogenosis and hepatocarcinogenesis. *Biochim. Biophys. Acta*, **605**, 217–45

26. Emmelot, P. and Scherer, E. (1980). The first relevant cell stage in rat liver carcinogenesis. A quantitative approach. *Biochim. Biophys. Acta*, **605**, 247–304

27. Farber, E. (1980). The sequential analysis of liver cancer induction. *Biochim. Biophys. Acta*, **605**, 149–66

28. Pitot, H. C. and Sirica, A. E. (1980). The stages of initiation and promotion in hepatocarcinogenesis. *Biochim, Biophys. Acta*, **605**, 191–216

29. Williams, G. M. (1980). The pathogenesis of rat liver cancer caused by chemical carcinogens. *Biochim. Biophys. Acta*, **605**, 167–89

30. Kalengayi, M. M. R. and Desmet, V. J. (1975). Sequential histological and histochemical study of the rat liver after single-dose aflatoxin B_1 intoxication. *Cancer Res.*, **35**, 2836–44

31. Hacker, H. J., Moore, M. A., Mayer, D. and Bannasch, P. (1982). Correlative histochemistry of some enzymes of carbohydrate metabolism in preneoplastic and neoplastic lesions in the rat liver. *Carcinogenesis*, **3**, 1265–72

32. Ehemann, V., Mayer, D., Hacker, H. J. and Bannasch, P. (1986). Loss of adenylate cyclase activity in preneoplastic and neoplastic lesions induced in rat liver by N-nitrosomorpholine. *Carcinogenesis*, **7**, 567–73

33. Klimek, F., Moore, M. A., Schneider, E. and Bannasch, P. (1988). Histochemical and microbiochemical demonstration of reduced pyruvate kinase activity in thioacetamide-induced neoplastic nodules of rat liver. *Histochemistry*, **90**, 37–42

34. Reinacher, M., Eigenbrodt, E., Gerbracht, U., Zenk, G., Timmermann-Trosiener, I., Bentley, P., Waechter, F. and Schulte-Hermann, R. (1986). Pyruvate kinase isoenzymes in altered foci and carcinoma of rat liver. *Carcinogenesis*, **7**, 1351–7

35. Moore, M. A., Nakamura, T. and Ito, N. (1986). Immunohistochemically demonstrated glucose-6-phosphate dehydrogenase, γ-glutamyltranspeptidase, ornithine decarboxylase and glutathione S-transferase enzymes: absence of direct correlation with cell proliferation in rat liver putative preneoplastic lesions. *Carcinogenesis*, **7**, 1419–24

36. Seelmann-Eggebert, G., Mayer, D., Mecke, D. and Bannasch, P. (1987). Expression and regulation of glycogen phosphorylase in preneoplastic and neoplastic hepatic lesions in rats. *Virchows Arch. (B)*, **53**, 44–51

37. Fischer, G., Domingo, M., Lodder, D., Katz, N., Reinacher, M. and Eigenbrodt, E. (1987). Immunohistochemical demonstration of decreased L-pyruvate kinase in enzyme altered rat liver lesions produced by different carcinogens. *Virchows Arch. (B)*, **53**, 359–64

38. Klimek, F., Eigenbrodt, E. Reinacher, M. and Bannasch, P. (1988). Pyruvate kinase in preneoplastic liver foci. Presented at the *51st Falk Symposium on Liver Cell Carcinoma*, June 5–8, Freiburg/Breisgau, FRG

39. Klimek, F., Mayer, D. and Bannasch, P. (1984). Biochemical microanalysis of glycogen content and glucose-6-phosphate dehydrogenase activity in focal lesions of the rat liver induced by N-nitrosomorpholine. *Carcinogenesis*, **5**, 265–8

40. Bannasch, P., Hacker, H. J., Klimek, F. and Mayer, D. (1984). Hepatocellular glycogenosis

and related pattern of enzymatic changes during hepatocarcinogenesis. *Adv. Enzyme Regul.*, **22**, 97–121

41. Fischer, G., Ruschenburg, J., Eigenbrodt, E. and Katz, N. (1987). Decrease in glucokinase and glucose-6-phosphatase and increase in hexokinase in putative preneoplastic lesions of rat liver. *J. Cancer Res. Clin. Oncol.*, **113**, 430–6

42. Müller, O. (1974). Der circadiane Glykogenrhythmus der Rattenleber (Biochemie, quantitative Histochemie, elekronenmikroskopische Morphometrie). *Acta Histochem.*, Suppl. XVI, 139–44

43. Roesler, W. J. and Khandelwal, R. L. (1986). The diurnal rhythm of liver glycogen phosphorylase: correlating changes in enzyme activity and enzymatic protein. *FEBS Lett.*, **195**, 344–6

44. Mayer, D., Moore, M. and Bannasch, P. (1982). Biochemical correlation of glycogen content and activity of some enzymes of carbohydrate metabolism in rat liver during early stages of carcinogenesis. *J. Cancer Res. Clin. Oncol.*, **104**, 99–108

45. Mayer, D., Moore, M. A. and Bannasch, P. (1983). Influence of phenobarbital on glycogen metabolism of rat liver pretreated with N-nitrosomorpholine. *Carcinogenesis*, **4**, 931–3

46. Mayer, D. and Schäfer, B. (1982). Biochemical and morphological characterization of glycogen-storing epithelial liver cell lines. *Exp. Cell Res.*, **138**, 1–14

47. Denis, C., Mayer, D., Trocheris, V., Viallard, V., Paris, H. and Murat, J. C. (1985). Study of carbohydrate metabolism in glycogen storing cell lines derived from cultured rat hepatocytes. *Int. J. Biochem.*, **17**, 247–51

48. Mayer, D. (1988). Regulation of carbohydrate metabolism in a glycogen-storing liver cell line. In Roberfroid, M. and Préat, V. (eds.) *Experimental Hepatocarcinogenesis*, pp. 283–96. (New York: Plenum)

49. Bannasch, P., Benner, U., Enzmann, H. and Hacker, H. J. (1985). Tigroid cell foci and neoplastic nodules in the liver of rats treated with a single dose of aflatoxin B₁. *Carcinogenesis*, **6**, 1641–8

50. Weber, E., Moore, M. A. and Bannasch, P. (1988). Enzyme histochemical and morphological phenotype of amphophilic foci and amphophilic/tigroid cell adenomas in rat liver after combined treatment with dehydroepiandrosterone and N-nitrosomorpholine. *Carcinogenesis*, **9**, 1049–54

51. Pearse, A. G. E. (1972). *Histochemistry, Theoretical and Applied*, p. 831. (Edinburgh and London: Churchill Livingstone)

52. Hacker, H. J. (1978). Histochemical demonstration of glycogen phosphorylase (EC 2.4.1.1) through the use of semipermeable membranes. *Histochemistry*, **58**, 289–96

53. Benner, U., Hacker, H. J. and Bannasch, P. (1979). Electron microscopical demonstration of glucose-6-phosphatase in native cryostat sections fixed with glutaraldehyde through semipermeable membranes. *Histochemistry*, **65**, 41–7

54. Mayer, D., Ehemann, V., Hacker, H. J., Klimek, F. and Bannasch, P. (1985). Specificity of cytochemical demonstration of adenylate cyclase in liver using adenylate-(ß,γ-methylene)diphosphate as substrate. *Histochemistry*, **82**, 135–40

55. Chatzipanagiotou, S., Nath, A., Vogt, B. and Jungermann, K. (1985). Alteration in the capacities as well as in the zonal and cellular distributions of pyruvate kinase L and M2 in regenerating rat liver. *Hoppe Seyler's Z. Biol. Chem.*, **366**, 271–80

56. Rappaport, A. M. (1976). The microcirculatory acinar concept of normal and pathological hepatic structure. *Beitr. Path.*, **157**, 215–43

57. Kitagawa, T., Watanabe, R., Kayano, T. and Sugano, H. (1980). *In vitro* carcinogenesis of hepatocytes obtained from acetyl-aminofluorene-treated rat liver and promotion of their growth by phenobarbital. *Gann*, **71**, 747–54

58. Kerler, R. and Rabes, H. M. (1988). Preneoplastic rat liver cells *in vitro*: Slow progression without promoters, hormones, or growth factors. *J. Cancer Res. Clin. Oncol.*, **114**, 113–23

59. Borenfreund, E., Higgins, P. J., Steinglass, M. and Bendich, A. (1975). Properties and malignant transformation of established rat liver parenchymal cells in culture. *J. Natl. Cancer Inst.*, **55**, 375–84

60. Montesano, R., Saint Vincent, L., Drevon, C. and Tomatis, L. (1975). Production of epithelial and mesenchymal tumours with rat liver cells transformed *in vitro*. *Int. J. Cancer*, **16**, 550–8

61. Kuroki, T., Drevon, C., Saint Vincent, L. and Montesano, R. (1979). Properties of the

IAR-series of liver epithelial cells transformed by chemical carcinogens. In Franks, L. M. and Wigley, C. B. (eds.) *Neoplastic Transformation in Differentiated Epithelial Cell Systems in vitro*, pp 173–85. (London, New York, Toronto, Sydney, San Francisco: Academic Press)

62. Iype, P. T., Turner, S. and Siddiqi, M.-S. (1980). Markers for transformation in rat liver epithelial cells in culture. *Ann. N.Y. Acad. Sci.*, **349**, 312–21

63. Tsao, M.-S., Grisham, J. W., Nelson, K. G. and Smith, J.-D. (1985). Phenotypic and karyotypic changes induced in cultured rat hepatic epithelial cells that express the 'oval' cell phenotype by exposure to N-methyl-N'-nitro-N-nitrosoguanidine. *Am. J. Pathol.*, **118**, 306–15

64. Tsao, M.-S., Grisham, J. W., Chou, B. B. and Smith, J. D. (1985). Clonal isolation of population of γ-glutamyltranspeptidase-positive and -negative cells from rat liver epithelial cells chemically transformed *in vitro*. *Cancer Res.*, **45**, 5134–8

65. Tsao, M.-S., Grisham, J. W. and Nelson, K. G. (1985). Clonal analysis of tumorigenicity and paratumorigenic phenotypes in rat liver epithelial cells chemically transformed *in vitro*. *Cancer Res.*, **45**, 5139–44

66. Tsao, M.-S. and Grisham, J. W. (1987). Phenotypic modulation during tumorigenesis by clones of transformed rat liver epithelial cells. *Cancer Res.*, **47**, 1282–6

67. Schaeffer, W. I. and Polifka, M. D. (1975). A diploid rat liver cell culture. III. Characterization of the heterodiploid morphological variants which develop with time in culture. *Exp. Cell Res.*, **95**, 167–75

68. Anderson, L. W. and Smith, H. S. (1979). Premalignancy *in vitro*: progression of an initially benign epithelial cell line to malignancy. *Br. J. Exp. Pathol.*, **60**, 575–81

69. Beckner, S. K., Reilly, T., Martinez, A. and Blecher, M. (1980). Alterations of cAMP metabolism and hormone responsiveness of cloned differentiated rat liver cells (RL-PR-c) upon spontaneous transformation. *Exp. Cell Res.*, **128**, 151–8

70. San, R. H. C., Shimida, T., Maslansky, C. J., Kreiser, D. M., Laspia, M. F., Rice, J. M. and Williams, G. M. (1979). Growth characteristics and enzyme activities in a survey of transformation markers in adult rat liver epithelial-like cell cultures. *Cancer Res.*, **39**, 4441–8

71. Larner, J. and Villar-Palasi, C. (1971). Glycogen synthetase and its control. *Curr. Top. Cell. Regul.*, **3**, 195–236

72. Krebs, E. G. (1972). Protein kinases. *Curr. Top. Cell. Regul.*, **5**, 99–133

73. Hers, H. G. (1976). The control of glycogen metabolism in the liver. *Annu. Rev. Biochem.*, **45**, 167–89

74. Cohen, P. (1980). Well established systems of enzyme regulation by reversible phosphorylation. In Cohen, P. (ed.) *Molecular Aspects of Cellular Regulation*, Vol. 1, pp 1–10. (New York: Elsevier North-Holland Biochemical Press)

75. Tan, A. W. H. (1982). Glycogen synthase R in livers of starved rats and starved rats given glucose. *J. Biol. Chem.*, **257**, 5004–7

76. Stalmans, W. (1976). The role of liver in the homeostasis of blood glucose. *Curr. Top. Cell. Regul.*, **11**, 51–97

29
Role of cell death in hepatocarcinogenesis

R. SCHULTE-HERMANN, W. BURSCH, L. FESUS, I. TIMMERMANN-TROSIENER, B. KRAUPP AND J. LIEHR

INTRODUCTION

Occurrence of cell death in tumours is a well-known phenomenon. It is generally accepted that hypoxia and depletion of nutrients may be responsible for cell death. The present paper will provide evidence for two points:

(a) There appears to exist a particular type of cell death in the liver (and in other organs) occurrence of which is controlled by hormones and tumour promoters.
(b) This promoter-controlled cell death is a major determinant of the growth rate of putative pre-neoplastic foci in rat liver and thereby a determinant of cancer development.

DISCREPANCY BETWEEN DNA SYNTHESIS AND GROWTH RATE OF PRE-NEOPLASTIC FOCI

Putative pre-neoplastic liver foci were induced in female Wistar rats by a single dose of N-nitrosomorpholine (250 mg/kg) ('initiation') and were identified in histological sections by means of a positive γ-glutamyltransferase (GGT) reaction and by cytological markers such as clearness of cytoplasm etc.[1-3]. To determine the proliferative activity of foci rats received a continuous infusion of [^{3}H]thymidine over 2 weeks, at 8 weeks after initiation. It was found that the number of proliferating cells was much higher in foci than in the normal parts of the liver tissue as noted previously[3,4]. When we plotted the size of individual foci against their DNA synthesis, large foci showed no higher DNA synthesis than small ones. Rather, large and small foci showed similar mean labelling indices (Figure 1).

Furthermore, we determined DNA synthesis in foci during long-term

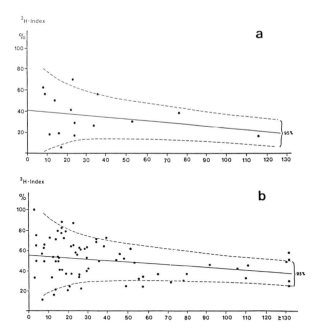

Figure 1 DNA synthesis in γ-glutamyltransferase-positive liver foci after infusion of [³H]thymidine for 2 weeks. (a) No promoting treatment; (b) 50 mg/kg phenobarbital daily, beginning simultaneously with thymidine infusion. Dashed lines: 95% confidence limits. ³H-Index = number of labelled cells. Abscissa: size of focus (cells/area)

treatment (12 months) with phenobarbital for promotion. As expected, liver foci showed accelerated growth. However, DNA synthesis — after an initial upsurge — was not enhanced over the control level at any time point investigated (Figure 2). These findings suggested that the enhanced proliferative activity in foci was partially counterbalanced by cell elimination.

CELL DEATH BY APOPTOSIS IN NORMAL LIVER

We studied cell death in a whole-liver-model. In normal rat liver, tumour promoters induce a hyperplasia as indicated by increases in DNA synthesis, mitotic activity and total DNA content[5,6]. Using high daily doses of cyproterone acetate (CPA), a synthetic steroid, and other agents, the hyperplasia was found to reach a plateau after a few days and to be fairly stable as long as application of the liver mitogen was continued. However, after cessation of treatment with CPA, part of the hyperplasia was readily reversible[2,6,7].

Histological analysis during regression of liver hyperplasia revealed the occasional presence of cells with highly condensed chromatin. Furthermore, eosinophilic bodies were found, many with pieces of chromatin, inside and

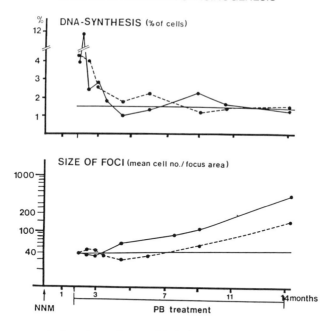

Figure 2 DNA synthesis and growth rate of foci. [³H]thymidine was given as pulses. Phenobarbital (PB) was at 50 mg/kg daily

outside hepatocytes. These morphological signs suggested the occurrence of a specific mode of cell death, 'apoptosis', as coined by Wyllie et al.[8].

Apoptosis is believed to proceed in certain stages, with more or less characteristic morphology, namely condensation of chromatin and separation from neighbouring cells, fragmentation, phagocytosis of fragments, partially by Kupffer cells, but mainly by hepatocytes; and finally intracellular degradation[8,9] (Figure 3). The presence of chromatin pieces in the cell fragments is important for discrimination from other eosinophilic particles, such as Mallory bodies or autophagosomes.

What is apoptosis? Apoptosis occurs under conditions where *no* major toxic injury can be identified as a cause of cell death. Apoptosis may also *not* be involved in cell death during terminal differentiation of cells such as in skin. In contrast, apoptosis does occur during removal of excessive tissues in embryo development, for instance removal of interdigit webs or of the Müllerian duct in the male embryo. It also occurs in adults during atrophy of hormone-dependent organs such as the adrenals or prostate. Apoptosis seems a phylogenetically old process since it was found in hydra, nematodes and insects[8,10]. Because of its occurrence under such specific physiological conditions, apoptosis was also called 'programmed' or 'controlled cell death'. However, this term can be misleading as it might suggest that other types of cell death would not occur in a programmed way. Therefore, in the present paper only 'apoptosis' or 'single cell death' will be used.

349

CELL DEATH (APOPTOSIS)

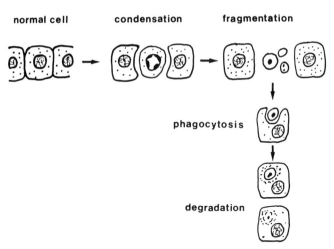

Figure 3 Hypothetical diagram of the process of apoptosis during regression of liver hyperplasia

There is not very much known about the biology of apoptosis. In lymphocytes and thymocytes apoptosis is triggered by glucocorticoids, and this effect is mediated by glucocorticoid receptors[11,12,15]. At least in the nematode *C. elegans*, apoptosis evidently is genetically encoded. Here mutants were found in which certain stages of cell death cannot occur[13]. Furthermore, Ucker identified a mammalian thymoma cell line in which a mutation resulted in the inability to undergo cell death[11].

Turning back to the liver, in the normal resting state apoptosis is very rare. We found an incidence of 1 per 1000 or less which probably reflects normal cell turnover[9]. The incidence is greatly enhanced during atrophy in response to severe starvation. During 8 days of starvation, liver DNA decreased by 25%. Concomitantly we found considerable numbers of apoptotic bodies ('AB'), especially on days 7 and 8 (Figure 4).

We also counted the incidence of apoptotic bodies in our model of drug-induced liver hyperplasia and involution. There was a massive upsurge in the period of DNA elimination[2,9,14]. How can we know that truly apoptosis — and not some other form of cell death — was involved? CPA determinations in the liver of the treated animals showed that the level of the mitogen dropped rapidly after cessation of treatment[7]. We wondered whether this drop might provide the signal for initiation of cell death.

To check this hypothesis we retreated the animals with CPA at the maximum of apoptotic activity. We found that retreatment dramatically decreased the incidence of apoptosis. And not only CPA was active. Other, chemically-unrelated mitogens (phenobarbital, α-hexachlorocyclohexane, nafenopin) also prevented cell death[2,9,14]. These findings strongly suggest that cell death does not occur in response to tissue damage that might have

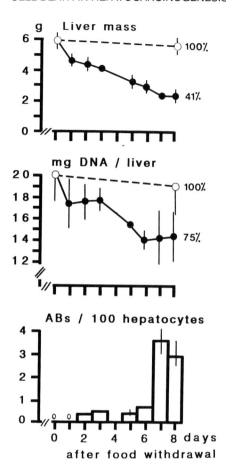

Figure 4 Effect of food withdrawal on liver mass, liver DNA content and incidence of apoptoses in rat liver. Female Wistar rats (150–160 g at food withdrawal) were killed between 1 and 8 days after food withdrawal. (Top) liver mass (g liver/rat); (centre) mg DNA/liver; top and centre, O---O fed rats, ●—● starved rats. (Bottom) number of apoptotic bodies (ABs) per 100 intact hepatocytes. Means of 3–5 animals are given. Vertical bars: for top and centre, S.D. (were not given smaller than symbols); (bottom) 95% confidence limits

occurred after CPA but rather is a regulatory phenomenon serving to eliminate the excessive hyperplasia.

It was also found that the apoptotic bodies disappeared very rapidly after application of the inhibitory signal. We followed the kinetics of disappearance more closely (Figure 5). Extra- and intra-hepatocellular apoptotic bodies both tended to disappear with linear kinetics in a semi-logarithmic plot. As would be predicted from the sequence of apoptotic stages (Figure 3), the extracellular apoptotic bodies disappeared first, with an approximate half-life of 30 min. Intracellular apoptotic bodies disappeared with a somewhat longer

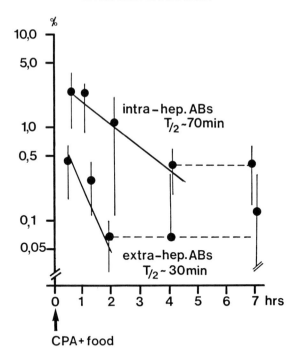

Figure 5 Time course of decrease of apoptotic bodies (ABs) incidence after cyproterone acetate (CPA) and food administration. Rats received CPA for 7 days as described in Figure 7. At 2 days after the last CPA dosing (i.e. at the peak incidence of ABs), rats were re-treated with a single dose of CPA (130 mg/kg). Additionally, rats received food according to the feeding schedule. Differentiation was made between extra- or intra-hepatocellular localization of the ABs. ●, CPA and food at time 0; 7000–8000 hepatocytes were scored per liver for determination of the AB incidence. Each point represents the mean ± S.D. of 5 or 6 animals

half-life of 70 min. Thus apoptosis in the liver is a rapid process; the visible stages may last on average about 2.5 hours. This can explain why at any given time point of observation only few apoptotic bodies can be found even when considerable amounts of DNA disappear from the liver.

The concept of apoptosis includes that fragments of dead cells (the apoptotic bodies) are phagocytosed by neighbouring hepatocytes. This was a point of concern because hepatocytes were not known to be capable of phagocytosis. To tackle this question we performed a two-step experiment[9] (Figure 6). In the first step, we induced liver growth with CPA and infused continuously [³H]thymidine. Thereby all proliferating, 'new' cells were labelled. In the second step we stopped CPA treatment, thus inducing apoptosis, and checked the labelling patterns of nuclei and apoptotic bodies within the same hepatocytes. In the majority of cases we found a labelled nucleus and an unlabelled apoptotic body in the same hepatocyte. This provides a clear proof that the chromatin in the apoptotic bodies was not derived from the host cell, i.e. it was from an extracellular source[9].

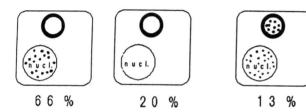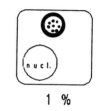

Figure 6 Occurrence of labelled DNA in nuclei and apoptotic bodies (ABs) of the same hepato-cytes. Continuous infusion of [³H]methyl-thymidine ([³H]TdR) was used to label all hepatocytes which proliferate during a cyproterone acetate (CPA) treatment for 7 days. Rats were killed 2 days after cessation of CPA (at the peak incidence of apoptosis in the liver) and [³H]TdR labelling of chromatin in hepatocytic nuclei and in ABs was determined by autoradiography of histological sections of the liver. The total number of intra-hepatocellular ABs with chromatin was taken as 100%; the data shown indicate the relative frequencies of ³H labelling of ABs as well as their occurrence in hepatocytes with or without ³H-labelled nuclei (for details see Bursch et al., 1985[9]). Nucl. = nucleus of intact hepatocyte apoptotic body (O); ☺ = labelled; O = unlabelled

Another interesting result of this experiment was that most intact hepato-cytes were labelled, but most apoptotic bodies were unlabelled. Thus, 'old', non-proliferating hepatocytes were apparently preferred for apoptosis[9]. The basis of this selectivity is unknown.

Table 1 presents a summary of markers of apoptosis. Since morphological criteria alone are not sufficient evidence of apoptosis, the importance of functional criteria, particularly the inhibition by liver mitogens, should be emphasized. In addition, the availability of biochemical markers would be helpful. So far the earliest discernible metabolic change during apoptosis is the activation of an endonuclease which degrades chromatin into nucleo-somes. Nucleosome formation has been studied as a marker in cultured cells[11,12,15,16], but to our knowledge not yet in the liver. One of us (L.F.) has recently detected that apoptotic cells contain high amounts of transglutamin-ase[17], an enzyme involved in cross-linking glutamine and lysine in proteins. Among hepatocytes only apoptotic bodies contain this enzyme as shown by immunocytochemistry. Further support for a correlation between transgluta-

Table 1 Indicators of apoptosis

(a)	*Morphological markers*
•	separation of cell
•	condensation of chromatin
•	occurrence of cell fragments ('apoptotic bodies')
•	phagocytosis of apoptotic bodies by neighbouring epithelial cells
(b)	*Functional markers*
•	occurrence during tissue involution
•	inhibition by growth stimuli
(c)	*Biochemical markers*
•	DNA fragmentation → nucleosomes
•	expression of transglutaminase (?)

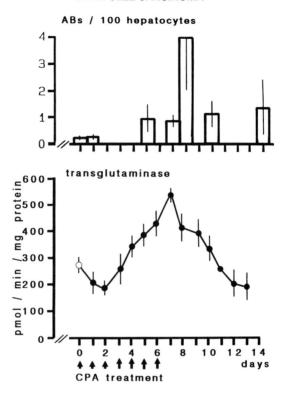

Figure 7 Time course of occurrence of apoptotic bodies (ABs) and of transglutaminase in rat liver during and after cyproterone acetate (CPA) treatment. Before commencing treatment, the rats (Wistar, female) were adapted for 2–3 weeks to an inverted light–dark rhythm (L:D 12:12 hours) with lights off from 9 a m. to 9 p.m. and lights on from 9 p.m. to 9 a.m.; food was available for 5 hours from 9 a.m. to 2 p.m. The animals were treated with CPA as indicated. Small arrows = 100 mg/kg/day, large arrows = 130 mg/kg/day. *Apoptoses* (ABs/100 hepatocytes): the number of apoptotic bodies (see Bursch *et al.*, 1985[9] for morphological description) found in histological sections is expressed as percentage of intact hepatocytes. *Transglutaminase*: The transglutaminase activity was determined as described elsewhere (Fesus *et al.*, 1986[17]). O, controls; ●, CPA-treated rats. Means ± S.D. of 3–5 rats are given

minase and apoptosis is provided by a roughly parallel increase and decrease of enzyme activity and apoptotic bodies during induction and regression of hyperplasia (Figure 7). The function of transglutaminase during apoptosis is unclear. Perhaps the most important aspect is that the enzyme may provide the first marker to label individual apoptotic cells.

APOPTOSIS IN PRE-NEOPLASTIC LIVER FOCI

We have found morphological signs of apoptosis in the foci, and the incidence was always higher than in normal liver[2]. We also tried to discriminate between 'persistent' and 'remodelling' foci on the basis of distinctness of their borders.

Apoptotic numbers were higher in the remodelling foci. In contrast, these two foci groups did not differ in their DNA synthesis[14]. Thus, in remodelling foci, cell proliferation and cell death may well balance each other, while 'persisting' foci (i.e. foci with distinct borders) may have an excess of cell proliferation[14].

Is cell death in foci truly due to apoptosis? It was found that phenobarbital, a model tumour promoter, indeed decreased the incidence of apoptotic bodies

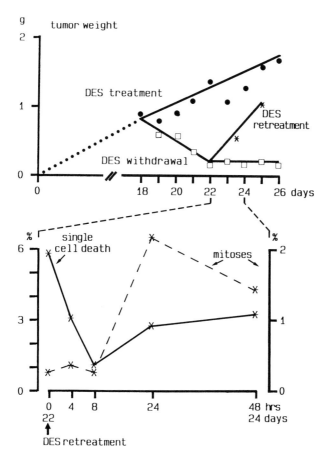

Figure 8 Growth, mitoses and cell death in an œstrogen-dependent hamster kidney tumour during diethylstilboestrol (DES) treatment, withdrawal and re-treatment. A 39-mg pellet consisting of 90% DES and 10% cholesterol was implanted subcutaneously in the back of male Syrian hamsters. The animals absorb 200–300 µg of DES/hamster/day from these pellets. Day 0: 1 day after implantation of the DES pellet 3.6×10^6 H-301 cells were inoculated subcutaneously into the area of the left posterior thorax. Day 0 until day 18: all hamsters were treated with DES and thereafter subjected to one of the following protocols. ●, Continued DES treatment until necropsy; □, DES withdrawal by removal of the pellet; *, DES withdrawal for 4 days, followed by re-administration of DES (one intraperitoneal injection of 25 µg DES/hamster and infusion of 0.21 µg DES/hamster/min by the means of Alzet osmotic minipumps, implanted subcutaneously). (Top) tumour weight. (Bottom) mitoses/100 tumour cells and single cell residues/100 vital tumour cells. Each point is the mean of 3 or 4 animals

355

in foci. Cessation of phenobarbital treatment after a longer period of promotion produced a striking increase of apoptotic bodies, and re-treatment depressed cell death again[2,14]. Thus both morphological and functional markers indicate the occurrence of apoptosis in foci. (This does of course not exclude the possibility of non-apoptotic cell death in foci, in addition to apoptosis.)

These findings lead to the following conclusions:

(a) Under the present experimental conditions, foci cells appear to have a shorter life-span than normal liver cells. This partially counterbalances the enhanced proliferative activity of early foci so that little net growth of foci occurs.

(b) A tumour promoter, by inhibiting apoptosis in foci, can accelerate foci growth in the absence of enhanced cell proliferation. This can explain the findings described above (Figure 2).

(c) Apoptosis may allow the liver to eliminate initiated or pre-neoplastic cells. It may therefore constitute one of the organism's defence lines against cancer development. Tumour promoters may interfere with this protective mechanism.

APOPTOSIS IN TUMOURS

Occurrence of apoptosis has been observed in liver cancer as well (unpublished observations). We have recently obtained quantitative data on apoptosis in another tumour model, namely an œstrogen-dependent hamster kidney tumour. This tumour shows rapid growth with diethylstilboestrol (DES); withdrawal of DES leads to tumour regression, re-treatment induces tumour growth again (Figure 8, top). In the regression period we found low mitotic activity and numerous single cell deaths. Upon re-treatment with DES mitoses increased while cell death decreased rapidly (Figure 8, bottom). Thus, also in this œstrogen-dependent tumour we find evidence of apoptosis.

These findings suggest that apoptosis may have general importance in the control of tumour development and growth. Closer analysis of the phenomenon may broaden our understanding of mechanisms and help develop new strategies for tumour therapy.

SUMMARY

Homeostasis of liver cell number involves control of cell proliferation as well as of cell death through apoptosis (sometimes also designated 'programmed' cell death or 'cellular suicide'). Apoptosis can be found during normal turnover of hepatocytes and at increased rates during liver atrophy following starvation and during regression of liver hyperplasia. Feeding and mitogen treatment can inhibit apoptosis.

Apoptosis seems to be a rapid process; its stages are histologically detectable for approximately 2.5 hours. The apoptotic bodies remaining after death and fragmentation of cells are phagocytosed by intact hepatocytes and by other neighbouring cells. The enzyme transglutaminase appears to be expressed in apoptotic hepatocytes.

In putative pre-neoplastic liver foci apoptosis appears to be a determinant of growth: enhanced rates of apoptosis seem to counterbalance partially the increased proliferative activity in these lesions. Remodelling foci contain more apoptoses than non-remodelling lesions. Thus, the incidence of apoptosis appears to be negatively correlated with the strength of expression of the altered phenotype in foci. Tumour promoters inhibit apoptosis in foci thereby accelerating growth of pre-neoplastic lesions and development of liver cancer.

Evidence of apoptosis was also found in an œstrogen-dependent hamster kidney tumour. In this tumour the incidence of single cell death was high after withdrawal of diethylstilboestrol and decreased dramatically upon re-treatment. Thus, also in this lesion hormone (promoter)-controlled cell death appears to be a determinant of tumour growth.

References

1. Institute of Laboratory Animal Resources (1980). Histological typing of liver tumors of the rat. *J. Natl. Cancer Inst.,* **64**, 179–206
2. Bursch, W., Lauer, B., Timmermann-Trosiener, I., Barthel, G., Schuppler, J. and Schulte-Hermann, R. (1984). Controlled cell death (apoptosis) of normal and putative preneoplastic cells in rat liver following withdrawal of tumor promoters. *Carcinogenesis,* **5**, 453–8
3. Schulte-Hermann, R., Timmermann-Trosiener, I. and Schuppler, J. (1986). Facilitated expression of adaptive responses to phenobarbital in putative pre-stages of liver cancer. *Carcinogenesis,* **7**, 1651–5
4. Schulte-Hermann, R., Ohde, G., Schuppler, J. and Timmermann-Trosiener, I. (1981). Enhanced proliferation of putative preneoplastic cells in rat liver following treatment with the tumor promoters phenobarbital, hexachlorocyclohexane, steroid compounds, and nafenopin. *Cancer Res.,* **41**, 2556–62
5. Schulte-Hermann, R. (1985). Tumor promotion in the liver. *Arch. Toxicol.,* **57**, 147–58
6. Schulte-Hermann, R., Hoffmann, V., Parzefall, W., Kallenbach, M., Gerhardt, A. and Schuppler, J. (1980). Adaptive responses of rat liver to the gestagen and anti-androgen cyproterone acetate and other inducers. II. Induction of growth. *Chem. Biol. Interact.,* **31**, 287–300
7. Bursch, W., Düsterberg, B. and Schulte-Hermann, R. (1986). Growth, regression and cell death in rat liver as related to tissue levels of the hepatomitogen cyproterone acetate. *Arch. Toxicol.,* **59**, 221–7
8. Wyllie, A. H., Kerr, J. F. R. and Currie, A. R. (1980). Cell death: the significance of apoptosis. *Int. Rev. Cytol.,* **68**, 251–306
9. Bursch, W., Taper, H. S., Lauer, B. and Schulte-Hermann, R. (1985). Quantitative histological and histochemical studies on the occurrence and stages of controlled cell death (apoptosis) during regression of rat liver hyperplasia. *Virch. Arch. Cell Pathol.,* **50**, 153–66
10. Schulte-Hermann, R., Bursch, W., Fesus, L. and Kraupp, B. (1988). Cell death by apoptosis in normal, preneoplastic and neoplastic tissue. In Feo, F., Pani, P., Columbano, A. and Garcea, R. (eds.) *Chemical Carcinogenesis: Models and Mechanisms.* (New York: Plenum Press), in press
11. Ucker, D. S. (1987). Cytotoxic T lymphocytes and glucocorticoids activate an endogenous suicide process in target cells. *Nature,* **327**, 62–4
12. Wyllie, A. H., Morris, R. G., Smith, A. L. and Dunlop, D. (1984). Chromatin cleavage in apoptosis: Association with condensed chromatin morphology and dependence on macromolecular synthesis. *J. Pathol.,* **142**, 67–77

13. Ellis, H. M. and Horvitz, H. R. (1986). Genetic control of programmed cell death in the *C. elegans. Cell,* **44**, 817–29

14. Schulte-Hermann, R., Bursch, W. and Timmermann-Trosiener, I. (1987). Liver tumour promoters. In Reutter, W., Popper, H., Arias, I. M., Heinrich, P. C., Keppler, D. and Landmann, L. (eds.) *Falk Symposium 43: Modulation of Liver Cell Expression*, pp 57–67. (Lancaster: MTP Press)

15. Wyllie, A. H. (1980). Glucocorticoid-induced thymocyte apoptosis is associated with endogenous endonuclease activation. *Nature,* **284**, 555–6

16. Duke, R. C. and Cohen, J. J. (1986). Il-2 adduction: withdrawal of growth factor activates a suicide program in independent T-cells. *Lymphokine Res.,* **5**, 289–99

17. Fesus, L., Thomazy, V. and Falsus, A. (1987). Induction and activation of tissue transglutaminase during programmed cell death. *FEBS Lett.,* **224**(1), 104–8

Section 5
Altered gene expression

30
Biochemical strategy of hepatocellular carcinoma

G. WEBER

INTRODUCTION

It is over 25 years since the ideas of the molecular correlation concept as a theoretical and experimental method for discovering the pattern of biochemical imbalance and its linking with transformation and progression in cancer cells were first introduced[1]. Progress in this programme involved collaboration with nearly 100 scientists. The results characterized the quantitative and qualitative alterations that occur in cancer cells which specifically distinguish the biochemistry of neoplastic tissues from that of normal, developing, or regenerating tissues[2,3].

The molecular correlation concept provided precise, testable predictions on the enzymic and metabolic pattern of cancer cells, and two major reviews outlined the main results and the propositions arising from the data[2,3]. In the majority of these studies, a continuum of hepatomas of different proliferative rates and malignancy was the biological model where the biochemical events were linked with transformation (occurring to the same extent in all tumours) or progression (expressed in increasing degrees of alterations in parallel with the growth rate).

METABOLIC IMBALANCES

Carbohydrate

The existence of key enzymes was discovered first in carbohydrate metabolism. The recognition of the key enzymes allowed testing of predictions. Our studies recognized the following quantitative alterations in carbohydrate metabolism of hepatomas. The activities of the three key enzymes of glycolysis increased, whereas those of key enzymes of gluconeogenesis decreased. These changes in the behaviour of antagonistic enzymes in the opposing pathways

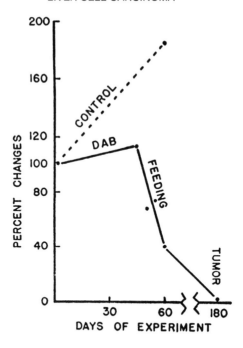

Figure 1 Glucose-6-phosphatase activity during carcinogenesis. Rats were on dimethylaminoazo-benzene diet for 150 days, then on fox chow for 30 days. Activity is expressed as per cent change from control fox chow-fed rats, killed at the same time. Each point represents the average of at least three animals

of glycolysis and gluconeogenesis served as a pattern for further discoveries in other metabolic pathways[2].

The first evidence for decrease of a liver enzymic activity during hepatocarcinogenesis leading to an absence of enzymic activity in the resulting hepatomas was reported in 1953 in identifying the behaviour of glucose-6-phosphatase (Figure 1)[4]. The analysis of the altered pattern of carbohydrate enzyme activities in liver cancer was completed in the 1960s (summarized in Figure 2)[5,6].

Our results have been confirmed by biochemical assays and histochemically in many laboratories. Most recently, the presence of the enzymic imbalance in carbohydrate metabolism has also been confirmed in pre-neoplastic nodules, which supports the view that these are very early changes[1-6]. On the basis of the studies carried out on the well-differentiated hepatomas, the biochemical alterations probably did indeed occur at the time of neoplastic transformation[3]. Confirmatory studies provided additional evidence of the testability of the molecular correlation concept. Furthermore, the biochemical alterations originally observed in chemically-induced transplantable hepatomas in the rat have been shown to apply to virally-induced hepatomas in the chicken, to many other types of murine tumours, and to primary neoplasms in human[3].

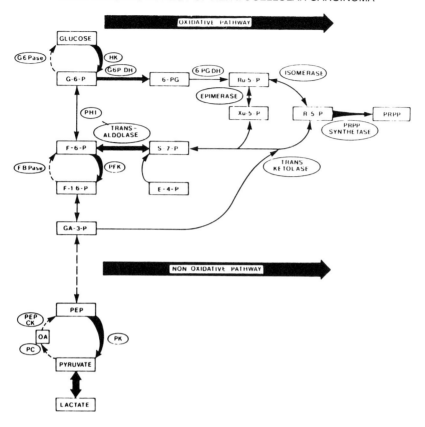

Figure 2 Enzymic imbalance in carbohydrate and pentose phosphate metabolism in hepatomas. The thick, straight arrows indicate transformation-linked alterations, the tapered arrows indicate progression-linked alterations. The dashed arrows indicate decreased activities
Abbreviations: E-4-P = erythrose-4-phosphate; F-1,6-P = fructose-1,6-phosphate; F-6-P = fructose-6-phosphate; FBPase, FDPase = fructose-bisphosphatase; GA-3-P = glyceraldehyde-3-phosphate; G-6-P = glucose-6-phosphate; G6Pase = glucose-6-phosphatase; G6PDH = glucose-6-phosphate dehydrogenase; HK = hexokinase; OA = oxaloacetate; PC = pyruvate carboxylase; PEP = phosphoenolpyruvate; PFK = 6-phosphofructokinase; 6-PG = 6-phosphogluconate; 6-PGDH = 6-phosphogluconate dehydrogenase; PHI = phosphohexose isomerase; PK = pyruvate kinase; PRPP = phosphoribosylpyrophosphate; R-5-P = ribose-5-phosphate; Ru-5-P = ribulose-5-phosphate; S-7-P = sedoheptulose-7-phosphate; Xu-5-P = xylulose-5-phosphate

It is of particular relevance that the extensively documented biochemical pattern of rat hepatomas applies to human primary hepatocellular carcinomas[3]. These alterations should provide targets for chemotherapy as outlined in our proposal for enzyme-pattern-targeted chemotherapy[3].

The following will concentrate on the biochemical imbalance in pyrimidine and purine metabolism because much of our current chemotherapeutic work centres in these areas.

Table 1 Enzymic markers of transformation in pyrimidine and DNA metabolism

Synthetic pathway	Degradative pathway
Increased activity	*Decreased activity*
Carbamoyl-phosphate synthase II[a]	Thymidine phosphorylase
Aspartate carbamoyltransferase[a]	Dihydrothymine
Dihydroorotase[a]	dehydrogenase[a]
Orotate phosphoribosyltransferase	
Orotidine-5'-phosphate decarboxylase	
UDP kinase	
CPT synthase[a]	
Ribonucleotide reductase[a]	
DNA polymerase[a]	
Uridine-cytidine kinase[a]	
Deoxycytidine kinase[a]	
Thymidine kinase[a]	

The relationship of enzymic activities with transformation and progression was determined in the rat hepatoma spectrum
[a]Also linked with progression

Pyrimidines and DNA

Table 1 shows the transformation- and progression-linked alterations in pyrimidine and DNA metabolism. In pyrimidine metabolism, the activities of key enzymes of *de novo* biosynthesis are increased, and those of degradation are decreased. The enzymes with the lowest activities, e.g. ribonucleotide reductase, are increased the most markedly.

It is important that the activities of the salvage enzymes are also increased. Table 1 indicates the linking of the enzymic activities with transformation and progression in the rat hepatoma spectrum.

The reciprocal alterations in enzymic activities, first observed for the behaviour of the enzymes of glycolysis and gluconeogenesis[2,5,6], now have been shown for the behaviour of the activities of thymidine kinase and dihydrothymine dehydrogenase. The behaviour of the activities of these pyrimidine enzymes closely correlated with that of the overall activity of the incorporation of thymidine into DNA and degradation of thymidine to CO_2. The good agreement between the behaviour of the activities of key enzymes measured in tissue extracts and that of the overall metabolic pathways determined in tissue slices indicates the biological relevance of these observations[2,3].

Purines

The enzymic alterations in purine metabolism in hepatomas are summarized in Table 2. The activities of ten enzymes in the pathways of purine and RNA biosynthesis are increased, and those of four enzymes of degradation are decreased. Adenylate kinase activity also decreased. In addition, ribonucleo-

Table 2 Enzymic markers of transformation in purine and RNA metabolism

Synthetic pathway	Degradative pathway
Increased activity	*Decreased activity*
Amidophosphoribosyltransferase	5'-Nucleotidase
Formylglycinamidine ribonucleotide synthase	Inosine phosphorylase
Adenylosuccinate synthase	Xanthine oxidase
Adenylosuccinate lyase	Uricase
AMP deaminase[a]	Adenylate kinase[a]
IMP dehydrogenase[a]	
GMP synthase[a]	
tRNA methylase	
Arginyl-tRNA synthase[a]	
RNA polymerase[a]	

The relationship of enzymic activities with transformation and progression was determined in the rat hepatoma spectrum
[a]Also linked with progression

tide reductase activity, already mentioned in pyrimidine biosynthesis, was elevated.

Additional areas where a biochemical imbalance has been observed include ornithine metabolism, pentose phosphate utilization, metabolism of membrane cyclic adenylate nucleotides[2,3] and histone metabolism. The biochemical imbalance in polyamine metabolism is yet another area. Altogether, over 50 enzymes were identified as transformation-linked (activities altered in all cancer cells), and at least 30 of these are also progression-linked (activities gradually altered in parallel with the malignancy of the tumours)[3].

QUALITATIVE ALTERATIONS IN CANCER CELLS: THE ISOZYME SHIFT

The qualitative changes are expressed in the gradual decrease in the activity of the liver-specific, regulatory, high K_m enzymes (e.g. glucokinase, liver-type pyruvate kinase), and the increase in activity of non-liver type, low K_m isozymes (e.g. hexokinase, muscle-type pyruvate kinase). An isozyme shift also occurs in enzymes of pyrimidine metabolism (uridine-cytidine kinase) and purine metabolism (adenylosuccinate lyase). The importance of the isozyme shift has been discussed elsewhere[3].

RE-PROGRAMMING OF GENE EXPRESSION IN CANCER CELLS: ENZYMIC AND IMMUNOLOGIC EVIDENCE

The enzymic pattern of ordered transformation- and progression-linked alterations in hepatoma cells was a manifestation of the re-programming of gene expression (Table 3). This interpretation of the altered biochemical

Table 3 Evidence for re-programming of gene expression in cancer cells: quantitative changes in enzyme amount in hepatoma 3924A

Pathways	Enzymes	Increased amount (x-fold)
Pentose phosphate	Glucose-6-phosphate dehydrogenase	5
Glycolysis	6-Phosphofructokinase	3
Pyrimidine synthesis	CTP synthase	11
de novo	Carbamoyl-P synthase II	8
salvage	Thymidine kinase	25
Purine synthesis	Amidophosphoribosyltransferase	2
	IMP dehydrogenase	10
Pyrimidine degradation	Dihydrothymine dehydrogenase	Decreased to 30%
Purine degradation	Xanthine oxidase	Decreased to 4%

phenotype is based on demonstration in cancer cells of changed amounts in the end products of gene expression, the concentrations of specific catalytic proteins, the enzymes. The enzyme amounts were measured by independent methods: (1) assay of enzyme activity, and (2) immunotitration of the enzyme protein amount by specific anti-enzyme serum. An increased enzyme amount was demonstrated for key enzymes of glycolysis (6-phosphofructokinase), pentose phosphate production (glucose-6-phosphate dehydrogenase), pyrimidine de novo biosynthesis (CTP synthase, carbamoyl-phosphate synthase II), pyrimidine salvage (thymidine kinase), and purine synthesis (amidophosphoribosyl transferase, IMP dehydrogenase). By contrast, in the degradative pathways there were decreased amounts of the pyrimidine enzyme, dihydrothymine dehydrogenase, and the purine enzyme, xanthine dehydrogenase. The evidence was that in all cases where it has been studied the altered enzymic activity indicated a change in the enzyme amount[7].

GENERALIZATION: STRONGLY CONSERVED PROGRAMME OF ALTERED GENE EXPRESSION

The data accumulated show that there is a strongly conserved segment of altered gene expression in chemically- or virally-induced or spontaneous neoplasms. The gene programme expressed in cancer cells transcends the species barrier, since it occurs in neoplasms in rodent, avian, and human organisms. It has been demonstrated that some or all aspects of the biochemical imbalance were present in 17 different animal and human malignant tumours[8].

SELECTIVE ADVANTAGES OF THE BIOCHEMICAL PHENOTYPE AND TARGETS FOR CHEMOTHERAPY

In all metabolic pathways examined in the hepatoma spectrum an imbalance was revealed in the reciprocal expression of the activities of the opposing key enzymes and of the synthetic and catabolic pathways. The alterations in carbohydrate metabolism provide an increased capacity for generating energy and through the elevated activities of glucose-6-phosphatase dehydrogenase, transaldolase, and phosphoribosyl pyrophosphate (PRPP) synthase to produce pentose phosphates and PRPP to be utilized in purine and pyrimidine biosynthesis[6]. In pyrimidine metabolism the increased activities of the synthetic enzymes and the decreased capacity of those in catabolism provide a heightened ability for the production of precursors for DNA biosynthesis. In purine metabolism the reprogramming of gene expression yielded an increased potential to produce IMP, ATP and particularly GMP, GDP and CTP, in presence of decreased capacity to degrade purines[2,3]. This biochemical imbalance should yield increased pools of dNTPs and our studies verified this prediction in that the concentrations of dCTP, dTTP, dATP, and dGTP were markedly increased in parallel with the elevation in the growth rates of the hepatomas[9]. The enzymic and metabolic imbalance in pyrimidine, purine and carbohydrate metabolism confers selective advantages to cancer cells.

Our evidence indicates that in cancer cells the number of genes which specify the production and regulation of opposing key enzymes in strategic metabolic pathways are closely co-adapted during evolution. The reprogramming of gene expression seems to reveal a pleiotropic programme of one or a family of master genes and integrative genomic elements. The molecular biology of the altered phenotype of cancer cells should account for biochemical alterations that occur in equal extent in all cancer cells irrespective of the extent of biological malignancy or degrees of differentiation. These transformation-linked, all-or-none, discontinuously-expressed biochemical markers of gene expression are stringently linked in the expression of neoplastic properties. The progression-linked enzymic and metabolic alterations should be accounted for by molecular biological events that provide the graded steps in gene expression that is stringently linked with the degrees of biological malignancy. In the meantime, since we have now identified much of the neoplastic phenotype of the biochemical commitment to replication, the most relevant components, the key enzymes, should be prime targets in the design of selective anti-cancer chemotherapy[2,3,10].

GENE LOGIC IN CANCER CELLS

Significant areas of gene logic were recognized as a result of our observations:
(1) Reciprocal control of activities of opposing key enzymes and pathways of synthesis and catabolism in various metabolic areas.
(2) The extent of rise in activities of key enzymes of purine and pyrimidine biosynthesis in rapidly-growing hepatomas was a function of the absolute activities of the enzymes in adult resting liver.
(3) The activities of purine and pyrimidine salvage enzymes in rapidly-growing hepatomas were 2- to 44-fold higher than those of the rate-limiting enzymes in the *de novo* synthetic pathways.
(4) The enzymic and metabolic alterations were stringently linked with transformation and progression.

(5) Activities of enzymes that were present in excess and never became limiting for a metabolic pathway changed in a random fashion.

(6) The ordered enzymic alterations were due to changes in enzyme amount, and thus they represented a re-programming of gene expression in cancer cells.

(7) The qualitative alterations in gene expression are indicated by the isozyme shift where the key enzymes which were subject to nutritional and hormonal regulation and had high K_m for their substrates were replaced, most markedly, in the rapidly-proliferating hepatomas, with an isozyme population that exhibited low K_m for substrates and was less or not at all subject to nutritional and hormonal controls.

(8) Since the re-programming of gene expression revealed in the enzymic and metabolic imbalance in the phenotype was present in 17 different types of cancer cells, including chemically- and virally-induced tumours in animals and primary neoplasias in humans, a strongly conserved segment of gene expression that is stringently linked with neoplastic transformation and progression has now been identified.

In consequence, investigations no longer need to be concerned with the apparent diversity of biochemical changes in cancer cells, because it has now been determined that what is important for cancer cells is highly ordered and what is not, is the randomness that is not stringently linked with the essence of neoplasia. Chemotherapy can now be targeted with confidence to the transformation- and progression-linked biochemical alterations that characterize the unique commitment of cancer cells to replication. Therefore, an approach has been provided for rationally designed enzyme-pattern-targeted chemotherapy[2,3,10].

DESIGN OF ENZYME-PATTERN-TARGETED CHEMOTHERAPHY

The following four concepts form the basis for the approaches of enzyme-pattern-targeted chemotherapy:

(1) The enzymic and metabolic imbalance in the phenotype of cancer cells provides selective reproductive advantages for cancer cells.

(2) By identifying the biochemical alterations that characterize the commitment of cancer cells for replication, we can pinpoint sensitive targets for drug treatment. These targets are the transformation- and progression-linked increased activities of key enzymes and the elevated pools of nucleotides and other metabolites.

(3) Selectivity of drugs against cancer cells will be the higher the more extensive is the biochemical difference from normal cells. The marked biochemical imbalance in cancer cells should indicate an increased dependence on the enzyme or the metabolic process involved.

(4) The amplified and stringently linked biochemical pattern of cancer cells should be more vulnerable to drug-induced perturbation than that of normal tissues which have a wider range of repair, adaptability, and capacity for recovery.

Our current studies with tiazofurin in human leukaemic patients provide an example of the rational design and use of inhibitors in an enzyme-pattern-targeted chemotherapy[10,11].

Enzyme-pattern-targeted chemotherapy of human leukaemia with tiazofurin

Systematic studies by Weber have provided evidence for the operation of an ordered biochemical imbalance in cancer cells which was due to a reprogramming of gene expression. Examination of the altered biochemical pattern indicated that such an integrated change in enzymic and metabolic capacity conferred selective advantages to cancer cells. It seemed clear that the increased activities of key enzymes should be sensitive targets for the design of anti-cancer chemotherapy.

There was another approach which offered a critical testing of the biological significance of the biochemical imbalance. This was the test suggested 30 years ago in our early studies[12]:

> It is possible that many of the biochemical changes described in cancer literature belong to a class which may be called 'concomitant and nonessential changes'. To determine the essentiality of a biochemical change in the neoplastic tissue the following rule may be applied: Does the re-establishment of corresponding normal tissue values inhibit the growth of tumor?

There were a number of studies, cited recently, which tested the validity of the above statement. In 1987 we started testing the validity of this approach by targeting tiazofurin against IMP dehydrogenase activity in patients suffering from refractory AML (acute myelocytic leukaemia). The rationale for these studies is summarized in the following:

(1) Increased IMP dehydrogenase activity in leukaemic cells.
(2) Inhibition of IMP dehydrogenase activity with tiazofurin should curtail GTP concentrations in leukaemic cells.
(3) Leukaemic cells produced much more tiazofurin adenine dinucleotide (TAD), the active metabolite of tiazofurin.
(4) A predictive test for sensitivity to tiazofurin was available.
(5) Blocking IMP dehydrogenase activity and decrease of GTP may induce differentiation.
(6) Impact of tiazofurin treatment can be monitored biochemically[10].

Experimental and conceptual background: IMP dehydrogenase and tiazofurin

Studies by Weber cited above indicate a marked imbalance in purine metabolism in cancer cells. Among the most significant alterations, we noted that IMP dehydrogenase, the rate-limiting enzyme of *de novo* GTP biosynthesis, increased in a transformation- and progression-linked fashion in the

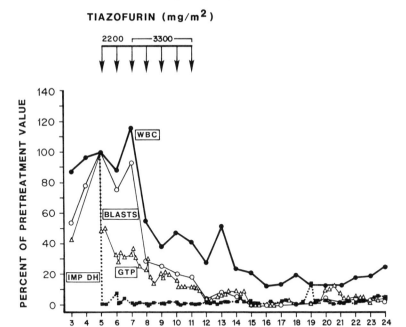

Figure 3 Effect of tiazofurin treatment in a case of refractory AML. The WBC and blast cell counts, the concentration of GTP per blast cells and the activity of IMP dehydrogenase (nmol/hour/mg protein) are given as percentages of the values observed before the beginning of tiazofurin treatment

hepatoma spectrum. This provided an increased capacity to make guanylates. GTP is a strategic precursor for DNA and RNA biosynthesis and dGTP is the rate-limiting precursor in the production of DNA. Moreover, GTP is required in protein biosynthesis and it plays a role in the expression of oncogenes that involve the function of the G-protein. The activity of IMP dehydrogenase increased in a number of other types of cancer cells, including human leukaemic cells[10]. On the basis of such considerations we suggested that IMP dehydrogenase should be a potentially sensitive target for the design of chemotherapy[2,3,13]. This idea was taken up by Robins[14] who prepared a number of compounds directed against IMP dehydrogenase. Two of these compounds proved to be good inhibitors of IMP dehydrogenase: ribavirin, a blocker of virus replication; and tiazofurin, an inhibitor of the growth of certain murine tumours.

Tiazofurin, a C-nucleoside, is activated in sensitive cells by a kinase to tiazofurin monophosphate which is converted by NAD phosphorylase into TAD, an NAD analogue. TAD is the active metabolite and it appears to be a determining factor in the anti-cancer action[15]. Tiazofurin has been in Phase I trials at the National Cancer Institute and a number of other centres, testing its toxicity and possible effectiveness in solid tumours in humans.

The clinical studies were not progressing well because of the toxicity of tiazofurin which was tested in the NCI treatment protocol. In this protocol, tiazofurin was given in a bolus once per day for 5 days or as a continuous i.v. drip for 5 days. The main toxicity was neurotoxicity and the NCI decided to hold off the trials because of this side effect.

We have however carried out preliminary studies to see whether tiazofurin might be useful in leukaemic patients, by designing a clinical trial which had the following novel features:

(1) The drug was given in a 1-hour infusion by pump to decrease the toxicity.
(2) Myelocytic leukaemia patients were treated because there was increased IMP dehydrogenase activity in leukaemic cells.
(3) Because our studies indicated that leukaemic cells formed 20-fold higher amounts of TAD from labelled tiazofurin than normal leukocytes, a predictive test was developed.
(4) The activity of IMP dehydrogenase and of the salvage enzyme, GPRT, and the concentration of GTP, the end product, were monitored in the blast cells.
(5) The tiazofurin concentration in the plasma was determined.
(6) The plasma hypoxanthine level was measured because all patients also received allopurinol, originally to decrease uric acid formation. Our Phase I/II trial was approved by NCI.

Tiazofurin in leukaemic patients inhibited IMP dehydrogenase activity and caused remission

The detailed results of the haematological and biochemical action of tiazofurin in refractory AML are published elsewhere[10,11] and here our report concentrates on the impact of this drug on the biochemical targets. Infusion of tiazofurin (2200 mg/m^2) decreased IMP dehydrogenase activity in the blast cells with a $t_{1/2}$ of 30 min and subsequently the GTP concentration fell with a $t_{1/2}$ of about 2 days. These biochemical events were followed by a decline of the blast count, whereas the granulocytes were selectively preserved (Figure 3). Bone-marrow examination showed a remarkable shift from myeloblasts to more mature myeloid elements, suggesting an *in vivo* differentiating action of tiazofurin[10,11].

Side effects with our daily 1-hour infusion, given for a period of 10–14 days, were less pronounced than in previous trials. During the course of treatment, we observed that allopurinol, given once in the morning (300 mg), failed to control hypoxanthine plasma level longer than a few hours. We decided to increase allopurinol dose and to give it in a divided fashion every 4–6 hours. This method succeeded in maintaining high plasma hypoxanthine levels in most patients.

Our studies indicated that hypoxanthine competitively inhibited the activity of the salvage enzyme, GPRT. In consequence, tiazofurin and allopurinol acted together to achieve enzyme-pattern-targeted chemotherapy in human leukaemia[10].

To date, a year after the study started, 16 patients have been treated. Out of these, 11 were evaluable, 2 were resistant to the treatment and 3 had early toxicities. The results include 1 complete remission now lasting over 7 months; other responses were haematological improvements, without reversal of cytogenetics, resulting in 2- to 10-month remissions.

From the point of view of the molecular correlation concept, these human studies demonstrated that the increased IMP dehydrogenase activity is indeed a suitable and sensitive target to chemotherapy. Our principle developed 30 years ago in testing the significance of an enzymic alteration by returning the enzyme activity to normal level indeed was a useful test for evaluating the biological significance of the metabolic alteration[4,10].

Our ideas on enzyme-pattern-targeted chemotherapy[10] have also been validated in the patients because the inhibition of the *de novo* biosynthesis of GTP through blocking IMP dehydrogenase activity (tiazofurin) and the inhibition of the salvage pathway through blocking the GPRT activity (hypoxanthine) provided a depletion of the end product, GTP, and a decline in the blast cell counts. These investigations have shown a good correlation in the behaviour of the biochemical parameters (IMP dehydrogenase activity, GTP concentration) and the haematological indicators (blast count)[10].

The treatment courses provided remissions of 2–8 weeks' duration and patients could be re-treated with the same dose protocol in some cases for many months. Our discovery that it is not necessary to increase the tiazofurin dose every time the patient returned with a relapse has provided a longer treatment possibility with decreased risk of toxicity.

Tiazofurin-induced differentiation and oncogene down-regulation

Induced differentiation *in vitro* by tiazofurin and by other inhibitors of *de novo* GTP biosynthesis has been observed in HL-60 tissue culture cells[16,17]. In these *in vitro* studies, if depletion of GTP was circumvented by providing high concentration of guanine in the tissue culture system, differentiation failed to occur even in presence of tiazofurin. Thus, the differentiation was due to depletion of GTP concentration.

However, our clinical studies are the first to demonstrate *in vivo* differentiation after tiazofurin administration in patients[10,11]. In our patients, the decrease in GTP concentration had to be 90% or more to provide a switch from expression of neoplasia to expression of the differentiation programme. Such a decrease in the GTP pool should curtail the expression of GTP-dependent oncogenes which might be responsible for switching off the cancer phenotype and permitting differentiation of the blast cells in the patient. This hypothesis is supported by our studies in K562 human leukaemic cells where tiazofurin decreased IMP dehydrogenase activity, and subsequently GTP concentration, followed by extinction of the expression of the c-Ki-*ras* oncogene. These molecular alterations were followed by expression of the differentiation programme as indicated by an increase in the production of haemoglobin[18]. If these results are directly applicable to our *in vivo* situation in the patient, then our studies have achieved pharmacological extinction of the action of oncogenes in human leukaemic cells by tiazofurin treatment.

SUMMARY

With the guide of the molecular correlation concept, a conceptual and experimental method, an ordered pattern of biochemical imbalance has been identified in carbohydrate, pyrimidine and purine metabolism. In these studies, strategic aspects of gene logic have been identified as follows.

(1) The activities of opposing key enzymes of antagonistic pathways of synthesis and degradation are reciprocally regulated. Activities of key enzymes of glycolysis and pyrimidine and purine biosynthesis increased, whereas those of gluconeogenesis and purine and pyrimidine catabolism decreased.

(2) Qualitative alterations in gene expression are characterized by a decrease in the activities of high K_m regulatory isozymes which are replaced by increased activities of low K_m isozymes which are not subject to nutritional or hormonal regulation.

(3) The enzymic pattern of ordered transformation- and progression-linked alterations in hepatoma cells is a manifestation of the re-programming of gene expression. This conclusion is based on demonstration in cancer cells of the changed amount in the end products of gene expression, the concentrations of specific catalytic proteins, the enzymes. In all cases where it has been studied, the altered enzymic activity was due to a change in the enzyme amount.

(4) There is a strongly conserved segment of altered gene expression in chemically- or virally-induced murine and avian hepatomas and in spontaneous hepatocellular carcinoma in human. Some, or all, aspects of biochemical imbalance discovered were present in 17 different animal and human tumours.

(5) The biochemical imbalance in hepatomas and other tumours conferred selective advantages to the neoplastic cells.

(6) On the basis of enzyme-pattern-targeted chemotherapy, the impact of tiazofurin was examined on the increased IMP dehydrogenase activity in human leukaemic patients.

Infusion of tiazofurin in 1-hour administration by pump decreased IMP dehydrogenase activity in the blast cells with a $t_{1/2}$ of about 2 days. These biochemical events were followed by a decline of the blast count, whereas the granulocytes were selectively preserved. Thus, the increased IMP dehydrogenase activity present in all hepatomas and other examined cancer cells is a suitable and sensitive target for chemotherapy. Our principle of testing the significance of an enzymic alteration by returning the enzymic activity to normal level through drug administration is a useful assay for the biological significance of the metabolic alterations.

Acknowledgements

This study was supported in part by Outstanding Investigator Grant no. CA42510 awarded by the USPHS National Cancer Institute to G.W.

References

1. Weber, G. (1961). Behavior of liver enzymes during hepatocarcinogenesis. *Adv. Cancer Res.*, **6**, 403–94
2. Weber, G. (1977). Enzymology of cancer cells. *N. Engl. J. Med.*, **296**, 486–93 and 541–51
3. Weber, G. (1983). Biochemical strategy of cancer cells and the design of chemotherapy. G. H. A. Clowes Memorial Lecture. *Cancer Res.*, **43**, 3466–92
4. Weber, G. and Cantero, A. (1955). Glucose-6-phosphatase activity in normal, precancerous, and neoplastic tissues. *Cancer Res.*, **15**, 105–8
5. Weber, G. (1968). Carbohydrate metabolism in cancer cells and the molecular correlation concept. *Naturwissenschaften*, **55**, 418–29
6. Weber, G. (1982). Differential carbohydrate metabolism in tumor and host. In *Molecular Interrelations of Nutrition and Cancer, UT System Cancer Center 34th Ann. Symp. Fundamental Cancer Res.*, pp 191–208. (New York: Raven Press)
7. Weber, G. (1987). Biochemical basis of cancer chemotherapy. Plenary Lecture. In Lapis, K. and Eckhardt, S. (eds.) *Lectures & Symposia of the 14th Intl. Cancer Congress*, **1**, pp 17–36. (Budapest, Hungary: Academia Publ.)
8. Weber, G. (1987). Strongly conserved segment of gene expression in cancer cells. In Reutter, W. *et al.* (eds.) *Modulation of Liver Cell Expression, Falk Symposia*, pp. 303–14 (Lancaster: MTP Press)
9. Jackson, R. C., Lui, M. S., Boritzki, T. J., Morris, H. P. and Weber, G. (1980). Purine and pyrimidine nucleotide patterns of normal, differentiating and regenerating liver and of hepatomas in rats. *Cancer Res.*, **40**, 1286–91
10. Weber, G., Jayaram, H. N., Lapis, E., Natsumeda, Y., Yamada, Y., Yamaji, Y., Tricot, G. J. and Hoffman, R. (1988). Enzyme-pattern-targeted chemotherapy with tiazofurin and allopurinol in human leukemia. *Adv. Enzyme Regul.*, **27**, 405–33
11. Tricot, G. J., Jayaram, H. N., Nichols, C. R., Pennington, K., Lapis, E., Weber, G. and Hoffman, R. (1987). Hematological and biochemical action of tiazofurin in a case of refractory acute myeloid leukemia. *Cancer Res.*, **47**, 4988–91
12. Weber, G. and Cantero, A. (1957). Glucose-6-phosphate utilization in hepatoma, regenerating and newborn rat liver, and in the liver of fed and fasted normal rats. *Cancer Res.*, **17**, 995–1005
13. Weber, G., Prajda, N. and Jackson, R. C. (1976). Key enzymes of IMP metabolism: Transformation- and proliferation-linked alterations in gene expression. *Adv. Enzyme Regul.*, **14**, 3–24
14. Robins, R. K. (1982). Nucleoside and nucleotide inhibitors of inosine monophosphate (IMP) dehydrogenase as potential antitumor inhibitors. *Nucleosides and Nucleotides*, **1**, 35–44
15. Jayaram, H. N. (1984). Biochemical mechanism of resistance to tiazofurin. *Adv. Enzyme Regul.*, **24**, 67–89
16. Lucas, D. L., Webster, H. K. and Wright, D. G. (1983). Purine metabolism in myeloid precursor cells during maturation. *J. Clin. Invest.*, **72**, 1889–1900
17. Sokoloski, J. A. and Sartorelli, A. C. (1987). Alterations in glycoprotein synthesis and guanosine triphosphate levels associated with the differentiation of HL-60 leukemia cells produced by inhibitors of inosine 5'-phosphate dehydrogenase. *Cancer Res.*, **46**, 2314–19
18. Olah, E., Natsumeda, Y., Ikegami, T., Kote, Z., Horanyi, M., Szelenyi, J., Paulik, E., Kremmer, T., Hollan, S. R., Sugar, J. and Weber, G. (1988). Induction of erythroid differentiation and modulation of gene expression by tiazofurin in K562 leukemia cells. *Proc. Natl. Acad. Sci. USA*, **85**, 6533–7

31
Serine metabolic imbalance in hepatocellular carcinoma

K. SNELL

THE METABOLIC ROLE OF SERINE

L-Serine is an amino acid and as such is utilized in all tissues for the synthesis of proteins. It is a dietary non-essential amino acid since animals have the capacity to synthesize serine *de novo* from the glycolytic intermediate, 3-phosphoglycerate (see below). In addition to the general role of all amino acids in protein synthesis, serine has a unique and essential role to play in the *de novo* biosynthesis of nucleotides for DNA replication and cell division. Every carbon and nitrogen atom of the three-carbon serine molecule is involved in this biosynthetic role. The hydroxymethyl moiety at carbon-3 supplies the one-carbon unit of 5,10-methylene tetrahydrofolate, which serves directly as a carbon donor for the pyrimidine nucleotide thymidylate and, via conversion to 10-formyl tetrahydrofolate, as two of the carbons of the purine ring in the transformylase reactions of *de novo* purine nucleotide biosynthesis. The remaining two-carbon atoms of serine, with the associated amino nitrogen atom, supply further atoms of the purine ring in the phosphoribosylglycinamide synthetase reaction of purine biosynthesis. The unique role of serine in acting as a precursor for nucleotide biosynthesis during cell proliferation was recognized by Eagle in 1959 in his studies to formulate a suitable and defined culture medium for the growth of mammalian cells *in vitro*[1]. He noted that as well as the dietary essential amino acids required for protein synthesis:

> There is another situation in which normally non-essential amino acids regularly become essential ... when a minute cell population is propagated in a relatively large volume of fluid. In most of the experiments the complete mixture of non-essential amino acids could be replaced by a single amino acid, *serine*.

There is an obvious analogy between the expansion of a minute cell population to a large cellular mass in culture conditions *in vitro*, and the clonal expansion of a transformed neoplastic cell(s) into a tumour in the pathogenesis of cancer. In this context the metabolism of serine in cancer cells compared to normal cells is of relevance to the pathogenesis of tumours and to the identification of strategic biochemical sites at which anti-cancer enzyme-targeted drugs could be directed. Conceptual reasons and experimental evidence for the importance of *de novo* nucleotide biosynthesis in the specific, genetically-programmed biochemical commitment of cancer cells to continual proliferation have been reviewed by Weber[2].

SERINE METABOLISM IN HEPATOMAS

In relation to hapatocellular carcinoma, it is essential to define the pattern of serine metabolism in the normal hepatocyte which is the presumed progenitor of the neoplastic transformed cell. The metabolism of serine in animal tissues, and particularly in liver, has been reviewed recently[3]. In liver, apart from the dissimilation of serine to glycine and methylene tetrahydrofolate by serine hydroxymethyltransferase, alternative metabolic routes include those initiated by serine dehydratase and by serine aminotransferase which relate to the important glucogenic function of this tissue. These alternative enzymes of hepatic serine utilization were measured in transplantable rat hepatomas of the Morris series (Table 1). The results show a retention, or increase in the case of the rapidly-growing 5123tc hepatoma, of serine hydroxymethyltrans-ferase accompanied by a deletion of serine dehydratase and serine aminotransferase. This pattern agrees with that found in a previous study of a different series of Morris hepatomas[5]. These enzymic changes in hepatomas signify a marked metabolic imbalance compared to normal liver, whereby the selective retention of serine hydroxymethyltransferase, in the absence of the alternative enzymes of serine utilization, preferentially channels the available intracellular serine into nucleotide precursor formation. In these studies

Table 1 Enzymes of serine utilization in rat hepatomas

Tissue	Enzyme activity (μmol/min/g wet wt)[a]		
	Serine hydroxy-methyltransferase	Serine dehydratase	Serine aminotransferase
Control liver for:			
20	1.84 ± 0.11	7.69 ± 0.37	0.21 ± 0.01
3924A	1.84 ± 0.08	6.85 ± 1.08	0.21 ± 0.01
5123tc	1.78 ± 0.02	7.73 ± 0.42	0.19 ± 0.01
Hepatoma:			
20	0.92 ± 0.05	<0.02	<0.01
3924A	0.35 ± 0.004	<0.02	<0.01
5123tc	3.09 ± 0.18	<0.02	<0.01

Values recorded as the mean ± S.E.M. of 3–5 determinations
[a]Enzyme activities were assayed as described by Snell[4]

enzyme assays showed proportionality between activity and enzyme amount, and mixing experiments of normal liver extracts with hepatoma extracts gave the expected additivity of enzyme activities. Thus, the enzymic changes represent alterations in the amounts of enzymes, which presumably reflect a specific and co-ordinated re-programming of gene expression in the hepatomas. The consequent re-orientation, or imbalance, of serine metabolism in hepatoma cells would confer on them a growth advantage over non-neoplastic hepatocytes in liver, by providing them with an increased biochemical capacity for DNA synthesis.

The intracellular serine which is preferentially channelled into *de novo* nucleotide biosynthesis in hepatomas could arise from a variety of sources. Uptake from the extracellular fluid is one possibility, and Sauer *et al.*[6] have shown large negative afferent–efferent concentration differences for serine across the vasculature of established transplantable rat hepatomas *in vivo*. However, mammalian liver is also equipped with the enzymic capacity for serine synthesis *de novo* from the glycolytic precursor 3-phosphoglycerate. Moreover, the enzymes involved in this pathway[7] — phosphoglycerate dehydrogenase, phosphoserine aminotransferase, and phosphoserine phosphatase — can be induced and repressed by hormonal factors and by dietary protein in normal liver[3]. The pathway enzymes are all increased in transplantable rat hepatomas, compared to normal liver tissue, and show increased amounts which are positively related to the growth rate of the tumours (Figure 1). These increases are quantitatively specific to the neoplastic state. For example, phosphoglycerate dehydrogenase activity is increased about 50-fold (on a tissue weight basis) in hepatoma 3924A, whereas in non-neoplastic proliferative states with very similar cellular doubling-times the increase is much less (2.6-fold for regenerating liver and about 10-fold for neonatal liver)[8]. The increase in hepatomas of enzymes of

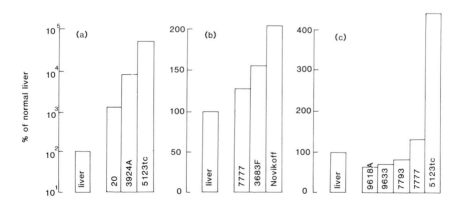

Figure 1 Enzymes of serine biosynthesis in transplantable rat Morris hepatomas. (a) 3-Phospho-glycerate dehydrogenase[8], (b) phosphoserine aminotransferase[5], and (c) phosphoserine phosphatase activities are expressed as the % of control values in normal liver on a units/mg tissue protein basis. The hepatomas are arranged from left to right in order of increasing growth rate

the serine biosynthesis pathway in concert with the enzymic imbalance in serine utilization which favours nucleotide precursor formation, suggests a co-ordinated modification of gene expression which serves to metabolically couple serine synthesis and utilization in this specific manner in cancer cells. The specificity of this genetic re-programming to the neoplastic state is further exemplified by the regenerating liver after partial hepatectomy where the increase in serine synthesis (phosphoglycerate dehydrogenase) is not coupled entirely to nucleotide precursor formation, since serine dehydratase is retained (unlike in hepatomas), presumably to maintain the essential glucogenic capacity of the renewing liver tissue[8].

COUPLING OF SERINE METABOLISM DURING HEPATOMA CULTURE *IN VITRO*

It was possible to test the hypothesis concerning the metabolic coupling of serine synthesis to its utilization for nucleotide precursor formation using a hepatoma 3924A-derived tumour cell line maintained in culture. Growing in monolayer culture conditions in McCoy's 5A medium, hepatoma cells pass from resting phase, through a lag phase into logarithmic phase, and then into a plateau phase. During this proliferative programme of the cancer cells, the already established enzymic imbalance present in the original 3924A solid tumour undergoes an expansive modulation through the logarithmic phase which returns to baseline values in the resting plateau growth phase[9]. In terms of nucleotide biosynthesis, the logarithmic growth phase involves a transient expansion of the intracellular ribonucleoside and deoxyribonucleoside triphosphate pools which correlates temporally with enzymes of purine and pyrimidine nucleotide *de novo* biosynthesis and with the metabolic fluxes of these pathways[9,10]. The enzyme of the serine synthesis pathway, phosphoglycerate dehydrogenase, and serine hydroxymethyltransferase showed a temporal association with the changes in nucleotide biosynthesis and with the incorporation of radioactivity from [3-^{14}C]serine into nucleotide bases of total cellular nucleic acids on a per cell basis[11]. The modulation of serine hydroxymethyltransferase[11] closely paralleled changes in the measured flux of *de novo* purine synthesis[10]. Moreover, incorporation from [3-^{14}C]serine into total purines was reduced in a dose-dependent manner by unlabelled formate due to dilution of the specific activities of 10-[^{14}C]formyl tetrahydrofolate[10]. These findings emphasize the essential role of serine as the endogenous pathway substrate for purine nucleotide biosynthesis *de novo*. The temporal association, during the proliferative growth phase in hepatoma cells in culture, of serine synthetic capacity with its utilization for nucleotide biosynthesis supports the hypothesis for a unique coupling of serine metabolism in cancer cells. The evidence suggests that the enzyme changes are alterations in amount of enzyme protein, presumably reflecting a specific and stringent re-orientation of gene expression to produce the metabolic imbalance in serine metabolism which favours the biochemical commitment to proliferation of these cancer cells.

INTRINSIC CONTROL OF SERINE BIOSYNTHESIS

The re-orientation of gene expression, which is manifest in the specific enzyme changes which accompany neoplastic transformation of the hepatocyte, can be viewed as a course control mechanism to up-regulate the whole system. It is important to establish in the new metabolic steady state where 'intrinsic' fine control of the pathway is exerted. Only in this way can those enzymes ('key enzymes') which have the greatest influence on total pathway flux be identified, to establish the strategic points at which anti-cancer chemotherapeutic agents should be directed. The development of control (strength) analysis in recent years has enabled the quantitative apportionment of the control strength or influence of individual enzymes in a pathway on the overall flux through that pathway to be defined[12,13]. The theoretical basis for this particular approach to the control analysis of pathways was established originally by Kacser and Burns[14] and by Heinrich and Rapoport[15], but the number of applications is still only a handful, mainly because of methodological difficulties in establishing the appropriate experimental conditions. The key features in the analysis are to determine the flux control coefficients (C_E^J) for the enzymes in a defined pathway, which is a systemic parameter quantitatively describing the incremental change in overall pathway flux ($\delta J/J$) as a ratio of a given incremental change in the enzyme under consideration ($\delta e/e$). The closer this ratio approaches unity, the greater the control influence that particular enzyme has on overall flux under a particular experimental steady-state situation. The summation theorem[12-15] requires that all of the enzymes in a defined pathway have control coefficients which aggregate to unity. In addition, each enzyme in a defined pathway has an elasticity coefficient (ϵ_X^e), which is a local parameter quantitatively describing the incremental change in enzyme rate ($\delta V_e/V_e$) as a ratio of a given incremental change in the concentration of some effector of the enzyme ($\delta X/X$) such as its substrate. The connectivity theorem[12-15] defines a relationship between elasticity coefficients and flux control coefficients which allows the latter to be derived from the former using matrix algebraic methods[16,17]. The elasticity coefficients of enzymes can be calculated relatively simply from either enzyme kinetic data and/or the value of the ratio between the mass action ratio (of the measured metabolic intermediates in the pathway) and the equilibrium constant for a near-equilibrium enzyme reaction[18]. From the elasticity coefficients and flux control coefficients it is possible to determine flux response coefficients (R_X^J) which define the influence of changes in effector concentrations on overall pathway flux by a ratio analogous to that indicated above for flux control coefficients.

We have applied such a control analysis to the serine biosynthetic pathway, in the first instance in normal rabbit liver *in vivo* under conditions of experimentally-varied pathway fluxes[19]. Our analysis involved the derivation of elasticity coefficients for the enzymes of the pathway from published enzyme kinetic data[20], and from the published measurements of concentrations of metabolic intermediates in the pathway[21] in order to calculate the mass action ratio. The result of the analysis relating to 'control' experimental conditions *in vivo*, in which there is a high serine biosynthetic flux, is shown in Figure 2. Because the concentration of 3-phosphohydroxypyruvate was below the

379

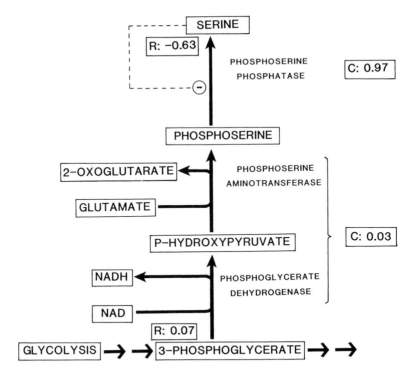

Figure 2 Control of the serine biosynthetic pathway. C represents the value of the flux control coefficient for the enzyme(s) indicated, and R represents the flux response coefficient for the metabolite indicated. Further details are given in the text. The data are taken from Fell and Snell[19] for normal rabbit liver *in vivo*

limits of analytical detection[21], separate elasticities could not be calculated for the first two steps of the pathway and a 'grouped' value was determined. These two steps in rabbit liver have been shown to operate close to thermo-dynamic equilibrium *in vivo*[21], so that it is legitimate on thermodynamic grounds to group the reactions as a single step. The flux control coefficient of phosphoserine phosphatase is 0.97; so close to unity that it behaves like a 'rate-limiting enzyme' for pathway flux under these conditions, albeit highly unusual in that it catalyses the *final* step of a biosynthetic pathway. Serine, the pathway product, feedback inhibits at this final pathway step, giving a flux response coefficient close to $-\frac{2}{3}$; i.e. a 3% rise in serine concentration will cause a 2% decrease in biosynthetic flux. This contrasts with the first two enzyme steps in the pathway, which despite having overall a relatively large elasticity coefficient, have a very low flux control coefficient resulting in a very small flux response coefficient, so that the overall pathway flux will be relatively unaffected by changes which might alter the concentration of 3-phosphoglycerate (such as alterations in glycolytic and/or gluconeogenic fluxes). This analysis shows that in rabbit liver *in vivo* under conditions of high biosynthetic flux, the pathway of serine biosynthesis is more responsive to product demand (serine concentration) than to precursor supply (3-phosphoglycerate concentration). Parenthetically, the analysis also highlights the danger of 'intuitively' assuming that the control of branched biochemical pathways is invariably exerted at the first enzyme step after the branch-point!

This analysis needs to be extended to hepatomas to define the control structure of the serine biosynthetic pathway in the neoplastic situation. If a similar structure is defined, and the discussion in earlier sections certainly indicates a greatly enhanced serine biosynthetic capacity compared to normal liver, then it follows that the utilization of serine will prove a highly effective self-regulating system for the 'metabolic coupling' of serine biosynthesis to nucleotide biosynthesis in a tandem pathway-control structure. This has implications for the strategy of a target-enzyme-directed anti-cancer agent in this metabolic area. The strategic significance of serine hydroxymethyltrans-ferase is highlighted: irreversible inhibition of this enzyme, leading to an accumulation of serine, would effectively attenuate serine biosynthetic flux reinforcing the pathway inhibition by substrate starvation.

SERINE HYDROXYMETHYLTRANSFERASE AS A TARGET FOR ANTI-CANCER DRUGS

As indicated above, metabolic flux from serine towards nucleotide precursor formation via serine hydroxymethyltransferase in hepatomas is favoured by the absence of some alternative enzymes of serine utilization. The increased flux into nucleobases of DNA was directly demonstrated in hepatoma 3924A during the expression of its proliferative programme in different phases of growth in culture. The alternative serine-utilizing enzymes are related to the glucogenic function of liver and are largely, or entirely, expressed only in this tissue[3,5]. Thus, in neoplasms of non-hepatic origin the increased capacity for channelling serine into nucleotide biosynthesis is manifest in absolute elevations of serine hydroxymethyltransferase in comparison to the cognate tissue of origin (Table 2). This pattern occurs in both rat and human tumours, and in sarcoma as well as carcinoma, indicating that it is a general feature of neoplastic transformation. The widespread distribution of serine hydroxy-methyltransferase in a variety of murine tumour cell types has also recently been reported[23]. Furthermore a positive correlation of enzyme activity with tumour growth rate was found in Friend leukaemia and Pliss rat lymphosarcoma models[24]. In human leukaemic patients, lymphocytic leukaemias had serine hydroxymethyltransferase activities which were 263–537% of those in normal lymphocytes, and granulocytic leukaemias had enzyme activities which were 259–350% of those in normal granulocytes[25].

It is noteworthy that serine hydroxymethyltransferase activity was markedly higher in a metastatic sub-clone ES/2 (216 nmol/hour/mg protein) of a mammary adenocarcinoma compared to its non-metastatic progenitor OES/5 (92 nmol/hour/mg protein) (K. Snell and S. A. Eccles, preliminary observations). This may reflect a higher capacity for *de novo* purine biosynthesis (guanylate synthesis) in transformed cells with metastatic

Table 2 Serine hydroxymethyltransferase activity in normal and neoplastic tissues

Tissue	Serine hydroxymethyltransferase activity (nmol/hour/mg protein) (% of control)[a]	
Rat kidney	63.6	
MK-1 renal carcinoma	157	(247)
Rat skeletal muscle	11.4	
Rat sarcoma	70.4	(618)
Rat mammary gland (non-lactating)	13.9	
Rat mammary gland (14 day lactating)	21.1	(152)
Rat mammary adenocarcinoma[b]	90.6	(652)
Human colon mucosa[c]	80.9	
Human colon adenocarcinoma[c]	378	(467)

Values recorded as the means of 5–10 determinations
[a]Enzyme activity was assayed as described by Snell[4]
[b]Mammary tumours were primaries of 'spontaneous' origin maintained by serial transplantation and assayed after the first passage stage. The tumours were generously made available by Dr. Suzanne A. Eccles, Institute of Cancer Research, Sutton, Surrey, U.K.
[c]Colon carcinomas and uninvolved normal colon tissue were obtained from patients undergoing surgical resection and were generously supplied by John N. Eble, M.D. and John L. Glover, M.D. of Indiana University School of Medicine, Indianapolis, U.S.A.[22]

potential and raises the intriguing possibility that elevated GTP levels may up-regulate the expression of a *ras* oncogene (which codes for a GTP-binding protein) as a component in the aetiology of the acquisition of metastatic potential. Two pieces of evidence suggest that this may be more than simply idle speculation, though speculation it certainly is! Firstly, inhibition of purine biosynthesis and a lowering of cellular GTP levels by the drug tiazofurin apparently leads to a down-regulation of *ras* oncogene transcript expression (E. Oláh, see Chapter 35). Secondly, it is known that the transfection of mammary carcinoma cells with an activated *ras* oncogene can confer metastatic properties on an already tumorigenic cell line[26,27]. Whether cellular GTP levels can operate as a direct metabolic switch for the trans-activation, or maintenance, of activated *ras* oncogene expression, and the relation of GTP levels to metastatic capacity, are matters for further investigation.

The strategic importance of serine hydroxymethyltransferase as a potential site for enzyme-directed anti-cancer agents lies not only in its role in providing precursors for purine nucleotide biosynthesis, but also in its role in the formation of the pyrimidine thymidylate (Figure 3). Inhibition of enzyme activity would therefore block DNA synthesis by a concurrent action on two parallel contributing biosynthetic pathways (purine and pyrimidine synthesis) and would result in a combination chemotherapeutic effect from a single enzyme-targeted inhibitory agent. In relation to pyrimidine synthesis, serine hydroxymethyltransferase is one of the trio of enzymes which constitute the

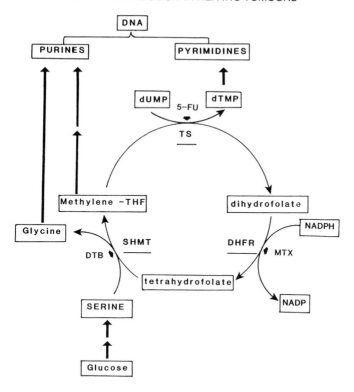

Figure 3 The role of serine in DNA synthesis and the thymidylate synthesis cycle.
Abbreviations: TS, thymidylate synthase; DHFR, dihydrofolate reductase; SHMT, serine hydroxymethyltransferase; 5-FU, 5-fluorouracil; MTX, methotrexate (amethoptrin); DTB, diaminodimethyltriazine benzene sulphonyl fluoride (NSC 127755). The scheme is adapted from that shown by Snell *et al.*[22]

thymidylate synthesis cycle, and it is noteworthy that each of the other two enzymes of this cycle has proved useful as a clinically-significant target for anti-cancer chemotherapeutic agents (Figure 3). The need for a further target in this metabolic area is indicated by the development of drug resistance in human tumour cell populations to agents directed at thymidylate synthase and dihydrofolate reductase.

Types of inhibitors which might be used to inhibit serine hydroxymethyltransferase include anti-folate analogues or serine antimetabolites. In addition, because of the role of pyridoxal 5'-phosphate as a bound cofactor of the enzyme, vitamin B$_6$ anti-metabolites such as D-cycloserine or 4-vinylpyridoxal[28], or more general pyridoxal-dependent-enzyme inhibitors like L-2-amino-4-methoxy-*trans*-3-butenoic acid[29], might be exploited. In fact these latter agents do not appear to be particularly useful, presumably because their actions are so non-specific and they can bind to many alternative amino acid metabolizing enzyme targets.

We have recently examined the inhibitory effect of one of the triazine group of anti-folates synthesized by Baker and his colleagues[30], 3-chloro-4-[4-[2-chloro-4-(4,6-diamino-1,2-dihydro-2,2-dimethyl-1,3,5-triazin-1-yl)phenyl]-butyl]benzene sulphonyl fluoride (Baker's Antifol II, NSC 127755). The agent exhibits anti-tumour activity against murine transplantable colon adenocarcinomas and the Dunning M5076 ovarian tumour[31]. Our studies used a mouse myeloma cell line (X63-Ag8.653) originally derived from a MOPC21 myeloma adapted for cell culture[32], and grown to a cell density of about 2×10^6 cells/ml in RPMI-1640 culture medium. Serine hydroxymethyltransferase activity in cell extracts (measured as detailed previously[11]) averaged 186 ± 51 nmol/hour/10^6 cells (360 nmol/hour/mg protein). NSC 127755 inhibited enzyme activity, in extracts preincubated for 1 hour at 37°C with varying concentrations of inhibitor, with an IC_{50} of 3.2×10^{-8} M. Pre-incubation of the intact cells for 1 hour at 37°C in 2.5 ml of fresh RPMI-1640 medium containing varying concentrations of inhibitor and at a cell density of 2×10^6 cells/ml, showed irreversible inhibition of serine hydroxymethyltransferase activity with an IC_{50} of 7.5×10^{-8}M. The effect of pre-incubation of intact cells for 1 hour with the inhibitor on thymidylate synthesis was assessed by subsequently measuring radioactivity incorporation from [6-^{3}H]deoxyuridine into DNA[33]. Any incorporation must proceed via the thymidylate synthase step and so is dependent on the availability of methylene tetrahydrofolate from the serine hydroxymethyltransferase reaction. NSC 127755 at a concentration of 10^{-7}M inhibited serine hydroxymethyltransferase activity by 56% in these experiments and inhibited [6-^{3}H]deoxyuridine incorporation into DNA by 61%. At an initial concentration of 10^{-3}M NSC 127755, sufficient to ensure 100% inhibition of serine hydroxymethyltransferase, myeloma cell cultures (seeded at a density of 3×10^5 cells/ml) failed to expand cell numbers and showed a 50% loss of viability (by trypan blue exclusion) by 18 hours of culture, a time identical to the doubling-time of control myeloma cell cultures. It is tempting to ascribe the inhibition of DNA synthesis and cytocidal action of NSC 127755 to the observed inhibition of serine hydroxy-methyltransferase in the myeloma cell culture. However, considerable caution is needed in such an interpretation. The substituted triazines, of which NSC 127755 is an example, were designed and shown to be irreversible active site inhibitors of dihydrofolate reductase[34,35]. Indeed the IC_{50} for inhibition of purified chicken liver dihydrofolate reductase was shown[35] to be about 3.5×10^{-8}M, a similar order of magnitude to the corresponding value for serine hydroxymethyltransferase in crude myeloma cell extracts. Inhibition of dihydrofolate reductase could indirectly have led to decreased deoxyuridine incorporation into DNA by decreasing tetrahydrofolate levels and attenuating the thymidylate synthesis cycle (Figure 3). Resolution of the site(s) of action of NSC 127755 in the myeloma cells requires measurements of folate cofactor levels and a knowledge of the relative active site affinities of purified dihydrofolate reductase and serine hydroxymethyltransferase for the inhibitor. Nevertheless, this is the first published report that serine hydroxy-methyltransferase can be inhibited in cells by triazine antifolates.

The use of serine anti-metabolites as inhibitors of serine hydroxmethyltransferase has received rather little attention. Cyclohexylserine has been shown to inhibit nucleic acid synthesis (but not protein synthesis) in human leukaemic cells, with a presumed action on serine hydroxymethyltransferase[36]. Acivicin, a glutamine analogue with structural resemblances also to serine, has potent anti-tumour actions[2,37] but did not inhibit rat sarcoma serine hydroxymethyl-transferase activity *in vitro* at concentrations up to 5 mM (K. Snell, unpublished observations). No inhibitory effects were found with azaserine under these conditions either (K. Snell, unpublished observations). A short series of alkyl α-substituted serines have been synthesized as potential irrever-sible suicide inhibitors of serine hydroxymethyltransferase but none was effective[38]. Perhaps the most successful attempt at the use of an anti-meta-bolite as an enzyme inhibitor is the irreversible suicide inhibitor D-fluoroalan-ine[39]. This takes advantage of the relatively unique ability of the enzyme to catalyse the transamination of the D-isomer of alanine. The ß-substi-tution of D-alanine with a reactive group determines that catalytic abstraction of the group will lead to alkylation of the enzyme at its active site[39]. Although irreversible inhibition of the enzyme was shown, the low affinity of D-fluoroalanine for serine hydroxymethyltransferase (10–60 mM)[39] unfortunately militates against its usefulness as an inhibitor *in vivo*. Nevertheless, the strategy of employing analogues of D-amino acid isomers is a promising one, since it should ensure specificity of action, with D-amino acid oxidase being the only other mammalian enzyme able to metabolize the isomer.

The potential for using optimal isomers as cytotoxic inhibitors was unwittingly first recognized over 100 years ago by Charles L. Dodgson who, writing under his pen-name of Lewis Carroll, has Alice speculate to her pet cat upon the properties of the inverted world *Through the Looking Glass:*[40]

How would you like to live in Looking-glass House, Kitty? I wonder if they'd give you milk in there? Perhaps Looking-glass milk isn't good to drink!

Kitty was never subjected to this experimental regimen! However, ironically Lewis Carroll died in 1898 in his sisters' house in Guildford, from the upstairs room of which he would have been able to see the author's laboratory at the University of Surrey — had the University been built at that time!

Acknowledgements

I am grateful and indebted to the following colleagues for their encourage-ment, assistance, and collaboration in different aspects of the work described: Dr. John N. Eble, Dr. Suzanne A. Eccles, Dr. David A. Fell, John L. Glover, M.D., Barbara Green, Professor W. Eugene Knox, Dr. Yutaka Natsumeda, Deborah Riches, Professor George Weber, M.D. I thank Dr. John A. Mead of the U.S. National Cancer Institute for providing NSC 127755. The studies were financially supported, in part, through USPHS grant AM-00567 to Professor W. E. Knox; USPHS-NCI grants CA-13526, CA-05034 and CA-42510 and an Outstanding Investigator Grant CA-642510 to Professor G. Weber; and by UICC (ICRETT) Fellowships to the author.

References

1. Eagle, H. (1959). Amino acid metabolism in mammalian cell cultures. *Science,* **130**, 432–7
2. Weber, G. (1983). Biochemical strategy of cancer cells and the design of chemotherapy: G. H. A. Clowes Memorial Lecture. *Cancer Res.,* **43**, 3466–92
3. Snell, K. (1984). Enzymes of serine metabolism in normal, developing and neoplastic rat tissues. *Adv. Enzyme Regul.,* **22**, 325–400
4. Snell, K. (1980). Liver enzymes of serine metabolism during neonatal development of the rat. *Biochem. J.,* **190**, 451–5
5. Snell, K. (1985). Enzymes of serine metabolism in normal and neoplastic rat tissues. *Biochem. Biophys. Acta,* **843**, 276–81
6. Sauer, L. A., Stayman, J. W. and Dauchy, P. T. (1982). Amino acid, glucose, and lactic acid utilization *in vivo* by rat tumours. *Cancer Res.,* **42**, 4090–7
7. Snell, K. (1986). The duality of pathways for serine biosynthesis is a fallacy. *Trends Biochem. Sci.,* **11**, 241–3
8. Snell, K. and Weber, G. (1986). Enzymic imbalance in serine metabolism in rat hepatomas. *Biochem. J.,* **233**, 617–20
8a. Knox, W. E., Herzfeld, A. and Hudson, J. (1969). Phosphoserine phosphatase distribution in normal and neoplastic rat tissues. *Arch. Biochem. Biophys.,* **132**, 397–403
9. Weber, G., Olah, E., Denton, J. E., Lui, M. S., Takeda, E., Tzeng, D. Y. and Ban, J. (1981). Dynamics of modulation of biochemical programs in cancer cells. *Adv. Enzyme Regul.,* **19**, 87–102
10. Natsumeda, Y., Ikegami, T., Murayama, K. and Weber, G. (1988). *De novo* guanylate synthesis in the commitment to replication in hepatoma 3924A cells. *Cancer Res.,* **48**, 507–11
11. Snell, K., Natsumeda, Y. and Weber, G. (1987). The modulation of serine metabolism in hepatoma 3924A during different phases of cellular proliferation in culture. *Biochem. J.,* **245**, 609–12
12. Kacser, H. and Porteous, J. W. (1987). Control of metabolism: what do we have to measure? *Trends Biochem. Sci.,* **12**, 5–14
13. Groen, A. K. and Tager, J. M. (1988). Control analysis provides a simple means of understanding the control structure of a metabolic pathway. *Biochem. J.,* **253**, 619–23
14. Kacser, H. and Burns, J. A. (1973). The control of flux. *Symp. Soc. Exp. Biol.,* **27**, 65–104
15. Heinrich, R. and Rapoport, T. A. (1974). A linear steady-state treatment of enzymatic chains. *Eur. J. Biochem.,* **42**, 89–95
16. Fell, D. A. and Sauro, H. M. (1985). Metabolic control and its analysis. Additional relationships between elasticities and control coefficients. *Eur. J. Biochem.,* **148**, 555 61
17. Sauro, H. M., Small, J. R. and Fell, D. A. (1987). Metabolic control and its analysis. Extensions to the theory and matrix method. *Eur. J. Biochem.,* **165**, 215–21
18. Groen, A. K., Van der Meer, R., Westerhoff, H. V., Wanders, R. J. A., Akerboom, T. P. M. and Tager, J. M. (1982). Control metabolic fluxes. In Sies, H. (ed.) *Metabolic Compartmentation.* pp 9–37. (New York: Academic Press)
19. Fell, D. A. and Snell, K. (1988). Control analysis of mammalian serine biosynthesis: feedback inhibition on the final step. *Biochem. J.,* **256**, 97–101
20. Nemer, M. J., Wise, E. M., Washington, F. M. and Elwyn, D. (1960). The rate of turnover of serine and phosphoserine in rat liver. *J. Biol. Chem.,* **235**, 2063–9
21. La Baume, L. B., Merrill, D. K., Clary, G. L. and Guynn, R. W. (1987). Effect of acute ethanol on serine biosynthesis in liver. *Arch. Biochem. Biophys.,* **256**, 569–77
22. Snell, K., Natsumeda, Y., Elbe, J. N., Glover, J. L. and Weber, G. (1988). Enzymic imbalance in serine metabolism in human colon carcinoma and rat sarcoma. *Br. J. Cancer,* **57**, 87–90
23. Tendler, S. J. B., Threadgill, M. D. and Tisdale, M. J. (1987). Activities of serine hydroxymethyltransferase in murine tissues and tumours. *Cancer Lett.,* **36**, 65–9
24. Bukin, Y. V. and Draudin-Krylenko, V. A. (1980). Regulation of serine hydroxymethyltransferase activity in normal, tumour and host cells. *Vestn. Akad. Med. Nauk., S.S.S.R.,* 67–9
25. Thorndike, J., Pelliniemi, T. and Beck, W. S. (1979). Serine hydroxymethyltransferase activity and serine incorporation in leukocytes. *Cancer Res.,* **39**, 3435–40
26. Vousden, K. H., Eccles, S. A., Purvies, H. and Marshall, C. J. (1986). Enhanced spontaneous metastasis of mouse carcinoma cells transfected with an activated c-Ha-*ras*-1 gene. *Int. J. Cancer,* **37**, 425–33

27. Waghorne, C., Kerbel, R. S. and Breitman, M. L. (1987). Metastatic potential of SP1 mouse mammary adenocarcinoma cells is differentially induced by activated and normal forms of c-H-*ras*. *Oncogenes*, **1**, 149–55

28. Bukin, Y. V., Draudin-Krylenko, V. A. and Korytnyk, W. (1979). Potentiating action of 4-vinylpyridoxal on inhibition of serine hydroxylmethyltransferase by D-cycloserine and its dimer. *Biochem. Pharmacol.*, **28**, 1169–73

29. Tisdale, M. J. (1981). The effect of L-2-amino-4-methoxy-*trans*-butenoic acid on serine hydroxymethyltransferase. *Chem.-Biol. Interact.*, **34**, 75–83

30. Baker, B. R. and Vermeulen, N. M. J. (1970). Irreversible enzyme inhibitors. Active-site-directed irreversible inhibitors of dihydrofolate reductase from L5178Y cells by substituted triazines and quinazolines. *Biochem. Pharmacol.*, **32**, 922–4

31. Corbett, J. H., Leopold, W. R., Dykes, D. J., Roberts, B. J., Grimswold, D. P. and Schnabel, D. M. (1982). Toxicity and anticancer activity of a new triazine antifolate (NSC 127755). *Cancer Res.*, **42**, 1707–15

32. Kearney, J. F., Radbruch, A., Liesegang, B. and Rajewsky, K. (1979). A new mouse myeloma cell line that has lost immunoglobulin expression but permits the construction of antibody-secreting hybrid cell lines. *J. Immunol.*, **123**, 1548–50

33. Perez, D. J., Slowicaczek, P. and Tattersall, M. H. N. (1984). Deoxyuridine metabolism in cultured human lymphoblasts treated with methotrexate. *Cancer Res.*, **44**, 457–60

34. Baker, B. R. and Vermeulen, N. M. J. (1970). Irreversible enzyme inhibitors. Irreversible inhibition of purified dihydrofolate reductase. *J. Med. Chem.*, **13**, 1143–50

35. Kumar, A. A., Mangum, J. H., Blankenship, D. T. and Freisheim, J. H. (1981). Affinity labelling of chicken liver dihydrofolate reductase by a substituted 4,6-diaminodihydrotriazine bearing a terminal sulfonyl fluoride. *J. Biol. Chem.*, **256**, 8970–6

36. Pazmino, N., Doherty, D. G. and Regan, J. D. (1973). Inhibition of DNA and RNA synthesis, but minimally of protein synthesis, in human leukaemia cells by a serine antimetabolite. *J. Natl. Cancer Inst.*, **51**, 761–5

37. Weber, G., Natsumeda, Y., Lui, M. S., Faderan, M. A., Liepniks, J. J. and Elliott, W. L. (1984). Control of enzymic programs and nucleotide pattern in cancer cells by acivicin and tiazofurin. *Adv. Enzyme Regul.*, **22**, 69–93

38. Tendler, S. J. B., Threadgill, M. D. and Tisdale, M. J. (1987). Structural studies on bioactive compounds, Part 7. The design and synthesis of α-substituted serines as prospective inhibitors of serine hydroxymethyltransferase. *J. Chem. Soc. Perkin Trans.*, I, 2617–23

39. Wang, E. A., Kallen, R. and Walsh, C. (1981). Mechanism-based inactivation of serine transhydroxymethylase by D-fluoroalanine and related amino acids. *J. Biol. Chem.*, **256**, 6917–26

40. Carroll, L. (1948). *Through the Looking Glass and What Alice Found There*. p. 37. (Harmondsworth: Penguin Books Ltd.)

32
Imbalance in polyamine metabolism in hepatocellular carcinomas

H. G. WILLIAMS-ASHMAN, S. BARDOCZ AND G. WEBER

INTRODUCTION

Sixteen years ago, at a time shortly after all of the enzymes for the major pathway for polyamine production in mammalian cells were discovered and characterized[1-5], Weber and Williams-Ashman, together with their co-workers in Indianapolis and Chicago, reported a series of investigations on polyamines and their biosynthetic decarboxylases in various Morris rat hepatomas[6-8]. These studies represented the first systematic examination of polyamine metabolism in relation to the widely different growth rates of a spectrum of malignant tumours that were all derived from the same type of untransformed cells. Meanwhile, numerous features of the turnover and potential functions of polyamines germane to the induction and proliferation of very many types of malignant tumours in experimental animals and man have been documented[9-13]. This presentation is a brief overview of just a few of the major findings and conclusions that have emerged from these studies with regard to relationships of polyamine metabolism to neoplastic growth, with special emphasis on hepatocellular carcinomas. Some key facts and concepts about the enzymology of mammalian polyamine metabolism and its physiologic and pharmacologic regulation will first be presented.

POLYAMINE TURNOVER IN MAMMALIAN CELLS

All nucleated mammalian cells synthesize and accumulate the polyamines spermine $[H_2N(CH_2)_3NH(CH_2)_4NH(CH_2)_3NH_2]$ and spermidine $[H_2N(CH_2)_3NH(CH_2)_4NH_2]$ in concentrations varying from roughly between 0.2 and 2.5 μmol/g fresh weight. Putrescine $[H_2N(CH_2)_4NH_2]$, the biosynthetic precursor of spermidine and spermine, is usually present intracellularly at much lower levels except in the case of certain highly malignant neoplasms. Although these three aliphatic amines can be transported into cells, nearly all

389

of the spermine, spermidine and putrescine in the organism is manufactured *de novo* in the cells that contain these molecules, and normally the concentrations of these polyamines in blood plasma and other extracellular fluids (except the seminal plasma of certain species) are kept exceedingly low in adult animals that do not have tissue damage or big tumour burdens. Under physiological circumstances, all of the nitrogen atoms in polyamines are largely protonated, so that the polyamines are strongly basic substances. Because of this, spermine and spermidine especially interact firmly but non-covalently with all sorts of biomolecules and particularly with all forms of DNA and RNA molecules. Innumerable enzymatic processes concerned with the synthesis, post-synthetic modification and degradation of various nucleic acids have been shown to be influenced directly by spermidine and spermine in either positive or negative directions. Spermine and spermidine also form non-covalent complexes with acidic phospholipids and a wide variety of membrane, enzymatic and other proteins, thereby influencing the functions of these biomolecules. And there are a few instances in which polyamines can act as substrates for enzymes catalyzing certain post-translational modifications of proteins.

It is frequently believed that the greatest physiological utility of spermidine and spermine may relate to their capacity to act as modifiers of the conformational status of various nucleic acids and proteins, and especially as regulators of key steps in polynucleotide and protein biosynthesis. However, these polyamines also can influence so many other sorts of intracellular biochemical processes *in vitro* that it may be hazardous to designate macro-molecular biosynthetic reactions as the most fundamental sites of polyamine action in all types of mammalian cells. An important aspect of the majority of such direct effects of polyamines demonstrable in cell-free systems is that they are clearly not due to non-specific increases in ionic strength brought about by addition of spermine or spermidine, and that they cannot be mimicked by replacement of the polyamines by inorganic metal ions. Furthermore, whereas alterations in the intracellular levels of inorganic metal ions depend on the transport of these ions into or out of cells, the big changes in the concentrations of polyamines that occurs when resting cells respond to many growth stimuli are mainly the result of swift alterations in the synthesis of enzymes that are rate-limiting for the production of spermidine and spermine.

Putrescine is synthesized by ornithine decarboxylase (ODC) which utilizes pyridoxal phosphate as co-enzyme. The second enzyme of polyamine biosynthesis is S-adenosylmethionine decarboxylase (AdoMetDC), the product of which contains an activated aminopropyl moiety. AdoMetDC contains covalently-bound pyruvoyl residues at the N-termini of both of its two identical protein subunits, which act as prosthetic groups. AdoMetDC is specifically activated by putrescine and inhibited by spermine. The third enzyme, spermidine synthase, transfers an aminopropyl group from decarboxylated AdoMet to putrescine to form spermidine. And the fourth enzyme is spermine synthase, which catalyzes a comparable transfer of an aminopropyl group to spermidine to produce spermine. Spermidine and spermine synthases are entirely different enzymes that do not require any co-enzyme or prosthetic group. ODC and AdoMetDC can be synthesized and degraded extremely rapidly *in vivo*, and the levels of either one or the other of these decarboxylases may be rate-limiting to spermidine and spermine synthesis, depending on the particular type of normal or malignant cell. By contrast, the content of spermidine and spermine synthases, which turn over much more slowly, is in nearly all cells from one to two orders of magnitude higher than that of the two decarboxylases of polyamine biosynthesis. The nucleoside 5'-methylthioadenosine (MTA) is the by-product of the spermidine and spermine synthase reactions. MTA concentrations in all normal cells are extremely low, and hardly ever greater than 5 nmol/g. This is because all non-malignant cells contain a highly active and specific MTA phosphorylase that splits MTA into adenine and methylthioribose-1-phosphate (MTR-1-P), as first discovered by Pegg and Williams-Ashman[14]. More recently it has been demonstrated that MTR-1-P can undergo a series of transformations whereby all but one of its ribose carbon atoms as well as its methylthio moiety can be converted to L-methionine[15,16]. Thus the ATP and L-methionine utilized for the synthesis of AdoMet required for spermidine and spermine production are effectively salvaged, since the adenine produced by the action of MTA phosphorylase on MTA can be converted to 5'-AMP by the action of the ubiquitous enzyme adenine phosphoribosyltransferase[15]. All of the afore-mentioned enzymes of polyamine biosynthesis are localized in the soluble fraction of the cytoplasm, and in every case the reactions they catalyze are essentially irreversible. The synthesis and activities of ODC and AdoMetDC are subject to regulation at transcriptional, translational and post-transla-tional levels[5,11-13].

SELECTIVE PHARMACOLOGIC INHIBITION OF POLYAMINE BIOSYNTHETIC ENZYMES

Many drugs that selectively and potently inhibit each enzyme of polyamine biosynthesis have been prepared over the last decade, as documented exten-sively in a recent comprehensive treatise[17].

α-Difluoromethyl-L-ornithine (DFMO), an enzyme-activated irreversible ('suicide') inhibitor of ODC has been studied most extensively. This drug is decarboxylated by ODC, and the reaction product, in the form of a Schiff base with pyridoxal phosphate, undergoes rearrangements that then result in formation of a catalytically inactive covalent adduct with the ODC enzyme protein. Continual treatment of intact animals or cultured cells with DFMO evokes dramatic decreases in intracellular putrescine and spermidine levels, but usually does not deplete the spermine content of cells very substantially. DFMO also elicits correspondingly immense increases in the intracellular concentrations of AdoMet. The latter phenomenon probably is a significant factor that contributes to the failure of ODC to reduce the cellular content of spermine, since in the presence of a big excess of AdoMet, pre-existing putre-scine and spermidine molecules may be efficiently converted to spermine. Addition of DFMO to a wide variety of normal and malignant cells in culture results in a striking depression of cell proliferation, and in some cases of terminal differentiation processes. The anti-proliferative actions of DFMO are generally cytostatic in nature, and can be reversed by supplying the DFMO-treated cells with putrescine. Inhibition of the growth of many types of experimental tumours *in vivo*, and also of the spread of metastases, has been observed after treatment of the host animals with DFMO, which can effectively be given in the drinking water and has surprisingly low toxicity. Nevertheless, extensive clinical trials of DFMO as a single anti-neoplastic agent in man have not been encouraging, perhaps in part because sufficient spermine remains in the tumours to satisfy the polyamine requirement for cell growth. Attempts to enhance the activity of certain cytotoxic anti-cancer drugs by concurrent administration of DFMO are currently under way in many laboratories and clinics, but it is too early to tell whether these chemotherapeutic maneuvers are of lasting value. Other potent and specific irreversible inhibitors of ODC have been discovered. Many of the more active of these drugs are ethynylated derivatives of putrescine, some of which suffer from the disadvantage that they are degraded to inactive products by the actions of certain amine oxidases[11,17].

The first inhibitor of AdoMetDC that does not directly inhibit ODC or either of the two polyamine synthases to be discovered was methylglyoxal bis (guanylhydrazone) (MGBG)[18,19]. Inhibition of AdoMetDC by MGBG is competitive with respect to the AdoMet substrate, and the direct inhibition of the enzyme by MGBG is much greater in the presence as compared to the absence of the activator putrescine. The inhibition by MGBG is reversible when the drug is removed by dialysis or gel filtration. If animals or cultured cells are exposed to MGBG for considerable periods and the drug is then removed from soluble cell-free extracts of tissues, the activity of AdoMetDC is strikingly increased by as much as 20-fold. This is hardly due to an increased synthesis of the enzyme resulting from MGBG treatment, but rather reflects stabilization of existing AdoMetDC molecules by the drug *in vivo*, as evidenced by immense prolongation of the apparent half-life of the enzyme in intact cells. Although MGBG potently inhibits the *de novo* synthesis of spermidine and spermine in living cells and elicits a profound rise in cellular putrescine levels, the drug exerts other actions that complicate interpretation of its effects on intracellular polyamine metabolism and cell growth, including inhibition of certain polyamine oxidizing enzymes, and induction of extensive damage to mitochondria[12,17,19]. MGBG is also a powerful inducer of spermidine/spermine N^1-acetyltransferase (see below). Very recently, several analogs of AdoMet containing reactive hydrazino, aminoxy or ethylhydroxylamine groups were shown to be potent irreversible inhibitors of AdoMetDC, and to cause an inhibition of L1210 leukemia cell proliferation that was associated with a decline in cellular spermidine and spermine content with massive increases in putrescine; cell growth was inhibited by these drugs after spermine and spermidine were lowered and could then be reversed by exogenous spermidine[13]. However, it is improbable that such analogs of AdoMet would have long lasting inhibitory actions on AdoMetDC in living cells because they may be rapidly degraded *in vivo*.

A number of synthetic compounds that selectively inhibit spermidine synthase (e.g. S-adenosyl-1,8-diamino-3-thiooctane) or spermine synthase (e.g. S-methyl-5'-thiomethyladenosine) have been reported[13]. Cyclohexylamine is another substance that selectively inhibits spermidine synthase. Application of the foregoing drugs alone or in combination with specific ODC or AdoMet inhibitors to the control of neoplastic cell growth is still in its infancy.

PATHWAYS FOR POLYAMINE INTERCONVERSIONS

It has long been known that liver and other organs can convert spermine to spermidine and also spermidine to putrescine at slow rates, and that these 'back conversions' of polyamines are greatly enhanced in liver after partial hepatectomy, or treatments with carbon tetrachloride, thioacetamide or growth hormone. Hölttä[20] discovered a novel flavoprotein polyamine oxidase (PAO), present in liver and many other tissues, that cleaves spermine to spermidine, and spermidine to putrescine, with stoichiometric production of 3-aminopropanal via oxidative reactions. Later studies by others (reviewed in ref. 11) showed that N^1-acetylspermine and N^1-acetylspermidine were much more effective substrates for PAO than are the corresponding non-acetylated polyamines. These N^1-acetylated polyamines are synthesized by the action of a specific spermidine/spermine N^1-acetyltransferase (SAT) that utilizes acetyl-CoA, and is found mainly in the cytoplasm. N^1-acetylspermine and N^1-acetyl-spermidine are oxidized respectively to spermidine and putrescine, plus 3-acetoamidopropanal. In all tissues, the activity of SAT is very much lower than that of PAO, even when SAT is induced. In liver and other tissues, SAT can be induced as much as 20-fold in response to regenerative stimuli and a variety of chemical agents. High concentrations of spermidine or spermine (but not putrescine), and also MGBG, serve as potent inducers of SAT. The half-life of SAT in living cells is remarkably short (<1 hour), comparable to that of ODC and AdoMetDC. Many lines of evidence[11,13] indicate that the N^1-acetyl-derivatives of spermine and spermidine are the physiological substrates for PAO *in vivo*; that the sequential actions of SAT and PAO convert spermine to spermidine, and spermidine to putrescine, *in vivo*; and that SAT activity is rate-limiting for this polyamine interconversion pathway that proceeds in many types of normal and malignant cells. Noteworthy is the fact that N^1-acetylation of spermine and spermidine reduces the net positive charge of the parent polyamines. N^1-acetylspermine and N^1-acetylspermidine are, therefore, bound to nucleic acids less firmly than the non-acetylated polyamines. (In living cells, the firm non-covalent complexing of spermidine and especially spermine with polynucleotides may effectively attenuate the availability of the bound polyamines as substrates for their enzymatic trans-formations.) The SAT–PAO pathway for polyamine interconversions may serve to salvage putrescine from spermidine, and spermidine from spermine, following the *de novo* synthesis of spermidine and spermine.

POLYAMINES AND THEIR BIOSYNTHETIC DECARBOXYLASES IN MORRIS RAT HEPATOMAS

Williams-Ashman *et al.*[7] measured the contents of polyamines and activities of ODC and AdoMetDC in seven well-standardized variants of transplanted Morris hepatomas in comparison with livers from appropriate strains of normal adult male rats that served as controls. The tumours and corresponding normal livers from well-fed rats were excised at the same time in the morning. The principal findings in these investigations may be summarized as follows. The ranges of the mean contents (nmol/g) of putrescine (19–28), spermidine (555–869) and spermine (834–1010) in normal control livers were reasonably narrow, and the mean of the ratios of spermidine/spermine in liver ranged from 0.55 to 0.84. In the two fastest-growing hepatomas examined, the steady-state concentrations of putrescine were strikingly higher than in control livers (286 and 142 nmol/g for hepatomas 392A and 3683F, respectively). All but one line (7800) of the hepatomas of slow or intermediate growth rates had significantly higher mean putrescine concentrations than the liver controls. The spermidine/spermine ratio tended to be significantly higher in all of the hepatomas, though the range of concentrations of these two polyamines for all of the tumours (spermidine, 588–1770 nmol/g; and spermine, 685–1560 nmol/g) was not very pronouncedly different from those in control livers. The ODC activities of the fast-growing hepatomas were several times higher than in normal livers, whilst in a number of slower-growing and more differentiated hepatomas the ODC activities were considerably less though significantly increased. Regardless of their *in vivo* growth rates, none of the hepatomas studied had greater AdoMetDC activities than the liver controls except for hepatoma 7777. The span of ranges of ODC/AdoMetDC activities in the normal livers (0.22–1.00) was smaller than that of the hepatomas (0.81–7.40); in most of the hepatoma lines the activity of AdoMetDC as determined in the presence of saturating levels of the putrescine activator was thus potentially more rate-limiting to spermidine and spermine biosynthesis than the activity of ODC. In these investigations[7], the activities of spermidine synthase and spermine synthase were not determined. However, many subsequent reports from other laboratories have indicated that the activities of these two polyamine synthases are usually in great excess over those of even fully induced ODC or AdoMetDC in a wide variety of normal tissues as well as in malignant cells derived therefrom[9,11–13]. In our early studies on Morris hepatomas[7], it was also shown that various properties of ODC and AdoMet in some hepatoma variants (most noticeably, very short half-lives *in vivo* of less than 1 hour, and the requirement for putrescine as activator of AdoMetDC) were essentially the same as those for the two polyamine biosynthetic decarboxylases in innumerable normal cells. The activity of ODC and AdoMetDC in regenerating remnants of liver after partial hepatectomy was not measured in our studies[7]. However, a large number of investigations have shown that immense (up to 400-fold) increases in ODC, and highly significant though lesser enhancements of AdoMetDC, spermidine synthase and spermine synthase activities occur transiently during liver regeneration following partial hepatectomy, or in the regenerating phase of liver growth that can follow acute treatment with certain hepato-toxins[5,11–13]. Elevations of ODC activities in any types of malignant tumours in comparison to the enzyme levels of their tissues of origin that are comparable to the tremendous increases in ODC in regenerating liver (or in livers of animals treated with certain chemical inducers of ODC) have never been described[11,13]. In this context it should be remembered that whereas there may be considerable synchrony of the transit through cell cycles of hepatocytes in various phases of liver regeneration, a comparable synchrony of proliferation of malignant cells in transplanted growing hepatomas is unlikely.

Two other enzymes besides ODC that utilize L-ornithine as substrate were measured in Morris hepatomas in the laboratory of George Weber. Both of these enzymes are in huge excess in comparison with the levels of ODC and AdoMetDC in normal adult liver, and are localized in mitochondria. The activity of ornithine carbamyltransferase (OCT) (a key enzyme of the urea cycle that catalyzes conversion of carbamylphosphate plus ornithine to citrul-line) was observed to be moderately decreased in various slow-growing and more differentiated hepatomas, and to be reduced to roughly 0.1–0.2% of the activity of liver in four lines of very rapidly-growing hepatomas[6]. The decline in OCT in the fast growing hepatomas was much greater than the diminution in their mitochondrial content. That OCT activity is almost obliterated in the rapidly proliferating Morris hepatomas is in sharp contrast to the finding of Sweeney et al.[21] that aspartate transcarbamylase (which catalyzes an important step in pyrimidine nucleotide biosynthesis and utilizes carbamyl phosphate) increases in activity in parallel with the growth rates of this spectrum of Morris hepatomas. Tomino et al.[22] reported that ornithine trans-aminase (which catalyzes formation of glutamic semialdehyde from ornithine) was not decreased in liver at 24 hours after partial hepatectomy but declined, independently of the tumour mitochondrial contents, in all fast-growing and highly de-differentiated Morris hepatomas to values that were less than 30% of normal liver controls.

SPERMIDINE/SPERMINE N¹-ACETYLTRANSFERASE ACTIVITIES IN MORRIS HEPATOMAS: COMMENTS ON THE POLYAMINE INTERCONVERSION PATHWAY IN MALIGNANT TUMOURS

As considered above, SAT (the enzyme responsible for N^1-acetylation of spermidine and spermine) is the rate-limiting and highly inducible enzyme for the SAT–PAO pathway for 'back' conversion of spermine to spermidine, and of spermidine to putrescine, which among other things might salvage sper-midine and putrescine, respectively, from spermine and spermidine that accumulate after the biosynthesis of the latter two polyamines via the *de novo* synthetic pathway. Bardocz and Weber (ref. 23 and unpublished observations) found that SAT activity, measured with either N^1-acetylspermidine or N^1-acetylspermine as substrates, progressively decreased to a nadir of less than 50% of the values found in 6-day-old rats in livers of developing animals as a function of increases in age over the range of 6–40 days. In a spectrum of Morris hepatomas, SAT activities varied from 1.5 to 5.5 times those of normal liver controls, but there was no parallelism between SAT activities and the growth rates of the tumours. The properties of SAT in normal liver were indistinguishable from those in the very fast-growing hepatomas 3924A. These results, although indicating an unequivocally high SAT activity in various Morris hepatomas, merit further investigation, because Pegg and Erwin[24] observed that not all of the basal activity in uninduced liver and other cells was immunoprecipitable SAT, whereas all of the greatly enhanced induced activities reacted completely with antibodies specifically directed against SAT. Liver and hepatoma PAO levels were not determined in the aforementioned studies of Bardocz and Weber. However, evidence that PAO is highly active in cultured HTC cells (derived from a Morris rat hepatoma) was forthcoming from observations that exposure of HTC cells to N^1,N^4-bis(allenyl)putrescine (MDL 72527) — a potent and specific 'suicide' inhibitor of PAO — evoked a dramatic accumulation of N^1-acetylspermidine in the HTC cells[25]. Comparable effects of the drug MDL 72527 were documented in studies on liver, spleen, L2110 leukemia cells, and Lewis lung carcinoma in mice[25]. MDL 72527 alone is not toxic and hardly affected growth of the tumours. Combined treatment with DFMO (to prevent *de novo* putrescine synthesis) and MDL 72527 (to attenuate 'back' conversion of spermine to spermidine and of spermidine to putrescine via inhibition of PAO) elicited a more pronounced depletion of the polyamine contents of L1210 leukemia and of Lewis lung carcinoma cells than was evoked by administration of either drug alone, with concomitant decreases in proliferation of these tumours being greater when both drugs were given[25]. The latter investigations indeed suggest that 'back' conversion of spermine to spermidine and of spermidine to putrescine by the SAT–PAO polyamine interconversion pathway can effectively salvage polyamines produced by *de novo* biosynthesis to cover the polyamine requirement for tumour growth. Obviously it would be of interest to examine the effects of administration of DFMO and MDL 72527, administered either alone or in combination, on the growth characteristics of a spectrum of Morris hepatomas, and on the content of polyamines and of the N^1-acetylated derivatives of spermine and spermidine in the tumours.

As Seiler[26] has pointed out, in non-dividing differentiated cells the uninhibited SAT–PAO polyamine interconversion pathway as such cannot change the combined total levels of putrescine, spermidine and spermine that are produced by the *de novo* biosynthetic pathway, but can only effect a re-distribution of the individual levels of each of these amines. Thus the polyamine interconversion pathway considered solely in the context of the actions of the polyamine biosynthetic enzymes might be regarded as a 'futile metabolic cycle'. Nevertheless, in rapidly proliferating cells such as Morris hepatomas that have not been treated with inhibitors of ODC or of PAO, the dynamics of polyamine production may be more complex. For example, it is established that N^1-acetylspermidine can be excreted out of certain cells, and, moreover, in rapidly growing tumours polyamines liberated from necrotic cells may be transported into visible tumour cells (for literature citations see refs. 9, 11, 25, 26). At all events, more extensive investigations on the role of

SAT- and PAO-catalyzed reactions in salvage of polyamines for the growth of Morris hepatomas and other malignant tumours need to be carried out before the biological significance of the polyamine interconversion pathway can be properly assessed.

SUMMARY AND CONCLUSIONS

In all tumours of a spectrum of rat hepatomas of widely divergent growth rates, the intracellular concentrations of putrescine, spermidine and spermine, as well as the activity of ornithine decarboxylase, were at least as high as in normal livers of rats of the same age, sex and dietary intake. Putrescine concentrations and ornithine decarboxylase activities were strikingly elevated in the more rapidly proliferating and dedifferentiated Morris hepatomas, whereas the ratio of activities S-adenosylmethionine decarboxylase/ornithine decarboxylase was decreased in all of the tumours examined, regardless of their growth rates. Ornithine transcarbamylase levels in comparison with normal liver were invariably lower in all of the Morris hepatomas and were almost obliterated in the very fast-growing tumours. These findings, together with many other lines of evidence, indicate that a capacity for vigorous *de novo* synthesis and accumulation of polyamines is retained in all of these rat hepatocellular carcinomas, as has been invariably found for an immense number of other types of malignant tumours in many species[27]. It seems inescapable that polyamine biosynthesis is essential for proliferation for all malignant as well as normal mammalian cells. This conclusion is in line with observations that various mutant cells that are unable to manufacture polyamines because of defects in polyamine biosynthetic enzymes exhibit an absolute requirement for exogenous polyamines in order to grow[11]. Thus adequate expression of genes coding for the enzymes of *de novo* polyamine synthesis is, according to the terminology of Weber[28,29], always linked to malignant transformations, and in some cases also to tumour progression. Recent observations on high activities of spermidine/spermine N^1-acetyltransferase in Morris rat hepatomas are also presented. The latter and other findings suggest that the pathway for 'back' (salvage) conversion of spermine to spermidine, and of spermidine to putrescine, via the sequential actions of the aforementioned polyamine acetyltransferase and of an intracellular flavo-protein polyamine oxidase, may be operative in Morris hepatomas, but insufficient evidence is currently available to decide whether this polyamine interconversion pathway plays a major role in the overall polyamine metabolism of these malignant tumours.

Acknowledgements

These studies were supported by an Outstanding Investigator Grant CA-42510 (G.W.) from the National Cancer Institute, NIH, USA.

References

1. Pegg, A. E. and Williams-Ashman, H. G. (1968). Biosynthesis of putrescine in the prostate gland of the rat. *Biochem. J.,* **108**, 533–9
2. Pegg, A. E. and Williams-Ashman, H. G. (1969). On the role of S-adenosyl-L-methionine in the biosynthesis of spermidine by rat prostate. *J. Biol. Chem.,* **244**, 682–93
3. Pegg, A. E. and William-Ashman, H. G. (1970). Enzymic synthesis of spermine in rat prostate. *Arch. Biochem. Biophys.,* **137**, 156–65
4. William-Ashman, H. G., Janne, J., Coppoc, G. L., Geroch, M. E. and Schenone, A. (1972). New aspects of polyamine biosynthesis in eukaryotic organisms. *Adv. Enzyme Regul.,* **10**, 225–45
5. William-Ashman, H. G. and Cannellakis, Z. (1979). Polyamines in mammalian biology and medicine. *Perspect. Biol. Med.,* **22**, 421–53
6. Weber, G., Queener, S. F. and Morris, H. P. (1972). Imbalance of L-ornithine metabolism in hepatomas of different growth rates as expressed in behaviour of L-ornithine carbamyl transferase activity. *Cancer Res.,* **32**, 1933–40
7. Williams-Ashman, H. G., Coppoc, G. L. and Weber, G. (1972). Imbalance in ornithine metabolism in hepatomas of different growth rates as expressed in formation of putrescine, spermidine and spermine. *Cancer Res.,* **32**, 1924–32
8. Williams-Ashman, H. G., Coppoc, G. L., Schenone, A. and Weber, G. (1973). Aspects of polyamine biosynthesis in normal and malignant eukaryotic cells. In Russell, D. H. (ed.) *Polyamines in Normal and Malignant Growth*, p. 161. (New York: Raven Press)
9. Pegg, A. E. and McCann, P. P. (1982). Polyamine metabolism and function. *Am. J. Physiol.,* **243**, C212–C221
10. Tabor, C. W. and Tabor, H. (1984). Polyamines. *Annu. Rev. Biochem.,* **53**, 749–90
11. Pegg, A. E. (1986). Recent advances in the biochemistry of polyamines in eukaryotes. *Biochem. J.,* **234**, 249–62
12. Porter, C. W. and Sufrin, J. R. (1986). Interference with polyamine biosynthesis and/or function by analogs of polyamines or methionine as a potential anticancer chemotherapeutic strategy. *Anticancer Res.,* **6**, 525–42
13. Pegg, A. E. (1988). Polyamine metabolism and its importance in neoplastic growth and as a target for chemotherapy. *Cancer Res.,* **48**, 759–74
14. Pegg, A. E. and Williams-Ashman, H. G. (1969). Phosphate-stimulated breakdown of 5′-methylthioadenosine by rat ventral prostate. *Biochem. J.,* **115**, 241–7
15. Williams-Ashman, H. G., Seidenfeld, J. and Galletti, P. (1982). Trends in the biochemical pharmacology and 5′-deoxy-5′-methylthioadenosine. *Biochem. Pharmacol.,* **31**, 277–88
16. Williams-Ashman, H. G. (1985). Metabolic significance of 5′-deoxy-5′-methylthioadenosine in relation to polyamine turnover in normal and malignant cells. In Selmeci, L., Brosnan, M. E. and Seiler, N. (eds.) *Recent Progress in Polyamine Research*, p. 231. (Budapest: Akademiai Kiado)
17. McCann, P. O., Pegg, A. E. and Sjoerdsma, A. (eds.) (1987). *Inhibition of Polyamine Metabolism*, pp 1–370. (New York: Academic Press)
18. Corti, A., Dave, C., Williams-Ashman, H. E., Mihich, E. and Schenone, A. (1974). Specific inhibition of the enzymic decarboxylation of S-adenosylmethionine by methylglyoxal bis(guanylhydrazone) and related substances. *Biochem. J.,* **139**, 351–7
19. Williams-Ashman, H. G. and Seidenfeld, J. (1986). Aspects of the biochemical pharmacology and methylglyoxal bis(guanylhydrazone). *Biochem. Pharmacol.,* **35**, 1217–25
20. Hölttä, E. (1977). Oxidation of spermidine and spermine in rat livers: purification and properties of polyamine oxidase. *Biochemistry,* **16**, 91–100
21. Sweeney, M. J., Hoffman, D. H. and Poure, G. A. (1971). Enzymes in pyrimidine biosynthesis. *Adv. Enzyme Regul.,* **9**, 51–61
22. Tomino, I., Katunuma, N., Morris, H. P. and Weber, G. (1974). Imbalance in ornithine metabolism in hepatomas of different growth rates as expressed in behaviour of L-ornithine: 2-oxo-acid aminotransferase (ornithine transaminase, EC. 2.6.1.13). *Cancer Res.,* **34**, 627–35
23. Bardocz, S. and Weber, G. (1986). Transformation-linked increase in activity of polyamine salvage enzymes in hepatomas. *International Conference on Polyamines in Life Sciences*, Lake Yamanaka, Japan, Abstr. No. P2.
24. Pegg, A. E. and Erwin, B. G. (1985). Induction of spermidine/spermine N′-acetyltransferase in rat tissues by polyamines. *Biochem. J.,* **231**, 285–9

25. Claverie, N., Wagner, J., Knodgen, B. and Seiler, N. (1987). Inhibition of polyamine oxidase improves the antitumoral effect of ornithine decarboxylase inhibitors. *Anticancer Res.,* **7**, 765–72

26. Seiler, N. (1987). Functions of polyamine acetylation. *Can. J. Physiol. Pharmacol.,* **65**, 2024–35

27. Scalabrino, G. and Ferioli, M. E. (1982). Polyamines in mammalian tumors. Part 2. *Adv. Cancer Res.,* **36**, 1–100

28. Weber, G. (1977). Enzymology of cancer cells, Parts 1 and 2. *New Engl. J. Med.,* **296**, 486 and 541

29. Weber, G. (1983). Biochemical strategy of cancer cells and design of chemotherapy: G. H. A. Clowes Memorial Lecture, *Cancer Res.,* **43**, 3466

33
Imbalance of histone metabolism in hepatocellular carcinoma: histone acetylation in normal rat liver and hepatomas

H. GRUNICKE, Y. YAMADA, Y. NATSUMEDA, W. HELLIGER, C. SCHLETTERER, H. TALASZ, G. WEISS, B. PUSCHENDORF AND G. WEBER

INTRODUCTION

The core histones H2A, H2B, H3 and H4 are subject to post-translational acetylation[1-3]. These reactions are directed by acetyltransferases which catalyse a transfer of acetyl moieties from acetyl-CoA to ε-amino groups of internal lysyl residues[4-6]. Despite considerable study the biological role of this post-translational modification has remained obscure[3,7]. Numerous reports describe correlations between histone acetylation and transcription[7]. Evidence for a role of histone acetylation in DNA replication and differentiation has also been presented[3,7,8]. It is unclear, however, whether the observations described so far indicate temporal or causal relationships. Perhaps the clearest situation is the massive hyperacetylation of histones which precedes histone replacement by protamines during spermatogenesis in several organisms[2,9,10]. With regard to the latter phenomenon it is tempting to speculate that the major role of histone acetylation is to labilize the binding between DNA and histone as a prerequisite for a histone replacement or alterations in nucleosomal structure which are necessary for transcription[11,12] and replication[3,7,8,12,13]. However, in spite of the fact that the detailed role of histone acetylation is still unclear, most authors agree that this reaction probably plays an important role in the regulation of DNA directed syntheses in eukaryotic nuclei. Reports describing differences in histone acetylation between malignant tumours and their tissues of origin are therefore of particular interest. Horiushi et al.[14] reported elevated levels of histone acetylation in hepatoma AH66 compared to foetal, regenerating or normal liver. Previous studies by our group yielded a higher extent of histone H4 acetylation in hepatoma AS30D when compared to normal, regenerating or foetal liver[15]. However, a systematic investigation in order to elucidate whether alterations in histone acetylation are merely coincidental phenomena or whether they represent growth related and/or transformation linked processes has not yet been performed. In this contribution these questions were addressed by studying histone acetyltransferase activity in a spectrum of hepatocellular carcinomas of low, intermediate and rapid growth rates and the results were compared with those observed in livers of normal animals of the same sex, strain, age and weight. In all tumours the acetyltransferase activity was higher than in corresponding normal livers and the rise correlated positively with the proliferation rates of the tumours. The acetyltransferase activity in tumours seems to represent a transformation — and progression — linked mechanism. The enzyme differs from the corresponding one in normal adult liver because anti-tumour agents which inhibit histone acetylation in tumours do not affect acetylation in host liver.

MATERIALS AND METHODS

Normal and hepatoma bearing ACI/N or Buffalo rats were maintained under standardized conditions[16]. Hepatomas were transplanted by s.c. inoculation in inbred male ACI/N or Buffalo strain rats as indicated. Tumour growth rate was defined by the time (in weeks) required to obtain a tumour diameter of 1.5 cm after s.c. inoculation of 10^7 cells. Hepatoma 3924A (growth rate 1.3 weeks) was grown s.c. in male inbred ACI/N rats. All other hepatomas (growth rates in parentheses) were propagated in male Buffalo strain rats: 20 (40–60); 7787 (25); 8999 (6.5); 7777 (2.2); 5123 TC (2.0); 7288 TC (1.5). Detailed descriptions of the biological and biochemical properties of these tumours have been published[16,17]. Control livers were obtained from normal inbred rats of the same sex, weight and strain as the tumour-bearing rats. Hepatomas and livers were harvested as described[18]. Hepatoma AS30D was grown i.p. and propagated by weekly i.p. transplantations. Tumour cells were harvested 6 days after inoculation.

NIH 3T3 fibroblasts were transfected with a c-myc oncogene construct. In this construct the oncogene was recombined *in vitro* with a MMTV–LTR sequence which subjects expression of the oncogene to transcriptional control by glucocorticoids. The transfected cells were kindly provided by Dr. B. Groner, Ludwig-Institute for Cancer Research, Bern, Switzerland. Cells were grown in Dulbecco's modified essential Eagle's medium in presence of 10% foetal calf serum.

Isolation of nuclei

Livers or hepatomas were rinsed with 0.15 M NaCl, 10 mM Na-butyrate and minced with scissors in the same solution. The supernatant was carefully decanted and the pellets were homogenized in 30 ml of buffer A (0.25 M sucrose; 0.05 M Tris, pH 7.9; 0.025 M KCl; 5 mM MgCl$_2$; 10 mM Na-butyrate) by 3 strokes (hepatomas 5 strokes) in a glass-teflon homogenizer. The homogenate was filtered through 4 layers of cheese cloth and centrifuged for 5 min at 750 × g. The pellets were resuspended in 20 ml of the same buffer and centrifuged at 2000 × g for 10 min. The pelleted nuclei were carefully resuspended in a small volume of buffer B (0.34 M sucrose; 0.1 M Tris, pH 7.9; 2 mM CaCl$_2$;0.1% Nonidet P-40 [NP-40]; 10 mM Na-butyrate). Volumes were adjusted to 20 ml per sample and centrifuged at 800 × g for 10 min. The pellets were washed in 20 ml buffer B and subsequently twice in 20 ml buffer B without NP-40. The final volume was adjusted to yield approximately 2 to 4 × 10^8 nuclei/ml. Purity of nuclei was checked by phase contrast microscopy. Nuclei were counted by microscopy under phase contrast in the Neubauer chamber. All steps were carried out at 0 to 4°C. Nuclei yield was calculated as percent of total DNA obtained in nuclear pellets.

Acetyltransferase activity assay

A modification of the procedure by Garcea and Alberts[19] was employed. The assay mixture contained in a total volume of 200 μl: 0.34 M sucrose; 0.1 M Tris pH 7.9; 2 mM CaCl$_2$; 10 mM Na-butyrate; 0.1% ß-mercaptoethanol; 100 μM [^{3}H]acetyl-CoA (0.5 Ci/mmol) and nuclei corresponding to 1.2 mg protein (approx. 1. 5 × 10^7 nuclei). Samples were pre-incubated for 5 min at 22°C in the absence of labelled acetyl-CoA. Incubation was started by addition of [^{3}H]acetyl-CoA and terminated after 1, 2, 4 and 8 min at 22°C by addition of 1 ml ice cold buffer B containing 200 μM unlabelled acetyl-CoA and subsequent centrifugation. Histones were extracted from the washed nuclei sediments with 200 μl of 0.4 N H$_2$SO$_4$ at 4°C for 1 hour. Proteins were precipitated with TCA (final concentration 20%), washed twice in 20% TCA redissolved in 0.1 N NaOH and the radioactivity was counted in a liquid scintillation counter. Uptake of label was linear with time up to 4 min. Specific activities are indicated as nmol/hour/mg total tissue protein. Protein concentration was determined in another aliquot of the same sample, employing the procedure by Lowry et al.[20] using bovine serum albumin as a standard.

Gel electrophoresis of histones

Histones were extracted from nuclei with 0.4 N H$_2$SO$_4$ as described before. Proteins were precipitated overnight at –20°C with 7 volumes of acetone. The precipitate was collected by centrifugation, washed with acetone, dried under vacuum and finally dissolved in cold H$_2$O. 30–40 μg of protein was applied to 0.075 × 14 × 16 cm acrylamide gels (12% polyacrylamide, 5% acetic acid, 8 M urea, 0.37% Triton-X-100) as described by Zweidler et al.[21] and run for 13.5 hours at 10 mA, 210 V. Proteins were stained with Coomassie brilliant blue R. Fluorography of [^{3}H]acetyl-labelled histone was carried out as described by Laskey and Mills[22]. DNA was determined employing the modifications of the Ceriotti procedure described by Keck[23].

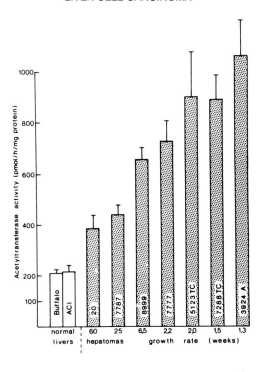

Figure 1 Histone actyltransferase activities in rat hepatomas and normal livers. Acetyltransferase activity was determined as described in the text. ACI/N normal liver was control for hepatoma 3924A and Buffalo for all the others. Vertical bars indicate SEM of 3 or more experiments in each group. Spearman's rank correlation coefficient ($\gamma s = 1 - [\frac{6 \Sigma d^2}{n(n^2 - 1)}]$) was calculated from the differences, d, between rankings, with $n - 7$ for orders of the 7 tumours of increasing growth rates and histone acetyltransferase activity for ranking growth rate against activity ($\gamma_s = 0.064$). The correlation was significant ($p \leq 0.05$). All differences between normal livers and tumours are statistically significant ($p < 0.01$)

RESULTS AND DISCUSSION

The specific activity of histone acetyltransferase in various hepatomas and the corresponding normal livers is shown in Figure 1. The results demonstrate that the enzyme activity is increased in all hepatomas and that the rise is proportional to the growth rates of the tumours. Statistical analyses yielded that the observed elevations are significant even in the case of slowest growing hepatomas.

The elevated activity of the histone acetyltransferase does not lead to an increase in the extent of histone acetylation. The concentrations of histone (and DNA) increase roughly in parallel with the specific activity of the enzyme (Table 1). Thus, the enzyme activities are about the same in all cases if the activity is based on milligrams of histone instead of milligrams of total protein. Accordingly, there are no persistent significant differences in the

Table 1 Histone and DNA contents in rat hepatomas and normal livers. For isolation of nuclei, preparation of histones and DNA determination see text. ACI/N normal liver is control of hepatoma 3924A and Buffalo is control of all the others

Tissues	Growth rate (weeks)	Histone		DNA	
		(mg/g protein)	(% of control)	(mg/g protein)	(% of control)
Normal livers					
Buffalo strain		13.6 ± 0.9	100	17.2 ± 0.8	100
ACI/N strain		15.2 ± 1.3	100	18.7 ± 0.3	100
Hepatomas					
20	60.0	30.9	227	26.0	151
7787	25.0	21.0	154	26.0	151
8999	6.5	37.4 ± 3.9 [a,b]	275	41.0 ± 3.5 [a,b]	238
7777	2.2	49.6 ± 1.4 [a,b]	365	56.2 ± 1.8 [a,b]	327
5123TC	2.0	58.3 ± 1.4 [a,b]	429	60.7 ± 2.9 [a,b]	353
7288TC	1.5	50.8 ± 1.4 [a,b]	374	55.9 ± 4.9 [a,b]	325
3924A	1.3	58.9 ± 5.3 [a,b]	388	58.5 ± 2.8 [a,b]	313

[a]Statistically significantly different from the respective normal livers ($p < 0.01$)
[b]Means ± S.E.M. of 3 or more experiments in each group

extent or the pattern of [^{3}H]acetate incorporation into core histones (data not shown). The fact that the specific activities of the acetyltransferase are roughly proportional to the elevated concentrations of histones may indicate that the enzyme activity in tumours represents a compensatory mechanism by the hepatomas to achieve an extent of histone acetylation similar to that in normal liver; since it occurs in proliferating cells, this process may indicate an acetylation of newly synthesized histones. Thus, the elevated histone acetyltransferase in hepatomas may represent a process which is related to chromatin replication in contrast to histone acetylation in adult liver. If this conclusion is valid one should postulate a similar replication-linked histone acetylation in regenerating liver. Table 2 demonstrates that this is indeed the case. Since the report by Pogo *et al.*[24] who described a peak in acetate incorporation in rat liver histones 3–4 hours following partial hepatectomy, histone acetylation in regenerating liver has been correlated mainly with RNA synthesis. The relationship between histone acetyltransferase activity and DNA synthesis, however, has not been thoroughly investigated. Table 2 demonstrates a sharp transitory peak in histone acetyltransferase activity 4 hours before the onset of replication (13–14 hours after hepatectomy). This peak is well beyond the first maximum in RNA synthesis which has been shown to occur between 6 and 8 hours after hepatectomy[24]. The elevated activity declines rapidly and reaches a minimum at the onset of DNA synthesis (16–18 hours after hepatectomy). Shortly after the onset of replication, the histone acetyltransferase activity riss again and reaches a new maximum at about 26 hours (approximately 6 hours before another round ot DNA synthesis occurs). If the activity of this enzyme is calculated per milligram of histone (instead of total protein), then the elevated activities during the peak of thymidine incorporation are diminished which may

Table 2 Histone acetyltransferase activity in regenerating rat liver. Male Sprague-Dawley rats (250–300 g) were partially hepatectomized as described by Higgins and Anderson[27]. Sham-operated animals served as controls. Acetyltransferase activities were determined in isolated nuclei as described in the text

Hours after partial hepatectomy	Relative activity[a] (per mg total protein)	Relative activity[a] (per mg histone)	Relative thymidine[b] incorporation
1.5	0	1.4	1
3	2 ± 9[c]	9 ± 2	1.25
5	–18	–23	1
6	16 ± 4	7 ± 5	1
12	–1 ± 0.5	8 ± 10	1
13	87 ± 32	84 ± 33	1
14	102 ± 15	35 ± 0.5	2.1 ± 0.3
15	11 ± 2	8 ± 1	2 ± 0.2
16	9 ± 8	16 ± 2	2.2 ± 0.05
18	–7.5 ± 1	17 ± 12	13 ± 4
19	25 ± 8	29 ± 5	–
20	47	8.1	103
23	49 ± 4	15 ± 12	67 ± 2
26	111 ± 42	138 ± 50	45 ± 2
29	41	21	27
34	5	14	19
36	19	21	53
39	–5.4	2.9	13.6

[a]Specific activity (nmol/g/mg protein) in regenerated liver/specific activity in sham-operated liver × 100
[b]Tdr incorporation (cpm/mg DNA) in regenerated liver/Tdr incorporation in sham-operated liver
[c]means ± S.E.M.

indicate that the activity in this time period represents acetylation of newly formed histones. The peak preceding DNA synthesis, on the other hand, may represent a histone acetylation which is involved in preparative steps leading to the onset of replication. A similar biphasic pattern of histone acetylation has been observed in *Physarum polycephalum* in which acetylation of pre-existing histones precedes DNA replication followed by an acetylation of newly synthesized histones during S-phase[8]. An elevated incorporation of labelled acetate into histones immediately before the onset of DNA replication is also observed after growth stimulation by v-myc in myc transfected fibroblasts (Figure 2). Thus, available evidence strongly suggests a replication linked type of histone acetylation.

The data in Figure 1 indicate a transformation and proliferation linked elevation of a histone acetyltransferase. Thus, this enzyme should be of interest in tumour chemotherapy. In fact, alkylating anti-tumour agents depress histone acetylation[25,26]. This effect was closely correlated with the anti-tumour effect of these drugs and it is reduced in resistant cells[26]. Whereas nitrogen mustard resistant and sensitive Walker cells exhibited equal capacities for repair of DNA interstrand cross-links (the presumed essential lesion after exposure to bifunctional alkylating agents), the inhibition of histone acetylation was significantly smaller in resistant cells compared to the

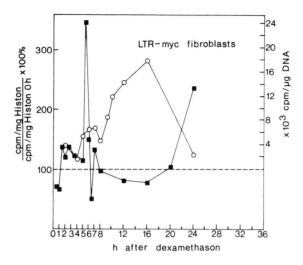

Figure 2 [³H]Acetate incorporation into core histones of fibroblasts following expression of c-myc by dexamethasone. ■, Histone acetylation; ○, thymidine incorporation. NIH 3T3 cells transfected with a MMTV–LTR c-myc construct (see text) were growth-arrested by reducing the serum concentration to 1% for 48 hours. At time 0, 1 μM dexamethasone was added and the incorporation of [³H]acetate and [³H]thymidine determined at the time points indicated. Labelled substrates (40 μCi [³H]acetate/ml (4 Ci/mmol) or 10 μCi [³H]thymidine (25 Ci/mmol) were added 20 min prior to harvesting cells. Histones were extracted with 0.25 N HCl from cell) pellets frozen in liquid nitrogen

sensitive counterparts[26]. All these observations emphasize the biological significance of the depression of histone acetylation. This conclusion is further supported by the finding that nitrogen mustard, while inhibiting histone acetylation in tumour cells, does not affect histone acetylation in the liver of the tumour-bearing animal (Figure 3). The selective sensitivity of histone acetylation in tumour and normal liver suggests a difference in the corresponding acetyltransferases. It is conceivable that proliferating tissues are characterized by elevated activities of a replication associated histone acetyltransferase which in contrast to the acetyltransferase activity in non-dividing tissues is sensitive to akylating agents.

It cannot be decided yet whether the elevated acetyltransferase activities observed in hepatomas correspond to any of the various types of this enzyme described so far[4-6] or whether it is related to any of the peaks in acetyltransferase activities observed in regenerating rat liver. Furthermore, since chromatin, the biological substrate, was employed as an acceptor rather than free histones, the rate of acetylation may be determined by the availability of the corresponding histone regions to the enzyme(s). Purification of the various acetyltransferases is required in order to discriminate between these alternatives.

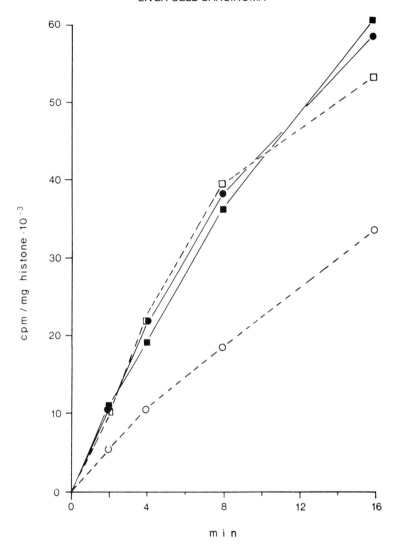

Figure 3 Effect of nitrogen mustard (HN2) on histone acetyltransferase activity in hepatoma AS30D and host liver. HN2 was administered i.p. to hepatoma AS30D-bearing animals at a final concentration of 2.5×10^{-5} mol/kg.
■, host liver; ● host liver + HN2; □, hepatoma, ○, hepatoma + HN2

SUMMARY

The behaviour of histone acetyltransferase (EC 2.3.1.48) activity has been investigated in normal rat liver and in a spectrum of rat hepatomas of slow, intermediate and rapid growth rates. In all hepatomas the acetyltransferase activity was higher than in the corresponding normal livers and the rise correlated positively with the proliferation rates of the tumours. Studies with regenerating liver and c-myc transfected fibroblasts revealed a type of histone acetylation which is in close temporal correlation with DNA synthesis. It is suggested that the elevated acetyltransferase activity in hepatomas corresponds to a replication associated type of histone acetylation. Treatment of tumour-bearing animals with therapeutic concentrations of alkylating agents depresses histone acetylation in the tumour (hepatoma AS30D) but not in host liver.

References

1. Allfrey, V. G. (1977). Postsynthetic modification of histone fractions: a mechanism for the control of chromosome structure by the modulation of histone-DNA interactions. In Lee, H. I. and Eckhardt, L. R. (eds.) *Chromatin and Chromatin Structure*, pp 167–91. (New York: Academic Press, Inc.)
2. Dixon, G. H., Candido, E. P. M., Honda, P. M., Louie, A. E., MacLeod, A. R. and Sung, M. D. (1977). The biological roles of post-synthetic modifications of basic nuclear proteins. In Fitzsimons, D. W. and Wolstenholme, G. E. W. (eds.) *The Structure and Function of Chromatin*, pp 229–58 (Amsterdam: Associated Publishers)
3. Doenecke, D. and Gallwitz, D. (1982). Acetylation of histones in nucleosomes. *Mol. Cell. Biochem.,* **44**, 113–28
4. Belikoff, E., Wong, L. J. and Alberts, B. M. (1980). Extensive purification of histone acetylase A, the major histone N-acetyltransferase activity detected in mammalian cell nuclei. *J. Biol. Chem.,* **255**, 11448–53
5. Böhm, I., Schlaeger, E. J. and Knippers, R. (1980). Acetylation of nucleosomal histones *in vitro. Eur. J. Biochem.,* **112**, 353–62
6. Yukioka, M., Sasaki, S., Qi, S. L. and Inoue, A. (1984). Two species of histone acetyltransferase in rat liver nuclei. *J. Biol. Chem.,* **259**, 8372–7
7. Reeves, R. C. (1984). Transcriptionally active chromatin. *Biochim. Biophys. Acta,* **782**, 343–93
8. Loidl, P. (1988). Towards an understanding of the biological function of histone-acetylation. *FEBS Lett.,* **227**, 91–5
9. Grimes, S. R. Jr. and Henderson, N. (1983). Acetylation of histones during spermatogenesis in the rat. *Arch. Biochem. Biophys.,* **221**, 106–16
10. Christensen, M. E., Rattner, J. B. and Dixon, G. H. (1984). Hyperacetylation of histone H4 promotes chromatin decondensation prior to histone replacement by protamines during spermatogenesis in rainbow trout. *Nucl. Acids. Res.,* **12**, 4575–92
11. Lorch, Y., LaPoint, J. W. and Kornberg, R. (1987). Nucleosomes inhibit the initiation of transcription but allow chain elongation with the displacement of histones. *Cell,* **49**, 203–10
12. Sterner, R., Boffa, L. C., Chen, T. A. and Allfrey, V. G. (1987). Cell-cycle dependent changes in conformation and composition of nucleosomes containing human histone gene sequences. *Nucl. Acids Res.,* **15**, 4375–91
13. Loidl, P. and Gröbner, P. (1987). Postsynthetic acetylation of histones during the cell cycle: A general function for the displacement of histones during chromatin rearrangements. *Nucl. Acids. Res.,* **15**, 8351–66
14. Horiuchi, K., Fujimoto, D., Fukushima, M. and Kanai, K. (1981). Increased histone acetylation and deacetylation in rat ascites hepatoma cells. *Cancer Res.,* **41**, 1488–91
15. Grunicke, H., Csordas, A., Helliger, W., Hauptlorenz, S., Loidl, A., Multhaup, I., Zwierzina, H. and Puschendorf, B. (1984). Depression of histone acetylation by alkylating antitumor agents: significance for antitumor activity and possible biological consequences. *Adv. Enzyme Regul.,* **22**, 433–46
16. Weber, G. (1983). Biochemical strategy for cancer cells and the design of chemotherapy. *Cancer Res.,* **43**, 3466–92

17. Weber, G. (1977). Enzymology of cancer cells. Parts 1 and 2. *New Engl. J. Med.,* **296,** 486–493 and 541–51
18. Lui, M. S., Faderan, M. A., Liepnieks, J. J., Natsumeda, Y., Olah, E., Jayaram, H. N. and Weber, G. (1984). Modulation of IMP dehydrogenase activity and guanylase activity by tiazofurin (2-ß-ribofuranosylthiazole-4-carboxamide). *J. Biol. Chem.,* **259,** 5078–82
19. Garcea, R. L. and Alberts, B. M. (1980). Comparative studies of histone acetylation in nucleosomes, nuclei and intact cells. *J. Biol. Chem.,* **255,** 11454–63
20. Lowry, O. A., Rosebrough, M. J., Farr, A. L. and Randall, R. J. (1951). Protein measurement with the Folinphenol reagent. *J. Biol. Chem.,* **193,** 265–75
21. Zweidler, A. (1978). Resolution of histones by polyacrylamide gel electrophoresis. *Methods Cell Biol.,* **17,** 223–33
22. Laskey, R. A. and Mills, A. B. (1957). Quantitative film detection of ^{3}H- and ^{14}C-polyacrylamide gels by fluorography. *Eur. J. Biochem.,* **56,** 335–41
23. Keck, K. (1956). An ultramicrotechnique for the determination of deoxypentosenucleic acid. *Arch. Biochem. Biophys.,* **63,** 446–67
24. Pogo, B. G. T., Pogo, A. O., Allfrey, V. G. and Mirsky, A. E. (1968). Changing patterns of histone acetylation and RNA synthesis in regeneration of the liver. *Proc. Natl. Acad. Sci. USA,* **59,** 1337–44
25. Zwierzina, H., Loidl, A., Fuith, L. C., Helliger, W., Puschendorf, B. and Grunicke, H. (1984). Depression of histone acetylation by alkylating antitumor agents in murine cells. *Cancer Res.,* **44,** 3336–9
26. Grunicke, H., Helliger, W., Hermann, B. J., Höck, W., Hofmann, J. and Puschendorf. B. (1986). Alkylating antitumor agents reduce histone acetyl-transferase activity. *Adv. Enzyme Regul.,* **25,** 87–97
27. Higgins, G. N. and Anderson, R. M. (1931). Experimental pathology of the liver: Restoration of the liver in the white rat following partial surgical removal. *Arch. Pathol.,* **12,** 186–202

34
Proliferating cell nucleolar antigens: a novel 120-kD PCNA

H. BUSCH, A. FONAGY, D. HENNING, R. K. BUSCH, J. FREEMAN,
J. HAZELWOOD, W. L. LIN AND A. B. REDDY

INTRODUCTION

In initial studies on distinctions between nuclear proteins of hepatomas and normal liver, it was demonstrated by two-dimensional gel electrophoretic techniques that the less differentiated the tumour, the greater the number of 'spot differences' that could be identified[1,2]. In these studies, it was shown that there were approximately 950 individual peptides in the nucleus of hepatoma or normal liver cells; many of these had similar migration characteristics.

Inasmuch as only a few nuclear proteins have been characterized, it seemed essential to devise techniques that would provide a more satisfactory differentiation which could be coupled with ultra-micro methods. Initially, for this purpose, polyclonal antibodies were developed in rabbits to nucleolar proteins. Following extensive absorption of these antibodies, it was demonstrated that nucleolar antigens were present in cancer cells that differed from those in normal liver cells and vice versa[3,4].

In the experimentally-produced antibodies directed against specific nucleolar products, the complexities of the antibodies produced increased with the duration of the immunization procedure as well as the complexity of the antigens. With the Novikoff rat hepatoma and human HeLa and Namalwa cell tumours, specific nucleolar antigens were purified and shown to be proteins (at least in part)[5-7]. These purified protein immunogens probably differ from the DNA-protein complexes utilized by Hnilica et al.[8] in their studies on DNP-specific antigens of a variety of tissues and tumours.

Although the initial goal of our experimental studies on nucleolar antigens was to define conditions that might permit an analysis of very minute amounts of proteins important to nucleolar functions, the results obtained with these studies became of particular interest for possible differentiation of human cancer cells and other cells.

Immunological[9-12] and biochemical[3,4,13] studies indicated that quantitative and qualitative differences exist in proteins of nucleoli of tumour cells compared to proteins from nucleoli of normal human tissues. These human tumour nucleolar antigens are of interest inasmuch as they may serve as potential targets for chemotherapy or immunotherapy, immunodiagnosis of cancer, and for obtaining useful information concerning tumour biology and particularly events in the phases of the cell cycle.

PROLIFERATING CELL NUCLEAR AND NUCLEOLAR PROTEINS (PCNAs)

In our initial studies[14], a proliferating cell nuclear antigen (PCNA) was identi-fied with autoantibodies from a patient with systemic lupus erythemato-sus[15-17]. Specific antibodies were purified by affinity chromatography in which Novikoff hepatoma nucleolar proteins were conjugated to Sepharose-4B. The purified anti-PCNA antibodies produced bright nucleolar fluorescence in tumour cells as shown by indirect immunofluorescence. This PCNA was found in nucleoli of human cell lines, HeLa, Hep-2, and Namalwa, and a solid human renal and a prostate carcinoma. Both strong and weak nucleolar fluorescence areas were found in the renal and prostate carcinoma indicating that there are varying degrees of proliferation among tumour cells. Two human colon carcinoma cell lines, Ω (an aggressive, fast-growing clone of human colon carcinoma cell line HCT 116) and CBS, a slow-growing human colon carcinoma cell line, were compared. The fast-growing colon carcinoma cells, Ω, exhibited a higher percentage of nucleolar fluorescence (28.5%) than that of the slow-growing colon cells (13.6%). By enzyme-linked immunosorbent assays (ELISA), the Ω cell extract had a higher PCNA antigen content (2.8-fold) than the CBS cell extract which, in turn, was higher than that of a normal human liver extract. This PCNA was also found in a human fetal lung fibroblast cell line (IMR-90). Very weak or negative nucleolar fluorescence was observed in several normal human tissues including liver, kidney, prostate and cheek cells. With this autoimmune antibody, nucleolar fluorescence was also observed in rat Novikoff hepatoma cells. Although normal rat liver did not have this PCNA nucleolar fluorescence, nuclear and nucleolar fluorescence were observed at 18 hours after partial hepatectomy.

The p145 antigen

In the previous studies in our laboratory which indicated the presence of nucleolar antigens in tumours that were not detected in normal tissues, some polyclonal antisera identified a 145-kD nucleolar antigen on immunoblots of tumour nucleoli but not in normal human liver nucleoli. A monoclonal antibody to a 145-kD nucleolar protein (p145) was produced by immunization of mice with a nucleolar extract of HeLa cells, which was enriched with this antigen[18]. This anti-p145 monoclonal antibody produced bright nucleolar immunofluorescence localization in a broad range of human tumours including cancers of the gastrointestinal tract, genito-urinary tract, lung, liver, breast, muscle, cartilage and blood. The p145 nucleolar antigen was not detected in most normal human tissues or in benign tumours; only weak nucleolar staining was observed in spermatogonia of the testes and in ductal regions of some hypertrophied prostates.

Nucleolar antigen p145 was readily and almost completely extracted from HeLa cell nucleoli by homogenization in a 0.01 M Tris buffer containing 0.2% deoxycholate. On sucrose density gradient centrifugation, the antigen sedimented with the nucleolar ribonucleoprotein (RNP) fraction. Nucleolar antigen p145 was released from RNPs following treatment with 4 M guanidinium hydrochloride or RNAse. Peptide mapping of nucleolar p145 antigen showed it was distinct from other known nucleolar antigens. Although it remains to be determined if the p145 antigen plays a role in cell transformation, maintenance of the malignant phenotype, or cell division, it now appears to have value as a tumour marker. It may also be a useful therapeutic target.

Nucleolar antigen p145, which is associated with growing cells and was found in a broad range of human cancers, was analysed in the human promyelocytic tumour cell line HL-60 which was induced to differentiate by retinoic acid[19]. Differentiation was monitored by morphological changes, [³H]uridine and [³H]thymidine uptake, the ability of cells to reduce nitroblue tetrazolium (NBT), and cell number. The monoclonal antibody to nucleolar antigen p145 produced bright immunofluorescence in all cycling interphase HL-60 cells; during mitosis only diffuse staining was detected. Nucleolar antigen p145 was undetected in HL-60 cells after 132 hours of treatment with retinoic acid. The absence of nucleolar antigen p145 was associated with a 81% and 70% decline in DNA and RNA synthesis, respectively, and apparent inactivation of ribosomal and non-ribosomal DNA transcription, as observed by electron microscopy. The loss in expression of the antigen also correlated with increased NBT-positive cells, appearance of morphologically distinct myeloid cells, and termination of cell proliferation. These data indicate that the expression of nucleolar antigen p145 occurred in cycling HL-60 cells but not in terminally-differentiated non-cycling HL-60 cells[19].

The p105 antigen

We also reported identification and partial characterization of a novel M_r 105000 nucleolar antigen (p105) identified by a monoclonal antibody[20]. This monoclonal antibody was obtained when a nucleolar protein extract, separated from the immunodominant protein C23, was used as the immunogen. Nucleolar antigen p105 was not detected in normal (resting) human liver, kidney, or peripheral blood lymphocytes, but was present in a variety of human malignant cells and tissues. Lymphocyte nucleoli also exhibited specific p105 staining at 72 hours after phytohaemagglutinin stimulation. Nucleolar antigen p105 was detected in growing and dividing HL-60 cells but was not detected in retinoic acid-induced differentiated HL-60 cells. When HeLa cells were made quiescent by 48 hours of serum starvation, the p105 antigen was not detected, but after re-feeding with serum-

Table 1 Preliminary nucleotide sequence of the p120 antigen

```
GGG AAG CTA CCA AAA GGG ATC TCT GCA GGA GCT GTC CAG ACA
GCT GGT AAG AAG GGA CCC CAG TCC CTA TTT AAT GCT CCT CGA
GGC AAG AAG CGC CCA GCA CCT GGC AGT GAT GAG GAA GAG GAG
GAG GAA GAC TCT GAA GAA GAT GGT ATG GTG AAC CAC GGG GAC
CTC TGG GGC TCC GAG GAC GAT GCT GAT ACG GTA GAT GAC TAT
GGA GCT GAC TCC AAC TCT GAG GAT GAG GAG GAA GGT GAA GCG
TTG CTG CCC ATT AGA ATC CAG GCT CGG AAG CAG AAG GCC CGG
GAA GCT GCT GCT GGG ATC CAG TGG AGT AAG GAG GAG ACC GAG
GAC GCT GAG GAA AAA GCA GAA GTG ACC CCT GAG TCA GCC CCC
CCA GAG GAG GAA GGG GCA GAT GGG AGC CTG CAG ATC GCC GTG
GAT GTG GTG CCA TTT GAT CTG CCC CCT GCT GTT GAG AAG GAG
CAG GAA GAA CAG GCT GTG GAC CAA CGA GCA GTT CAC CCA CGG
ATC GCC GAT ATT GTG CGT ATT CGT GAT CGT TTT GGG AAC CAG
CGG GAG GAA GGG CGG GAA CGT GAA TAC GAT CTG AAC GAC CTC
AAG GAG GAT CTG GCC TAC TAC TCT TCC GGA TCT GAC GAG GTG
CTT GGC AAG CTC ATG CTC CTC TTC CCT TAT CCC GTC GAG CTC
GAG TTA GAA GAA GCT GAG GAG GTG GCT CGG GAC CTT ACC CAG
CGG ACC AAT ACC TTG ACC GTT CGA CGC CGA CGA TCT GCA AAG
GCT CTA ATC AAT CGT GTT GGG AAC CTG GAT CTG TCT CTG GGC
TGG TCA AAG ACT GGA GGG CTA GTG CTG GAT TAT CAT GTG GTG
TTG GTG AAG CCC CGA CTA GTA CCT TGG GCA GCA GGA CAT CGT
GGG AGC CTA CAG CAT CAG GTT GCC CAT GGC CGG CTA CTG CCC
GAA CAT GAG CGG ATC GCC CTG GAC GAC TGT AAG CTA GGA CAG
AAG ACC AGC TAC ATG GCC ATG ATG CAG ATG AAG ACG GGT CAG
ATC CTT GCC AAT GAT GCC AAT CTG CAG GAG GCT AAG AGT GTT
GTG GGC AAC TTG GAC CGG CTG GGA GCC ACG AAC GTC ACC ATC
AGC CAC TAT GAT GGG CGC CAG TTC CCC AAG GTG GTG GGG GGC
```

```
TTT  GAC  CGA  GTA  CTG  CTG  GTA  GAT  GCT  CCC  TGC  AGT  GGC  GGG
GTC  ATC  TCC  AAG  GAT  CCA  GCC  GCC  GTG  AAG  ACT  AAC  AAG  GAG
AAG  GAC  ATC  CTG  CGC  TGT  CGT  GCT  CAC  CTC  CAG  AAG  GAG  CTC
CTG  AGT  GCT  ATT  GAC  TCT  GAC  GTC  AAT  GCG  ACC  TCC  AAG  GGA
GGC  TAC  GCT  GTT  TAC  TGC  TAC  ACC  TGT  TCT  ATC  ACA  GTA  GAG
AAT  GAG  CTG  GTG  GTA  GAC  GTA  TAT  GCT  CTG  AAA  AAG  AGG  GTG
CGA  CTG  TGG  CCC  ACG  GGC  CTA  CGC  GAC  TTT  GGC  CAG  GAA  TTT
ACC  CGC  GTG  CGA  GAA  AGG  GAA  CGC  TTC  CAC  CCC  AGT  CTG  TCT
ACC  CGA  GTG  TTT  TAC  CCT  TTC  CAT  ACC  CAC  AAT  ATG  GAT  TTC
TTC  ATT  TTT  AAG  TTC  AAG  TAC  AAA  TTT  TCC  AAT  TCT  ATC  CAG
TCC  CAG  CGC  GGA  AAT  TCT  AAT  GAA  ACA  GCC  ACA  CCT  ACA  GTA
GAC  TTG  GCC  CAG  GTC  ATC  GTC  GTC  AAG  TCT  GAG  AAC  AGC  CAG
CCA  GCC  ACA  AAA  GCC  AAG  CCA  CCA  GCT  GCA  AAG  ACA  AAG  CAG
CTG  CAG  CCT  AAA  CAA  CAT  CAA  AAA  AAG  AAG  GCC  TCC  TTC  AAG
GTA  AAT  AGT  CAG  TCC  AAA  TCC  GGG  GCA  GAC  TCA  GAA  TTG  ACT
GAT  CCT  AGT  CAG  ACA  AAG  ACA  CCC  AAA  GCT  TCC  TCC  AGC  CAG
CCA  AGC  GTG  AAA  CCA  GCT  CCA  GGA  AAG  CAA  GAA  GGG  ATC  GAG
CAG  ACA  TCC  ACA  GGG  AAG  GGG  CTA  TCC  CTC  CGA  TCA  CCT  TTA
CAA  GAC  TCA  CAC  AAA  GTT  AAA  GCT  CAC  CGG  AGG  CAG  ACA  CTC
TTT  TTG  GGC  CAC  GGG  CAC  ACA  AAA  CTA  AGG  CTG  TGT  AGC  ATC
CCT  GCC  TCA  GGC  GCT  CAC  CAC  GAA  AAG  AGG  ACC  ATC  GAG  CCC
AAG  TTT  GCA  CAA  CTC  CTA  GGG  GAG  CAG  AGG  CAG  TTG  ACC  CAG
GCC  GGC  TCA  AAA  CTC  AGC  GCT  TTC  CAG  AGG  CCA  AAT  CCA  CAG
ACA  CCC  AGC  AGC  CAC  AGC  CCA  CTG  TGT  CAG  CCA  TCC  CAG  GCA
GTG  GCT  AGC  AGC  CAC  AGG  AGA  GGA  AGA  CAG  CCA  AGT  ATG  CGG
GTG  GCC  AGC  CTT  ATG  CTT  TAT  TGT  AGA  TGC  ACT  AAA  CAT  TCT
ACA  CAT  TTT  AAA  CCC  AAA  TGC  CCT  CAG  C                     AAT
```

Table 2 Preliminary amino acid sequence of the p120 antigen

Gly	Lys	Pro	Asp	Asp	Glu	Ala	Asp	Val	Phe	Asp	Arg	Leu	Phe	Glu	Asn	Arg	Val	Trp	Leu	Gly	Ile	Asn
Lys	Lys	Ala	Gly	Thr	Gly	Arg	Glu	Glu	Val	Leu	Asp	Asn	Leu	Phe	Thr	Gly	Val	Ala	Gly	Gly	Leu	Leu
Leu	Gly	Pro	Met	Val	Glu	Glu	Glu	Glu	Leu	Gln	Phe	Arg	Leu	Leu	Leu	Val	Tyr	Leu	Pro	Lys	Ala	His
Pro	Pro	Gly	Val	Asp	Ala	Ala	Glu	Ala	Pro	Arg	Gly	Leu	Gly	Glu	Lys	Asn	Asp	His	Gln	Thr	Asn	Arg
Lys	Gln	Ser	Asn	Asp	Leu	Ala	Lys	Asp	Pro	Val	Ala	Lys	Lys	Ala	Thr	Leu	Ser	Arg	Glu	Ser	Asp	Leu
Gly	Ser	Asp	His	Tyr	Leu	Ala	Lys	Gly	Ala	His	Gln	Lys	Lys	Asn	Arg	Asp	Ser	Arg	His	Tyr	Ala	Gly
Ile	Leu	Gly	Gly	Gly	Pro	Gly	Gly	Gly	Lys	Arg	Asp	Met	Glu	Arg	Pro	Val	Gly	Glu	Met	Asn	Val	
Ser	Phe	Glu	Asp	Ala	Ile	Ile	Val	Leu	Glu	Arg	Glu	Leu	Asp	Val	Arg	Leu	Pro	Ser	Arg	Ala	Ala	Thr
Ala	Asn	Glu	Leu	Asp	Glu	Gln	Thr	Gln	Met	Ile	Glu	Gln	Ile	Glu	Asp	Gly	Leu	Leu	Ile	Gln	Glu	Asn
Gly	Ala	Glu	Trp	Ser	Arg	Trp	Pro	Ile	Glu	Gln	Gly	Ile	Phe	Arg	Leu	Lys	Val	Gln	Leu	Leu	Arg	Thr
Ala	Pro	Glu	Gly	Asn	Ala	Ser	Glu	Asn	Gln	Asp	Arg	Tyr	Pro	Pro	Ala	Trp	Leu	His	Asp	Met	Leu	Ile
Val	Arg	Glu	Ser	Ser	Ala	Glu	Val	Asp	Ile	Ser	Tyr	Leu	Val	Gln	Ser	Pro	Val	Met	Lys	Lys	Ile	
Gln	Gly	Asp	Glu	Glu	Arg	Gly	Asp	Ala	Val	Arg	Ser	Ser	Thr	Ala	Lys	Arg	Ala	Cys	Asn	Ser	Ser	
Thr	Lys	Ser	Asp	Asp	Lys	Glu	Pro	Glu	Gln	Gly	Ser	Tyr	Glu	Leu	Leu	Thr	Val	Arg	Cys	Thr	Val	His
Ala	Lys	Glu	Asp	Glu	Gln	Thr	Pro	Glu	Ala	Ile	Glu	Gly	Leu	Arg	Ile	Gly	Pro	His	Ala	Gly	Val	Tyr
Gly	Arg	Glu	Ala	Glu	Lys	Glu	Lys	Pro	Pro	Leu	Tyr	Asp	Val	Thr	Asn	Leu	Gly	Gly	Pro	Val	Gly	Asp

Gly	Arg	Gln	Phe	Pro	Lys	Val	Val	Gly	Gly	Phe	Asp	Arg	Val	Leu	Leu
Asp	Ala	Pro	Cys	Ser	Gly	Thr	Gly	Val	Ile	Ser	Lys	Asp	Pro	Ala	Val
Lys	Thr	Asn	Lys	Asp	Glu	Lys	Asp	Ile	Leu	Arg	Cys	Ala	His	Leu	Gln
Lys	Glu	Leu	Leu	Leu	Ser	Ala	Ile	Asp	Ser	Val	Asn	Ala	Thr	Ser	Lys
Thr	Gly	Gly	Tyr	Leu	Val	Tyr	Cys	Thr	Cys	Ser	Ile	Thr	Val	Glu	Glu
Asn	Glu	Trp	Val	Val	Asp	Tyr	Ala	Leu	Lys	Lys	Arg	Asn	Val	Arg	Leu
Val	Pro	Thr	Gly	Leu	Asp	Phe	Gly	Gln	Glu	Gly	Phe	Thr	Arg	Phe	Arg
Glu	Arg	Arg	Phe	His	Pro	Ser	Leu	Arg	Ser	Thr	Arg	Arg	Phe	Tyr	Pro
His	Thr	His	Asn	Met	Asp	Gly	Phe	Phe	Ile	Ala	Lys	Phe	Lys	Lys	Phe
Ser	Asn	Ser	Ile	Pro	Gln	Ser	Gln	Thr	Gly	Asn	Ser	Glu	Thr	Ala	Thr
Pro	Thr	Asn	Val	Asp	Leu	Pro	Gln	Val	Ile	Pro	Lys	Leu	Gln	Lys	Gln
Gln	His	Pro	Lys	Lys	Ala	Ser	Phe	Gln	Lys	Leu	Asn	Gly	Ile	Ser	Lys
Gly	Ala	Asp	Ser	Glu	Leu	Ser	Thr	Val	Pro	Ser	Val	Thr	Lys	Thr	Gln
Ala	Ser	Ser	Ser	Phe	Gln	Asp	Ser	Ser	Gln	Pro	Ala	Gly	Lys	Ala	Glu
Gly	Ile	Arg	Glu	Pro	Lys	Val	Thr	Gly	Lys	Leu	Lys	Gln	Arg	Ser	Pro
Lys	Leu	Gln	Ser	Ser	Lys	Lys	Val	Ala	Ser	Leu	Arg	Gln	Asn	Ala	Leu
Pro	Arg	Ala	Gln	Thr	His	Lys	His	Arg	Leu	Cys	Tyr	Pro	Ile	Gln	Asp
Ser	Gly	His	Pro	Glu	Leu	Arg	Thr	Ile	Ile	Ser	Pro	Phe	Gly	Gly	Gln
Gly	Val	Glu	Lys	Gln	Gln	Leu	Pro	Glu	Gln	Pro	Phe	Glu	Lys	Ala	Ala
Phe	Gln	Lys	Gln	Asn	Asp	Thr	Pro	Lys	Gly	Leu	Ser	Leu	Pro	Leu	Cys
Leu	Pro	Ser	Val	Pro	Ala	Ala	Pro	His	Gln	Gln	Arg	Gly	Arg	Asn	Leu
Ser	Pro	Gly	Ala	Thr	Ala	Ser	Cys	Cys	Tyr	Leu	Arg	Trp	Leu	Lys	Thr
Arg	Arg	Val	Ala	His	Cys	His	Cys	His	Gln	Val	Gly	Thr	Leu	Ala	Ser
Val	Arg	Met	Pro	Ser	Leu	Leu	Cys	Ile	Pro	Met	Lys	Phe	Asn	Thr	His
Phe	Lys	Thr	Ser	Ala											

containing medium, the antigen p105 was detected in the HeLa nucleoli within 2 hours. These results indicate that nucleolar antigen p105 is a proliferating cell nuclear and nucleolar antigen-like molecule which appears early in the G_1–S phase of the cell cycle[20].

The p120 antigen

Tumour nucleoli were treated with polyclonal antisera to normal human tissue nucleoli to block some determinants common to tumour and normal tissue nucleoli. Immunization of mice with these complexes resulted in the development of a monoclonal antibody (FB2) to a novel M_r 120 000 nucleolar proliferation-associated antigen[21]. By indirect immunofluorescence, antibody FB2 produced bright nucleolar staining in a variety of malignant tumours, including cancers of the breast, liver, gastrointestinal tract, genito-urinary tract, blood, lymph system, lung and brain. Although specific nucleolar immunofluorescence was not detected in most normal tissues, it was detected in some proliferating non-malignant tissues including spermatogonia of the testes, ductal regions of hypertrophied prostate, and phytohaemagglutinin-stimulated lymphocytes. The M_r 120 000 antigen was not detected in 48-hour serum-deprived HeLa cells but was readily detectable (within 30 min) following serum re-feeding. The M_r 120 000 antigen was not detected in retinoic acid-treated HL-60 cells following morphological differentiation but was detected in 48-hour phytohemagglutinin-treated lymphocytes. These studies suggest that the M_r 120 000 antigen is a proliferation-associated antigen which plays a role in the early G_1 phase of the cell cycle[21].

Localization of the 120-kD PCNA antigen

The human proliferation-associated nucleolar antigen p120 was localized to substructures within HeLa cell nucleoli by immunofluorescence and immuno-electron microscopy of cells whose nucleoli were segregated by drug treatment or extracted with nucleases[22]. By indirect immunofluorescence, protein p120 was localized diffusely throughout. EM microscopy demonstrated that protein p120 staining delineated a network of 20–30 nm diameter beaded fibrils distributed throughout the nucleolus. This distribution was unique compared to that of the nucleolar proteins p145, RNA polymerase I, or B23 which were examined simultaneously. Drug-induced segregation of nucleoli by actinomycin D or dichlorobenzimidazole riboside, followed by immuno-electron microscopy, indicated that protein p120 was concentrated at the periphery of the granular region in segregated nucleoli. *In situ* nuclease digestion of cells with DNase I and/or RNase A did not release p120 from the nucleolus. Instead, p120 immunoreactivity was retained within phase-dense residual nucleoli. These results provide evidence that protein p120 is associated with, and in fact delineates, a network of fibrils which is retained in the nucleolar residue fraction of proliferating cells[21,22].

cDNA Sequence of the p120 antigen

Using standard methods for identification and isolation of the cDNA and sequence analysis based on the restriction maps, the preliminary nucleotide sequence of the p120 antigen is shown in Table 1. From the cDNA sequence, the derived preliminary amino acid sequence indicates a number of interesting features of this molecule as shown in Table 2.

One of the most notable regions is the series of acidic clusters in the amino terminal portion of the molecule. Glutamic acid sequences up to six in length flanked by two aspartic acid residues were identified. Some of these sequences are possible 'nucleolus recognition signals' since they are also present in nulceolar proteins B23 and C23. The centre of the molecule is rich in aromatic amino acid and methionine residues. The C-terminal portion of the molecule is notable for the relatively large number of cysteine residues and the presence of cysteine dimers. In addition, this portion of the molecule is rich in proline.

An important feature of the molecule is the Pro–Ala–Lys–Lys–Ala–Lys which is a nuclear recognition signal. A search for homologies has not found any molecule in the protein bank with a similar sequence. However, very limited homologies were identified for N-myc and C-myc as well as two virion proteins.

DISCUSSION

A major goal of the research in our laboratory has been the identification of 'the final common pathway of cancer'. It is by recognition of such elements that we can begin the progress of selective and specific anti-cancer therapy. It is not yet known whether any of the antigens identified with four monoclonal antibodies are 'cancer specific', but it is important that p120 is the earliest antigen we have identified that is present in most of the human cancers studied and not in most non-tumour tissues. Accordingly, its epitope may be useful as a drug target in the manner indicated in the accompanying figure, which details the alignment of drug modelled in red on the structure of an epitope or a peptide (Figure 1A, B).

Epitopes as drug targets

Can we utilize the information derived from epitopes to develop new drugs? Inasmuch as an epitope is a small portion of a protein or other macromolecule which is recognized by a specific antibody, it has attachment sites for the antibody which offer specificity of interaction. When the protein or macromolecule is properly cleaved with proteases or specific cleavage reagents, these epitopes can be preserved intact with high immunoreactivity for the antibodies. The epitope content of a given peptide can be quantitated by immunochemical assays such as the ELISA or radioimmunoassay.

In addition, the antibodies can be utilized for 'affinity' binding for the peptides containing the epitopes. Purification of the epitopes on ion-exchange

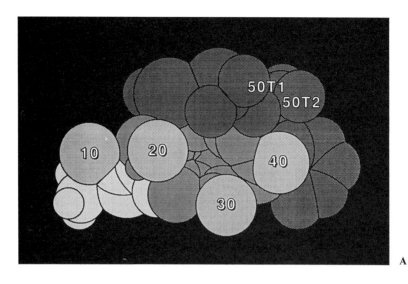

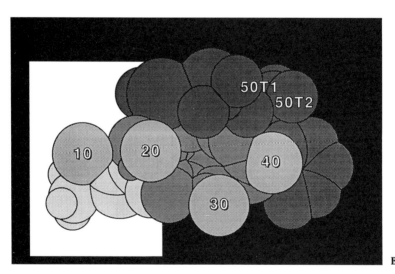

Figure 1A Schematic peptide showing hydrophic regions in dark tint and hydrophilic residues in light and medium tints.
Figure 1B Shows interaction of a theoretical drug indicated by the white rectangle, which binds to both hydrophilic and hydrophobic residues on the left-hand side of the peptide. The goal of the future is to identify critical peptides of the p120 protein, which on binding with drugs will result in cessation of p120 function

columns, thin-layer chromatography and affinity techniques can be followed with the aid of immunochemical procedures.

Information on the amino acid sequence of the epitope is essential for development of potential therapeutic information. The goal of such procedures is to precisely position reactive groups. Just how important such sequence information is becomes apparent when one thinks of the numbers of possible di-, tri- and tetrapeptides. Assuming that each position in a peptide sequence could be filled by 1 of 20 amino acids, there are 400 possible dipeptides, 8000 possible tripeptides and 160000 possible tetrapeptides. For the chemist to produce replicas of such structures, on a hit or miss basis, would be impossible. Even defining the NH_2- and C-terminals would be an advantage for such synthesis although the more information that becomes available about conformation and sequence, the more satisfactory the chemistry that can be applied.

More information is developing about the epitopes of protein p120, and from their structure as well as the overall structure of this molecule, drug design should be possible utilizing novel three-dimensional imaging techniques.

These sequences will permit deductions of the functional types of structures that offer specific spatial and functional orientations for binding the epitopes. As compounds are developed, their structure–activity relationships (SAR) can be tested by immunological and enzymatic methods to select optimum therapeutic agents.

Whether such approaches will offer a quicker path to success in cancer treatment than the 'empirical' or 'screening' approaches used for evolution of the current series of anti-cancer drugs[23] is only speculative at present. One would hope that tests of the feasibility of the approach would not be in the too far distant future. If success is obtained, there will be opportunity to amplify epitope directed therapy to 'cancer related' products and potentially 'cancer specific' products, when these are identified and characterized.

Acknowledgement

These studies were supported by the Cancer Research Center Grant CA-10893, P1, awarded by National Cancer Institute, Department of Health and Human Services, Public Health Service; The DeBakey Medical Foundation; H. Leland Kaplan Cancer Research Endowment; Linda & Ronald Finger Cancer Research Endowment; and The William S. Farish Fund.

References

1. Takami, H. and Busch, H. (1979). Two-dimensional gel electrophoretic comparison of proteins of nuclear fractions of normal liver and Novikoff hepatoma. *Cancer Res.*, **39**, 507–18
2. Takami, H., Busch, F. N., Morris, H. P. and Busch, H. (1979). Comparison of salt-extractable nuclear proteins of regenerating liver, fetal liver, and Morris hepatomas 9618A and 3924A. *Cancer Res.*, **39**, 2096–105

3. Busch, R. K. and Busch, H. (1977). Antigenic proteins of nucleolar chromatin of Novikoff hepatoma ascites cells. *Tumori*, **63**, 347–57

4. Davis, F. M., Busch, R. K., Yeoman, L. C. and Busch, H. (1978). Differences in nucleolar antigens of rat liver and Novikoff hepatoma ascites cells. *Cancer Res.*, **38**, 1906–15

5. Chan, P.-K., Feyerabend, A., Busch, R. K. and Busch, H. (1980). Identification and partial purification of tumor nucleolar antigens: Human tumor antigen 54/6.3. *Cancer Res.*, **40**, 3194–201

6. Lischwe, M. A., Roberts, K. D., Yeoman, L. C. and Busch, H. (1982). Nucleolar specific acidic phosphoprotein C23 is highly methylated. *J. Biol. Chem.*, **257**, 14600–2

7. Lischwe, M. A., Ochs, R. L., Reddy, R., Cook, R. G., Yeoman, L. C., Tan, E. M., Reichlin, M. and Busch, H. (1985). Purification and partial characterization of a nucleolar scleroderma antigen (M_r = 34000; pI 8.5) rich in N^G,N^G-dimethylarginine. *J. Biol. Chem.*, **260**, 14304–10

8. Hnilica, L., Chiu, J., Hardy, K., Furitani, H. and Briggs, R. (1978). In Busch, H. (ed.) *The Cell Nucleus*, Vol. 5, pp 307–31. (New York: Academic Press)

9. Busch, H., Gyorkey, F., Busch, R. K., Davis, F. M. and Smetana, K. (1979). A nucleolar antigen found in a broad range of human malignant tumor specimens. *Cancer Res.*, **39**, 3024–30

10. Busch, H., Busch, R. K., Chan, P.-K., Isenberg, W., Weigand, R., Russo, J. and Furmanski, P. (1981). Results of a 'blind' study on the presence of the human tumor nucleolar antigen in breast carcinomas, benign breast tumors and normal breast tissues. *Clin. Immunol. Immunopathol.*, **18**, 155–67

11. Busch, H., Busch, R. K., Chan, P.-K., Kelsey, D. and Takahashi, K. (1982). Nucleolar antigens of human tumors. *Methods Cancer Res.*, **19**, 109–78

12. Davis, F. M., Gyorkey, F., Busch, R. K. and Busch, H. (1979). A nucleolar antigen found in several human tumors but not in nontumor tissues. *Proc. Natl. Acad. Sci. USA*, **76**, 892–6

13. Yeoman, L. C., Jordan, J. J., Busch, R. K., Taylor, C. W., Savage, H. and Busch, H. (1976). A fetal protein in the chromatin of Novikoff hepatoma and Walker 256 carcinosarcoma tumors that is absent from normal and regenerating rat liver. *Proc. Natl. Acad. Sci. USA*, **73**, 3258–62

14. Chan, P. K., Frakes, R., Tan, E. M., Brattain, M. G., Smetana, K. and Busch, H. (1983). Indirect immunofluorescence studies of proliferating cell nuclear antigen in nucleoli of human tumor and normal tissues. *Cancer Res.*, **43**, 3770–7

15. Takasaki, Y., Deng, J. and Tan, E. (1981). A nuclear antigen associated with cell proliferation and blast transformation. *J. Exp. Med.*, **154**, 1899–909

16. Almendral, J. M., Huebsch, D., Blundell, P. A., Macdonald-Bravo, H. and Bravo, R. (1987). Cloning and sequence of the human nuclear protein cyclin: Homology with DNA-binding proteins. *Proc. Natl. Acad. Sci. USA*, **84**, 1575–9

17. Bravo, R., Frank, R., Blundell, P. A. and Macdonald-Bravo, H. (1987). Cyclin/PCNA is the auxiliary protein of DNA polymerase-δ. *Nature*, **326**, 515–20

18. Freeman, J. W., McRorie, D. K., Busch, R. K., Gyorkey, F., Gyorkey, P., Ross, B. E., Spohn, W. H. and Busch, H. (1986). Identification and partial characterization of a nucleolar antigen with a molecular weight of 145000 found in a broad range of human cancers. *Cancer Res.*, **46**, 3593–8

19. Freeman, J. W., Dowell, B. L., Ochs, R. L., Ross, B. E. and Busch, H. (1987). Effect of differentiation on the expression of nucleolar antigen p145 in HL-60 cells. *Cancer Res.*, **47**, 586–91

20. Freeman, J. W. and Busch, H. (1987). Identification and partial characterization of a M_r 105000 nucleolar antigen associated with cell proliferation. *Cancer Res.*, **47**, 6329–34

21. Freeman, J. W., Busch, R. K., Gyorkey, F., Gyorkey, P., Ross, B. E. and Busch, H. (1988). Identification and characterization of a human proliferation-associated nucleolar antigen with a molecular weight of 120000 expressed in early G_1 phase. *Cancer Res.*, **48**, 1244–51

22. Ochs, R. L., Reilly, M. T., Freeman, J. W. and Busch, H. (1988). Intranucleolar localization of human proliferating-cell nucleolar antigen p120. Submitted for publication

23. Maness, P. F., Perry, M. E. and Levy, B. T. (1983) P^1,P^4-di(adenosine-5')tetraphosphate inhibits phosphorylation of immunoglobulin G by Rous sarcoma virus $pp60^{src}$. *J. Biol. Chem.*, **258**, 4055–8

35
Pattern of oncogene expression in hepatoma cells

E. OLÁH

INTRODUCTION

Altered gene expression is a common feature of neoplastic cells. Rat liver tumours have been thoroughly investigated and convincing evidence for reprogramming of gene expression has been presented. This has been reflected (1) in transformation- and/or progression-linked quantitative enzymic and metabolic alterations that support the molecular correlation concept[1] (see Weber, Chapter 30; (2) in altered isozyme composition[2] and (3) in altered expression of particular proto-oncogenes[3].

Much of the recent progress in understanding the origin and maintenance of malignant phenotype has derived from the study of cellular genes, termed proto-oncogenes. These can induce unregulated proliferation when 'activated' by several mechanisms yielding quantitative or qualitative alterations in their expression.

Proteins encoded by different proto-oncogenes and oncogenes have been claimed[4,5] to act in the mitogenic signal pathways in various ways (Figure 1): as growth factors; as receptors for these growth factors; or as signal-transducing proteins that generate second messengers which then regulate two separate ionic changes leading to increases in intracellular calcium and pH and to subsequent activation of certain genes (including the *myc* and *fos* proto-oncogenes). The activation of these genes has been supposed to play a major role in initiating the sequence of events which culminates in DNA synthesis and cell proliferation[5,6].

Evidence that many, if not all, of the oncogene products may be involved in the mitogenic signal pathways has come from recent work linking oncogenes and growth factors[7].

More than 40 different proto-oncogenes and oncogenes have now been identified, yet so far we know of only four biochemical mechanisms through which the protein products of these genes may act[4,6], namely (1) protein phosphorylation (tyrosine or serine and threonine as substrate amino acids);

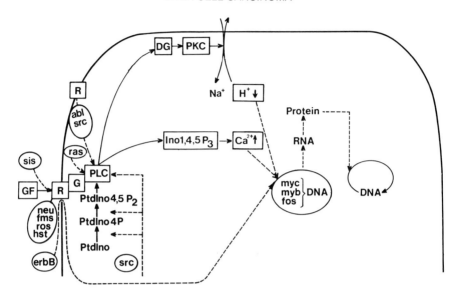

Figure 1 The main components of mitogenic signal pathways. Dashed arrows indicate the positions where different oncogenes might participate in signaling. *Abbreviations:* GF = growth factor; R = receptor; G = G protein; PLC = phospholipase C; PtdIno = phosphatidylinositol; P = phosphate; DG = diacylglycerol

(2) metabolic regulation by proteins that bind GTP in the manner of the G or N proteins; (3) post-transcriptional control of gene expression, e.g. influencing the biogenesis of mRNA; (4) participation in replication of DNA.

The great variety of alterations of cellular genes (such as inappropriate, enhanced or decreased levels of expression, gene amplification, point mutations, chromosomal translocation and rearrangements) may interfere with any of these mechanisms leading to the development of malignant transformation.

This chapter describes the oncogene pattern of experimental and human hepatomas. There is special emphasis on Morris hepatomas and an example of the modulation of oncogene expression by interfering with some of the key metabolic processes such as the activity of IMP dehydrogenase (E.C. 1.1.1.205) and the concentration of GTP is given.

MORRIS HEPATOMAS AND OCCURRENCE OF ONCOGENES

Biological systems

Morris hepatomas are one of the most meaningful model systems in cancer research. These chemically-induced, transplantable rat-liver tumours are histopathologically classified[8], and their growth, kinetics and cytogenetics have been analysed[9-11]. The utilization of the hepatoma spectrum of different

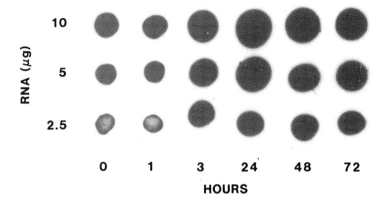

Figure 2 Expression of c-*myc* transcripts in total RNA prepared from hepatoma 3924A cells at different periods of growth. Dot-blot analysis was carried out as described in text

growth rates facilitated the discovery of the biochemical imbalance in cancer cells[1]. This imbalance entails reciprocally regulated, transformation- and/or progression-linked quantitative alterations of the opposing metabolic pathways and key enzyme activities[1,9,10].

The hepatoma 3924A cell line was established from the solid tumour and has been maintained in tissue culture for 21 years. The culture conditions, chromosome pattern, proliferation kinetic parameters and drug sensitivity have been reported[11-14].

Our earlier work showed that the transition of resting cell cultures into the proliferating phase provides a biological system of altered gene expression that is convenient for elucidating displays of enzymic and metabolic programs linked with neoplastic cell proliferation[14,15].

Utilization of the same model system has enabled us to explore the following questions about oncogene expression. (1) Do changes in oncogene transcript level accompany different phases of growth? (2) Are the genomic structures and oncogene transcripts in normal rat liver and in hepatoma cells different? (3) Are the patterns of oncogene expression which characterize these hepatoma cells similar to patterns which occur in other hepatomas?

Oncogene expression in hepatoma 3924A cells

A dot-blot analysis of c-*myc* expression was carried out in total RNA prepared from hepatoma 3924A cells at different phases of growth, using a ^{32}P-labelled c-*myc* probe.

Increased levels of c-*myc* transcripts were observed in every phase of growth, except for a 1.8-fold lower level observed 1 hour after reseeding the cells. A pronounced and sustained elevation of the c-*myc* expression was detected from 3 hours onward throughout exponential and plateau phases of growth (Figure 2). In the tumour there is an 11-fold abundance of c-*myc*

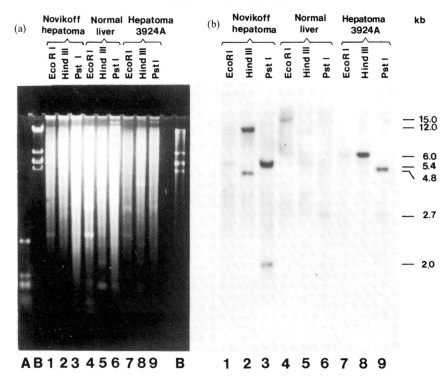

Figure 3 Analysis of c-*myc*-related sequences in hepatomas and normal rat liver. High-molecular-weight DNAs were digested with restriction enzymes and subjected to agarose gel electrophoresis (a). The fractionated DNA was then transferred to nitrocellulose filter and hybridized to [³²P]-nick translated c-*myc* probes. Amplified and rearranged c-*myc* sequences were seen in Novikoff and Morris hepatoma 3924A (b)

transcripts over that of normal liver even when RNA samples were taken from late plateau-phase hepatoma cells (data not presented). Previously, we have reported the ASG banding karyotype of the 3924A solid tumour and of its cell line culture which exhibited numerous rearranged marker chromosomes. The hepatoma 3924A tumour contains a marker chromosome carrying a homogeneously staining region, which is a cytogenetic marker of gene amplification. Further studies were designed to reveal the presence of amplified c-*myc* sequences in 3924A cells. EcoRI, HindIII and PstI digested normal adult rat liver and hepatoma 3924A DNAs (Figure 3a) were analysed by Southern blotting. The results (Figure 3b) indicate specific amplification and rearrangements of c-*myc* sequences. The extent of c-*myc* amplification in hepatoma 3924A cells was estimated by densitometric analysis indicating a 10–14–fold increase compared to normal rat liver. The figure also shows amplified and rearranged c-*myc* sequences in the chemically-induced, transplantable Novikoff hepatoma. The members of the *ras* family, unlike nuclear c-*myc* oncogene, exhibit quantitative alterations, rather than an increased

Table 1 Oncogenes in Morris hepatomas[33,34]

Hepatoma	Histological classification	Carcinogen	Alterations of oncogenes in hepatomas (compared to normal rat liver)[a]			
			myc	Ha-ras	Ki-ras	src
3924A	PD	FdiAA	++	+	none	none
8994	HD	4'-F-4-BAA	+	+	+	none
7288 C	WD	2,7-FAAF$_6$	+	+	+	none
7777	WD	FPA	+	+	+	none
5123 TC	WD	FPA	+	+	+	none
7800	HD, WD	FPA	+	+	+	none
5123 D	WD	FPA	+	N.I.	N.I.	N.I.
7136 A	WD	TMA	+	N.I.	N.I.	N.I.
7794 A	WD	FPA	++	N.I.	N.I.	N.I.

[a] + = increased expression; ++ = increased expression and amplification
Abbreviations: HD = highly differentiated; WD = well differentiated; PD = poorly differentiated; 4'-F-4-BAA = 4'-fluoro-4-biphenylacetamide; 2,7-FAAF$_6$ = N,N'-2,7-fluorenylenebis-2,2,2-trifluoroacetamide; FPA = N-2-fluorenylphthalamic acid; TMA = 2,4,6-trimethylaniline; FdiAA = N-2-fluorenyldiacetamide. N.I. = not investigated.

expression of normal gene products. Our results show that the c-Ha-*ras* gene is expressed in normal rat liver and there is a 2-fold elevation in expression of the c-Ha-*ras* gene in hepatoma 3924A samples compared to normal rat liver. However, the relative abundance of this transcript was not as pronounced as for that of c-*myc* (data not presented).

Oncogene pattern in Morris hepatomas (solid tumours)

The pattern of c-*myc* expression for hepatoma 3924A was found to be similar in other Morris hepatomas (Table 1). The increased expression of c-*myc* sequences in these liver tumours is a recurrent observation.

Table 2 Abnormalities of c-*myc* gene that result in increased expression

	Alteration	Tumour	References
1.	Integration of a proviral sequence near the c-*myc* gene	chicken B-cell lymphomas	16
2.	Gene amplification	several human tumours	17
3.	Translocation or rearrangements	Burkitt lymphoma, mouse plasmacytomas	18
4.	Alterations in a normal transcriptional repressor	Burkitt's lymphoma	19
5.	Deletions (involving the untranslated first exon)	mouse plasmacytoma	18
6.	Alterations in the utilization of the normal c-*myc* promoter sequences	human hepatoma	20

The c-*myc* oncogene is one of the most convincing examples of an oncogene implicated in tumour aetiology. Several types of abnormality involving c-*myc* indicate its role in tumour formation (Table 2). The consensus is that these various rearrangements lead to the constitutive expression of relatively high levels of c-*myc* mRNA and protein. Despite intensive studies however, it is still unclear how each of these DNA rearrangements relates to the altered regulation and level of expression of the normal c-*myc* gene.

Amplifications may play a role in the growth of cancer cells, different from the other lesions, since amplification involves an intact c-*myc* gene rather than structural alterations produced by other mechanisms. Also, the aetiological significance for cancer can be attributed to amplifications because amplified DNA persists in mammalian cells only if it confers selective advantage to the cells[59].

The cause of gene amplification in mammalian cells and the mechanisms by which it persists remain to be solved, but amplification of *myc* genes has been most frequently associated with the more aggressive forms of several neoplasias[60].

Oncogene pattern in rodent hepatomas

There have been several reports on the activation of oncogenes belonging to the *ras* gene family in rodent liver tumours induced by chemical carcinogens (Table 3). While *ras* oncogene transcripts were present at different levels in the tumours induced in rats, a majority of the hepatomas in mice contained activated Ha-*ras* oncogenes. The concept that *ras* oncogenes can be the targets of chemical carcinogens has been supported by new evidence on carcinogen-specific, activating mutations of the Ha-*ras* locus[21]. When these hepatocellular carcinomas are induced by carcinogen treatment, a mutation of *ras* locus specific to various carcinoma–DNA adducts has been accomplished. For example, treatment of B6C3F mice with N-hydroxy-2-acetyl-amino-fluorene generates Ha-*ras* oncogenes activated by C→A transversions in the first base of codon 61[22].

It is generally accepted that *ras* oncogenes participate in the initiation of neoplastic development. However, there are studies suggesting that activation of *ras* genes may play a part in the progression of some tumours toward a more malignant phenotype[23]. In addition, successful transformation of a variety of normal mammalian cells has been achieved *in vitro* by utilizing single mutated members of the *ras* family[21,24–26].

The involvement of the c-*myc* oncogene in the formation and/or maintenance of hepatocellular carcinoma has been clearly established, yet the contribution of the *myc* gene to the malignant phenotype is still unresolved. To date, much evidence suggests that qualitative alterations in the amino acid-coding sequences may not play a major role in the transforming potential of the c-*myc* gene[27]. In fact, quantitative alterations, such as increased and/or deregulated expression of the normal gene product may be associated with the transforming capacity of this gene. However, since c-*myc*

Table 3 Oncogenes in induced hepatocellular carcinomas

Species	Carcinogen	Oncogene (alteration)	Incidence	Reference
Rat	DBN + BHT	N-*ras* (point mutation)	5	36
	IQ	N-*ras* (point mutation)	11	37
	Aflatoxin B₁	Ki-*ras* (point mutation)	20	38
		Ha-*ras* (elevated expression)	100	39
		c-*myc* (elevated expression)	100	39
	CDE diet	Ha-*ras* (point mutation) +	85	40
		c-*myc* (elevated expression)	+ 15	
Mouse	HoAFF	Ha-*ras*-1 (point mutation)	100	41
	VC	Ha-*ras*-1 (point mutation)	100	41
	HODE	Ha-*ras*-1 (point mutation)	100	41
		Ha-*ras*-1 (amplification and/or rearrangement) +	95	22
		K-*ras* (point mutation)	+ 5	
	DEN	c-*myc* (increased expression)	100	42
		c-*myc* (increased expression)	100	35
	3-Me-DAB	Ha-*ras* (increased expression)	100	33
		c-*myc* (increased expression)	100	33
Woodchuck	Woodchuck hepatitis virus	c-*myc* (increased expression)	33	43

Abbreviations: DBN = dibuthylnitrosamine; BHT = butylated hydroxytoluene; IQ = 2-amino 3-methylimidazo [4,5-f] quinoline; CDE diet = choline-deficient diet containing 0.1% ethionine; HoAFF = N-hydroxy-2-acetylaminofluorene; VC = vinyl carbamate; HODE = 1'-hydroxy-2'-3'-dehydrooestragole; DEN = diethylnitrosamine; 3-Me-DAB = 3'-methyl-4-dimethylaminoazobenzene

is expressed in virtually all proliferating cells, it seems most likely that the same mechanism(s) of mitogenic signal pathways have been used to promote tumour cell growth, whereas dosage and cellular background seem to determine how this activity is expressed[4,18].

The c-*myc* expression seems to be more frequently associated with the final stage of tumour progression but early alterations in hepatoma formation associated with increased c-*myc* expression have also been reported[29,30].

Other data indicate that the c-*myc* gene may be essential but not sufficient for hepatocyte transformation[31]. These results are consistent with the proposal that activation of another, cytoplasmic proto-oncogene (e.g. *ras*) is necessary to transform normal cells to malignant phenotype[32].

Altered expression of *ras* genes is also common in hepatomas, although the biological significance of these changes with respect to the process of neoplastic proliferation is currently unclear.

Previous studies have indicated increases in the level of c-Ha-*ras* in 'perineoplastic' hepatocytes and in regenerating rat liver[3,33]. Further studies are required to determine whether these alterations relate to hepatocarcinogenesis or to compensatory cell proliferation that is known to occur during the early period of some carcinogen treatments.

There are some indications that the expression of c-*raf*, c-*fos* homologue transcripts increases in carcinogen-induced mouse and rat hepatic tumours[29,35]. No concurrent changes in c-*src*, c-*abl* and c-*mos* sequences were detected in rodent hepatomas.

ONCOGENES IN HUMAN HEPATOMAS

The actual incidence of oncogenes in human tumours is difficult to assess. Available information has been obtained from *in vitro* DNA transfection–transformation assays. This method has been accepted for comparing relative transforming efficiencies of a variety of oncogenes. However, because of several shortcomings of the NIH/3T3 cell line, the relevance of this assay to naturally-occurring neoplasia has been challenged. These shortcomings include the infinite growth potential and the lack of functional correlation between transformation *in vitro* and tumorigenicity *in vivo*. To overcome this problem some workers replaced NIH/3T3 cells with primary strains of normal mammalian fibroblasts in DNA transfection–transformation assays and used the combined *in vivo* tumorigenicity and the *in vitro* focus assay.

So far, transforming *ras* genes are the oncogenes most frequently identified in human cancer. Their overall incidence in common types of human cancer is estimated to be between 5 and 40%[21]. Point mutation, which appears to be the most frequent form of *ras* gene activation, is not the sole modifier of the gene.

The abnormally high expression of normal *ras* products as a consequence of perturbation of the regulatory sequences or gene amplification is also suggested to contribute to malignancy[21]. Contrary to the frequent involvement of the *myc* gene in amplification, the incidence of *ras* gene amplification in human tumours is as low as 1%.

Despite several efforts, the detection of transforming genes by *in vitro* DNA transfection–transformation assay in human hepatocellular carcinomas has not proved too successful[44,45].

N-*ras* activation has been observed in human liver cancer and Hep-G2 human hepatoma cell line[46]. This hepatoma cell line has also been shown to have high steady-state levels of c-*myc* transcripts. The constitutive activity of c-*myc* gene was attributed to an alteration in normal promoter utilization[20]. On the other hand, consequent alteration in c-*myc* transcript level was not seen in liver samples from seven hepatoma patients[47].

The transforming *hst* gene, that was originally identified in DNA from stomach cancer, has been detected in 2 out of 12 human hepatocellular carcinomas[48].

Recently a transforming DNA, named *lca*, was identified in primary human hepatocellular carcinoma utilizing the transfection assay[49]. In addition to the increased c-*myc* and Ha-*ras* expressions, elevated mRNA levels were seen for *erb* B, *fos* and *fms* oncogenes, respectively, in human hepatoma samples[50].

Among the frequently detected oncogenes, c-*abl*, c-*fes*, c-*fms*, c-*myc*, c-Ha-*ras* and c-*sis* gene were expressed in the PLC/(PRF)5 human hepatoma cell line[51].

MODULATIONS OF ONCOGENE EXPRESSION

The four biochemical mechanisms by which oncogene products act provide direct targets for the modulation of oncogene expression. The components of mitogenic signal pathways offer indirect targets. There is still little evidence for effectively influencing oncogene expression. Examples mostly come from cancer cells that underwent induced differentiation.

Teratocarcinoma cells induced to differentiate with interferon suppressed their c-*myc* RNA levels at least 20-fold, without any change in transcription rate[52]. Similar conclusions have been obtained by independent studies utilizing lymphoma cells[53]. In the promyelocytic leukemia HL-60, reduction of the expression of the amplified c-*myc* oncogene after induction by DMSO or retinoid acid to the granulocyte–macrophage differentiation has been described[54].

Contrary to these observations no change in c-*myc* transcript levels was seen during hemin or sodium butyrate induced erythroid differentiation of K562(S) cells. But a decreased expression of c-*abl* oncogene that related to a decrease in the proliferation capacity has been reported[55,56]. In contrast to these inducers, cytostatic concentrations of 1-ß-D-arabinofuranosylcytosine induced early decreases in c-*myc* mRNA expression in K562 cells[56]. In our recent studies, we used an inhibitor against the activity of IMP dehydrogenase, the rate-limiting enzyme of *de novo* GTP biosynthesis, to induce differentiation of K562 human leukemia cells. Tiazofurin treatment in concentrations that induced erythroid differentiation increased the doubling

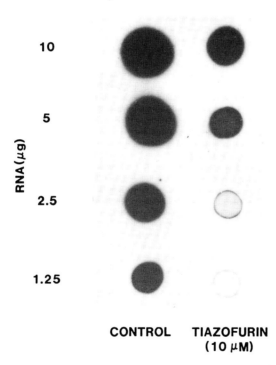

Figure 4 Dot-blot analysis of c-*myc* transcripts in total RNA prepared from control untreated and from tiazofurin-treated cells. Cells were exposed to 10 μM tiazofurin for 12 hours. Procedure was as described in text

time. The accomplishment of differentiation was preceded by the early inhibition of IMP dehydrogenase activity, the decrease in GTP concentration and in down-regulation of c-Ki-*ras* and c-*myc* genes[57].

Our knowledge of the structure and function of the G proteins and *ras* proteins prompts speculative comparison of their biochemical roles, i.e. participation in signal transduction. Like the G proteins, the normal c-*ras* proteins are associated with plasma membrane and bind GTP. The GTP-bound form is supposed to be the active form of both regulatory G- and *ras* proteins.

Our studies provided evidence that decreased levels of guanine nucleotides are fundamentally involved in the tiazofurin-initiated differentiation. Down-regulation of the c-*ras* gene was suggested to relate to the decrease in GTP concentration[57].

In the present studies experiments were carried out to determine whether tiazofurin would control oncogene expression in hepatoma 3924A cells in culture. Tiazofurin exposure (10 μM, 12 hours) resulted in a marked decrease in the c-*myc* (Figure 4) and in the c-Ha-*ras* (data not presented) RNA levels. These results are in agreement with our demonstration that tiazofurin induced a very rapid decrease in IMP dehydrogenase activity (by 50% in 15 min) and a subsequent decline in the end product of the pathway (GTP concentration decreases by 50% in 1 hour).

The previously surveyed data gained in experimental hepatomas provided independent evidence that *ras* and *myc* genes may participate in the formation and/or maintenance of hepatocellular carcinomas, although the full significance of these genes for hepatocarcinogenesis is still unclear. However, if these oncogenes do play a basic role in the expression and/or the maintenance of transformed phenotype in these cells, our results might be the first on the action of an anticancer chemotherapeutic drug tiazofurin, through down-regulation of *myc* and *ras* oncogenes.

CONCLUSIONS AND FUTURE EXPECTATIONS

A limited variety of oncogenes has been observed in experimental hepatomas. To date, no specific hepatoma-associated oncogenes have been discovered. However, the actual incidence of the members of *ras* and *myc* families proved to to be significantly frequent. From the available information we have learned that *ras* and *myc* oncogenes have both transforming and immortalizing activities that are exerted via mutated and/or overexpressed *ras* and via over-expressed and/or amplified *myc* genes. We succeeded in demonstrating the presence of amplified and rearranged *myc* genes in hepatoma 3924A and in Novikoff hepatoma cells. This alteration generally occurs in experimental hepatomas indicating the possible 'cooperation' of the nuclear and cytoplasmic genes in maintaining the malignant phenotype. Studies to elucidate the contribution of pathophysiological states, such as acute hepatotoxicity, liver regeneration and development of hepatic fibrosis to the elevation of the expression of certain oncogenes have also been conducted in order to outline the relevance of over-expression of certain genes for hepatocarcinogenesis.

The integration of the results on the human hepatomas is still in the preliminary stages and systematic expansion of this research utilizing better experimental systems for detecting oncogenes will be needed. Evidence for the modulation of oncogene expression has been presented in our studies. The use of tiazofurin as an inhibitor of IMP dehydrogenase activity resulted in a substantial decrease in GTP concentration. As a probable consequence, down-regulation of c-*myc* and c-Ha-*ras* genes was achieved, providing the first traces of evidence that an anti-cancer agent can be used to modulate oncogene expression in hepatoma cells.

Acknowledgements

This work was supported in part by Hungarian Research Foundation Grant OTKA 9/754/1988.

References

1. Weber, G. (1983). Biochemical strategy of cancer cells and the design of chemotherapy: G. H. A. Clowes memorial lecture. *Cancer Res., 43*, 3466–92
2. Weinhouse, S. (1983). Isozyme alterations, gene regulation and the neoplastic transformation. *Adv. Enzyme. Regul., 21*, 369–86
3. Corcos, D., Defer, N., Raymondjean, M., Paris, B., Corral, M., Tichonicky, L., Kruh, J., Glaise, D., Saulnier, A. and Gaguen-Guillouzo, C. (1984). Correlated increase of the expression of the c-*ras* genes in chemically induced hepatocarcinomas. *Biochem. Biophys. Res. Commun., 122*, 259–64
4. Bishop, J. M. (1987). The molecular genetics of cancer. *Science, 235*, 305–11
5. Berridge, M. J. (1986). Inositol lipids and cell proliferation. In Kahn, P. and Graf, T. (eds.) *Oncogenes and Growth Control*, pp 145–153. (Berlin, Heidelberg, New York, London, Paris: Springer Verlag)
6. Varmus, H. E. (1984). The molecular genetics of cellular oncogenes. *Annu. Rev. Genet., 18*, 553–612
7. Goustin, A. S., Leof, E. B., Shipley, G. D. and Moses, H. L. (1986). Growth factors and cancer. *Cancer Res., 46*, 1015–29
8. Morris, H. P. and Wagner, B. P. (1968). Induction and transplantation of rat hepatomas with different growth rate (including 'minimal deviation' hepatomas). *Methods Cancer Res., 41*, 125–52
9. Weber, G. (1977). Enzymology of cancer cells, Part I. *N. Engl. J. Med., 296*, 486–93
10. Weber, G. (1977). Enzymology of cancer cells, Part 2. *N. Engl. J. Med., 296*, 541–61
11. Oláh, E. and Weber, G. (1979). Giemsa banding karyotype of rat hepatomas of different growth rates. *Cancer Res., 39*, 1708–17
12. Oláh, E., Lui, M. S., Tzeng, D. Y. and Weber, G. (1980). Phase and cell cycle specificity of pyrazofurin action. *Cancer Res., 40*, 2869–75
13. Lui, M. S., Faderan, M. A., Liepnieks, J. J., Natsumeda, Y., Oláh, E., Jayaram, H. N. and Weber, G. (1984). Modulation of IMP dehydrogenase activity and guanylate metabolism by tiazofurin (2-ß-D-ribofuranosylthiazole-4-carboxamide). *J. Biol. Chem., 259*, 5078–82
14. Weber, G., Oláh, E., Lui, M. S., Kizaki, D. Y. and Takeda, E. (1980). Biochemical commitment to replication in cancer cells. *Adv. Enzyme Regul., 18*, 3–26
15. Oláh, E. (1983). Biochemistry of cycling and resting cancer cells. In Mirand, E. A., Hutchinson, N. B. and Mihich, E. (eds.) *Biology of Cancer 2, Part C*, pp 179–88. (New York: Alan R. Liss Inc.)
16. Hayward, W. S., Neel, B. G. and Astrin, S. M. (1981). Activation of cellular oncogenes by promoter insertion in ALV-induced lymphoid leukosis. *Nature (London), 296*, 475–9

17. Yokota, J., Tsunetsugu-Yokota, Y., Battifora, H., LeFevre, C. and Cline, M. J. (1986). Alterations of *myc, myb* and *ras*[Ha] proto-oncogenes in cancers are frequent and show clinical correlation. *Science,* **231**, 261–4

18. Cole, M. D. (1986). The *myc* oncogene: its role in transformation and differentiation. *Annu. Rev. Genet.,* **20**, 361–84

19. Leder, P., Battey, J., Lenoir, G., Moulding, C., Murphy, W., Potter, H., Stewart, T. and Taub, R. (1983). Translocations among antibody genes in human cancer. *Science,* **222**, 765–71

20. Huber, B. E. and Thorgeirsson, S. S. (1987). Analysis of c-*myc* expression in a human hepatoma cell line. *Cancer Res.,* **47**, 3413–20

21. Barbacid, M. (1987). *ras* genes. *Annu. Rev. Biochem.,* **56**, 779–827

22. Wiseman, R. W., Stowers, S. J., Miller, E., Anderson, M. W. and Miller, J. A. (1986). Activating mutations of the c-Ha-*ras* protooncogene in chemically induced hepatomas of the male B6C3 F_1 mouse. *Proc. Natl. Acad. Sci. USA,* **83**, 5825–9

23. Balmain, A. (1985). Transforming *ras* oncogens and multistage carcinogenesis. *Br. J. Cancer,* **48**, 1–15

24. Spandidos, D. and Wilkie, N. (1984). Malignant transformation of early passage rodent cells by a single mutated human oncogene. *Nature (London),* **315**, 469–75

25. Yoakum, G. H., Lechner, J. F., Gabrielson, E. W., Korba, B. E., Malan-Shibley, L., Willey, J. C., Valerio, M. G., Shamsuddin, A. M., Trump, B. F. and Harris, C. C. (1985). Transformation of human bronchial epithelial cells transfected by Harvey *ras* oncogene. *Science,* **227**, 1174–9

26. Shwartz, S. A., Shuler, C. F. and Feebeck, P. (1988). Transformation of normal homologue cells by a spontaneously activated Ha-*ras* oncogene. *Cancer. Res.,* **48**, 3470–7

27. Battey, J., Moulding, C., Taub, R., Murphy, W., Stewart, T., Potter, H., Lenoir, G. and Leder, P. (1983). The human c-*myc* oncogene: structural consequences of translocation into the IgH locus in Burkitt lymphoma. *Cell,* **34**, 779–87

28. Beer, D., Coloma, J., Schwartz, M., Sawada, N. and Pitot, H. (1986). Proto-oncogene expression in isolated gamma-glutamyl transpeptidase-positive hepatocytes. *Proc. Am. Assoc. Cancer Res.,* **27**, 79

29. Huber, B. E., Heilman, C. A. and Thorgeirsson, S. S. (1986). Gene expression in the progressive development of hepatocellular carcinoma in the rat. *Proc. Am. Assoc. Cancer Res.,* **27**, 7

30. Keath, E. J., Caimi, P. G. and Cole, M. D. (1984). Fibroblast lines expressing activated c-*myc* oncogenes are tumorigenic in nude mice and syngeneic animals. *Cell,* **39**, 339–48

31. Leder, A., Pattengale, P. K., Kuo, A., Stewart, T. A. and Leder, P. (1986). Consequences of widespread deregulation of the c-*myc* gene in transgenic mice: multiple neoplasms and normal development. *Cell,* **45**, 485–95

32. Land, H., Parada, L. F. and Weinberg, R. A. (1983). Tumorigenic conversion of primary embryo fibroblasts requires at least two cooperating oncogenes. *Nature (London),* **304**, 596–602

33. Makino, R., Hayashi, K., Sato, S. and Sugimura, T. (1984). Expression of the c-Ha-*ras* and c-*myc* genes in rat liver tumors. *Biochem. Biophys. Res. Comm.,* **119**, 1096–102

34. Cote, G. J. and Chiu, J. -F. (1987). The expression of oncogenes and liver-specific genes in Morris hepatomas. *Biochem. Biophys. Res. Comm.,* **143**, 624–9

35. Dragani, T. A., Manenti, G., Della Porta, G., Gattoni-Celli, S. and Weinstein, I. B. (1986). Expression of retroviral sequences and oncogenes in murine hepatocellular tumors. *Cancer Res.,* **46**, 1915–19

36. Funato, T., Yokota, J., Sakamoto, H., Kameya, T., Fukushima, S., Ito, N., Terada, M. and Sugimura, T. (1987). Activation of N-*ras* gene in a rat hepatocellular carcinoma induced by dibutylnitrosamine and butylated hydroxytoluene. *Jpn. J. Cancer Res. (Gann),* **78**, 689–94

37. Ishikawa, F., Takaku, F., Nagao, M., Ochiai, M., Hayashi, K., Takayama, S. and Sugimura, T. (1985). Activated oncogenes in a rat hepatocellular carcinoma induced by 2-amino-3-methylimidazo [4,5-f]quinoline. *Jpn. J. Cancer Res. (Gann),* **76**, 425–8

38. McMahon, G., Hanson, L., Lee, J-J. and Wogan, G. N. (1986). Identification of an activated c-Ki-*ras* oncogene in rat liver tumours induced by aflatoxin B_1. *Proc. Natl. Acad. Sci. USA,* **83**, 9418–22

39. Tashiro, F., Morimura, S., Hayashi, K., Makino, R., Kawamura, H., Horikoshil, N.,

Nemoto, K., Ohtsubo, K., Sugimura, T. and Ueno, Y. (1986). Expression of the c-Ha-*ras* and c-*myc* genes in aflatoxin B_1-induced hepatocellular carcinomas. *Biochem. Biophy. Res. Comm.*, **138**, 858–64

40. Yaswen, P., Goyette, M., Shank, P. R. and Fausto, N. (1985). Expression of c-Ki-*ras*, c-Ha-*ras* and c-*myc* in specific cell types during hepatocarcinogenesis. *Mol. Cell. Biol.*, **5**, 780–6

41. Garte, S. J., Hood, A. T., Hochwalt, A. E., D'Eustachio, P., Snyder, C. A., Segal, A. and Albert, R. E. (1985). Carcinogen specificity in the activation of transforming genes by direct-acting alkylating agents. *Carcinogenesis*, **6**, 1709–12

42. Hsieh, L. L., Hsiao, W.-L., Peraino, C., Maronpot, R. R. and Weinstein, I. B. (1987). Expression of retroviral sequences and oncogenes in rat liver tumors induced by diethylnitrosamine. *Cancer Res.*, **47**, 3421–4

43. Möröy, T., Marchio, A., Etiemble, J., Trépo, C., Tiollais, P. and Buendia, M.-A. (1986). Rearrangement and enhanced expression of c-*myc* in hepatocellular carcinomas of hepatitis virus infected woodchucks. *Nature*, **324**, 276–9

44. Perucho, M., Goldfarb, M., Shimizu, K., Lama, C., Fogh, J. and Wigler, M. (1981). Human-tumor-derived cells contain common and different transforming genes. *Cell*, **27**, 467–76

45. Pulciano, S., Santos, E., Lauver, A. V., Long, L. K., Aaronson, S. A. and Barbacid, M. (1982). Oncogenes in solid human tumors. *Nature*, **300**, 539–42

46. Huber, B. E., Dearfield, K. L., Williams, J. R., Heilman, C. A. and Thorgeirsson, S. S. (1985). Tumorigenicity and transcriptional modulation of c-*myc* and N-*ras* oncogenes in a human hepatoma cell line. *Cancer Res.*, **45**, 4322–9

47. Su, T-S., Lin, L-H., Lui, W. Y., Chang, C., Chou, C. K., Ting, L-P., Hu, C-P., Han, S-H. and P'eng, F-K. (1985). Expression of c-*myc* gene in human hepatoma. *Biochem. Biophys. Res. Comm.*, **132**, 264–8

48. Nakagama, H., Ohnishi, S., Imawari, M., Hirai, H., Takaku, F., Sakamoto, H., Terada, M., Nagao, M. and Sugimura, T. (1987). Identification of transforming genes as *hst* in DNA samples from two human hepatocellular carcinomas. *Jpn. J. Cancer Res. (Gann)*, **78**, 651–4

49. Ochiya, T., Fujiyama, A., Fukushige, S., Hatada, I. and Matsubara, K. (1986). Molecular cloning of an oncogene from a hepatocellular carcinoma. *Proc. Natl. Acad. Sci. USA*, **83**, 4993–7

50. Zhang, X-K., Huang, D-P., Chiu, D-K. and Chiu J-F. (1987). The expression of oncogenes in human developing liver and hepatomas. *Biochem. Biophys. Res. Comm.*, **142**, 932–8

51. Motoo, Y., Nahmoudi, M., Osther, K. and Bollon, A. P. (1986). Oncogene expression in human hepatoma cells PLC/PRF/5. *Biochem. Biophys. Res. Comm.*, **135**, 262–8

52. Dony, C., Kessel, M. and Gruss, P. (1985). Posttranscriptional control of *myc* and p53 expression during differentiation of the embryonal carcinoma cell line F9. *Nature*, **317**, 636–9

53. Knight, E. Jr., Anton, E. D., Fabey, D., Friedland, B. K. and Jonak, G. J. (1985). Interferon regulates c-*myc* gene expression in Daudi cells at the posttranscriptional level. *Proc. Natl. Acad. Sci. USA*, **82**, 1151–4

54. Westin, E. H., Wong-Staal, F., Gelman, E. P., Dalla-Favera, R. and Papas, T. (1982). Expression of cellular homologues of retroviral oncogenes in human hematopoietic cells. *Proc. Natl. Acad. Sci. USA*, **79**, 2490–4

55. Gambari, R., del Senno, L., Piva, R., Barbieri, R., Amelotti, F., Bernardi, F., Marchetti, G., Citarella, F., Tripodi, M. and Fantoni, A. (1984). Human leukemia K562 cells: relationship between hemin-mediated erythroid induction, cell proliferation and expression of c-*abl* and c-*myc* oncogenes. *Biochem. Biophys. Res. Comm.*, **125**, 90–6

56. Scarra, G. L. B., Romani, M., Coviello, D. A., Garré, C., Ravazzolo, R., Vidali, G. and Aimar, F. (1986). Terminal erythroid differentiation in the K562 cell line by 1-ß-D-arabinofuranosylcytosine: accompaniment by c-*myc* messenger RNA decrease. *Cancer Res.*, **46**, 6327–32

57. Oláh, E., Natsumeda, Y., Ikegami, T., Köte, Zs., Horányi, M., Szelényi, J., Paulik, E., Kremmer, T., Hollán, Zs., Sugár, J. and Weber, G. (1988). Induction of erythroid differentiation and modulation of gene expression by tiazofurin in K562 leukemia cells. *Proc. Natl. Acad. Sci. USA*, **85**, 6533–7

58. Hurley, J. B., Simon, M. I., Teplow, D. B., Robinshaw, J. D. and Gilman, A. G. (1984).

Homologies between signal transducing G-proteins and *ras* gene products. *Science, 226,* 860–2

59. Stark, G. R. and Wahl, G. M. (1984). Gene amplification. *Annu. Rev. Biochem., 53,* 447–91
60. Schimke, R. T. (1982). *Gene Amplification* (New York: Cold Spring Harbor Lab., Cold Spring Harbor)
61. Gu, J. R., Hong, J. X., Hu, L. F., Tian, P. K., Wan, T. F. and Yu, X. S. (1986). N-*ras* oncogene in human liver cancer and monoclonal antibodies against its product p21. *14th International Cancer Congress,* Vol. 3, p. 1140. (Budapest: Karger and Akadémiai Kiadó)

Section 6
Diagnosis and Therapy
of Liver Cell Carcinoma

36
Early recognition of liver cell tumours

K. OKUDA

INTRODUCTION

Primary liver cell carcinoma or hepatocellular carcinoma (HCC) is prevalent in South Africa and Southeast Asia where this cancer is endemic among cirrhotics. Benign liver cell adenoma is extremely rare in the Far East and it occurs almost exclusively in non-cirrhotic livers. In this presentation, the strategy and methodology for early detection of HCC will be discussed.

FOLLOW-UP OF PATIENTS WITH CHRONIC LIVER DISEASE

With the exception of South African blacks[1,2], more than 80% of the patients with HCC have an underlying chronic liver disease, notably cirrhosis[3], before they develop the cancer. In other words, HCC develops mainly in patients with cirrhosis and pre-cirrhosis, or progressive chronic liver disease. It has been shown that hepatitis B surface antigen (HBsAg) positive patients

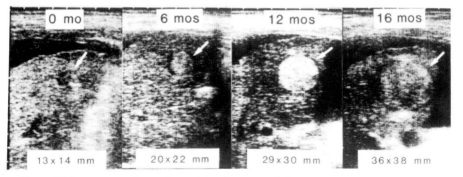

Figure 1 Measurement of growth speed by ultrasound. This 13 × 14 mm lesion found in a cirrhotic liver surrounded by ascites (0 months) grew to the size of 20 × 22 mm in 6 months with a change from hypoechoic to isoechoic in the internal echo. At 12 months, the internal echo is hyperechoic suggesting a subsequent rapid growth

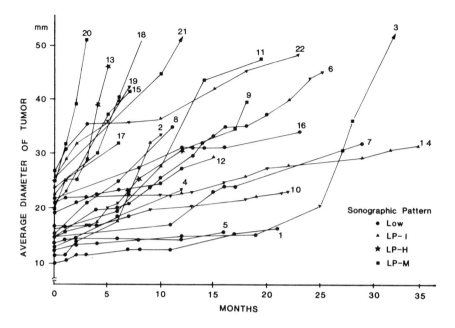

Figure 2 Growth speed of HCC (smaller than 3 cm) measured by ultrasound in 22 cases. Note the great variation in the growth speed, and low echo of the interior in the majority of the cases. LP-I, low periphery-isoechoic interior; LP-H, low periphery-hyperechoic interior; LP-M, low periphery-mixechoic interior.

(carriers) are more prone to hepatocarcinogenesis, but more recent data in Japan suggest that non-carriers with cirrhosis are almost just as susceptible to HCC as carriers[4]. Therefore, at least in Japan, all patients with chronic liver disease should be treated similarly. The degree of risk of developing HCC may vary between post-hepatic and alcoholic cirrhosis, the latter being less likely to develop cancer. However, it is also well known that alcoholic micronodular cirrhosis will change to macronodular cirrhosis upon abstinence and predisposes to hepatocarcinogenesis[5]; in fact, and ironically, those with alcoholic cirrhosis in Japan die either from cirrhosis or from HCC that frequently follows abstinence.

How frequently should the patient be followed and how? The current practice in Japan is to follow high risk patients with abdominal ultrasound examination and measurement of serum alpha-fetoprotein (AFP) at an interval of 2–4 months depending upon the degree of risk. There have been two studies in which the speed of growth of small HCC was measured. Our study[6] showed that a 2 cm lesion took 3 months to expand by 1 cm (Figure 1 and 2), and the Taiwan study[7] demonstrated that a fastest growing 1 cm HCC took 4.6 months to become 3 cm in size. The cost of examination is also to be considered. The health insurance system in Japan has been arguing whether the expensive radioimmunoassay for AFP be paid every 3 months. So far, however, the test has been covered by the insurance. Serum AFP levels are

Tumor size
∠3 cm
3-5 cm
100
50
0
Number of patients (%)
0-19
20-199
200-1000
1000-3000
3000-10⁴
10⁴∠
AFP (ng/ml)

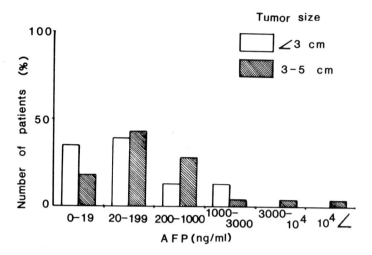

Figure 3 Serum AFP levels in 51 cases of small HCC (less than 5 cm). Note that about 35% of HCC smaller than 3 cm show normal AFP levels and that about 50% show levels between the upper normal limit and 1000 ng/ml. When these mildly elevated levels do not return to normal, suspicion should mount

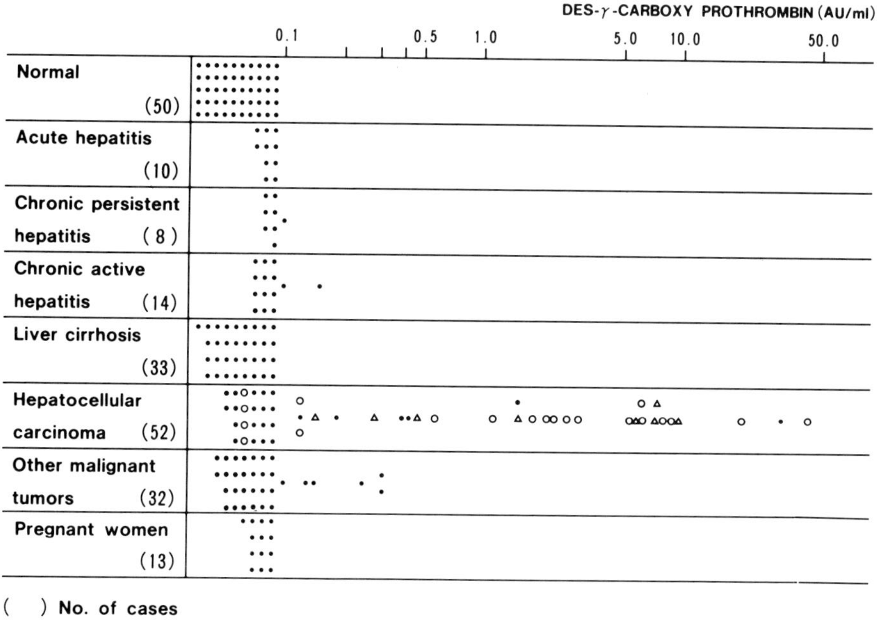

DES-γ-CARBOXY PROTHROMBIN (AU/ml)
0.1
0.5
1.0
5.0
10.0
50.0
Normal (50)
Acute hepatitis (10)
Chronic persistent hepatitis (8)
Chronic active hepatitis (14)
Liver cirrhosis (33)
Hepatocellular carcinoma (52)
Other malignant tumors (32)
Pregnant women (13)
( ) No. of cases

Figure 4 Des-γ-carboxy prothrombin levels in various diseases. Note that this test has very few pseudopositives in diseases other than HCC. With AFP, there are many more pseudopositive tests in chronic liver disease and other malignancies (H. Okuda *et al., J. Hepatol.*, 1987, **4**, 353, with permission from Elsevier)

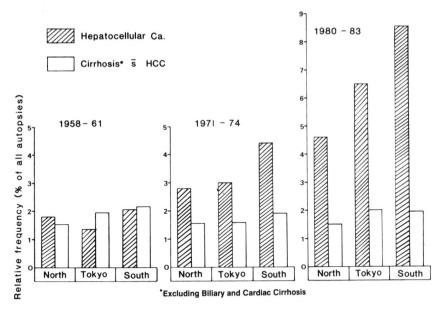

Figure 5 Time trends and geographic differences in the frequency of HCC and cirrhosis in Japan. Data are based on autopsies done at the university hospitals in Hokkaido (north), the Tokyo-Chiba area and Kyushu (south). In the period of 1958–61, the numbers of HCC and cirrhosis without HCC were about the same at the autopsy table. HCC steadily increased in number whereas no such increase occurred with cirrhosis, and more recently (1980–83), the number of HCC far exceeds that of cirrhosis

usually low or normal in patients with small HCC, seldom alarmingly high (Figure 3). However, levels continuously above the normal limit should arouse suspicion. The recently developed marker, des-γ-carboxy prothrombin[8] may prove complementary to AFP (Figure 4), but is less sensitive.

How high is the risk among those with chronic liver disease? In early 1960s, HCC was found in about 20% of all autopsies for cirrhosis in Japan, but it is now found in more than 70% of the comparable autopsy material (Figure 5)[4]. Why such a change? The recent studies in Japan indicate a marked and progressive increase of HBsAg negative HCC cases[9,10]; perhaps the prolonged life span of cirrhotic patients is another cause. Whatever the explanation, the fact remains that the majority of patients with cirrhosis will eventually develop HCC[4]. In a short follow-up study many evolutions of HCC would not be experienced, but following a large number of cirrhotics for a longer period, a considerable number of HCCs emerging in cirrhotic livers will be detected. In the prospective study of Okuda et al.[11], 8/34 (23.5%) HBsAg-positive or high anti-HBc cirrhotics developed HCC during a 4.5 year follow-up period. The Taiwan study by Beasley et al.[12] showed a figure of approximately 3000 HCC cases per 100 000 HBsAg-positive cirrhotics per year. Clearly, B-positive cirrhotics have a very high risk. In Japan, the age at which HCC develops is younger in B-positive subjects compared to B negative

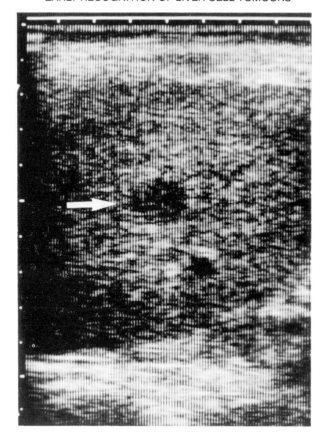

Figure 6 A small 11 × 14 mm lesion seen by real-time ultrasound (at arrow) in the S_{IV} region of the middle lobe

ones[13]. It seems that non-A,non-B cirrhosis gives rise to HCC at older ages (taking a longer time) than B cirrhosis. We have seen more than 20 patients who developed HCC after a lapse of 20–35 years from a major surgery that required blood transfusion. In one study in Tokyo, 40% of HCC cases had a history of past blood transfusion[14]. Chronic non-A,non-B hepatitis appears benign or not progressive, but it frequently progresses to cirrhosis after a lapse of many years and then gives rise to HCC. The rate of HBsAg positivity among HCC cases has steadily declined in Japan[8-10] suggesting a diluting-out of HBsAg-positive cases by negative (non-A,non-B) ones.

IMAGING OF SMALL HCC

Real-time ultrasonography revolutionized imaging diagnosis of small mass lesions within the liver. The previous colloid scintigraphy was not sensitive,

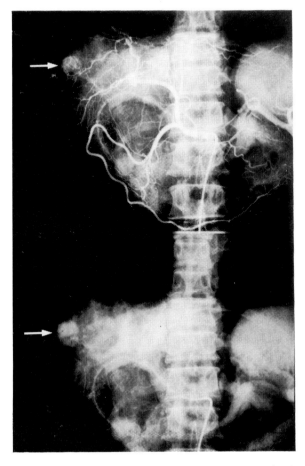

Figure 7 Celiac arteriography demonstrates a 17 × 20 mm hypervascular lesion (at arrow) in the S_V region of the right lobe (upper). It remains as a tumour stain in the late phase. HCC lesions smaller than this one seldom display neovasculature

incapable of identifying lesions small than 3 cm or so. Except for diffusely-spread HCC, masses larger than 1 cm clearly demarcated from the parenchyma will be discerned by ultrasonography in the hands of well-trained personnel (Figure 6). It does not involve radiation, and can be performed on the out-patient basis. Coeliac angiography is an established imaging for HCC which will show hypervascularity and neovasculature (Figure 7)[15]. However, angiography is less diagnostic for small lesions which are not too much different from hyperplastic nodules grossly[16]. Unlike large HCC, small HCC seldom demonstrates neovasculature or hypervascularity and the only abnormal finding is staining (Figure 8). To demonstrate tumour stains, infusion arteriography is perhaps most useful[17]. However, even with infusion

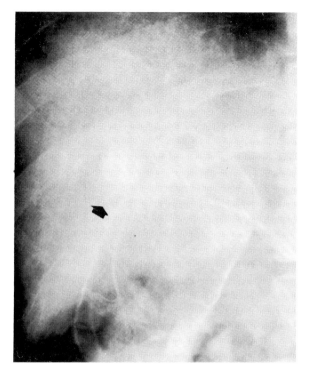

Figure 8 A 15-mm tumour stain seen in the right lobe (S$_{VI}$ region) in the late phase of celiac arteriography (at arrow).

arteriography, distinction between small HCC and stains of hyperplastic regenerative nodules is difficult[16]. X-ray computed tomography is just as diagnostic as angiography. However, plain unenhanced computed tomography is less diagnostic and will miss small lesions. Dynamic enhancement computed tomography is clearly more diagnostic and it will also serve in the differential diagnosis from hemangioma. Following bolus injection of contrast medium, HCC is quickly enhanced and de-enhanced (Figure 9), whereas hemangioma is slowly enhanced starting from the periphery of the mass and enhancement remains significantly longer (Figure 10). In our experience, combined plain and dynamic computed tomography scans made diagnosis of HCC in 87% of HCC greater than 2 cm, but only 25% of the lesions smaller than 1.5 cm. Magnetic resonance imaging is perhaps more diagnostic than plain computed tomography, but less so compared to dynamic computed tomography, depending upon the strength of the magnetic field. With a very strong superconductive magnet, some of the cirrhotic nodules are discerned, and diagnosis of small HCC may be just as good as dynamic computed tomography. Magnetic resonance imaging is also useful in the differential diagnosis of HCC and hemangioma; the latter displays significantly larger T_2 values. It also provides certain information of

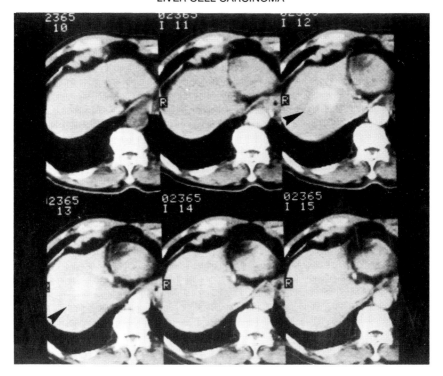

Figure 9 Dynamic computed tomography obtained following intravenous bolus injection of contrast medium. This 4.5-cm HCC is isodense and not recognizable on plain computed tomography, but was rapidly and homogeneously enhanced (at arrowhead). The contrast medium also disappeared quickly (frames I14 and 15). Quick enhancement and deenhancement are characteristic of HCC

tissue histology[18]. Cancer necrosis following therapy such as arterial embolization is clearly recognizable on magnetic resonance imaging (Figure 11).

At this moment, the most sensitive way of delineating small HCC lesions is the use of Lipiodol, an oily contrast medium[19]. If several milliliters of Lipiodol are injected into the hepatic artery before withdrawing the catheter on completion of angiography, and a computed tomography scan performed after 10 days or 2 weeks, HCC lesions will be seen as densely opacified spots, as shown in Figure 12. Lipiodol goes to the liver parenchyma as well, but it is cleared from there in due time whereas the HCC tissue is incapable of clearing it. The exact mechanism whereby Lipiodol is cleared from parenchyma but not from HCC is not known, but this author suspects that the Kupffer cells and lymphatic system of the parenchyma expedite clearance of Lipiodol and the same are not operative in HCC tissue. Lipiodol also serves as a vehicle to deliver a chemotherapeutic agent to the lesion where it remains and releases the agent continually. Lipiodol remains in the mass almost indefinitely, sometimes interfering with the subsequent assessment of the therapeutic effect.

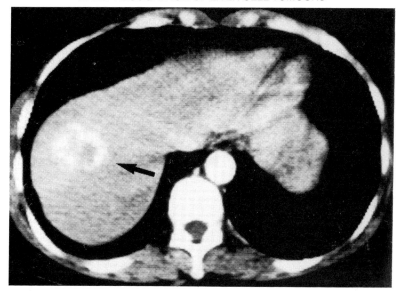

Figure 10 A medium-sized benign hemangioma which was slowly enhanced following bolus injection of contrast medium. The enhancement characteristically occurs from the periphery of the mass toward the centre

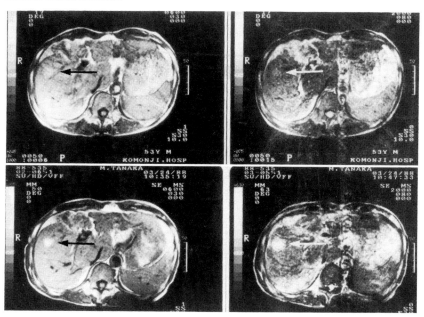

Figure 11 Magnetic resonance images of small HCC. The left two panels are T_1 weighted images and the right two panels T_2 weighted images. The upper two images were made before arterial embolization and the lower two after the embolization. This 2-cm HCC is seen as a bright lesion in both T_1 and T_2 weighted images, but following arterial embolization it has become much brighter suggesting necrosis. In the right lower panel, the capsule around the mass is recognizable.

447

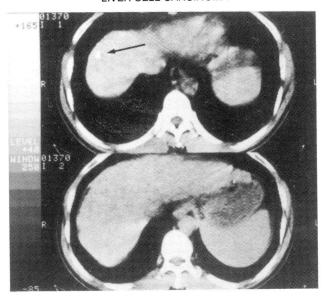

Figure 12 Lipiodol computed tomography showing a 6 × 8 mm HCC. Several milliliters of Lipiodol, an oily contrast medium, is injected into the hepatic artery and computed tomography scan is made 10 days to 2 weeks later. The HCC lesion keeps Lipiodol whereas the liver parenchyma clears it during this period, leaving HCC as a distinctly contrasted lesion. As small as a 5-mm HCC is discerned despite the partial volume phenomenon

HISTOLOGICAL DIAGNOSIS

In the actual clinical setting in the Far East where HCC is prevalent and early detection is possible with efforts, histological diagnosis of a very small lesion found in a cirrhotic liver is not a simple task. In the past five years or so, the Japanese hepatologists and pathologists have learned that some of the small lesions detected by imaging appear benign histologically yet they become overt HCC or the same liver from which such lesions have been surgically removed develops overt HCC within a year or so[20].

With many resected materials, Arakawa *et al.* conducted careful studies with clinical data, imaging and follow-up. Such studies have revealed that a very early lesion does not show classical malignant histological features such as mitosis, nuclear atypism, large nuclei, etc. The only changes that have been discerned are occasional acinar formations (Figure 13), nuclear crowding and cytoplasmic basophilia (Figure 14). Malignant transformation seems to occur in a hyperplastic nodule (Figure 15), and the early lesions are extremely well differentiated (Figure 16), within which more clearly malignant clones develop as nodules-in-nodules (Figure 17)[21]. From the clinical point of view, the conventional histological criteria do not or should not apply to such lesions, and an intra-hepatic lesion found in a cirrhotic liver as a discrete area should be regarded as an equivalent of an early HCC.

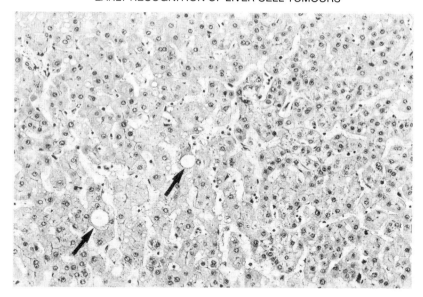

Figure 13 Extremely well-differentiated HCC (left half of this high power field) seen in a hyperplastic nodule detected by ultrasound in a cirrhotic liver. Cells are one or two cell thick in arrangement and lack malignant histological features. However, occasional acinar formation (at arrow) is seen. The cells in the right half of the field are more basophilic with nuclear crowding and could perhaps represent HCC (H & E, × 100)

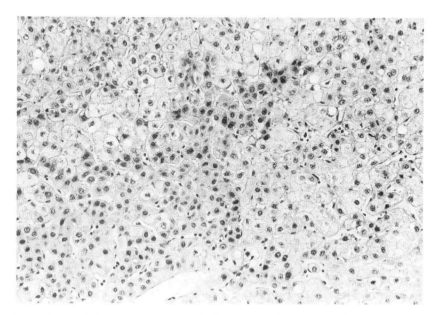

Figure 14 Basophilic cells are seen within a benign appearing hyperplastic nodule. They are more likely to have undergone malignant transformation (H & E, × 200)

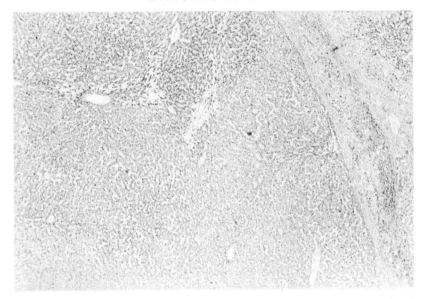

Figure 15 Lower magnification view of an adenomatous hyperplastic nodule found by imaging in a cirrhotic liver. Note a thin pseudocapsule and the lack of typical portal triad (H & E, × 40)

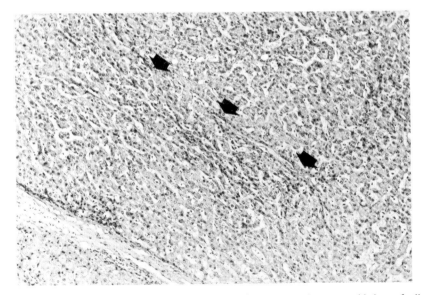

Figure 16 A new clone of cells growing while compressing (at arrows) upon an old clone of cells within an adenomatous hyperplasic nodule found in a cirrhotic liver. The new growing tissue displays occasional acinar formation and perhaps represents an extremely well-differentiated HCC of Edmondson–Steiner's Grade I (H & E, × 100)

It has also been shown that within an early lesion which is usually extremely well differentiatated, more malignant lesions appear and replace the earlier better differentiated cancer cells[22]. By the time the mass becomes 3–5 cm in size, the mass itself or most part of the mass is less well differentiated (Edmondson–Steiner's grade II to III). It is not clear whether the same process occurs in the early HCC lesions occurring in a liver with alcoholic cirrhosis.

PROBLEMS AND PERSPECTIVES

From the above discussion, it is clear that an early HCC lesion in a liver with post-hepatic cirrhosis is histologically almost indistinguishable from large benign regenerative nodules. In other words, there is little room for further improvement of sensitivity in imaging diagnosis for small HCC. The key issue for the future in terms of early diagnosis, is determination of the nature of nodules found by imaging, whether they are already transformed, doomed to transform, or will remain benign. To distinguish these lesions in the future, one needs perhaps molecular biological techniques to quantitate expression of certain oncogenes and their products.

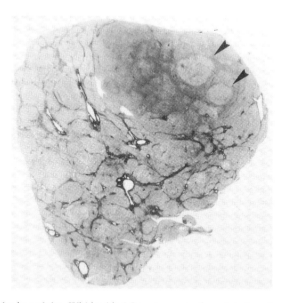

Figure 17 Nodules-in-nodules. Within this 1.7-cm hyperplastic nodule two clearly-demarcated small lesions have evolved (arrowheads). Histologically, both are overt HCC, suggesting that the mother nodule was already a cancer, but of an extremely well-differentiated one (× 3). (M. Arakawa *et al., Gastroenterology,* 1986, **91**, 198, reproduced with permission from Elsevier)

SUMMARY

Early detection and diagnosis is most desirable in the treatment of hepatocellular carcinoma (HCC). In the past, discovery of small HCC was a rare incidental event. A systematic way of detecting small HCC is to follow patients with chronic liver disease, particularly cirrhosis, at regularly spaced intervals with special attention to the liver. For that purpose, abdominal ultrasound and AFP measurement are most important. Japan and Taiwan have been successful in the detection of small HCC in recent years using such a strategy. If a small lesion is found by ultrasound in a cirrhotic liver, a more definitive diagnosis is required. Usually, a computed tomography scan, then celiac angiography and biopsy are carried out. With these modalities, the diagnosis is established in most cases except in patients in whom biopsy of the space occupying lesion detected by imaging is interpreted as 'benign or not malignant' histologically. Such lesions are more likely extremely well differentiated HCC. Differential diagnosis between HCC and benign hemangioma is sometimes difficult by ultrasound and plain computed tomography. For this reason, dynamic enhancement computed tomography is desirable beside plain computed tomography. Despite these considerations, there have been some inadvertent resections done for hemangioma in Japan. Magnetic resonance imaging may prove helpful in the differential diagnosis of hemangioma and HCC. Positive AFP tests are rather infrequent in patients with small HCC, and the recently developed tests for des-γ-carboxy prothrombin may prove complementary to AFP in the screening for HCC.

References

1. Steiner, P. E. (1960). Cancer of the liver and cirrhosis in trans-Saharan Africa and the United States of America. *Cancer,* **13**, 1085–166
2. Okuda, K., Peters, R. L. and Simson, I. W. (1984). Gross anatomical features of hepatocellular carcinoma from three disparate geographic areas. Proposal of new classification. *Cancer,* **54**, 2165–73
3. Shikata, T. (1976). Primary liver carcinoma and liver cirrhosis. In Okuda, K. and Peters, R. L. (eds.) *Hepatocellular Carcinoma.* pp 53–72. (New York: Wiley)
4. Okuda, K., Fujimoto, I., Hanai, A. and Urano, Y. (1987). Changing incidence of hepatocellular carcinoma in Japan. *Cancer Res.,* **47**, 4967–72
5. Lee, F. I. (1966). Cirrhosis and hepatoma in alcoholics. *Gut,* **7**, 77–95
6. Ebara, M., Ohto, M., Shinagawa, T., Sugiura, N., Kimura, K., Matsutani, S., Morita, M., Saisho, H., Tsuchiya, Y. and Okuda, K. (1986). Natural history of minute hepatocellular carcinoma smaller than three centimeters complicating cirrhosis. A study in 22 patients. *Gastroenterology,* **90**, 289–98
7. Sheu, J. C., Sung, J. L., Chen, D. S., Yang, P. M., Lai, M. Y., Lee, C. S., Hsu, H. C., Chuang, C. N., Yang, P. C., Wang, T. H., Lin, J. T. and Lee, C. Z. (1985). Growth rate of asymptomatic hepatocellular carcinoma and its clinical implications. *Gastroenterology,* **89**, 259–66
8. Okuda, H., Obata, H., Nakanishi, T., Furukawa, R. and Hashimoto, E. (1987). Production of abnormal prothrombin (des-γ-carboxy prothrombin) by hepatocellular carcinoma. A clinical and experimental study. *J. Hepatol.,* **4**, 357–63
9. Okuda, K., and the Liver Cancer Study Group of Japan (1980). Primary liver cancers. *Cancer,* **54**, 2663–9
10. The Liver Cancer Study Group of Japan (1986). Survey and follow-up of primary liver cancer in Japan. Report 7. *Acta Hepatol. Jpn.,* **27**, 1161–9

11. Obata, H., Hayashi, N., Motoike, Y., Hisamitsu, T., Okuda, H., Kobayashi, S. and Nishioka, K. (1980). A prospective study on the development of hepatocellular carcinoma from liver cirrhosis with persistent hapatitis B virus infection. *Br. J. Cancer*, **25**, 741–7

12. Bealsey, R. P., Blumberg, B., Popper, H. and Wain-Hobson, S. (1982). Hepatitis B virus and hepatocellular carcinoma. In Okuda, K. and Mackay, I. (eds.) *Hepatocellular Carcinoma*, pp 60–93 (Geneva: UICC)

13. Okuda, H., Obata, H., Motoike, Y. and Hisamitsu, T. (1984). Clinicopathological features of hepatocellular carcinoma — comparison of hepatitis B seropositive and seronegative patients. *Hepato-Gastroenterol.*, **31**, 64–8

14. Ohbayashi, A., Tanaka, S., Ohtake, H., Harada, H., Komachiya, K., Kodama, T., Okada, Y. Y., Takahashi, K. and Tanaka, N. (1983). Clinico-pathological observations on relationship of blood transfusion to liver cirrhosis and hepatocellular carcinoma. *Acta Hepatol. Jpn.*, **24**, 521–5

15. Okuda, K., Obata, H., Jinnouchi, S., Kubo, Y., Nagasaki, Y., Shimokawa, Y., Motoike, Y., Muto, H., Nakajima, Y., Musha, H., Yamazaki, T., Sakamoto, K., Kojiro, M. and Nakashima, T. (1977). Angiographic assessment of gross anatomy of hepatocellular carcinoma: comparison of celiac angiograms and liver pathology in 100 cases. *Radiology*, **123**, 21–9

16. Sumida, M., Ohto, M., Ebara, M., Kimura, K., Okuda, K. and Hirooka, N. (1986). Accuracy of angiography in the diagnosis of small hepatocellular carcinoma. *Am. J. Roentgen.*, **147**, 531–6

17. Takashima, T. and Matsui, O. (1980). Infusion hepatic angiography in the detection of small hepatocellular carcinoma. *Radiology*, **136**, 3321–5

18. Ebara, M., Ohto, M., Watanabe, Y., Kimura, K., Saisho, H., Tsuchiya, Y., Okuda, K., Arimizu, N., Kondo, F., Ikehira, H., Fukuda, N. and Tateno, Y. (1986). Diagnosis of small hepatocellular carcinoma: Correlation of MR imaging and tumor histological studies. *Radiology*, **159**, 371–7

19. Yumoto, Y., Jinno, K., Tokuyama, K., Arai, Y., Ishimitsu, T., Maeda, H., Konno, T., Iwamoto, S., Ohnishi, K. and Okuda, K. (1985). Hepatocellular carcinoma detected by iodized oil. *Radiology*, **154**, 19–24

20. Arakawa, M., Sugihara, S., Kenmochi, K., Kage, M., Nakashima, T., Nakayama, T., Tashiro, S., Hiraoka, T., Suenaga, M. and Okuda, K. (1986). Small mass lesions in cirrhosis: transition from benign adenomatous hyperplasia to hepatocellular carcinoma? *J. Gastroenterol. Hapatol.*, **1**, 3–14

21. Arakawa, M., Kage, M., Sugihara, S., Nakashima, T., Suenaga, M. and Okuda, K. (1986). Emergence of malignant lesions within an adenomatous hyperplastic nodule in a cirrhotic liver. *Gastroenterology*, **91**, 198–208

22. Okuda, K. and Kojiro, M. (1987). Small hepatocellular carcinoma. In Okuda, K. and Ishak, K. G. (eds.) *Neoplasms of the Liver*. pp 215–26 (Tokyo: Springer-Verlag)

37
Imaging techniques for the diagnosis of hepatic tumours

M. A. ROTHSCHILD, M. ORATZ, S. S. SCHREIBER AND H. KAUFMAN

INTRODUCTION

There are numerous techniques currently available to image the liver. These include angiography, radionuclide studies, cholangiography, endoscopic retrograde cholangiography, single photon emission computerized tomography (SPECT), computerized axial tomography (CAT), magnetic resonance imaging (MRI), positron emission tomography (PET) and ultrasound techniques. Many of these technical procedures are available in most hospitals. However, if the purpose of these imaging techniques is to define the presence of a liver tumour early enough in the development of the changing pattern of cell growth to be able to provide effective long-term treatment, then each procedure has fallen short of this goal. However we can employ these studies in a rational fashion so that an appropriate intervention may be made as early as possible during the cancer's initial growth stage.

ANGIOGRAPHY

Angiography is the injection of significant quantities, up to 150 ml, of concentrated organic iodide contrast material into the circulation[1-4] (Figure 1A,B). This procedure is fraught with potential allergic reactions and these reactions occur frequently enough to suggest that the prophylactic use of two doses of steroids within 12 hours prior to the study be utilized as a routine procedure. The hepatic arteriogram is the most important aspect of angiography because of the arterial blood supply to the tumour. The image depends on where the injection is made. A direct injection into the hepatic arterial tree will image specifically the vasculature of that area, and the early blush and vessel filling fades rapidly. A celiac artery injection will give a two-phased distribution: an early arterial phase and a later returning portal phase due to the return of dye that has circulated through the venous side.

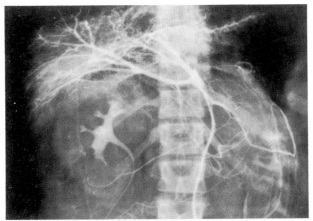

Figure 1A

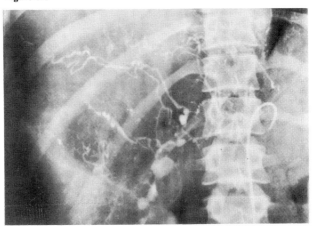

Figure 1B

Figure 1 Angiographic studies. On the angiogram, note a large hypovascular mass with multiple abnormal vessels and macroaneurysms. Angiogram demonstrates displacement of the normal hepatic vasculature without abnormal vessels, which indicates the presence of a large avascular undifferentiated embryonal sarcoma. (Reproduced with permission from Ros *et al.* (1986), 'Undifferentiated (embryonal) sarcoma of the liver: radiologic–pathologic correlation', *Radiology,* **160**, 141–5)

The third type of infusion or injection would result in an examination of the portal system directly. With very rapid imaging sequences and an injection through a wedged hepatic catheter a sinusoidal image may be obtained and these areas fill and refill very rapidly giving a changing picture. This is due to the rapid washout via the portal circulation. In a tumour with a good arterial supply the tumour stain may persist much longer due to the lack of portal inflow. The presence of tumour invasion of the portal vein or of segments of the portal vein can be determined from celiac injections.

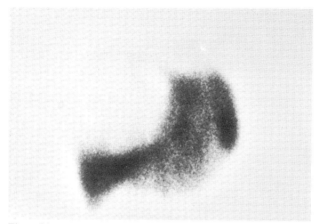

Figure 2A

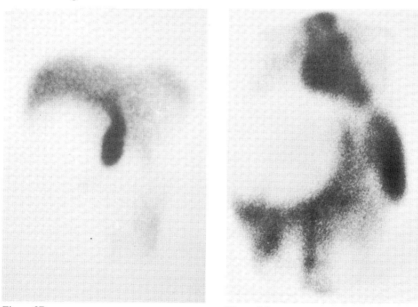

Figure 2B   **Figure 2C**

Figure 2 Nuclear radiology studies. (A) A liver scintiscan obtained with sulphur colloid^{99m} Tc shows a large (14-cm diameter), well-defined defect in the right lobe of the liver. Note smooth margins and rim of functioning tissue around the mass. (B) Liver scintiscan obtained 45 min after injection with^{99m} Tc iminodiacetic acid shows no accumulation of activity within the mass. The gall baldder is displaced medially by tumour. Bowel activity indicated no obstruction of the biliary tree. (C) On a blood pool scintiscan, obtained with ^{99m} Tc labelled autologous red blood cells, a large defect is seen which indicates the avascular nature of this undifferentiated embryonal sarcoma. (Reproduced with permission from Ros *et al.* (1986), 'Undifferentiated (embryonal) sarcoma of the liver: radiologic–pathologic correlation', *Radiology,* **160**, 141–5)

RADIONUCLIDE IMAGING

Radionuclide imaging of the liver for the detection of hepatic tumours has been employed for many years and can still contribute to the follow-up of lesions detected by other means as well as screening procedures on acutely ill subjects[5-10]. Use of this technique depends upon the clearance of the tracer doses of radiolabelled colloidal material by the reticuloendothelial cell system. However, since both the radioactivity and the colloidal material are at tracer levels, the rate-limiting factor in any of the colloidal scans is blood flow to the liver. This is why, for example, in cirrhosis of the liver, the underlying condition predisposing to hepatocellular carcinoma in many cases, reveals such a poor hepatic image. Blood flow has been diverted away from the liver due to portal hypertension allowing the colloidal material to be retained in the reticuloendothelial cell functioning system of other areas of the body such as the bone marrow and spleen. In a patient with a normal haemodynamic system, a photopenic area indicates a space-occupying lesion. The colloidal scan cannot differentiate between pathogenic processes, but signals for further investigation. These studies may be performed at the bedside. The limit of detection is about 1.5 cm unless the lesion is at the surface of the liver. If hepatomegaly is used as a criterion for hepatic malignancy in the absence of a well-defined area of absent uptake, then the scan will be falsely positive a high percentage of the time and the accuracy of diagnosis will be very poor. However employing a definite cold area the scan is 80% accurate for intra-abdominal malignancies metastasizing to the liver (Figure 2A–C).

GALLIUM

Gallium studies have been utilized to search for hepatocellular carcinoma. The gallium is transported in the blood bound to transferrin. Hepatocellular carcinoma has been shown to involve an increased number of transferrin receptors. Perhaps this is the mechanism whereby gallium will concentrate in the tumour as opposed to the photopenic area seen employing the standard colloidal scan. There are many complications however to the interpretation of gallium studies. The gallium is concentrated normally in the liver, spleen and bone marrow as well as other organs. It is cleared early during the first 24 hours, partially by the kidneys and the majority is secreted in the gastro-intestinal tract so that there is a considerable overlay of background activity. The tumour-to-background ratio may not be high enough to be of any practical use in many cases. Further, the gallium studies are also positive in local as well as diffuse deposition of inflammatory cells, as well as in lymphomas.

SPECT

Single photon emission computerized tomography (SPECT) is an advance over the two-dimensional planar routine radionuclide imaging pro-

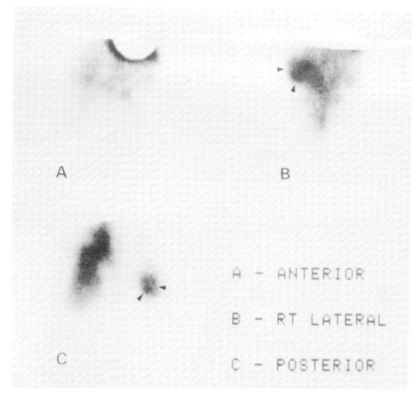

Figure 3 Cavernous haemangioma (A–C) are routine images obtained with labelled red cells. (A) anterior, (B) right lateral, (C) post area. Arrows indicate activity on the dome of the right lobe. H, haemangioma; S, spleen

cedures[11-13]. This technique depends upon the appropriate concentration of a radiopharmaceutical or biochemical within a functioning area of the liver. The single energy photon permits localization of the decay event by rotating the camera about the patient. A three-dimensional image may be obtained. This technique is more sensitive in diagnosing small intra-hepatic lesions than is routine planar scintigraphy with a detection rate of 72%, compared to 36% with single-plane scintigraphy, 80% with ultrasound, computed tomography (64%) and angiography (88%) in the same study. The main problem in terms of sensitivity of utilizing this as well as all routine radionuclide scanning procedures lies in the tissue attenuation of the radiopharmaceutical γ-emission by overlying tissue. The main advantage and one which will, we feel certain, be exploited to its fullest in the future, is the utilization of a functioning scan as opposed to an anatomic localization. All lesions including haemangiomas and other vascular lesions are imaged with greater accuracy than with planar scinitigraphy. However lesions < 1 cm are not detected by either method. SPECT is more sensitive than ultrasound. Another use of SPECT is in defining hepatic size. If this technique can be applied either to

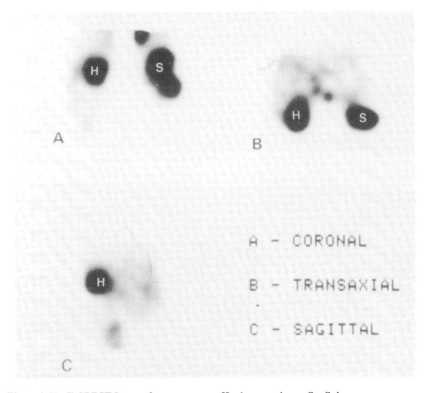

Figure 4 (A–C) SPECT Images from same case. H = haemangioma, S = Spleen

the photon deficicnt oı photon-accumulated areas, then tumour size could be accurately determined (Figures 3–5).

[99m]Tc

The use of the lidocaine derivatives, or iminodiacetic acid derivatives labelled with pertechnetate have become important radionuclide functioning studies for biliary transport and hepatic function[14,15]. These agents which are cleared through the liver by the hepatocyte are rapidly transported into the biliary system and secreted into the bile and are primarily used for studies of acute cholecystitis and following biliary or gastro-intestinal surgery. However, these agents will result in photopenic areas in the absence of normal functioning hepatocytes such as in tumours, primary or metastatic. These studies are also limited of course by the same degree of sensitivity of the instrumentation, namely tumours < 1–1.5 cm are highly unlikely to be visualized by this technique. The single exception would be carcinoma of the gall bladder where a marked irregularity to the gall bladder bed is highly suggestive of this condition.

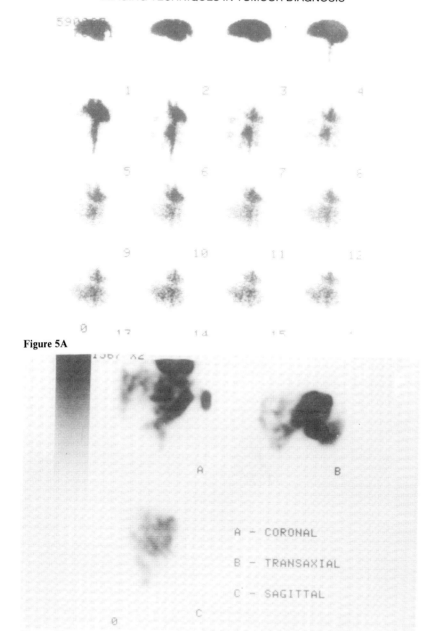

Figure 5A

Figure 5B

Figure 5 Metastatic renal cell carcinoma proven at biopsy and pathologic examination. (A) Flow study of blood pool scan demonstrates increased early flow to multiple foci in the liver. (B) SPECT images from same study reveal multiple photopenic foci that correspond to foci of increased flow. (Figures 3–5 reproduced with permission from Tumeh *et al.* (1987), 'Cavernous hemangioma of the liver: detection with single proton emission computed tomography', *Radiology,* **164**, 353–6)

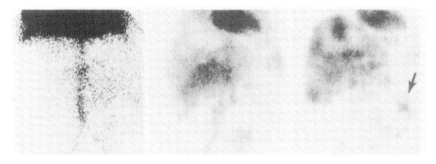

Figure 6 Hepatic angiosarcoma. Image from ^{99m}Tc red blood cell study. Early dynamic sequence on the left center, early blood pool image demonstrates areas of decreased uptake and right 3-hour delayed study, shows increased uptake in same areas and an extra-hepatic site in the small bowel indicated by the arrow. This type of picture may be seen in other lesions with an increase in blood pool but a decrease in arterial in flow. (Reprinted from Ferris *et al.* (1986), 'Hepatic angiosarcoma: mimicking of angioma on three-phase technetium-99m red blood cell scintigraphy', *Journal of Nuclear Medicine*, **27**, 1861–3)

The use of ^{99m}Tc pertechnetate-labelled tin-sensitized red blood cells has achieved an important diagnostic role in the study of vascular tumours[16–18] (Figure 6). The test is more efficient if the patient's red cells are labelled *in vitro* as opposed to the intravenous injection of the tracer dose of tin and radioactivity shortly thereafter in this procedure some free pertechnetate remains and activity in the stomach may obscure or degrade the clarity of the image. This technique may be done at the bedside and applying a computer program, early images during the first few circulations through the liver may be obtained giving information concerning the blood flow to the tumour area.

Usually the blood flow is decreased while, within a half to one hour, the activity over the tumour area is increased. Utilizing this procedure, hepatic haemangiomas are clearly diagnosable for they give either a decreased or normal blood flow but a highly increased area of activity in the tumour because of its increased blood volume. Smaller areas of tumour blood flow abnormality cannot be identified again because of the lack of sensitivity of the imaging instrument. Hepatoma likewise will demonstrate an increased late uptake over the lesion and because of the good arterial supply may also demonstrate an increase in flow seen during the early time periods. Any tumour with these characteristics will give these results and thus the test is not completely diagnostic.

CAT

Computerized axial tomography (CAT) imaging procedures remain the gold standard and the most frequently and most effectively employed technique to define small intra-hepatic lesions[19–27]. Utilizing the very best of circumstances, lesions as small as a few millimetres may be suggested by this technique. The technique frequently utilizes the intravenous infusion of organic iodide solutions to provide contrast material to increase the pathologic-to-normal tissue ratio. However, sometimes just the opposite occurs (Figure 7A,B). An advance in this procedure has been to utilize dynamic CAT imaging procedures in which very rapid sequences are obtained following intra-arterial contrast material injection (Figure 8A–F). This technique while being able to define vascular abnormalities associated with intra-hepatic tumours is subject to the same potential hazards as those mentioned for routine angio-graphy of the liver. As much as 50 g of contrast material must be injected over a 2-min period. This technique was reported to reduce the false-negative routine CAT study rate from 31/155 studies to 2/155. The CAT scan is more sensitive than planar scintigraphy or SPECT. For patients whose condition does not permit even short periods away from support systems only radio-nuclide studies are possible. However for all other patients and for the search for any intra-hepatic tumour, the CAT scan is the procedure of choice. The CAT scan cannot however differentiate between the various forms of tumours, and other lesions such as abscesses and cysts which may give similar pictures. Entirely different from the radionuclide study, the CAT scan utilizes the tissue attenuation of the externally-applied radiation in order to define tissue differentiation and the anatomic sensitivity of this procedure is excellent.

MRI

Magnetic resonance imaging (MRI) is one of the newest procedures available for hepatic imaging[28–39]. This procedure depends upon the innate magnetism of nuclei with an uneven number of protons and neutrons in the nucleus. The nucleus of any atom will be magnetic if it has 'non-zero' spin or angular momentum. Consequently, about half of all elements have magnetic nuclei and in particular the naturally-occurring isotopes ^{1}H, ^{23}Na, ^{31}P and ^{13}C. The nucleus of a hydrogen atom is a single proton which possesses both a positive charge and intrinsic angular moment or spin with the result that it has a magnetic dipole moment and can be treated like a small bar magnet. When a large number of such spin magnets are placed in an external magnetic field, the majority align in the direction of the field or parallel, while others align in an opposite direction or anti-parallel. It requires energy to turn a magnet over in a magnetic field; thus, the opposed orientation is a higher energy state than the aligned. Since there are two energy levels available to each nucleus, transitions may take place from one level to another. All MRI imaging involves inducing transitions between the two states by absorption or emission of energy. A radiofrequency is superimposed on the magnetic field for a certain duration to alter the populations of parallel and anti-parallel nuclei. Following cessation of this pulse the system tends to revert back to equilibrium, referred to as 'spin–lattice relaxation' or T_1. The transition of a nucleus from a higher energy to a lower energy level may be accompanied by a transition of another nucleus to a higher energy state, a process called 'spin–spin relaxation' or T_2. T_1 images portray water content differences. Many tumours have drastically increased relaxation times, cirrhosis increases

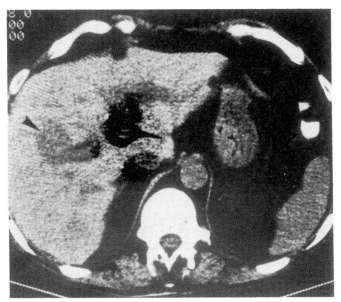

Figure 7A

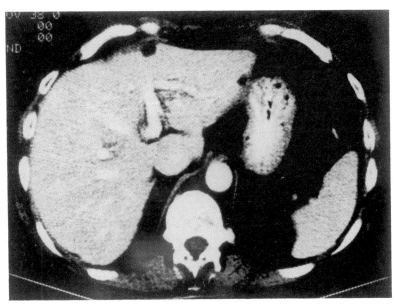

Figure 7B

Figure 7 (A) There is a decrease in the tumour-to-normal tissue differentiation following the injection of contrast material. (B) A patient with metastatic carcinoid tumour. (Reprinted with permission from Bressler *et al.* (1987), 'Hypervascular hepatic metastases: CT evaluation', *Radiology*, **162**, 49–51)

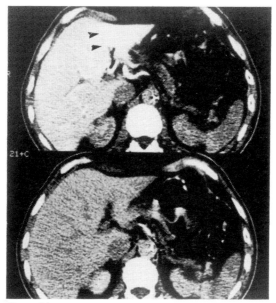

Figure 8A

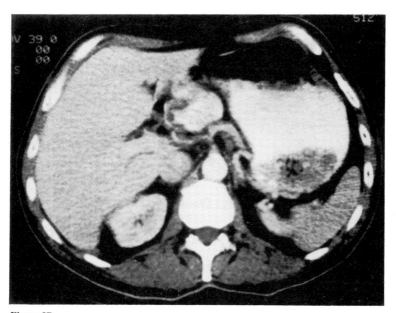

Figure 8B

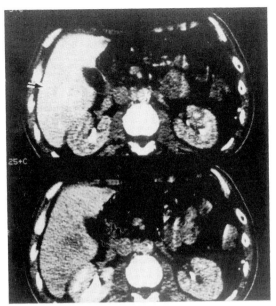

Figure 8C

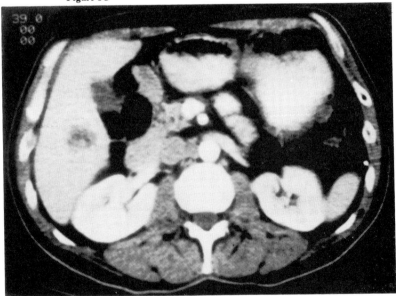

Figure 8D

Figure 8 Colon carcinoma metastasis and perfusion abnormality. (A) CAT scan (top) shows discrete hyperperfusion of the lateral segment of the left lobe (arrowheads). Delayed scan (bottom) at 15 min shows isodense lateral segment. (B) Intravenous bolus dynamic (IVBD) computed tomography scan at same level showing isodense lateral segment. (C) CAT scan (top) at a lower level shows metastasis in the right lobe (arrow) and a discrete, ovel sub-segmental hyperperfusion abnormality in the medial segment of the left lobe (arrowheads). Delayed scan

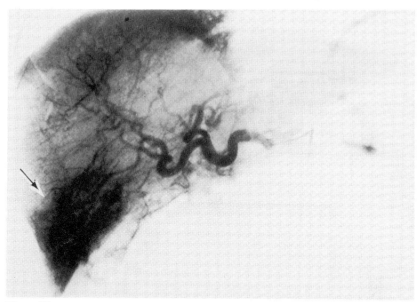

Figure 8E

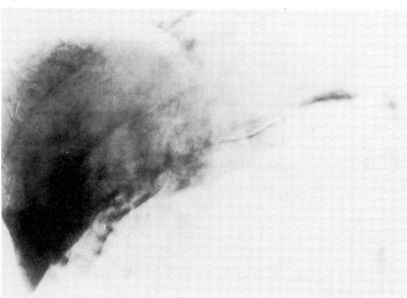

Figure 8F

(bottom) at 15 min shows metastasis to be hypodense; the area of the perfusion abnormality is isodense. (D) IVBD scan at same level as (B) shows metastasis. No abnormalities seen in the medial left lobe segment. (E) Selective hepatic angiogram (subtraction) shows right lobe metastasis (arrow). (F) Hepatogram phase shows dense staining of metastasis; left lobe is normal. (Reproduced with permission from Freeny and Marks (1986), 'Hepatic perfusion abnormalities during CT angiography: detection and interpretation', *Radiology,* **159**, 685–91)

467

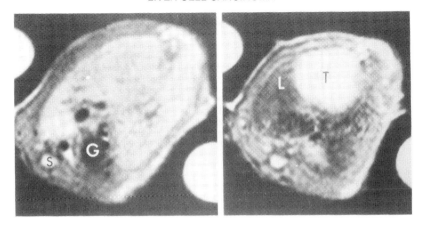

Figure 9 Enhanced detection of tumour after injection of ferrite (20 μmol Fe/kg) in a rat. (Left) Before injection, tumour and liver are isointense and indistinguishable (S, spine, G, gastric fundus). (Right) After injection, there is loss of signal from normal liver (L), which allows a large tumour nodule (T) to be identified easily. (Reproduced with permission from Saini *et al.* (1987), 'Ferrite particles: a superparamagnetic MR contrast agent for enhanced detection of liver carcinoma', *Radiology,* **162**, 217–22)

T_1 of the liver, while primary biliary cirrhosis and haemochromatosis both shorten liver T_1 because of accumulation of paramagnetic substances. As with the CAT scan there has been an attempt made to improve the image by utilizing paramagnetic substances which will alter the relaxation time of the magnetized nuclei (Figure 9). These paramagnetic substances, injected intravenously, have been shown to enhance, in many instances, the tumour to normal tissue signal ratios and thus provide a better anatomic localization. Dynamic MRI scans can be obtained utilizing an intra-arterial injection of a paramagnetic contrast agent such as gadolinium DTPA. This procedure appears to be about as sensitive as the dynamic CAT scan to image vascular abnormalities. The length of time required to obtain the images and the motion artifacts due to respiration are major problems. While MRI has proven to be outstanding in terms of the CNS, imaging of the liver has so far proven to be not necessarily any more precise or accurate than the CAT scan even though there are numerous anecdotal instances of MRI studies which are positive in the face of a prior negative investigation. MRI is outstanding for hepatic haemangioma — but then all other diagnostic modalities are equally diagnostic. The MRI study is expensive, requires a prolonged period of steady and quiet breathing (upwards of an hour), to obtain a single set of images. Furthermore, there are no standardized techniques so that each laboratory is currently utilizing its own imaging sequences and thus the data are difficult to compare. In order to determine where MRI fits in a diagnostic work-up for the future, in terms of tumour diagnosis, pathological functioning and imaging studies must be correlated. At present, it is fair to state that if the suspicion of an intra-hepatic lesion remained high, even with a negative work-up, an MRI study may be indicated. However, in an acutely-ill subject, or one who can cooperate only partially, such a technique will not be successful.

PET

Positron emission tomography (PET) is a new functioning imaging procedure[40–42]. This procedure depends upon the intra-hepatic concentration of a radiopharmaceutical which emits a positron. The positron collides with a negative electron, both are annihilated, and energy is emitted at exactly 180° from this annihilation event. Thus, the ability to localize this intra-hepatic emission of γ-rays can be done with precision and the hypo- or perhaps the hyper-functioning tumour tissue can be so localized. The problem with this technique is again that the instrumentation is nowhere near as precise in terms of anatomic identification as are the CAT scan or MRI procedures. Further, this technique requires cyclotron production of very short-lived high-specific-activity radionuclides which then must be incorporated into an appropriate radiopharmaceutical or biochemical. This biochemical then must be made suitable for intravenous injection into the patient, the imaging instrumentation must be at hand, and the personnel, capable of handling this highly technical procedure, available. Obviously the expense of such an imaging procedure means that the technique is investigative at best and is one which only the future can indicate as to its effectiveness in routine clinical evaluation of hepatic tumours.

ULTRASONOGRAPHY

Ultrasonography has proven to be a safe, inexpensive, rapid, effective means of diagnosing intra-hepatic masses or cysts which alter the echo of the externally-applied sound waves[43–47]. There appears to be no contraindication to the use of this technique and the only problem is that overlying tissue or air-containing structures significantly degrade the image. The employment of the echo and the Doppler techniques simultaneously permits evaluation of vascular flow and of vascular structures which could be impinged upon during the growth of a tumour. The tumour resulting in cystic areas could likewise be diagnosed effectively with the echo technique. A recent advance has been the intra-operative use of the echo scanning procedure and this technique has proven to be effective in diagnosing intra-hepatic tumours where all other procedures have been negative including intra-operative examination and palpation (Figure 10 A,B). This technique looks most effective in assisting the planning and staging of intra-operative procedures and postoperative follow-up of patients with intra-hepatic neoplasms.

OTHER TECHNIQUES

Tumour-seeking antibodies have been used to localize tumour tissue via scanning the patient following intravenous administration of labelled

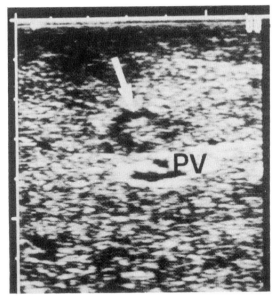

Figure 10A

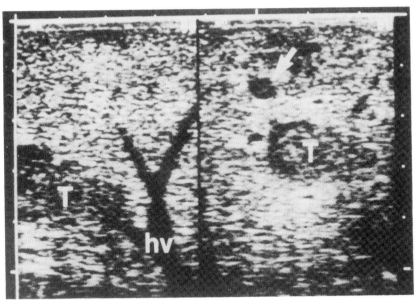

Figure 10B

Figure 10 (A) Operative sonogram revealing a solitary metastatic tumour which was not previously noted. (B) Operative sonogram of multiple metastatic tumours. Two large tumours (T) were diagnosed pre-operatively, while a smaller one (arrowed) was identified by this technique. (Reproduced from Machi *et al.* (1987), 'Intraoperative ultrasonography in screening for liver metastases from colorectal cancer: comparative accuracy with traditional procedures', *Surgery*, **101**, 678–84)

antibodies.[131]I, ^{123}I, ^{111}In and ^{99m}Tc have been employed to label either complete or fragments of the antibodies. Mono- or polyclonal antibodies may be utilized and 24–72 hours following the injection have been chosen as the imaging times. Tumour-to-background ratios must be high in order to assure any sensitivity. Sensitivities from 40 to 90% have been reported but the false-positive rate is nearly 33%. Much further investigation will be required before this promising technique will be clinically useful.

CONCLUSION

This summary of available procedures for the diagnosis of intra-hepatic tumours has pointed out the advantages and disadvantages of the vast array of options open to the clinician and researcher alike in the evaluation of intra-hepatic disease. Unfortunately, these techniques cannot as yet be precise enough to diagnose disease very early where progression of the altered DNA is defining a tumor line of cells. However the earlier the tumor or beginning cell accumulation can be identified then the progress could be improved. It is hoped that the investigation which has been reported at this Conference and occupies the early portion of this text will be utilized so that an appropriate imaging procedure can be identified. It appears that the simple anatomic localization of masses, even as small as a few millimeters, cannot necessarily improve the longevity of these patients unless the tumor area per se is resectable and further studies will have to prove just how effective surgical resection is in terms of longevity. What is needed is an ability to utilize tracer radionuciloe studies, to be able to diagnose alterations within the cells prior to the development of actual mass lesions. Perhaps the rates of hepatic accumulation or the plasma disappearance of a labeled antibody may provide one such avenue for future investigation.

Acknowledgement

This work was supported in part by the Louise and Bernard Palitz Research Fund.

References

1. Freeny, P. C. (1983). Angiography of hepatic neoplasms. *Sem. Roentgen.*, **18**, 114–22
2. Stanley, P. (1986). Angiography for abdominal pediatric tumors. *Crit. Rev. Oncol./ Hematol.*, **6**, 71–95
3. Chuang, V. P. (1987). Hepatic angiography. In Okuda, K. and Ishak, K. G. (eds.), *Neoplasms of the Liver.* pp 259–77 (Berlin: Springer-Verlag)
4. Takayasu, K. and Okuda, K. (1987). Celiac angiography in the diagnosis of small hepatocellular carcinoma. In Okuda, K. and Ishak, K. G. (eds.), *Neoplasms of the Liver.* pp 279–87 (Berlin: Springer-Verlag)
5. Kew, M. C. and Levin, J. (1987). Scintigraphy in the diagnosis of hepatocellular carcinoma. In Okuda, K. and Ishak, K. G. (eds.), *Neoplasms of the Liver.* pp 239–49. (Berlin: Springer-Verlag)

6. Hayes, R. L. (1978). The medical use of gallium radionuclides: A brief history with some comments. *Sem. Nucl. Med.,* **8**, 183–91

7. Larson, S. M. (1978). Mechanisms of localization of gallium-67 in tumors. *Sem. Nucl. Med.,* **8**, 193–203

8. Hauser, M. F. and Alderson, P. O. (1978). Gallium-67 imaging in abdominal disease. *Sem. Nucl. Med.,* **8**, 251–70

9. Ogihara-Umeda, I. and Kojima, S. (1988). Increased delivery of gallium-67 to tumors using serum-stable liposomes. *J. Nucl. Med.,* **29**, 516–23

10. Serafini, A. N., Jeffers, L. J., Reddy, K. R., Heiba, S. and Schiff, E. R. (1988). Early recognition of recurrent hepatocellular carcinoma utilizing gallium-67 citrate scintigraphy, **29**, 712–16

11. Tumeh, S. S., English, R. J. and Holman, B. L. (1985). The complementary role of SPECT in the diagnosis of cavernous hemangioma of the liver. *Clin. Nucl. Med.,* **10**, 884–6

12. Kudo, M., Hirasa, M., Takakuwa, H., Ibuki, Y., Fujimi, K., Miyamura, M., Tomita, S., Komori, H., Todo, A., Kitaura, Y., Ikekubo, K. and Torizuka, K. (1986). Small hepatocellular carcinomas in chronic liver disease: detection with SPECT. *Radiology,* **159**, 697–704

13. DeLand, F. H. and Shih, Wei-Jen (1984). The status of SPECT in tumour diagnosis. *J. Nucl. Med.,* **25**, 1375–9

14. Chervu, L. R., Nunn, A. D. and Loberg, M. D. (1982). Radiopharmaceuticals for hepatobiliary imaging. *Sem. Nucl. Med.,* **12**, 5–17

15. Ros, P. B., Olmstead, W. W., Dachman, A. H., Goodman, Z. D., Ishak, K. G. and Hartman, D. S. (1986). Undifferentiated (embryonal) sarcoma of the liver: Radiologic-pathologic correlation: *Radiology,* **160**, 141–5

16. Ginsberg, F., Slavin, J. D. and Spencer, R. P. (1986). Hepatic angiosarcoma: mimicking of angioma on three-phase technetium-99m red blood cell scintigraphy. *J. Nucl. Med.,* **27**, 1861–3

17. Rabinowitz, S. A., McKusick, K. A. and Strauss, H. W. (1984). ^{99m}Tc red blood cell scintigraphy in evaluating focal liver lesions. *Am. J. Radiol.,* **143**, 63–8

18. Moinuddin, M., Allinson, J. R., Montgomery, J. H., Rockett, J. F. and McMurray, J. M. (1985). Scintigraphic diagnosis of hepatic hemangioma: Its role in the management of hepatic mass lesions. *Am. J. Radiol.,* **145**, 223–8

19. Takayasu, K., Muramatsu, Y., Shima, Y., Moriyama, N., Yamada, T. and Makuuchi, M. (1986). Hepatic lobar atrophy following obstruction of the ipsilateral portal vein from hilar cholangiocarcinoma. *Radiology,* **160**, 389–93

20. Mathiew, D., Guinet, C., Bouklia-Hassane, A. and Vasile, N. (1988). Hepatic vein involvement in hepatocellular carcinoma. *Gastrointest. Radiol.,* **13**, 55–60

21. Muramatsu, Y., Takayasu, K., Moriyama, N., Shima, Y., Goto, H., Ushio, K., Yamada, T., Hasegawa, H., Koyama, Y. and Hirohashi, S. (1986). Peripheral low-density area of hepatic tumors: CT–pathologic correlation. **160**, 49–52

22. Titelbaum, D. S., Burke, D. R., Meranze, S. G. and Saul, S. H. (1988). Fibrolamellar hepatocellular carcinoma: Pitfalls in nonoperative diagnosis. *Radiology,* **167**, 25–30

23. Alpern, M. B., Lawson, T. L., Foley, W. D., Perlman, S. J., Reif, L. J., Arevalos, E. and Rimm, A. A. (1986). Focal hepatic masses and fatty infiltration detected by enhanced dynamic CT. *Radiology,* **158**, 45–9

24. Fevery, J., Baert, A. L., Marchal, G. M., Broeckaert, L., De Groote, J. and Vantrappen, G. (1985). The value of computed tomography, ultrasonography, and peritoneoscopy with biopsy in the detection of liver metastases secondary to gastro-enterological tumors. *Acta Gastro-Enterol. Belg.,* **18**, 105–10

25. Bressler, E. R., Alpern, M. B., Glazer, G. M., Francis, I. R. and Ensminger, W. D. (1987). Hypervascular hepatic metastases: CT evaluation. *Radiology,* **162**, 49–51

26. Glazer, G. M., Aisen, A. M., Francis, I. R., Gross, B. H., Gyves, J. W. and Ensminger, W. D. (1986). Evaluation of focal hepatic masses: A comparative study of MRI and CT. *Gastrointest. Radiol.,* **11**, 263–8

27. Itai, Y. (1987). Imaging diagnosis with computed tomography. In Okuda, K. and Ishak, K. G. (eds.) *Neoplasms of the Liver,* pp 289–300. (Berlin: Springer Verlag)

28. Greif, W. L., Buxton, R. B., Lauffer, R. B., Saini, S., Stark, D. D., Wedeen, V. J., Rosen, B. R. and Bradyl, T. J. (1985). Pulse sequence optimization for MR imaging using a

paramagnetic hepatobiliary contrast agent. *Radiology, 157*, 461–6
29. Sigal, R., Lanir, A., Atlan, H., Naschitz, J. E., Simon, J. S., Enat, R., Front, D., Israel, O., Chisin, R., Krausz, Y., Zur, Y. and Kaplan, N. (1985). Nuclear magnetic resonance imaging of liver hemangiomas. *J. Nucl. Med., 26*, 1117–22
30. Anderson-Berg, W. T., Strand, M., Lempert, T. E., Rosenbaum, A. E. and Joseph, P. M. (1986). Nuclear magnetic resonance and gamma camera tumor imaging using gadolinium-Labeled monoclonal antibodies. *J. Nucl. Med., 27*, 829–33
31. Carr, D. H., Graif, M., Niendorf, H. P., Brown, J., Steiner, R. E., Blumgart, L. H. and Young, I. R. (1986). Gadolinium–DTPA in the assessment of liver tumours by magnetic resonance imaging. *Clin. Radiol., 37*, 347–53
32. Bernardino, M. E., Steinberg, H. V., Pearson, T. C., Gedgaudas-McClees, R. K., Torres, W. E. and Henderson, J. M. (1986). Shunts for portal hypertension: MR and angiography for determination of patency. *Radiology, 158*, 57–61
33. Glazer, G. M. (1988). MR imaging of the liver, kidneys, and adrenal glands. *Radiology, 166*, 303–12
34. Tsang, Yuk-Ming, Stark, D. D., Chen, M. C., Weissleder, R., Wittenberg, J. and Ferrucci, J. T. (1988). Hepatic micrometastases in the rat: Ferrite-enhanced MR imaging. *Radiology, 167*, 21–4
35. Ohtomo, K., Itai, Y., Yoshikawa, K., Kokubo, T., Yashiro, N., Iio, M. and Furukawa, K. (1987). Hepatic tumors: dynamic MR imaging. *Radiology, 163*, 27–31
36. Reinig, J. W., Dwyer, A. J., Miller, D. L., White, M., Frank, J. A., Sugarbaker, P. H., Chang, A. E. and Doppman, J. L. (1987). Liver metastasis detection: comparative sensitivities of MR imaging and CT scanning. *Radiology, 162*, 43–7
37. Stark, D. D., Wittenberg, J., Edelman, R. R., Middleton, M. S., Saini, S., Butch, R. J., Brady, T. J. and Ferrucci, J. T. (1986). Detection of hepatic metastases: Analysis of pulse sequence performance in MR imaging. *Radiology, 159*, 365–70
38. Moss, A. A. and Stark, D. D. (1987). Magnetic resonance imaging of liver tumors. In Okuda, K. and Ishak, K. G. (eds.) *Neoplasms of the Liver.* pp 301–19 (Berlin: Springer-Verlag)
39. Hamm, B., Wolf, Karl-Jurgen and Felix, R. (1987). Conventional and rapid MR imaging of the liver with Gd–DTPA. *Radiology, 164*, 313–20
40. Myers, W. G., Bigler, R. E., Benua, R. S., Graham, M. C. and Laughlin, J. S. (1983). PET tomographic imaging of the human heart, pancreas, and liver with nitrogen-13 derived from [^{13}N]-L-glutamate. *Eur. J. Nucl. Med., 8*, 381–4
41. Fukuda, H., Matsuzawa, T., Tada, M., Takahashi, T., Ishiwata, K., Yamada, K., Abe, Y., Yoshioka, S., Sato, T. and Ido, T. (1986). 2-Deoxy-2-[^{18}F]-fluoro-D-galactose: A new tracer for measurement of galactose metabolism in the liver by positron emission tomography. *Eur. J. Nucl. Med., 11*, 444–8
42. Knapp, W. H., Helus, F., Sinn, H., Ostertag, H., Georgi, P., Brandeis, W.-E. and Braun, A. (1984). N-13 L-glutamate uptake in malignancy: its relationship to blood flow. *Radiochem. Radiopharm., 25*, 989–97
43. Alpern, M. B., Rubin, J. M., Williams, D. M. and Capek, P. (1987). Portal hepatis: duplex Doppler US with angiographic correlation. *Radiography, 162*, 53–6
44. Moriyasu, F., Ban, N., Nishida, O., Nakamura, T., Soh, Y., Miura, K., Sakai, M., Miyake, T. and Uchino, H. (1986). Portal hemodynamics in patients with hepatocellular carcinoma. *Radiology, 161*, 707–11
45. Matsuda, Y. and Yabuuchi, I. (1986). Hepatic tumors: US contrast enhancement with CO_2 microbubbles. *Radiology, 161*, 701–5
46. Taylor, K. J. W., Riley, C. A., Hammers, L., Flax, S., Weltin, G., Garcia-Tsao, G., Conn, H. O., Kuc, R. and Barwick, K. W. (1986). Quantitative US attenuation in normal liver and in patients with diffuse liver disease: importance of fat. *Radiology, 160*, 65–71
47. Machi, J., Isomoto, H., Yamashita, Y., Kurohiji, T., Shirouzu, K. and Kakegawa, T. (1987). Intraoperative ultrasonography in screening for liver metastases from colorectal cancer: comparative accuracy with traditional procedures. *Surgery, 101*, 678–84

38
Radiolabelled antibodies in the treatment of non-resectable hepatocellular cancer: Johns Hopkins and Radiation Therapy Oncology Group experience

S. E. ORDER, G. B. STILLWAGON, S. A. LEIBEL, S. O. ASBELL, J. L. KLEIN AND P. L. LEICHNER

THEORETICAL BASIS FOR FERRITIN PRODUCTION IN HEPATOCELLULAR CANCER

Hepatocellular cancer produces ferritin[1]. Ferritin production is theoretically related to messenger RNA and the similarity of the promoter regions both for viral protein synthesis and ferritin[2]. The presumed viral background of ferritin producing malignancies includes Kaposi's sarcoma in AIDS, Hodgkin's disease and hepatocellular cancer (hepatitis B). Ferritin produced by hepatocellular cancer is an apoferritin lacking iron. It is not clear whether this ferritin is a unique isoferritin, although circulating, unique isoferritins have now been identified in Hodgkin's disease and in neuroblastoma[3,4].

BIOLOGICAL BASIS OF [131I]ANTIFERRITIN TUMOUR TARGETING

Studies comparing [131I]antiferritin and [131I]normal IgG in intact rodents showed identical deposition in normal organs, including ferritin-bearing organs[5-7]. Thus, the failure of radiolabelled antiferritin to target specifically normal ferritin-bearing tissues is likely due to the insufficiency of antibody–antigen binding due to the reduced vascular permeability of normal vasculature. Hepatocellular cancer, however, has neovasculature and produces ferritin, allowing radiolabelled antibody to target the tumour[5-7].

The distinguishing characteristics necessary for [131I]antiferritin targeting and radiolabelled antibody deposition in hepatocellular cancer were defined in studies with syngeneic rat hepatomas[5-7]. In addition to the required ferritin production by the tumour, tumour neovasculature was also a necessary

Table 1 RTOG results

Dose of [¹³¹I]Antiferritin[a] (mCi)	Chemotherapy (mg)	White cell/platelet counts
Day 0–30	Adriamycin (15)	>4000/>100000
Day 5–20	5-Fluorouracil (500)	
Day 0–20	Adriamycin (15)	3000–3999/75000–99999
Day 5–10	5-Fluorouracil (500)	
Day 0–20	No drugs	2000–29999/50000–74999
Day 5–10	No drugs	<2000/<50000 (no R$_x$)

$Dose\ of\ [^{131}I]Antiferritin$ rendered in table as displayed.

[a]Rabbit, pig, baboon and horse antibodies were used in sequence. Radioimmunoassay, if negative, allows further cycles of treatment with non-immunoreactive immunoglobulins. Baboon antiferritin to date has been the least immunogenic[13]

component for antibody deposition. Tumour neovasculature allows the 150000 molecular weight IgG to permeate the blood vessels and to enter the tumour interstices. Relative to tumour size, neovasculature is more abundant in small tumours, becoming reduced in proportion to tumour mass as lesions grow. *In vivo* targeting studies using [¹³¹I]antiferritin in four rat hepatocellular cancers (H4IIe, 7800, 7777 and 3924), with equal ferritin content but with varying neovasculature, demonstrated the importance of neovasculature. The greater the vascular content, the greater the tumour targeting by radiolabelled antibody. Other features of tumour targeting by radiolabelled antibody include reduced neovascularity in necrotic tumour centres which also have reduced ferritin concentration due to reduced synthesis and, thus, evidence limited tumour targeting.

Nude rats bearing a human hepatocellular cancer, HepG2, demonstrated similar tumour targeting with radiolabelled antiferritin. These studies additionally demonstrated the superiority of antiferritin monoclonal antibody chelated with ¹¹¹In or ⁹⁰Y, suggesting the possibility of an increased tumour dose achievable with an isoferritin antibody[8].

CLINICAL PHASE I–II STUDY

Prior to determining a clinical response to radiolabelled [¹³¹I]antiferritin in the initial phase of these studies, an induction therapy of external radiation in 300 rad fractions X 7 (4 fractions/week) was used in conjunction with 15 mg Adriamycin and 500 mg 5-fluorouracil (5-FU), the latter used on alternating treatment days[9]. Remission/progression analysis was carried out with a special computerized reconstruction from serial computerized axial tomographs as previously reported[10]. A 25% increase in tumour volume was considered to be evidence of progression, and a 30% reduction in tumour volume was considered to be partial remission[1]. Response to the induction therapy of external beam irradiation and chemotherapy resulted in a 15% remission. Effects of [¹³¹I]antiferritin were evaluated beginning with the tumour volume observed 1 month after induction therapy, and required two cycles of [^{131}I]antiferritin to determine response.

Dose escalation studies were performed with 30 to 100 mCi [^{131}I] antiferritin, labelled at 8–10 mCi/mg IgG; 30 mCi bound all available labelled at 8–10 mCi/mg IgG; 30 mCi bound all available ferritin sites in hepatocellular cancer, saturating the tumour[9,11]. Additional doses above 30 mCi led to increased haematologic toxicity. While no acute toxicity was observed, white cell count levels, and more often, platelet levels, were reduced 4 weeks after administration. There was no other organ toxicity. The most dramatic result for this first group of patients was a complete remission of 3 years, who on relapse due to new developments, received cyclic treatment for a total of 7.5-year survival. In this patient pancytopenia inhibited further therapy. The latter parts of these studies were incorporated into the U.S. National Cooperative Group known as RTOG, the Radiation Therapy Oncology Group (RTOG Protocol 79–28).

The observation of haematologic toxicity led to efforts to take advantage of the tumour effective half-life, both physical and biological half-lives, by developing a schedule of two radioimmunoglobulin infusions per week, later adding sensitizing doses of Adriamycin and 5-FU. Cyclic treatment using a series of animal species as sources for immunoglobulin production were also developed in these studies, providing 3–4 days tumour effective half-lives (RTOG Protocol 83–01)[9,11]. Composite results of this dose scheduling and species of derivation for immunoglobulin administration are shown in Table 1.

Of 105 patients treated with two cycles of radiolabelled antibody in these results, 41% had partial remission, 7% complete remission. Other important observations included the stratification of alpha-fetoprotein (AFP) positive and negative patients. In these initial studies[11] half of the patients were AFP+ and half were AFP–. [^{131}I]Antiferritin could not be given more often than bimonthly due to concern for haematologic recovery. Thus, rapidly dividing AFP+ tumours, although responsive, progressed between therapeutic infusions due to rapid cell division and the prolonged treatment intervals. Two-thirds of the remissions occurred in AFP– patients. The median survival of AFP+ patients without previous treatment or metastasis was 5 months, while in contrast the median survival for AFP– patients was 10.5 months.

Additional information from animal studies and the first phase III randomized trial comparing chemotherapy and [^{131}I]antiferritin indicate that pre-irradiation with as little as 600 rad to 900 rad increased radiolabelled antibody deposition up to 5-fold both in experimental animals and in patients[12,13]. Newer tissue culture data indicate that radiation at the low dose rates caused by [^{131}I]antiferritin, combined with Adriamycin exposure, shifts cells into G_2 and M phases where they are most radiosensitive. The ideal clinical doses of [^{131}I]antiferritin may well be 20 mCi day 0, and 10 mCi day 5, with 15 mg Adriamycin and 500 mg 5-FU based on response with reduced haematologic toxicity.

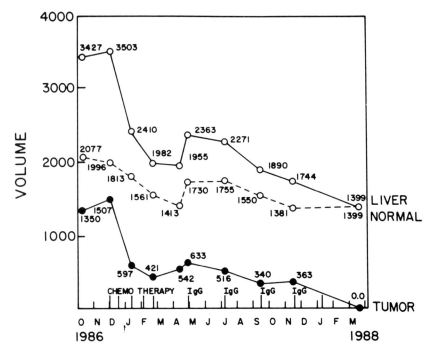

Figure 1 Tumour volumetrics applied to a patient with a non-resectable AFP– hepatocellular cancer. The patient first remitted, then progressed on chemotherapy, then remitted with radio-labelled antibody, finally achieving sufficient tumour reduction for surgical resection

PHASE III RANDOMIZED PROSPECTIVE STUDY

The patient population for this study was composed of non-resectable hepatocellular cancer patients not previously treated and without known metastasis. All patients received external radiation and chemotherapy induction as previously described. Patients were stratified into AFP+ and AFP– groups and randomized through the national cooperative group, RTOG (Protocol 83–19).

The 5-month median survival rate for AFP+ patients reported previously was replicated in these studies. No difference was observed in survival between chemotherapy, Adriamycin (60 mg/m^2 and 5-FU (500 mg/m^2) and the previous schedule of [^{131}I]antiferritin (Table 1). One AFP+ patient treated with [^{131}I]antiferritin has been converted from the non-resectable state to resection, and has achieved 3 years complete remission.

In the AFP– patients to date, there is a 20% survival advantage for radio-labelled antibody; the 10.5 months median survival rate for the antibody treated patients was replicated as in the phase I–II studies. The differences between chemotherapy and [^{131}I]antiferritin survival statistics would be even greater were it not for the fact that the study allows radiolabelled antibody

478

treatment for patients who have failed chemotherapy, or who have cardiac toxicity limiting further chemotherapy. Of 8 patients allowed to receive radiolabelled antibody under these conditions, 6 have remitted, 3 have been resected and 2 of these remain disease free for more than 2 years (Figure 1). One patient who failed to respond to radiolabelled antibody therapy was originally AFP– before becoming AFP+. A second patient would not allow in-patient therapy and received less than the optimal dose. This patient remitted 27% after two cycles of radiolabelled antibody with a 30% study requirement for partial remission.

These crossover remissions have suggested that prior chemotherapy with Adriamycin and 5-FU may shift more tumour cells into a radiosensitive phase of the cell cycle and/or cause sublethal damage which is carried to complete cytotoxic damage by radiolabelled antibody therapy. Although an extensive report of the randomized trial is presently in preparation, it is clear that only radiolabelled antibody treated patients were converted to surgical resectability; one AFP+ and two AFP– patients have been completely resected. Our total recent experience in converting non-resectable to resectable hepatocellular cancer, including the use of ^{90}Yttrium antiferritin antibody therapy, resulted in 10 patients becoming surgically resectable[14].

FUTURE POSSIBILITIES

Our studies with [^{131}I]antiferritin will seek to reduce cycle time by integrating two cycles of chemotherapy and one of radiolabelled antibody. Such an integrated regimen would both optimize shifts in the cell cycle and reduce treatment time to monthly therapy.

An interesting approach to increasing tumour binding has been demonstrated by a Chinese research team under the leadership of Professor Tang at the Shanghai Liver Cancer Hospital. These workers infused [^{131}I]antiferritin directly into the hepatic artery, with a proposed rationale that all the injected antibody would initially pass through the tumour[15]. This approach raises the possibility of increased tumour binding on the first pass, potentially improving tumour targeting. Another approach to enhance targeting of the tumour relative to normal tissue is the use of chelates of different chemical structure. Our studies with chelated ^{90}Y antiferritin indicated excessive reticuloendothelial tissue binding, particularly in the liver and spleen; this reduced the tumour dose. This phenomenon of antibody retention by the reticuloendothelial system may be exaggerated in hepatocel-lular cancer, for it less critical in Hodgkin's disease patients, where more dramatic results are observed in tumour uptake of antibody with subsequent remission. A major determinant of deposition in normal tissue appears to be the chemical nature of the chelate used to join the antibody and the radioisotope. Studies in our laboratory have indicated that altered patterns of biodistribution occur when different types of chelates are used. Improved chelates may further enhance hepatocellular cancer deposition compared to normal liver deposition. Exploratory studies with these chelates are under way in our laboratories.

Another important avenue of research is the integration of radioimmuno-globulin therapy and chemotherapy. There are few studies that have attempted to integrate chemotherapeutic agents with low dose rate, protracted radiation. To date Adriamycin has been shown to shift cells in the cycle to G_2 and M where they are more radiosensitive (J. R. Williams and L. Dillehay, pers. commun.). Fu[16] of the University of California at San Francisco has demonstrated enhanced tumour response when low dose rate irradiation is combined with cisplatin. These two studies indicate that combination therapy with protracted radiation and drugs may prove promising for research and eventual clinical application.

Although the worldwide incidence of liver cancer may be reduced through vaccination against hepatitis B, the lack of previous hepatitis in the US Caucasian population indicates the need for improved therapy. Of our study population, 10% was hepatitis B antigen or antibody positive[17]. This hepato-cellular cancer will remain a clinical challenge. Beyond the limited therapeutic benefit demonstrated for some patients with hepatocellular carcinoma, the experience with radiolabelled antibody represents an important step toward the application of these antibodies in the treatment of malignant disease. As basic studies better characterize those aspects of hepatocellular cancer that make it susceptible to this therapy, it should allow adaptation of these principles of therapy for other human malignancies.

Acknowledgements

This work was supported by NIH grants CA-43791 and CA-06973, by Hybritech, Inc., and by RTOG (protocols 79–28 and 83–01)

References

1. Richter, G. W. (1965). Comparison of ferritins from neoplastic and non-neoplastic human cells. *Nature*, **207**, 616–18
2. Drysdale, J. W. (1983). Ferritin as a tumor marker. *J. Clin. Immunoassay*, **6**, 234–40
3. Hann, H. L., Lange, B. J., Stahlhut, M. W. and McGlynn, K. A. (1988). Prognostic importance of serum transferrin and ferritin in childhood Hodgkin's disease. *Proc. Am. Soc. Clin. Onc.*, **7**, 263 (abst.)
4. Hann, H. L., Evans, A. E., Cohen, I. V. and Leitmeyer, J. E. (1981). Biologic differences between neuroblastoma: stages IV–S and IV. Measurements of serum ferritin and E-rosette inhibition in 30 children. *New Engl. J. Med.*, **305**, 425–9
5. Rostock, R. A., Leichner, P. K., Kopher, K. A. and Order, S. E. (1983). Selective tumor localization in experimental hepatoma by radiolabelled antiferritin antibody. *Int. J. Radiat. Oncol. Biol. Phys.*, **9**, 1345–50
6. Rostock, R. A., Klein, J. L., Kopher, K. A. and Order, S. E. (1984). Variables affecting the tumor localization of I-131 antiferritin in experimental hepatoma. *Am. J. Clin. Oncol.*, **6**, 9–18
7. Rostock, R. A., Klein, J. L., Leichner, P. K. and Order, S. E. (1984). Distribution of physiologic factors that affect I-131 antiferritin tumor localization in experimental hepatoma. *Int. J. Radiat. Oncol. Biol. Phys.*, **10**, 1135–41
8. Zhang, X., Klein, J. L. and Order, S. E. (1988). Quantitative comparison of tumor dose of radiolabelled monoclonal and polyclonal antibodies in an experimental tumor model.

Antibody, Immunoconj. Radiopharm., **1**, 35–41

9. Order, S. E., Klein, J. L., Ettinger, D., Alderson, P., Siegelman, S. and Leichner, P. (1980). Phase I–II study of radiolabelled antibody integrated in the treatment of primary hepatic malignancies. *Int. J. Radiat. Oncol. Biol. Phys.,* **6**, 703–10

10. Yang, N. C., Leichner, P. K., Fishman, E. K., Siegelman, S. S., Frenkel, T. L., Wallace, J. R., Loudenslager, D. M., Hawkins, W. G. and Order, S. E. (1986) CT volumetrics of primary cancers. *J. Comp. Asst. Tomgr.,* **160**, 175–8

11. Order, S. E., Stillwagon, G. B., Klein, J. L., Leichner, P. K., Siegeman, S. S., Fishman, E. K., Ettinger, D. S., Haulk, T., Kopher, K. and Leibel, S. A. (1985) I-131 antiferritin: a new treatment modality in hepatoma: An RTOG study. *J. Clin. Oncol.,* **3**, 1573–82

12. Leichner, P. K., Yang, N. C., Frenkel, T. L., Loudenslager, D. M., Hawkins, W. G., Klein, J. L. and Order, S. E. (1988). Dosimetry and treatment planning for 90-Y labelled antiferritin in hepatoma. *Int. J. Radiat. Oncol. Biol. Phys.,* **14**, 1033–44

13. Msirikale, J. S., Klein, J. L., Schroeder, J. and Order, S. E. (1987). Radiation enhancement of radiolabelled antibody deposition in tumors. *Int. J. Radiat. Oncol. Biol. Phys.,* **13**, 1839–44

14. Sitzmann, J. V., Order, S. E., Klein, J. L., Leichner, P. K., Fishman, E. K. and Smith, G. W. (1987). Conversion by new treatment modalities of non-resectable to resectable hepatocellular cancer. *J. Clin. Oncol.,* **5**, 1566–73

15. Tang, Z., Liu, K., Guo, Y., Ma, Z., Yu, D., Yu, Z., Bao, Y., Lu, J., Lin, Z., Yu, Y., Zhao, H., Chen, K., Qian, F., Yuan, A. and Wu, Z. (1986). Tumor imaging and targeting therapy for hepatocellular carcinoma: preliminary results of experimental and clinical studies. *Chinese Med. J.,* **11**, 855–60

16. Fu, K. K., Lam, K. N. and Rayner, P. A. (1985). The influence of time sequence of cisplatin administration and continuous low dose rate irradiation (CLDRI) on their combined effects on a murine squamous cell carcinoma. *Int. J. Radiat. Oncol. Biol. Phys.,* **11**, 2119–24

17. Di Biscegli, A. M., Sjogren, M., Klein, J., Waggoner, J. G. and Order, S. E. (1988). The role of hepatitis B virus infection in hepatocellular carcinoma in the United States. *Falk Symposium: Liver Cell Carcinoma, Germany* (abst.)

39
Surgery for hepatic tumours

R. A. MALT

INTRODUCTION

Some masses in the liver should be removed. Many should be ignored. The appropriate action depends on the balance among the patient's symptoms, the predicted outcome of the disease left untreated, and the surgeon's skill.

The secrets of hepatic surgery are knowing that a border of 2cm of uninvolved liver around any neoplasm is more than enough and that the normal liver is generally compressed or displaced by the tumour, not destroyed. Even when the parenchyma is infiltrated with cancer, compensatory hyperplasia (regeneration) of remaining normal liver usually takes place[1]. Surgery removes the disease. The patient survives on the good liver he had been living on all along. As estimated by imaging techniques, removal of half the liver mass (including the neoplasm) is replaced in 3–6 months[2,3].

ASSESSMENT

Because the location, anatomy, and invasiveness of a neoplasm can be assessed by computed tomography enhanced with intravascular radio-paque contrast medium or by a magnetic resonance image enhanced with intravascular ferrite[4], a transcutaneous biopsy specimen seldom needs to be obtained. Although hepatic arteriography may help in diagnosis, it is not mandatory for a safe operation.

The chief reasons for a biopsy examination are not to decide which treatment is best, but to establish that a neoplasm is too widespread to allow its complete removal or that the liver parenchyma is too diseased to tolerate surgery. Moreover, malignant cells can be implanted into the needle track and into the peritoneal cavity during removal of the specimen, and the tumour may bleed uncontrollably. Even a large specimen obtained at the operating table can be non-representative, misleading, and bloody.

BENIGN NEOPLASMS

Cholangioadenomas and haemangiomas

Cholangioadenomas (bile-duct adenomas) and *haemangiomas* are the commonest benign neoplasms, occurring in 27% and 20% of men, respectively, in 95 consecutive medico-legal autopsies conducted in Finland[5]. The diameters of these tumours were in the range 0.3–15.5 mm, and their frequency increased with age. Cholangioadenomas never need removal or biopsy examination except when indistinguishable from the dangerous neoplasms: for example, when palpation at the operating table engenders confusion about whether an hepatic tumour is benign or malignant.

On the whole, haemangiomas also deserve neglect. Their bright appearance on a T_2-weighted spin-echo magnetic resonance image is 90% diagnostic in separating haemangioma from carcinoma[6]. Rupture is so rare that fewer than 50 examples are recorded — almost all of them tumours over 10 cm in diameter[7]. Although subcapsular leakage is more common, it, too, seldom needs treatment unless the patient or the physician is oversensitive. Long-term oestrogen administration may be responsible for three of the four instances in which giant haemangiomas have recurred after radiation treatment or resection[8].

Hepatoadenomas

Hepatoadenomas are solitary, scattered, or confluent. Even before the days of birth-control pills, they were nearly twice as frequent in women as in men. In the 1960s, when long-term use of oral contraceptives was common, the balance toward women became even more lop-sided. Fortunately, the number of patients now requiring treatment for this neoplasm, which has a tendency to undergo haemorrhagic infarction and rupture, is much decreased.

Because the bulk of the hepatic mass is in the right liver, and neoplasms should be randomly distributed, most solitary hepatoadenomas are in the right liver, often deep. Rupture is a catastrophe requiring an impromptu major hepatectomy.

Despite this worrisome scenario, neoplasms suspected of being hepatoadenomas should not be removed electively until the effects of removing sources of steroidal stimulation are observed[9]. When the tropic stimulus is gone, the tumour or tumours may regress. If the mass of a hepatoadenoma decreases by 50%, removal is seldom required. Absence of regression means that surgery should be considered.

When there is massive involvement of the liver with multiple hepatoadenomas, leaving some adenomas and enough liver tissue to support life is more important than rooting out every adenoma and creating hepatic insufficiency in the process. A malignant potential for hepatoadenomas has often been discussed, but never unequivocally established.

TUMOUR-LIKE CONDITIONS

Chief among the pseudo-tumours is *focal nodular hyperplasia*. Except when physicians become overly concerned, it is a harmless mass of hepatic tissue and scar, producing symptoms mainly when its bulk displaces adjacent structures. Current thought is that focal nodular hyperplasia is a hyperplastic reaction to a vascular ingrowth and that ingrowth stops when counter-balanced by the resistance of normal hepatic tissue[10,11].

Because focal nodular hyperplasia has no malignant potential, it does not have to be removed unless it is large enough to produce disabling symptoms or is indistinguishable from a malignancy. Although focal nodular hyperplasia is probably not caused by hormonal imbalances, androgens and oestrogens may nonetheless be tropic[12]. As with hepatoadenoma, signs of regression after removal of all steroidal therapy should be assessed before surgery is recommended.

Focal nodular hyperplasia is most simply distinguishable from hepatoadenoma by its uptake of ^{99m}Tc-sulphur colloid. Until recently, this dichotomy was attributed to the presence of Kupffer cells in foci of nodular hyperplasia and their absence from hepatoadenoma. This explanation cannot be correct, however, since all 13 hepatoadenomas examined by modern microscopical techniques had Kupffer cells, and three adenomes took up radioactive sulphur colloid to yield a positive scintigram[13]. Magnetic resonance images can sometimes also make identification of focal nodular hyperplasia nearly certain[14].

Both a *regenerating nodule* in the liver of a cirrhotic liver and a localized *hematoma* can be mistaken for a neoplasm. Although tense *cysts* used to be confused with a solid neoplasm, this masquerade is scarcely possible in the era of diagnostic ultrasonography and computed imaging. Cystadenomas are rare.

Hamartoma, a name once given to virtually all hepatic tumours, is properly restricted to a specific, large benign neoplasm usually manifesting itself in the first 2 years of life[15].

PRIMARY MALIGNANT NEOPLASMS

Hepatocellular carcinoma

In areas across the 'hepatic-cancer belt' of China and Africa, hepatitis B-induced *hepatocellular carcinoma* is overwhelmingly the most frequent malignancy; resection is the most expeditious treatment when enough normal hepatic tissue can be spread to permit life[16]. In the temperate regions, most hepatocellular cancer is multifocal, on a substrate of alcoholic cirrhosis, making the bearers poor surgical candidates because of associated portal hypertension and defective synthesis of serum proteins.

Some patients are fortunate in that their cancers are indolent, small and unifocal, induced by specific substances, or susceptible to embolic infarction under angiographic control.

The indolent cancer is the so-called fibrolamellar variant of hepatocellular carcinoma[17,18]. Found mostly in patients less than 25 years old, often women, fibrolamellar hepatocarcinomas tend to be compact and do not notably metastasize until late in their course. They compose about 7% of all hepatic cell cancers and, obviously, a larger proportion of those in young patients. Although 5-year survival rates after resection are about 40% versus 20% for the usual hepatocellular carcinoma, these data must be tempered by recognition that better results are likely to be obtained when the population is skewed towards young patients in relatively good health.

'Minimal' hepatic cancers are localized neoplasms under 3 or 4 cm in diameter[19-24]. They are usually suspected as a result of screening programmes designed to detect high levels of alpha-fetoprotein in residents of endemic areas who are already suspected of being at risk of cancer because of a positive assay for hepatitis B antigen. The doubling time of the serum alpha-fetoprotein titre is close to that of the neoplasm, and real-time ultrasonography permits monitoring the actual rate of growth of the suspected neoplasm. Because the median period before the neoplasm can be found by imaging techniques is about 3.2 years, in the population at high risk screening is recommended every 4–5 months.

In Japan 19% of patients with primary hepatocellular cancer have neoplasms under 3 cm in diameter, and all have intrinsic hepatic parenchymal dysfunction. Nonetheless, the mortality rate from removing these minimal cancers in patients with diseased livers is only 10.5%. The 4-year survival rate is 59%, as compared with a survival rate of about 18% following removal of the usual large Oriental hepatocellular neoplasm[20]. Cancers < 5 cm in diameter having a pseudo-capsule can be resected with a 35% 5-year survival rate versus 8% for the common hepatocarcinoma[22]. In Taiwan, a 4-year survival rate of 44% is documented[24].

Safe removal of small neoplasms from patients with cirrhosis or hepatitis is often feasible because direct-contact intra-operative ultrasonography permits sensitive and accurate localization of an otherwise imperceptible neoplasm, removal of the neoplasm with the least infringement on major vascular structures, and loss of the least hepatic tissue[25]. Indeed, the exact region to be removed can be defined by sonographically guided injection of methylene blue into the branch of the portal vein supplying the region. Loss of blood can be kept low by occlusion of the same branch of the portal vein with a balloon catheter.

Growth of cancers that are induced or promoted by steroids can potentially be inhibited by removal of the promoter: namely, œstrogens and progestins in women who have taken those substances for birth control or other reasons, and androgens in hypopituitary men, in children being treated for aplastic anaemia or Fanconi's syndrome, in patients taking them for paroxysmal nocturnal haemoglobinuria, and in athletes using anabolic steroids for dubious reasons[26-29]. Aside from inhibited growth when steroids are removed, there is a suggestion that steroid-induced or steroid-promoted neoplasms do not behave malignantly, even though their histological appearance is nominally that of a cancer[26]. Furthermore, some are susceptible to chemotherapy, unlike most hepatocellular carcinoma.

Symptoms of pain or pressure on other organs produced by a large, localized hepatocellular carcinoma in an otherwise normal liver can some-times be alleviated by producing ischaemic infarction under angiographic control. The survival rate is 42% at 15 years[30]. If compensatory hyperplasia of the normal remnant occurs, the necrotic neoplasm can sometimes be resected without compromise of hepatic function.

Cell proliferation inherent in cirrhosis, haemochromatosis, and injury from hepatitis B virus provides a substrate for development of hepatocellular carcinoma[31]. But why do some people with ostensibly normal livers get cancer? Perhaps these sporadic cancers are potentiated in human beings as they are in rats and mice by substances in the environment apparently as innocuous as *p*-dichlorobenzene (mothballs)[32], some benzodiazepines[33,34], nitrosodiethanolamine (in cosmetics and cutting oil)[35], and methylpyrilene (until recently sold without a prescription as an hypnotic).

Cholangiocarcinomas

Cholangiocarcinomas exist in both a parenchymal form responsible for masses in the liver like other hepatic cancers and a central form that blocks bile ducts (the Altemeier–Klatskin tumour at the confluence of the bile ducts). Although parenchymal cholangiocarcinoma can often be resected, cure is rare and palliation uncertain.

Resection of the bile ducts for cholangiocarcinoma is feasible only about 10% of the time and must give the best results, because resectable neoplasms have a cancer-free plane around them somewhere. More typically, infiltrative ductal adenocarcinoma permits at best a biliary–enteric bypass to relieve obstructive jaundice and the symptoms it produces (75% of cases)[36-40]. Despite the occasional and habitually reported survival of a few patients for several years or even a decade after resection or bypass — and that is the stimulus for aggressive surgery in the absence of other effective forms of treatment — the mean survival time is less than 9 months.

Sarcomas

Sarcomas are the least frequent of hepatic cancers in the adult. When they are local, all should be resected if feasible because there is no other effective form of treatment[41-45]. Fibrosarcomas are occasionally associated with hypogly-caemia, the cause of which is still uncertain. *Leiomyosarcomas* probably arise from the vascular structures of the liver and from the vena cava. With conspicuous exception, only palliation is possible, and that not often. The incurable *malignant haemangioendothelioma (angiosarcoma)* follows exposure to Thorotrast (an obsolete radioactive contrast substance for the reticuloendothelial system), arsenicals, vinyl chloride, or methyltestosterone therapy in children with aplastic anaemia or Fanconi's syndrome. Although *rhabdomyosarcomas* are unsuccessfully treated in adults, chemotherapeutic cure is possible in children with unifocal disease after the bulk of the neoplasm is resected to leave only microscopic areas of disease as targets for chemotherapy.

METASTATIC CANCERS

Because their numbers are often few, the best results are from resection of metastases from cancers of the left colon. Cancers from the right colon tend to be multifocal. There is no predilection of metastases for either side of the liver, colorectal metastases being distributed in proportion to the relative mass of any part of the liver[46]. Although most statistics show that the best chance for 25% 5-year survival is defined when colorectal metastases are no more than 3 or 4 cm and are no larger than 5 cm in diameter, huge metastases from slow-growing primaries can sometimes be cured (for example, mesonephric duct carcinoma). For purposes of resection a metastasis surrounded by small satellites is empirically the same as a solitary metastasis. Massive resections for palliation of symptoms caused by the mass are indicated for highly selected, young, vigorous patients, despite their having the right or left liver full of metastases and micrometastases elsewhere[47-51].

Inasmuch as the period of delay — weeks or months — before the metastasis is resected is not a determinant of success, clinical common sense should be invoked. Metastases at the leading edge of the liver discovered at the time of a colon resection can be removed impromptu. Large, deep ones should be removed at another time, after verification of their size, assessment of macroscopic satellites, and consideration of the surgeon's track record.

Metastases from carcinoids are resected mainly to relieve hormonal effects of the neoplasm when long-acting somatostatin analogue is ineffective or unavailable and when angiographically-guided embolization of the liver is unsuccessful in reducing the discomfort of an enormous, rigid mass.

References

1. Bucher, N. L. R. and Malt, R. A. (1971). *Regeneration of Liver and Kidney.* (Boston: Little, Brown)
2. Zoli, M., Marchesnini, G., Melli, A., Viti, G., Marra, A. and Pisi, E. (1986). Evaluation of liver volume and liver function following hepatic resection in man. *Liver,* **6**, 286–91
3. Nagasue, N., Yukaya, H., Ogawa, Y., Kohno, H. and Nakamura, T. (1987). Human liver regeneration after major hepatic resection: A study of normal liver and livers with chronic hepatitis and cirrhosis. *Ann. Surg.,* **206**, 30–9
4. Weissleder, R., Stark, D. D., Rummeny, E. J., Compton, C. C. and Ferrucci, J. T., Jr. (1988). Splenic lymphoma: Ferrite-enhanced MR imaging in rats. *Radiology,* **166**, 423–30
5. Karhunen, P. J. (1986). Benign hepatic tumours and tumour like conditions in men. *J. Clin. Pathol.,* **39**, 183–8
6. Stark, D. D., Felder, R. C., Wittenberg, J., Saini, S., Butch, R. J., Edelman, R. R., Mueller, P. R., Simeone, J. F., Cohen, A. M. *et al.* (1985). Magnetic resonance imaging of cavernous hemangioma of the liver. *Am. J. Roentgenol.,* **145**, 213–22
7. Takagi, H. (1985). Diagnosis and management of cavernous hemangioma of the liver. *Sem. Surg. Oncol.,* **1**, 12–22
8. Conter, R. L. and Longmire, W. P., Jr. (1988). Recurrent hepatic hemangiomas: Possible association with estrogen therapy. *Ann. Surg.,* **207**, 115–19
9. Bühler, H., Pirovino, M., Akovbiantz, A., Altorfer, J., Weitzel, M., Maranta, E. and Schmid, M. (1982). Regression of liver cell adenoma: A follow-up study of three consecutive patients after discontinuation of oral contraceptive use. *Gastroenterology,* **82**, 775–82
10. Wanless, I. R., Mawdsley, C. and Adams, R. (1985). On the pathogenesis of focal nodular hyperplasia of the liver. *Hepatology,* **5**, 1194–200

11. Pirovino, M., Triller, J. and Steffen, R. (1987). Die fokale noduläre Hyperplasie der Leber. *Schweiz. Med. Wochenschr.*, **117**, 1165–73
12. Alberti-Flor, J. J., Iskandarani, M., Jeffers, L., Zeppa, R. and Schiff, E. R. (1984). Focal nodular hyperplasia associated with the use of a synthetic anabolic androgen. *Am. J. Gastroenterol.*, **79**, 150–1
13. Lubbers, P. R., Ros, P. R., Goodman, Z. D. and Ishak, K. G. (1987). Accumulation of technetium-99m sulfur colloid by hepatocellular adenoma: Scintigraphic–pathologic correlation. *Am. J. Roentgenol.*, **148**, 1105–8
14. Butch, R. J., Stark, D. D. and Malt, R. A. (1986). MR imaging of hepatic focal nodular hyperplasia. *J. Comput. Assist. Tomogr.*, **10**, 874–7
15. Stocker, J. T. and Ishak, K. G. (1983). Mesenchymal harmartoma of the liver: Report of 30 cases and review of the literature. *Ped. Pathol.*, **1**, 245–67
16. Olweny, C. L. M., Katongole-Mbidde, E., Bahendeka, S., Otim, D., Mugerwa, J. and Kyalwazi, S. K. (1980). Further experience in treating patients with hepatocellular carcinoma in Uganda. *Cancer*, **46**, 2717–22
17. Nagorney, D. M., Adson, M. A., Weiland, L. H., Knight, C. D., Jr., Smalley, S. R. and Zinsmeister, A. R. (1985). Fibrolamellar hepatoma. *Am. J. Surg.*, **149**, 113–19
18. Hodgson, H. J. F. (1987). Fibrolamellar cancer of the liver. *J. Hepatol.*, **5**, 241–7
19. Sheu, J.-C., Sung, J.-L., Chen, D.-S., Yang, P.-M., Lai, M.-Y., Lee, C.-S., Hsu, H.-C., Chuang, C.-N., Yang, P.-C., Wang, T.-H., Lin, J.-T. and Lee, C.-Z. (1985). Growth rate of asymptomatic hepatocellular carcinoma and its clinical implications. *Gastroenterology*, **89**, 259–66
20. Nagasue, N., Yukaya, H., Chang, Y. C., Ogawa, Y., Ota, N., Kimura, N. and Nakamura, T. (1987). Appraisal of hepatic resection in the treatment of minute hepatocellular carcinoma associated with liver cirrhosis. *Br. J. Surg.*, **74**, 836–8
21. Bismuth, H., Houssin, D., Ornowski, J. and Meriggi, F. (1986). Liver resections in cirrhotic patients: A Western experience. *World J. Surg.*, **10**, 311–17
22. Nagao, T., Inoue, S., Goto, S., Mizuta, T., Omori, Y., Kawano, N. and Morioka, Y. (1987). Hepatic resection for hepatocellular carcinoma: Clinical features and long-term prognosis. *Ann. Surg.*, **205**, 33–40
23. Lin, T.-Y., Lee, C.-S., Chen, K.-M. and Chen, C.-C. (1987). Role of surgery in the treatment of primary carcinoma of the liver: A 31-year experience. *Br. J. Surg.*, **74**, 839–42
24. Lee, C.-S., Sung, J.-L., Sheu, J.-C., Chen, D.-S., Lin, T.-Y. and Beasley, R. P. (1986). Surgical treatment of 109 patients with symptomatic and asymptomatic hepatocellular carcinoma. *Surgery*, **99**, 481–90
25. Traynor, O., Castaing, D. and Bismuth, H. (1988). Peroperative ultrasonography in the surgery of hepatic tumours. *Br. J. Surg.*, **75**, 197–202
26. Malt, R. A., Galdabini, J. J. and Jeppsson, B. W. (1983). Abnormal sex-steroid milieu in young adults with hepatocellular carcinoma. *World J. Surg.*, **7**, 247–52
27. McCaughan, G. W., Bilous, M. J. and Gallagher, N. D. (1985). Long-term survival with tumor regression in androgen-induced liver tumors. *Cancer*, **56**, 2622–6
28. Forman, D., Vincent, T. J. and Doll, R. (1986). Cancer of the liver and the use of oral contraceptives. *Br. Med. J.*, **292**, 1357–61
29. Porter, L. E., Van Thiel, D. H. and Eagon, P. K. (1987). Estrogens and progestins as tumor inducers. *Semin. Liver Dis.*, **7**, 24–31
30. Lin, D.-Y., Liaw, Y.-F., Lee, T.-Y. and Lai, C.-M. (1988). Hepatic arterial embolization in patients with unresectable hepatocellular carcinoma — A randomized controlled trial. *Gastroenterology*, **94**, 453–56
31. Farber, E. (1987). Possible etiologic mechanisms in chemical carcinogenesis. *Environ. Hlth Perspect.*, **75**, 64–70
32. Rall, D. P. (1987). Carcinogenicity of p-dichlorobenzene. *Science*, **236**, 897
33. Diwan, B. A., Rice, J. M. and Ward, J. M. (1986). Tumour-promoting activity of benzodiazepine tranquillizers, diazepam and oxazepam, in mouse liver. *Carcinogenesis*, **7**, 789–94
34. Préat, V., de Gerlache, J., Lans, M. and Roberfroid, M. (1987). Promoting effect of oxazepam in rat hepatocarcinogenesis, *Carcinogenesis*, **8**, 97–100
35. Lijinsky, W. and Kovatch, R. M. (1985). Induction of liver tumors in rats by nitrosodiethanolamine at low doses. *Carcinogenesis*, **6**, 1679–81

36. Bengmark, S., Ekberg, H., Evander, A., Klofver-Stahl, B. and Tranberg, K. -G. (1988). Major liver resection for hilar cholangiocarcinoma. *Ann. Surg.,* **207**, 120–5
37. Miyazaki, K., Nagafuchi, K. and Nakayama, F. (1988). Bypass procedure for bile duct cancer. *World J. Surg.,* **12**, 64–7
38. Pichlmayr, R., Ringe, B., Lauchart, W., Bechstein, W. O., Gubernatis, G. and Wagner, E. (1988). Radical resection and liver grafting as the two main components of surgical strategy in the treatment of proximal bile duct cancer. *World J. Surg.,* **12**, 68–77
39. White, T. T. (1988). Skeletization resection and central hepatic resection in the treatment of bile duct cancer. *World J. Surg.,* **12**, 48–51
40. Bismuth, H., Castaing, D. and Traynor, O. (1988). Resection or palliation: Priority of surgery in the treatment of hilar cancer. *World J. Surg.,* **12**, 39–47
41. Forbes, A., Portmann, B., Johnson, P. and Williams, R. (1987). Hepatic sarcomas in adults: A review of 25 cases. *Gut,* **28**, 668–74
42. Ishak, K. G. and Malt, R. A. (1989). Sarcomas of the liver and spleen. In Raaf, J. H. (ed.) *Management of Soft-Tissue Sarcomas.* (Chicago: Year Book Medical Publishers) (In press)
43. Tamburro, C. H., Makk, L. and Popper, H. (1984). Early hepatic histologic alterations among chemical (vinyl monomer) workers. *Hepatology,* **4**, 413–18
44. Maki, H. S., Hubert, B. C., Sajjad, S. M., Kirchner, J. P. and Kuehner, M. E. (1987). Primary hepatic leiomyosarcoma. *Arch. Surg.,* **122**, 1193–6
45. Horowitz, M. E., Etcubanas, E., Webber, B. L., Kun, L. E., Rao, B. N., Vogel, R. J. and Pratt, C. B. (1987). Hepatic undifferentiated (embryonal) sarcoma and rhabdomyosarcoma in children: Results of therapy. *Cancer,* **59**, 396–402
46. Schulz, W., Hagen, C. and Hort, W. (1985). The distribution of liver metastases from colonic cancer: A quantitative postmortem study. *Virchows Arch. (A),* **406**, 279–84
47. Cady, B. and McDermott, W. V. (1985). Major hepatic resection for metachronous metastases from colon cancer. *Ann. Surg.,* **201**, 204–9
48. Sesto, M. E., Vogt, D. P. and Hermann, R. E. (1987). Hepatic resection in 128 patients: A 24-year experience. *Surgery,* **102**, 846–51
49. Adson, M. A. (1987). Resection of liver metastases — When is it worthwhile? *World J. Surg.,* **11**, 511–20
50. Cobourn, C. S., Makowka, K., Langer, B., Taylor, B. R. and Falk, R. E. (1987). *Surg., Gynecol. Obstet.,* **165**, 239–46
51. Registry of Hepatic Metastases. (1988). Resection of the liver for colorectal carcinoma metastases: A multi-institutional study of the indications for resection. *Surgery,* **103**, 278–88

40
Indications for liver grafting in hepatic tumours

R. PICHLMAYR

The main indication for liver grafting today is end-stage benign liver disease, mainly on the basis of cirrhosis. But the first decade of clinical hepatic transplantation has been characterized particularly by performing this procedure in tumour patients. Frequent and early tumour occurrences soon raised the question of justification and worth of this complex procedure in tumour patients. This question still has not been answered, and such an answer will always be preliminary; developments in non-surgical or surgical–oncologic therapies will alter this indication in an unpredictable way. At present, a limited field of indication for liver grafting in tumour patients seems to exist[1–3]. The main argument for this view is the well-known proof that long survival after liver grafting in tumour patients can be obtained, although in hitherto relatively few patients. A second argument might be the palliation which can be obtained more regularly by liver grafting in patients severely suffering from the tumours which are frequently huge and highly painful. A third argument could be a prolongation of life, although burdened by the high probability of tumour recurrence. The second and third arguments will not be accepted generally as long as the survival time of those 'palliatively' transplanted patients is as short as it is, in the majority of experience within a few months. Thus, only patients with a curative chance will probably be selected for liver grafting.

It has been tried to work out the characteristics of tumours and tumour stages which might give the chance of a curative, or at least long-lasting, palliative effect by re-evaluating the literature and our own experience in 98 liver grafts in tumour patients[1,4].

Liver grafts have been performed in a variety of tumour types, predominantly in hepatocellular carcinoma (HCC) with or without underlying cirrhosis (Table 1). The relative frequency of the tumour indication, which was high in the previous years, declined; but we still continue with this indication (Table 2).

The overall results are burdened by two facts: first, during the time period,

Table 1 Histological classification of liver tumours for which liver transplantation has been performed

Histopathologic diagnosis	n
Hepatocellular carcinoma	21
Hepatocellular carcinoma + cirrhosis	28
Cholangiocellular carcinoma	9
Cholangiocellular carcinoma + cirrhosis	3
Hepatoblastoma	2
Haemangiosarcoma	2
Haemangioendothelioma	1
Adenocarcinoma of the bile duct	20
Metastases[a]	8

[a]Colorectal carcinoma (3), carcinoid (2), melanoma (2), and teratoma (1)

when the majority of transplantations for tumour had been performed, there was a high post-operative mortality due to various reasons, particularly in combined tumour, cirrhotic patients. Secondly, and mainly, tumour recurrence is frequent. Thus, operative mortality declined in more recent years, but still long survival expectancy is limited: the overall actual survival rates are as follows: *1972 to 1984*, 6 months, 43%; 1 year, 23%; 3 years, 10%; and 5 years, 10%. *1985 to 1987*, 6 months, 96%; 1 year, 68%; and 2 years, 57%.

Table 2 Development of indication for liver transplantation in Hannover in 313 patients (25.11.1972–30.04.1988)

Year	Benign diseases	Malignant diseases	Total patients	Retrans- plantations	Total transplantations
1972	1	–	1	–	1
1975	–	1	1	–	1
1976	1	1 (1)[c]	2	–	2
1977	1	2	3	–	3
1978	1 (1)[a]	–	1	–	1
1979	5	2	7	–	7
1980	1	7 (1)[a](2)[b]	8	–	8
1981	8 (2)[a]	15 (2)[a](2)[b](4)[c]	23	2 (1)[d]	25
1982	14 (3)[a]	14 (4)[c]	28	3	31
1983	21 (9)[a]	6 (2)[b](3)[c]	27	3	30
1984	25 (7)[a]	8 (2)[b](3)[c]	33	5	38
1985	33 (6)[a]	8 (5)[b](1)[c]	41	5	46
1986	42 (6)[a]	22 (4)[b](9)[c]	64	19 (17)[d]	83
1987	46(14)[a]	9 (3)[b](4)[c]	55	10 (9)[d]	65
1988 (April)	17 (4)[a]	2	19	2	21
Total	216(52)[a]	97 (3)[a](20)[b](29)[c]	313	49	362

[a]Children
[b]Central bile-duct carcinoma
[c]Tumour in cirrhosis
[d]Number of patients

Table 3 Survey of 'long-term' survival after hepatic transplantation for malignant liver tumours in 7 European centres[a] (1.9.87)

Histological diagnosis	Number of patients transplanted	Survival			Longest survival	Currently alive
		> 1 year	> 2 years	> 5 years		
Hepatocellular carcinoma (HCC)	73	29	18	7	11 years 9 months	21
HCC in cirrhosis	84	19	9	2	12 years	16
Cholangiocellular carcinoma with/without cirrhosis	42	11	4	1	6 years 6 months	7
Other primary liver tumours[b]	16	4	4	1	5 years 9 months	4
Bile-duct carcinoma	38	15	6	–	3 years 11 months	8
Metastases[c]	43	12	6	–	4 years 10 months	12
Total	296	90	47	11		68

[a]Data compiled from a present inquiry with the following contributing centres: Berlin, Birmingham, Cambridge, Hamburg, Hannover, Innsbruck and Vienna
[b]Angiosarcoma (7), haemangioendothelioma (4), hepatoblastoma (3), sarcoma (2)
[c]Colorectal carcinoma (30), mammary carcinoma (4), carcinoid (4), melanoma (2) phaeochromocytoma (1), sarcoma (1), teratoma (1)

493

Although these results are not very different from those obtained in patients after radical and extensive tumour surgery for gastric or for lung cancer and certainly better than those for pancreatic cancer, the limited overall results will more and more raise the question of the value and justification of this therapy. The extent of the procedure has to be taken into account, the costs of treatment, the disappointment of many of those patients after a period of exaggerated hope and the restriction of organs, possibly needed for other patients with a better prognosis. But all these arguments are somewhat problematic and should stand back, if life-saving or significant life prolongation in a good state of health could possibly be achieved.

TUMOUR CHARACTERISTICS

How can we select patients whose tumours have a chance of profiting from transplantation?

First, histology of the tumour is important: In evaluating the criteria of 7 European centres with a total of 296 liver grafts in tumour patients 1987 (Table 3), apparently HCC may be the most suitable tumour type. But it has to be mentioned, that individual long-term survival could be achieved in each individual tumour type. Similar are the results in our 98 patients (Figure 1).

Again, it has to be emphasized that these results include all patients — that also means the more complicated first series in the earlier years of experience, and thus mortality is not only caused by tumour. Thus — with caution — one can draw the preliminary conclusion about the pattern of suitability of tumour types for transplantation (Table 4).

TUMOUR STAGES

In accordance with general oncology, the tumour stage also plays a major and decisive role in liver grafting for tumours. At least retrospectively it has

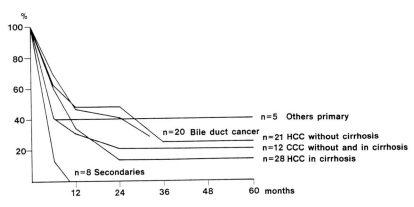

Figure 1 Hepatic transplantation in malignant liver tumours. Different kinds of tumours. Actuarial survival

Table 4 Liver transplantation for malignancies. Preliminary sequence of suitability

Primary malignancies of the liver	
HCC without cirrhosis	favourable, esp. when solitary
HCC in cirrhosis	partly suitable
CCC	altogether unfavourable
others, esp. sarcoma	possibly
Liver metastases	
of endocrine tumours	possibly
of sarcoma	possibly
of colorectal tumours	possibly (?)
Bile-duct carcinoma	
central (Klatskin)	possibly
gall bladder	possibly not

become clear that many of the tumours which have been classified pre- and also intra-operatively as those without extra-hepatic spread, histologically have turned out to have positive lymph nodes, at least in the hilar region. None of those patients with positive lymph nodes survived our studies for more than 1 or exceptionally for 2 years. Thus, in differentiating the results according to lymph node-negative and lymph node-positive stages — or similarly according to TNM classification — large differences in the results become evident. This is true particularly for HCC and for the central bile-duct tumours (Figures 2 and 3). From these results we justify liver grafting particularly in these two tumour types, provided that there are no signs of extra-hepatic tumour manifestations. Additional parameters, as for example solitary or multiple tumour spread, have to be evaluated further in larger series. It has to be mentioned that liver grafting in central bile-duct carcinoma is still debatable, as previous results of others have failed to show significant life prolongation[2,3].

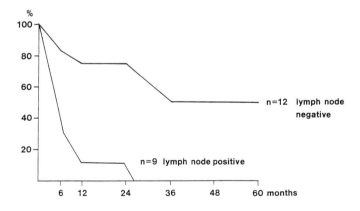

Figure 2 Hepatic transplantation in malignant liver tumours. HCC without cirrhosis. Lymph-node negative or positive

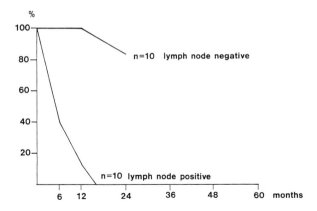

Figure 3 Hepatic transplantation in malignant liver tumours. Proximal bile-duct tumours. Lymph node positive or negative

In addition to histological tumour types and tumour stages, one should probably try to elaborate more specific tumour characteristics about the individual tumour biology. Thus, differences in macroscopic and microscopic growth characteristics are well known, particularly the encapsulated and the diffusely infiltrating type. At least in resectional treatment, the former apparently shows a better prognosis. This may also be true in liver grafting, although it has not been worked out yet. Similarly, we found the tendencies at particularly high alpha-fetoprotein values are an unfavourable prognostic index[4] — but this may be correlated with the tumour extent.

On the other hand, there seems to be no difference in the prognosis of HCC tumours in, or without, underlying cirrhosis — apart from a higher operative mortality in the former; at least in our group of patients and without further separation into tumour stage.

Specific biological tumour markers may be relevant for decisions about the individual usefulness of liver grafting in a tumour patient. Certainly, here we still have a wide field of investigation and research.

The argument for justification of the value of liver grafting in selected tumour patients, which is at least in wide concordance, particularly with the leading groups in Pittsburgh and in Cambridge, is valid only on the pre-requisite that all chances for a conventional surgical or non-surgical treatment have been used or are excluded. Advances in liver resection for tumours of the liver parenchyma and the bile-duct system, particularly also the central bile duct areas, have to be mentioned[5,7,8].

In order to extend resectional therapy to hitherto unresectable tumour stages, we recently introduced the approach or the *ex situ* operation of the liver[9]. The feasibility of this procedure is thus shown; its therapeutic place has to be worked out consequently. It may open resectability to hitherto unresect-able conditions — thus perhaps reducing the need for liver grafting — and may furthermore offer more radical and hopefully better combined oncologic and surgical strategies for liver tumour patients.

Acknowledgement

The following centres contributing data are thanked: Berlin, Birmingham, Cambridge, Hamburg, Hannover, Innsbruck and Vienna.

References

1. Pichlmayr, R. (1988). Is there a place for liver grafting for malignancy? *Transplant. Proc.,* **20**, 478–82
2. Iwatsuki, S., Gordon, R. D., Shaw, B. W., and Starzl, T. E. (1985). Role of liver transplantation in cancer therapy. *Ann. Surg.,* **202**, 401–7
3. O'Grady, J. G., Polson, R. J., Rolles, K., Calne, R. Y. and Williams, R. (1988). Liver transplantation for malignant disease: Results in 93 consecutive patients. *Ann. Surg.,* **207**, 373–9
4. Ringe, B., Wittekind, C., Bechstein, W. O., Bunzendahl, H. and Pichlmayr, R. (1989). The role of liver transplantation in hepatobiliary malignancy. A retrospective analysis of 95 patients with particular regard to tumour stage and recurrence. *Ann. Surg.* **209**, 88–98
5. Iwatsuki, S., Shaw, B. W. and Starzl, T. E. (1983). Experience with 150 liver resections. *Ann. Surg.,* **197**, 247–53
6. Bismuth, H., Castaing, D. and Houssin, D. (1985). Die Leberresektion. *Chirurg,* **56**, 203–10
7. Pichlmayr, R., Ringe, B., Bechstein, W. O., Lauchart, W. and Neuhaus, P. (1988). Approach to primary liver cancer. Recent results. *Cancer Res.,* **110**, 65–73
8. Pichlmayr, R., Ringe, B., Lauchart, W., Bechstein, W. O., Gubernatis, G. and Wagner, E. (1988). Radical resection and liver grafting as the two main components of surgical strategy in the treatment of proximal bile duct cancer. *Wld J. Surg.,* **12**, 68–77
9. Pichlmayr, R., Bretschneider, H. J., Kirchner, E., Ringe, B., Lamesch, P., Gubernatis, G., Hauss, J., Niehaus, K. J. and Kaukemüller, J. (1988). *Ex situ* Operation an der Leber. Eine neue Möglichkeit in der Leberchirurgie. *Langenbecks Arch. Chir.,* **373**, 122–6

41
Liver transplantation for hepatocellular carcinoma

D. H. VAN THIEL, V. DINDZANS, J. S. GAVALER, L. MAKOWKA AND T. E. STARZL

According to the U.S. National Cancer Institute, 13 600 new cases of malignant tumours of the liver and biliary tree were expected to occur within the United States in calendar year 1986[1]. This incidence is rather low compared to many other more populous areas of the world such as Southeast Asia and Japan (Table 1) where the incidence of hepatitis B virus (HBV) infection and, as a result hepatocellular carcinoma (HCC), is more common. HBV is responsible for greater than 80% of the cases of HCC worldwide such that HBs Ag-positive carriers have a 200-fold greater risk of developing HCC than do Ag-negative controls and as many as 50% of all carriers may develop HCC. The risk of becoming a carrier for HBV is inversely related to the age at which the HBV infection occurs, being > 85% for infected newborns and < 10% for adults. Chronic hepatitis B viral infection with macronodular cirrhosis and integration of the hepatitis B virus DNA into the liver cell genome is not the only cause of hepatocellular carcinoma in the world, however. Hepatoma is a rather common consequence of a larger number of chronic liver diseases and occurs in such diseases at a variable rate between 1 and 100% depending upon the type of cirrhosis and the nature of the underlying liver disease (Table 2).

Table 1 Annual incidence of hepatocellular carcinoma

Rate	Incidence (per 100 000)	Location
Very high	> 20	China, Southeast Asia, South Africa (Blacks)
High	10–20	Japan, Southern Europe, Switzerland, Bulgaria
Intermediate	5–9	East Europe, France, Germany, Yugoslavia
Low	5	Great Britain, United States, Australia, New Zealand, Latin America, India, Sri Lanka

Table 2 Rate of hepatocellular carcinoma as a consequence of cirrhosis

Disease	Rate
Macronodular cirrhosis	40–55%
Micronodular cirrhosis	3–10%
Alcoholic cirrhosis	15%
Haemochromatosis	17–25%
Alpha-1-antitrypsin deficiency	1%
Tyrosinaemia	100%
Wilson's disease	1%
Primary biliary cirrhosis	1%

Environmental factors other than viral infection also contribute importantly to the prevalence of hepatocellular carcinoma worldwide. These additional environmental factors include the therapeutic use of sex steroids, particularly oral contraceptives, nutritional deficiency states, fungal mycotoxin contamination of cereal products and of industrial exposures experienced in the workplace (Table 3).

The optimal treatment for hepatocellular carcinoma is partial or subtotal hepatectomy with preservation of as much normal residual hepatic tissue as is possible. This can be accomplished by experienced surgeons with a quite low mortality rate[2]. Mortality rates, however, vary considerably in various series and range between 5 and 30%[3]. The extent of the resection as well as the indication for the resection and the severity of the underlying liver disease present in a given patient importantly affect the mortality experienced with

Table 3 Environmental factors contributing to the development of hepatocellular carcinoma

- Oestrogens
  Especially oral contraceptive agents, with an estimated 500-fold increased risk after 85 months of use
- Available steroids
- Dietary restriction
  Protein
  Methionine
  Selenium
  Zinc
  Folic acid
  Vitamin B_{12}
- Aflatoxins
- Industrial Exposure
  Arsenic
  Vinyl chloride
  Other agents less well-characterized

Table 4 Types of hepatic resections

• Right on left hepatic lobectomy — gall bladder fossa and IVC

• Left lateral segment — falciform ligament

• Right trisegmentectomy — all of true right lobe and medial segment of left lobe

• Left trisegmentectomy — all of true left lobe and the anterior segment of the right lobe

• Total hepatectomy with orthotopic transplantation

• Wedge resection — does not follow anatomic planes; usually reserved for benign lesions

---

such resections. The various types of hepatic resection possible are shown in Table 4 and Figure 1. Unfortunately, although hepatic resection is the only curative procedure for hepatocellular carcinoma, < 50% of cases explored are resectable either because of underlying cirrhosis or the size and/or location of the tumour and < 20% of explored cases are totally resectable despite the application of new surgical techniques such as intra-operative ultrasonic localization and dissection of the tumour, the hepatic vessels and the biliary tree.

Total hepatectomy followed by orthotopic liver transplantation is currently the only hope for cure in those patients with underlying cirrhosis or with extensive tumour burdens that preclude standard large hepatic resections (Table 4 and Figure 1). Liver transplantation has been applied to the problem of hepatic malignancy ever since the first clinical applications of the procedure[4-6]. Shown in Figure 2 is the accumulative survival rate for more than 800 adult transplant recipients operated upon at the University Health

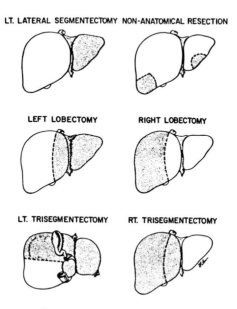

LT. LATERAL SEGMENTECTOMY   NON-ANATOMICAL RESECTION

LEFT LOBECTOMY   RIGHT LOBECTOMY

LT. TRISEGMENTECTOMY   RT. TRISEGMENTECTOMY

Figure 1 Schematic representation of the types of major hepatic resections possible with good survival

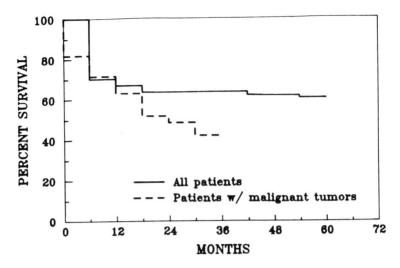

Figure 2 Kaplan–Meier survival curves for 800 adult liver transplant recipients (————) and a subset of 70 recipients transplanted because of a hepatic malignancy (- - - -)

Center of Pittsburgh for all indications except hepatic malignancy and the 70 patients transplanted for a malignant tumour of the liver at the same institution by the same surgeons, using the same immunosuppressive regimens[7].

The percentage of patients transplanted for hepatic malignancy at a given institution varies markedly depending upon a variety of factors including the longevity of the programme, the approach of the institution to patients with HBsAg positivity and cholangiolar carcinoma and the numbers of patients being referred for transplantation for other indications[6-9]. In the Denver–Pittsburgh experience during the pre-cyclosporine era, 13.5% of all recipients had hepatic malignancy as the indication for their procedure. In more recent times, following the introduction of cyclosporine and as a result of more cases being referred for indications other than hepatic malignancy, the percentage of cases transplanted for hepatic malignancy has fallen by 50% to 6.8%[10]. In contrast to the experience in the United States, the experience in Europe has included a larger percentage (29%) of cases with hepatic malignancy as the indication for transplantation. In some European centres, a full one-third of the patients transplanted have had a hepatic malignancy as the indication[9].

The experience with hepatic transplantation for malignancy at these various centres throughout the world has been very similar to that reported by the Pittsburgh group with long-term survival (> 3 years after transplantation) being between 20 and 30% (Figure 2). This survival figure is one-half to one-third that experienced for all other indications for which liver transplantation has been applied but is nonetheless considerably better than that experienced with any other type of therapy, particularly medical therapy where no survivors exist after one year[11].

Table 5 Co-existent liver disease in 21 patients with incidental primary liver neoplasms

Disease	Number of patients
Cirrhosis	5
Tyrosinaemia	4
Biliary atresia	4
Sclerosing cholangitis	4
Alpha-1-antitrypsin deficiency	2
Familiary cholestasis	1
Sea-blue histiocyte syndrome	1

The experience with liver transplantation applied for hepatocellular carcinoma is not entirely grave. Individuals who have been transplanted for other conditions in which a hepatic malignancy typically < 5 cm in diameter was found (Table 5) have done very well and have had a survival rate similar to that experienced by those transplanted for the same condition not complicated with a hepatic cancer (Figure 3). Of the 14 such cases, all but one has survived without re-occurrence of their hepatocellular carcinoma with the duration of follow-up ranging from 3 to 73 months and with 6 of these 13 long-term survivors being free of recurrent disease beyond 3 years.

In contrast to the experience with hepatocellular carcinoma occurring 'incidentally' in a liver at the time of hepatic transplantation, the clinical course of those transplanted solely because of hepatocellular carcinoma has

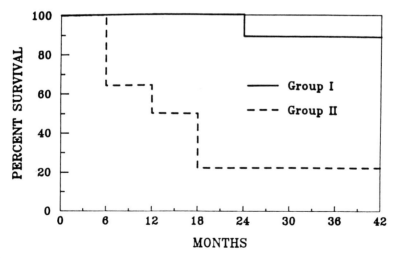

Figure 3 Kaplan–Meier survival curves for liver graft recipients to have an incidental hepatic neoplasm in a liver removed for another reason (———) and those transplanted for hepatic malignancy (– – – –)

been quite different. Among 20 such patients transplanted during the cyclosporine era, 5 (25%) died during the immediate post-operative period (within 2 months of transplantation); 8 of the remaining 15 (53%) developed recurrent disease at intervals of 4–12 months following transplantation. Recurrence of the hepatoma in the allograft was the first evidence of disease recurrence in 50% of the cases, in 38% of recurrent cases the recurrence occurred first in the lungs and 12% it occurred first in bone. Of the remaining 8, 2 have survived for only 1 and 8 months, respectively, while 6 have survived free of recurrent disease for intervals ranging from 6 to 54 months.

A recent report extracted from the European Liver Transplant Registry reported a 30% survival for patients transplanted for hepatocellular carcinoma at 2 years[8]. The data compiled by Pichlmayr[9] from 7 major European centres is quite similar to that experienced in Pittsburgh with 30% of the patients surviving for 1 year but only 17% surviving free of disease for > 2 years.

These results from Europe and the United States clearly document that despite the elimination of patients with extra-hepatic malignancy detected by a careful screening of each candidate for metastatic disease with computed-tomography scans of the chest, abdomen, and head as well as with bone scanning techniques, that microscopic metastasis, unrecognized either before surgery and at the time of the transplant procedure itself persists in such cases despite resection of the gastro-hepatic and hepato-duodenal ligaments, skeletalization of all vascular structures as well as the common bile duct and resection of the bile duct as it crosses behind the duodenum with the creation of a roux-en-Y choledochojejunostomy.

At this point in time, the results with the application of adjuvant chemotherapy after the hepatectomy during the anhepatic phase of the transplant procedure and in the first several months following liver transplantation for hepatoma are not yet available. The experiences with such modifications of current techniques are either being formulated now, or at least in some cases are only beginning to be accumulated.

The exception to the rule of a poor prognosis with hepatic transplantation for hepatocellular carcinoma is the experience with fibrolamellar carcinoma[14]. Typically, this tumour occurs in young adults and in the absence of any underlying liver disease. Moreover, it reportedly grows slowly, has a high resectability rate, and therefore, a longer survival rate than that experienced with other types of hepatocellular carcinoma[12–14]. A total of 9 patients with this variant of hepatocellular carcinoma have been treated by the Pittsburgh group during the cyclosporine era with orthotopic liver transplantation. None of them had distant metastasis at the time of transplantation although 2/9 had tumour infiltrating the diaphragm which necessitated excision of a part of the diaphragm with the liver and the tumour; 3 of the tumours (33%) showed some degree of vascular invasion of the resection specimen. One-third of these patients died early as a result of one or another non-tumour-related surgical problems. Of the remaining 6, 2 have died as a result of recurrent disease at 32 and 33 months post-transplant, while 4 are alive with only 1 having evidence of recurrent disease with a mean duration in survival of 30 months.

There has been no reported experience with the particular tumour variant in the data available from the European Liver Transplant Registry[8,9]. The available American experience however, suggests that a limited number of pulmonary metastases may not be a contraindication for liver transplantation in this sub-group and that an aggressive approach to recurrent disease with additional resectional surgery and chemotherapy may be possible[14].

Yet another unique type of hepatic malignancy that may be amenable to liver transplantation is the recently relatively recognized epithelioid haemangioendothelioma[15-17]. Characteristically, this tumour grows slowly like the fibrolamellar variant with a natural history that spans 5–10 years despite metastasis to bone, lungs, pleura and lymph nodes: 6 cases of this tumour have been transplanted in Pittsburgh; 2 had known distant metastatis (1 to the lung and 1 to a rib) prior to transplantation; 4 had extra-hepatic intra-abdominal disease recognized at surgery but not pre-operatively (3 in lymph nodes and 1 involving the diaphragm). All 6 have survived with follow-ups ranging from 10 to 49 months (mean 22 months). The 2 with distant metastasis have had their disease remain stable. Because the natural history of this disease is so unusual, it is not yet possible to make a definitive statement about the role of transplantation in such cases.

Bile-duct cancers comprise 16% of the tumours for which liver transplantation has been applied in the Pittsburgh experience. On average, these patients are older than the other tumour patients and 72% have had primary sclerosing cholangitis as the underlying chronic liver disease. Half have also had ulcerative colitis. In 55% of the cases, particularly those with sclerosing cholangitis, the tumour was not identified prior to hepatic resection despite an extensive pre-operative evaluation including brushing of the bile ducts for cytologic examination being obtained from the involved biliary tree whenever possible. Overall, 11% of the cases transplanted for sclerosing cholangitis had not been cholangiolar carcinoma[18]: 18% of these patients died early in the post-operative course; 78% of the survivors however, developed clinically-evident recurrent disease on mean at 8.5 months post-transplantation. Only 22% have survived > 15 months without recurrent disease. The experience of the Cambridge group with this tumour has been similar to that experienced in Pittsburgh[19]. The data of Pichlmayr suggest that those with nodal metastasis at the time of transplantation do very poorly, with only 13% being alive at 1 year and none at 2 years, while 100% of those without nodal metastasis are alive at 1 year and 83% are alive at 2 years following transplantation[9].

It is clearly evident from the above data that the results with total hepatectomy and orthotopic liver transplantation for the treatment of hepatic malignancy currently are less than ideal. Increasing surgical experience with the procedure and the use of cyclosporine has resulted in fewer immediate post-operative deaths such that the application of this mode of therapy can be more clearly evaluated. In general, particularly when compared to the results experienced with non-malignant diseases of the liver, the results have been poor, with only 20–30% of the patients surviving for periods > 1 year. Progress in this area awaits the development of new chemotherapeutic agents that are effective against hepatocellular carcinoma or the development of means of targeting and destroying microscopic metastatic foci of malignant disease once the bulk of the tumour load is removed as a result of the total hepatectomy.

Current recommendations are that liver transplantation be applied to those patients with hepatic malignancy such as the fibromellar variant and the more unusual epithelioid haemangioendothelioma and occasionally for those with other types of hepatocellular but not biliary epithelial tumours, who have extra-hepatic malignancy ruled out by means of computed tomography scanning of the chest, abdomen and head and a bone scan followed either by a careful staging laparotomy or with a back-up candidate available for the allograft should the potential recipient be found to have extra-hepatic disease at the time of operation.

Despite such caution, transplants are still likely to occur in patients with undetected extra-hepatic malignancy. The use of adjuvant chemotherapy may be effective in such cases. Currently, however no good data relative to this point exist.

Acknowledgement

This work was supported in part by grants from NIDDK 2R01 DK32556-05 and NIAAA 5R01 AA06601-03.

References

1. *Cancer Statistics* (1986). *CA,* **36**, 9–25
2. Iwatsuki, S., Shaw, B. W. Jr. and Starzl. T. E. (1982). Experience with 150 liver resections. *Ann. Surg.,* **197**, 247–53
3. Foster, J. H. and Berman, M. M. (1977). *Solid Liver Tumors,* 1st edn. (Philadelphia: W. B. Saunders)
4. Starzl, T. E. (with the assistance of Putnam, C. W.) (1969). *Experience in Hepatic Transplantation,* 1st edn. (Philadelphia: W. B. Saunders)
5. Starzl, T. E., Porter, K. A., Putnam, C. W., Schroter, G. P. J., Halgrimson, C. G., Weil, R., Hoelscher, M. and Reid, H. A. S. (1976). Orthotopic liver transplantation in 93 patients. *Surg. Gynecol. Obstet.,* **142**, 487–505
6. Starzl, T. E., Iwatsuki, S., Van Thiel, D. H., Gartner, J. C., Zitelli, B. J., Malatack, J. J., Schade, R. R., Shaw, B. W. Jr., Hakala, T. R., Rosenthal, J. J. and Porter, K. A. (1982). Evaluation of liver transplantation. *Hepatology,* **2**, 614–36
7. Iwatsuki, S., Starzl, T. E., Todo, S., Gordon, R. D., Esquivel, C. O., Tzakis, A. G., Makowka, L., Marsh, J. W., Koneru, B., Stieber, A., Klintmalm, G. and Husberg, B. (1988). Experience in 1000 liver transplants under cyclosporine–steroid therapy: A survival report. *Transpl. Proc.,* **20**, 498–504
8. Bismuth, H., Castaing, D., Ericzon, B. G., Otte, J. B., Rolles, K., Ringe, B. and Sloof, M. (1987). Hepatic transplantation in Europe. First Report of European Liver Transplant Registry. *Lancet* (Sept. 19), **2**(8560), 674–6
9. Pichlmayr, R. (1987). Is there a place for liver grafting for malignancy? Presented at the *International Organ Transplant Forum*, September 8–11, Pittsburgh, Pennsylvania
10. Koneru, B., Tzakis, A. G., Bowman, J., Cassavilla, A., Zajko, A. B. and Starzl, T. E. (1988). Postoperative surgical complications. In Makowka, L. and Van Thiel, D. H. (eds.) *Gastroenterology Clinics of Norhtern America.* pp 71–91. (Philadelphia: W. B. Saunders)
11. Bassendine, M. F. (1987). Aetiological factors in hepatocellular cancer. In Williams, R. and Johnson, P. J. (eds.) *Clinical Gastroenterology.* pp 1–16. (Philadelphia: Bailliére Tindall)

12. Craig, J. R., Peters, R. L., Edmondson, H. A. and Omata, M. (1980). Fibrolamellar carcinoma of the liver. A tumor of adolescents and young adults with distinctive clinico-pathologic features. *Cancer,* **46**, 372–9
13. Berman, M. M., Libbey, P. and Foster, J. H. (1980). Hepatocellular carcinoma. Polygonal cell type with fibrous stroma. *Cancer,* **46**, 1148–55
14. Starzl, T. E., Iwatsuki, S., Shaw, B. W., Nalesnik, M. A., Farhi, D. C. and Van Thiel, D. H. (1986). Treatment of fibrolamellar hepatoma with partial or total hepatectomy and transplantation of the liver. *Surg. Gynecol. Obstet.,* **162**, 145–8
15. Weiss, J. W. and Enzinger, F. M. (1982). Epithelioid hemangioendothelioma: A vascular tumor often mistaken for a carcinoma. *Cancer,* **50**, 970–81
16. Weldon-Linne, C. M., Victor, T., Christ, M. L. and Fry, W. A. (1981). Angiogenic nature of the intravascular bronchio-alveolar tumor of the lung. An electron microscopic study. *Arch. Pathol. Lab. Med.,* **105**, 174–9
17. Ishak, K. G., Sesterheen, I. A., Goodman, M. Z. D., Rabin, L. and Stromeyer, W. (1984). Epithelioid hemangioendothelioma of the liver; A clinicopathologic and follow-up study of 32 cases. *Human Pathol.,* **15**, 839–52
18. Marsh, J. W., Iwatsuki, S., Makowka, L. and (1988). Orthotopic liver transplantation for primary sclerosing cholangitis. *Ann. Surg.* (in press)
19. Rolles, K., Williams, R., Neuberger, J. and Calne, R. (1984). The Cambridge and King's College Hospital experience of liver transplantation, 1968–1983. *Hepatology,* **4** (Suppl. 1), Jan.–Feb., 50S–55S

42
Strategies in prevention of hepatocellular carcinoma by vaccination

F. DEINHARDT AND W. JILG

INTRODUCTION

Hepatocellular carcinoma (HCC) is one of the most frequent, fatal malignancies of man, particularly in the Far East and in Africa. In a recent international meeting it was reported that worldwide 250 000–1 000 000 deaths yearly resulted from HCC[1]. There is now overwhelming evidence that chronic hepatitis B virus (HBV) infection is the major risk factor for the development of HCC, and this evidence takes the form of epidemiological observations, and studies in laboratory animals as well as biochemical and molecular biological investigations: the geographical distribution of high HBV endemicity and high prevalence of HCC is identical[2]; the risk of HCC in HBs-antigen carriers is more than 200-fold higher than in individuals without any HBV markers[3]; HCC can be induced experimentally in woodchucks by inoculation with woodchuck hepatitis virus (WHV), an hepadna virus closely related to HBV[4]; and integration of viral DNA into host cellular DNA is observed almost invariably in liver tumour cells[5]. Thus, HCC is a human cancer for which a viral aetiology is very likely; consequently, like any other infectious disease, it should be preventable and the most efficient way of prevention is probably vaccination. Considerable efforts have been made to develop effective and safe vaccines against hepatitis B and strategies for their economic use, the aim being to control and prevent chronic hepatitis B virus infection and thus eliminate a major cause not only of chronic debilitating and often fatal liver failure but also of HCC. We give here a brief overview of the present status of hepatitis B vaccination and the strategies for its use in preventing HCC.

HEPATITIS B VACCINES

First generation vaccines are produced from plasma of chronic carriers of HBV. They consist of the major surface antigen of HBV (HBsAg) which is

Table 1 Seroconversion rates after vaccination with three doses of hepatitis B vaccine (at months 0, 1, and 6) in 108 healthy young adults

Months after first vaccination	Anti-HBs positive		GMT[a]
	(n)	(%)	(IU/litre)
1	39	36	2.5
2	85	78	18.9
3	97	89	59.4
4	97	89	71.4
5	97	89	87.4
6	96	88	88.3
7	102	94	1560

[a]Geometric mean titre of *all* individuals

produced in high amounts mainly in the form of small particles with a diameter of about 22 nm in the livers of chronically infected individuals. Several purification steps, including different inactivation procedures, ensure the absence of HBV as well as of other infectious agents in these vaccines. Such plasma-derived vaccines are effective and safe[6]; they induce antibodies against HBsAg (anti-HBs) in protective levels in $> 90\%$ of healthy individuals

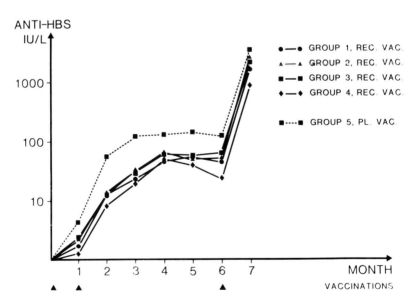

Figure 1 Immune response of healthy young adults to plasma derived hepatitis B vaccine (group 5, $n = 72$) and to 4 lots of recombinant vaccine (group 1, $n = 30$; group 2, $n = 82$; group 3, $n = 86$, group 4, $n = 16$). Seroconversion rates were 97–100% in all groups

Table 2 Immune response to three doses of hepatitis B vaccine in different age groups

| Age (years) | n | Sex (f/m) | Anti-HBs | | |
			Positive (%)	> 10 IU/litre (%)	GMT[a] (IU/litre)
10–19	21	15/6	100	100	820
20–29	62	43/19	97	95	481
30–39	46	30/16	98	89	565
40–49	40	29/21	96	92	538
50–59	17	15/2	71	65	34

[a]Geometric mean titre of *all* individuals

after three vaccinations (Table 1). Inadequate supply of human plasma containing the HBsAg used in these vaccines limits production, and so second-generation vaccines have been developed by using recombinant DNA technology. These vaccines contain HBsAg produced in recombinant baker's yeast in which the HBV gene coding for HBsAg has been inserted[7]. Recently, a recombinant vaccine produced in mammalian cell lines has been developed[8]. Yeast-derived vaccines studied for several years and licensed in many countries have been shown to have immunogenicity comparable to the plasma-derived vaccines (Figure 1) and they are tolerated equally well[9].

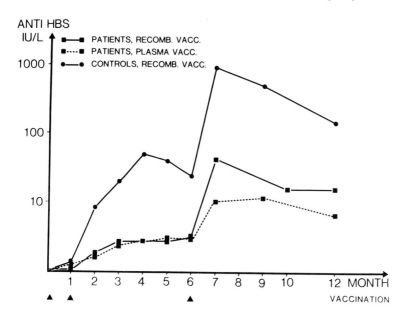

Figure 2 Immune response of dialysis patients to plasma-derived hepatitis B vaccine (*n* = 75) and recombinant hepatitis B vaccine (*n* = 49), compared with healthy controls (*n* = 16) vaccinated with recombinant vaccine. Patients were immunized with 40 μg HBsAg per dose; healthy persons received 10 μg HBsAg per dose

Use of current hepatitis B vaccines

For full protection, either three or four vaccinations are recommended by different manufacturers; vaccinations are given at 0, 1, and 6 months or 0, 1, 2, and 12 months; 90–95% of vaccinees respond with protective antibody levels, i.e. with anti-HBs concentrations > 10 IU/litre, but the immune responses to hepatitis B vaccination depend on sex, age, and immune status of the vaccinee. Females respond better than males[10], although the difference does not seem to be of any practical importance. The influence of age on the immune response is more pronounced, especially in individuals aged > 50 years (Table 2)[11]. Children and even newborns respond very well to hepatitis B vaccination; only half of the normal dose in adult vaccinees is needed for those aged < 12 years. Immunocompromised individuals respond poorly to hepatitis B vaccination, as demonstrated in transplant recipients and in haemodialysis patients[12–14]. Only 50–60% of these patients respond to vaccination, usually with significantly lower titres than normal healthy individuals (Figure 2). The route of administration of vaccine also influences the immune response, with injections of the vaccine into the upper arm (*m. deltoideus*) leading to better results than intra-gluteal vaccination[15].

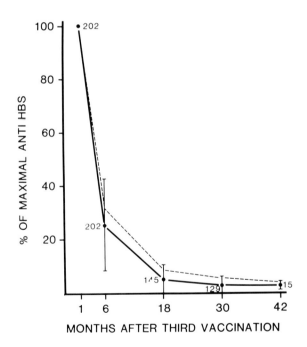

Figure 3 Percentage decrease of anti HBs after immunization with hepatitis B vaccine. Individuals vaccinated with recombinant vaccine (———) (standard deviations and number of individuals tested are indicated) compared to individuals after plasma derived vaccine (– – – –)

Duration of protection

Protection against HBV infection achieved by vaccination is due to the presence of anti-HBs; the minimum protective concentration is assumed to be about 10 IU/litre. The kinetics of antibody decrease after the completion of a course of vaccination are similar in all vaccinees, irrespective of sex, age or maximum antibody titre[16] (Figure 3): the persistence of specific antibodies above the 10 IU level depends mainly on the maximum anti-HBs value reached 4 weeks after the last (third or fourth) vaccination[16-19]. However, long-term follow-up studies after vaccination in groups with high risk of HBV infection showed that the protection against clinically-apparent disease outlasts the presence of specific antibodies[6,20,21]. This agrees well with recent re-vaccination studies demonstrating a good immunological memory in all individuals who reacted well to the initial vaccination; even 30 months after disappearance of specific antibodies, an anamnestic response to re-vaccination was seen in these subjects and led to a rapid increase of anti-HBs to high levels[22] (Figure 4). Nevertheless, as the duration of this kind of protection (against disease) is unknown, it seems wise at present to re-vaccinate all individuals whose antibody levels have decreased to $\leq$ 10 IU/litre. The time of re-vaccination can be estimated from the maximum anti-HBs concentration after the full course of immunization[17]; if this information is unavailable, re-vaccination should be performed after 5–7 years.

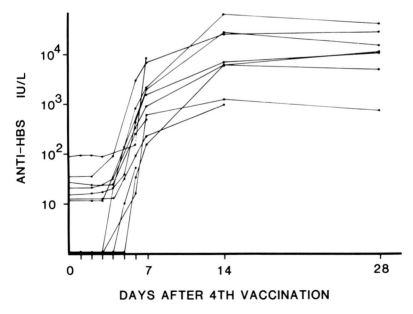

Figure 4 Anti-HBs response after a fourth dose of hepatitis B vaccine in 11 individuals vaccinated 2–5 years earlier whose anti-HBs values had fallen to 0–80 IU/litre[22]

VACCINATION STRATEGIES FOR PREVENTING HCC

Vaccination strategies for preventing HCC must take into account the age in which most individuals become infected by HBV. In Southeast Asia, most children are infected at birth, so the best regimen to interrupt an infection which might have occurred even shortly before birth is passive–active immunization, i.e. the combination of specific hepatitis B immunoglobulin and active vaccination[23]. However, the high cost of immunoglobulin makes this approach impracticable on a larger basis. Fortunately, recent studies in newborns as well as studies in experimentally-infected chimpanzees have shown that properly timed vaccination alone is nearly as effective as the passive–active regimen (C. Stevens, personal communication)[24,25]. Thus, in areas with high HBV prevalence and transmission often occurring at birth, vaccination should be performed in newborns as soon as possible, i.e. immediately after birth. As a minimum all newborns of carrier mothers should be vaccinated but ideally vaccine should be given to all newborns in such areas because testing of the mothers is also costly and often impracticable, and all children in these areas will be at risk for hepatitis B later. The same approach could be followed also in countries with different epidemiological situations, e.g. Africa where transmission at birth is very rare and children usually become infected during the first one or two years of life. However, another strategy is possible and perhaps preferable: although newborns respond to HBV vaccine, this response is considerably better after the first three months of life and hepatitis B vaccination could be given at this time, allowing combination with other vaccinations such as tetanus, diphtheria, and polio and thus simplifying the logistics considerably.

There is some concern that reaching all children in high risk areas might be difficult, especially for the third immunisation and for re-vaccinations, so that a high proportion will be insufficiently protected. However, this is no reason to delay starting this vaccination programme as soon as possible. It has been shown that after only two injections of hepatitis B vaccine most and particularly young vaccinees already develop antibodies against HBsAg in the protective range (Jilg, Schmidt and Deinhardt, in preparation). Although the titres are usually low, they are long-lasting and provided most individuals with an immunological memory, as it was shown that these individuals react 6–12 months after the last vaccination with anamnestic responses. Thus, after two vaccinations they would probably also react to a natural infection in a similar way so that they would be protected at least against disease and the development of a carrier state. In areas with high prevalence of HBV, children come into contact with natural virus very soon, and this leads to natural boosters and thus to long-lasting immunity.

Thus the main hindrances to mass immunization programmes in high-risk areas like Southeast Asia and Africa is the high cost of, and the lack of, the infrastructure needed for conducting large vaccination campaigns. Lower-priced vaccines are already available but many countries in endemic areas cannot afford even these vaccines; furthermore, the proper storage and distribution of the vaccine cannot be guaranteed. However, the eradication of smallpox showed that even in these areas, mass immunization campaigns are possible. Alternative hepatitis B vaccines with higher immunogenicity, so that a single dose would suffice, and a higher stability might be necessary for these countries, and in many laboratories efforts are being made to develop such vaccines. However, this is no reason to delay mass vaccinations. Success in preventing HCC will not be seen for a very long time; twenty to fifty years usually pass between infection with HBV and the development of HCC, and failure to begin vaccination programmes now will condemn large numbers of people to unnecessary suffering.

References

1. Popper, H. (1988). Pathobiology of hepatocellular carcinoma. In Zuckerman, A. J. (ed.) *Viral Hepatitis and Liver Disease*. pp 719–22. (New York: Alan R. Liss)
2. Szmuness, W. (1978). Hepatocellular carcinoma and the hepatitis B virus: evidence for a causal association. *Prog. Med. Virol.*, **24**, 40–69
3. Beasley, P., Hwang, L. Y., Lin, C. C. and Chien, C. S. (1981). Hepatocellular carcinoma and hepatitis B virus. A prospective study of 22707 men in Taiwan. *Lancet*, **2**, 1129–33
4. Popper, H., Roth, L., Purcell, R. H., Tennant, B. C. and Gerin, J. L. (1987). Hepatocarcinogenicity of the Woodchuck hepatitis virus. *Proc. Natl. Acad. Sci. USA*, **84**, 866–70
5. Brechot, C. (1987). Hepatitis B virus (HBV) and hepatocellular carcinoma. HBV DNA status and its implications. *J. Hepatol.*, **4**, 269–79
6. Stevens, C. E., Taylor, P. E., Tong, M. J., Toy, P. T. and Vyas, G. N. (1984). Hepatitis B vaccine: an overview. In Vyas, G. N., Dienstag, J. L. and Hoofnagle, J. H. (eds.) *Viral Hepatitis and Liver Disease*. pp 275–91. (Orlando, Florida: Grune and Stratton)
7. McAleer, W. J., Buynak, E. B., Maigetter, R. Z., Wampler, D. E., Miller, W. J. and Hilleman, M. R. (1984). Human hepatitis B vaccine from recombinant yeast. *Nature*, **307**, 178–80
8. Adamowicz, P., Tron, F., Vinas, R., Mevelec, M. N., Diaz, I., Couroucé, A. M., Mazert, M. C., Lagarde, D. and Girard, M. (1988). Hepatitis B vaccine containing the S and PreS-2 antigens produced in Chinese hamster ovary cells. In Zuckerman, A. J. (ed.) *Viral Hepatitis and Liver Disease*. pp 1087–90. (New York: Alan R. Liss)
9. Jilg, W., Schmidt, M. and Deinhardt, F. Four years experience with a recombinant hepatitis B vaccine. *Infection*.
10. Zachoval, R., Jilg, W., Lorbeer, B., Schmidt, M. and Deinhardt, F. (1984). Passive–active immunization against hepatitis *J. Inf. Dis.*, **150**, 112–17
11. Deinhardt, F. and Jilg, W. (1988). Vaccination in old age. In Bianchi, L., Holt, P., James, O. F. W. and Butler, R. N. (eds.) *Aging and the Liver*. pp 371–6 (Lancaster: MTP Press)
12. Lauchart, W., Feuerhake, A., Meiners, G., Pichlmayr, R. and Müller, R. (1983). Low response to active hepatitis-B vaccination in kidney allograft recipients. *Transplant. Proc.*, **15**, 1092–3
13. Grob, P. J., Binswanger, U., Zarubu, K., Joller-Jemelka, H. I., Schmid, M., Häckl, W., Blumberg, A., Abplanalp, A., Herwig, W., Iselin, H. and Descoeudres, C. (1983). Immunogenicity of a hepatitis B subunit vaccine in hemodialysis and in renal transplant recipients. *Antiviral. Res.*, **3**, 43–52
14. Jilg, W., Schmidt, M., Weinel, B., Küttler, Th., Brass, H., Bommer, J., Müller, R., Schulte, B., Schwarzbeck, A. and Deinhardt, F. (1986). Immunogenicity of recombinant hepatitis B vaccine in dialysis patients. *J. Hepatol.*, **3**, 190–5
15. Centers for Disease Control (1985). Suboptimal response to hepatitis B vaccine given by injection into the buttock. *Morbid. Mortal. Wkly Rep.*, **8**, 105–13
16. Jilg, W., Schmidt, M. and Deinhardt, F. (1988). Persistence of specific antibodies after hepatitis B vaccination. *J. Hepatol.*, **0**, 201–7
17. Jilg, W., Schmidt, M., Deinhardt, F. and Zachoval, R. (1984). Hepatitis B vaccination: how long does protection last? *Lancet*, **2**, 458

18. Laplanche, A., Couroucé, A. M., Jungers, P., Benhamou, E. and Crosnier, J. (1984). Hepatitis B vaccination: how long does protection last? *Lancet*, **2**, 866
19. Grob, P. J., Dufek, A. and Joller-Jemelka, H. I. (1985). Hepatitis-B-Impfung — Wann ist eine Booster-Injektion nötig? *Schw. Med. Wochenschr.*, **115**, 394–402
20. Hadler, S. C., Francis, D. P., Maynard, J. E., Thompson, S. E., Judson, F. N., Echenberg, D. F., Ostrow, D. G., O'Malley, P. M., Penley, K. A., Altman, N. L., Braff, E., Shipman, G. F., Coleman, P. J. and Mandel, E. J. (1986). Long-term immunogenicity and efficacy of hepatitis B vaccine in homosexual men. *N. Engl. J. Med.*, **315**, 209–14
21. Coursaget, P., Chotard, J., Vincelot, P., Diop-Mar, I., Yvonnet, B., Sarr, M., N'doye, R. and Chiron, J. P. (1986). Seven-year study of hepatitis B vaccine efficacy in infants from an endemic area (Senegal). *Lancet*, **2**, 1143–5
22. Jilg, W., Schmidt, M. and Deinhardt, F. (1988). Immune response to hepatitis B revaccination. *J. Med. Virol.*, **24**, 377–84
23. Stevens, C. E., Taylor, P. E., Tong, M. J., Toy, P. T., Vyas, G. N., Zang, E. A. and Krugman, S. (1988). Prevention of perinatal hepatitis B virus infection with hepatitis B immune globulin and hepatitis B vaccine. In Zuckerman, A. J. (ed.) *Viral Hepatitis and Liver Disease*. pp 982–8. (New York: Alan R. Liss)
24. Chung, W. K., Choi, K. Y., Shim, K. S., Chung, J. W., Sun, H. S., Chung, K. W., Kim, B.S., Chun, C. S., Sung, I. K., Cho, K. H., Kang, J. W., Kim, S. J. and Prince, A. M. (1988). Safety, immunogenicity, and efficacy of a new heat-inactivated hepatitis B vaccine in the newborn. In Zuckerman, A. J. (ed.) *Viral Hepatitis and Liver Disease*. pp 1014–16 (New York: Alan R. Liss)
25. Iwarson, S., Wahl, M., Ruttimann, E., Snoy, P., Seto, B. and Gerety, R. J. (1988). Successful postexposure vaccination against hepatitis B in chimpanzees. *J. Med. Virol.*, **25**, 433–9

Index